HERD HEALTH

A TEXTBOOK OF HEALTH AND PRODUCTION MANAGEMENT OF AGRICULTURAL ANIMALS

O.M. RADOSTITS, D.V.M., M.Sc.

Professor, Department of Veterinary Internal Medicine
Western College of Veterinary Medicine
University of Saskatchewan
Saskatoon, Saskatchewan, Canada

D.C. BLOOD, O.B.E., B.V.Sc., M.V.Sc., F.A.C.V.S., Hon. L.L.D. (Sask.), Hon. A.R.C.V.S.

Professor of Veterinary Medicine
School of Veterinary Medicine
University of Melbourne, Australia

1985

W.B. SAUNDERS COMPANY

PHILADELPHIA   LONDON   TORONTO   MEXICO CITY   RIO DE JANEIRO   SYDNEY   TOKYO

W. B. Saunders Company: West Washington Square
                           Philadelphia, PA 19105

                           1 St. Anne's Road
                           Eastbourne, East Sussex BN21 3UN, England

                           1 Goldthorne Avenue
                           Toronto, Ontario M8Z 5T9, Canada

                           Apartado 26370—Cedro 512
                           Mexico 4, D.F., Mexico

                           Rua Coronel Cabrita, 8
                           Sao Cristovao Caixa Postal 21176
                           Rio de Janeiro, Brazil

                           9 Waltham Street
                           Artarmon, N.S.W. 2064, Australia

                           Ichibancho, Central Bldg., 22-1 Ichibancho
                           Chiyoda-Ku, Tokyo 102, Japan

Library of Congress Cataloging in Publication Data

Radostits, O.M.
    Herd Health: A Textbook of Health and Production
    Management of Agricultural Animals

    Includes bibliographies.
    1. Veterinary hygiene. 2. Livestock. 3. Veterinary medicine. I. Blood, D.C. (Douglas
Charles) II. Title. SF757.R28 1985   636.089'3   84-13858
ISBN 0-7216-1237-7

Herd Health: A Textbook of Health and Production
Management of Agricultural Animals   ISBN   0-7216-1237-7

Last digit is the print number: 9   8   7   6   5   4   3   2   1

Dedicated to our families
for their understanding
of our interest
in veterinary medicine

"And he gave it for his opinion that whoever could make two ears of corn or two blades of grass grow on a spot of ground where only one grew before would deserve better of mankind and do more service to his country than the whole race of politicians put together"

JONATHAN SWIFT
The Voyage to Brobdingnag
in *Gulliver's Travels*

Preface

This book is about the role of the veterinarian in the efficient production of livestock. It is our conviction that the present rapid growth of health maintenance services to herds and flocks will continue and that within a decade this form of veterinary activity will dominate food animal practice. The net economic gains from successful herd health programs are large and the techniques for the examination of herds and flocks and the delivery of the necessary services are available. More articles on planned health and production programs appear in journals each year and relevant conferences are devoting an increasing proportion of their schedules to the subjects of preventive veterinary medicine and production techniques for individual herds and flocks. Rural veterinary practitioners world-wide are recognizing the need to change their attitudes about the services they provide. For this reason, the traditional role as a healer of individual sick animals is gradually being replaced by the delivery of totally integrated animal health and production management. Many veterinary colleges are now revising their curricula to meet this new challenge.

One of the difficulties confronting the teachers of the present generation, and the veterinarians already involved in professional work and who wish to embark on a herd health endeavor, has been the absence of a textbook. This book has been written in an attempt to fill that need. However, it is brought forward with some hesitation because much of the ground that the book covers is still unmapped and the programs and surveillance methods used are exploratory. We are quite sure that if the book succeeds as a manual of applied preventive veterinary science, it will be very different in its second edition from this early tentative presentation.

The book is written for undergraduate veterinary students who are interested in working with agricultural animals. We hope that it will serve as a beginning for veterinary courses in health management. The text describes the management of animal health in dairy and beef cattle herds, beef feedlots, swine herds, and sheep flocks. It also contains a chapter on the historical development of herd health and a chapter on the use of computers in herd health. The common thread we have tried to weave throughout the book is the management of animal health and production that will result in the most efficient production of livestock.

We hope too that undergraduates in animal science and veterinarians already in practice will find some useful information in these pages.

The most difficult part of the preparation of the book has been to avoid rewriting existing textbooks on veterinary medicine, animal husbandry, and nutrition, while at the same time selecting appropriate information. One of the megatrends of today and the future is the information explosion. The volume of literature on the health and production of food-producing animals is very large and involves many disciplines, of which we have been very conscious while writing this book.

Becoming a species specialist would appear to be the only hope of mastering a small part of the literature, and it is our hope that future editions of this book will be written by authors who are veterinary species specialists. We believe that this edition represents a beginning.

Many thanks are given to Mrs. Penny Yung and Mrs. Carol Kettles, who typed the manuscript with interest and smiling faces. We also acknowledge that many of the ideas that are incorporated in Chapter 2 were contributed by Sandra Lamb and F.H.W. Morley during an exercise aimed at producing a computer simulation program for a dairy farm.

Thanks are also extended to many former students—now practicing veterinarians—who encouraged us to continue our interest in herd health.

O.M. RADOSTITS
D.C. BLOOD

Contents

General Principles

INTRODUCTION

The most important need of humans is a dependable food supply. The efficient production of livestock that yield meat and milk is a major concern of human society in general and sociologists, animal scientists, and animal specialists in particular. The veterinarian has always been concerned with the effects of health on the production of herds of animals.

In 1975, The Committee of Inquiry into the Veterinary Profession in the U.K. under the chairmanship of Sir Michael Swann examined the role of the veterinarian in the future. The Committee indicated that the profession will

1

be increasingly concerned with preventive medicine on the farm, including advice on husbandry and management for the purpose of maintaining and improving animal health and welfare, the productivity and profitability of the farm business, and the hygiene of its products (Report 1975).

This book is about the role of the veterinarian in planned animal health and production in farm animals, particularly cattle, sheep, and swine.

A planned animal health and production program, commonly known as herd health, is a combination of regularly scheduled veterinary activities and good herd management designed to maintain optimum animal health and to achieve optimum production (Blood 1979). Herd health programs vary from simple ones in which the veterinarian visits the herd on a regular basis to examine animals and their performance and to make recommendations for the control of disease and improvement of production, to intensive programs in which the veterinarian—with the assistance of other animal specialists—makes detailed recommendations about the daily management of the animal health production program. This may include recommendations on nutrition, breeding programs, the purchase of breeding stock, and the selling of animals ready for market and advice on cash flow. Some veterinarians are now employed as resident herd managers and are responsible for ensuring maximum utilization of all available resources by coordinating the services and advice provided by all the agricultural advisors who are involved with the herd.

OBJECTIVES

The primary objective in a herd health program is to maintain animal health and production at the most efficient level that will provide maximum economic returns to the animal owner (Schnurrenberger 1979). The ever-present goal is to control and manage animal health and production at a high level of efficiency and at the same time to seek and introduce new techniques that will continue to improve efficiency (Blaxter 1979).

Some equally important secondary objectives include the provision of comfortable animal housing commensurate with reasonable animal welfare, the minimization of pollution of the environment by animal wastes, and the prevention of diseases that are transmissible from animals to man (the zoonoses).

TARGETS OF PERFORMANCE

The objectives of herd health are achieved by application of the concept of target of performance. A target of performance is the level of animal health and production that is considered to be optimum and will yield the best economic returns on investment. The targets of performance are determined from the performance found on a sample of farms that are considered to be representative of the economically conscious commercial farm population.

In a herd health program, the actual performance of animal health and production is determined on a regular basis and compared with the targets of performance. The differences between the targets of performance and actual performance are the shortfalls. The reasons for failure to achieve the targets of performance are then identified, recommendations for improvement are made, and performance is monitored continuously to assess the effectiveness of the action taken. The cycle is then repeated on a continuous basis.

HISTORICAL ASPECTS OF PREVENTIVE VETERINARY MEDICINE

The historical development of preventive veterinary medicine can be divided into four phases of activity (Table 1–1).

In Phase 1, which began about 100 years ago, national and state governments were involved in the eradication of diseases such as brucellosis and tuberculosis that were transmissible from cattle to man. These diseases have already been eradicated in some countries, and real progress is being made toward eradication in others. Other countries have been involved in the control of contagious diseases such as foot and mouth disease, rinderpest, and trypanosomiasis in order to reduce livestock losses, which lead to widespread nutritional deficiencies among the human population. These national disease eradication programs have been directed toward effective control in the animal population on a geographical area basis. As each area became free of the disease, only disease-free animals were allowed to enter. In this way, the disease could theoretically be eradicated from the entire country. These programs have been successful because the diagnostic tests were reliable, the testing was compulsory, and the financial resources necessary to do the job were made available from the public treasury.

Table 1-1. HISTORICAL DEVELOPMENT OF PREVENTIVE VETERINARY SERVICES

Phase	Principal Preoccupation	Principal Mode of Action	Principal Agent	Support Mechanism
1	Area problems. Protection of all herds by control of disease on area basis.	Government-sponsored health programs on area basis, brucellosis and tuberculosis eradication programs	Government veterinary officer	Trouble-shooter from government agency
2	Treatment of individual animals gives rise to enquiries about preventive programs	Incidental preventive programs, e.g., mastitis control, fertility, maintenance, parasitic disease status	Private practitioner	Private, university, or government consultant
3	Positive action via herd programs to maintain health status, e.g., reproductive efficiency, quarter infection rate	Packaged herd disease preventive programs, planned actions at programmed visits	Private practitioner (or government or employed veterinarian)	Consultants as above with specialties in individual diseases
4	Integration of health maintenance plans with production and management plans to give whole farm best effect	Positive action via herd programs as above with control data handling for all participating herds. Data bank makes production planning and prediction possible	Private practitioners (or employed veterinarian) May be in conjunction with husbandry advisor	Disease consultants and husbandry advisors *BUT* Data lab most important to provide statistical and financial analysis

In Phase 2, beginning about 1940, meat-, milk-, and fiber-producing animals (cattle, swine, and sheep) became valuable when animal farms began to sell livestock and livestock products off the farm as a source of net income. Prior to this time, most practicing veterinarians were involved in equine practice, which consisted largely of seasonal routine work (Henderson 1960). With the decline of the horse as a source of power on the farm, the veterinarian turned his activity to cattle, swine, and sheep practice. Between 1945 and 1965, there was an exceptionally large growth in rural large animal practice. This period coincided with a sharp increase in the standard of living in the developed countries, which created an unprecedented demand for meat and milk. The law of supply and demand increased the price of meat to the consumer, and in turn farm animals became valuable. When animals became ill, it was economical to call the veterinarian to treat them on an individual basis. During this period, modern veterinary education was also born, and veterinary graduates possessed the knowledge and skills to treat a wide variety of animal diseases with remarkable success. Antibiotics and chemotherapeutics were also introduced during this period, and veterinarians could treat a wide variety of the common infectious diseases such

as pneumonia and enteritis with spectacular results. Veterinary graduates were taught how to perform aseptic surgery, and the cesarean section in cattle, for example, became a common surgical procedure in veterinary practice. This created a tremendous demand for veterinarians and veterinary service. However, because of a shortage of veterinarians, those veterinarians who were in practice were very busy and spent most of their time treating individual sick animals. This activity resulted in the term "fire-engine practice." Because of a lack of time there was little effort made to control or prevent diseases on a herd basis. The emphasis was on the individual animal affected with clinical disease. Efforts to control or prevent disease consisted mainly of large-scale testing programs for diseases such as brucellosis and vaccination programs. Veterinarians spent considerable time vaccinating pigs for hog cholera and cattle for brucellosis.

In Phase 3, beginning about 1965, veterinarians and farmers began to appreciate the value of taking positive action to maintain a high level of animal health and efficient production on a herd basis. Farmers themselves gradually learned how to recognize and treat the common diseases of farm animals. In the earliest stages of this phase, preventive medicine consisted of recommendations for the control or prevention of specific diseases. For example, an outbreak of blackleg in young cattle was followed by a recommendation to vaccinate all susceptible animals with a clostridial vaccine. This was later followed by the veterinarian's recommendations for control of specific diseases that were likely to occur in the herd. As veterinarians became more involved and more familiar with the herd and the farmer on a regular basis, the presence of subclinical disease and inadequacies in management that resulted in poor animal performance were recognized. Subclinical disease in its broadest sense was recognized as the major cause of economic loss in food-producing animal herds. Diseases such as infertility and subclinical mastitis in dairy cows and intestinal helminthiasis in sheep, for example, responded dramatically and economically to strategic prophylactic procedures or changes in management.

During this phase, the use of the word *disease* was expanded to include not only clinical and subclinical disease but also management inefficiency, all three of which can result in suboptimal performance.

The recognition that economic benefits could be derived by taking positive action against subclinical disease was then followed by the development of planned herd health programs. Veterinarians began to make regularly scheduled visits to farms to examine the animal health and production status of the herd and to make recommendations for improvement. Herd health began to evolve. Between 1970 and 1980, there was considerable activity in the development of herd health programs for dairy cattle (Harrington 1979; Goodger and Ruppanner 1982a Lesch et al. 1980; Heider et al. 1980), beef breeding herds, beef feedlots, swine herds, and sheep flocks. Considerable progress has been made in dairy (Barfoot et al. 1971) and swine herd health (Becker 1979; Muirhead 1980). Programs for beef breeding herds and feedlots (Cope 1979) and for sheep flocks (Bailey 1979) are in the developmental stages. Health management is now an important component of a modern equine practice (Haines 1979).

During this phase, farmers and veterinarians recognized the value of keeping good records of animal health and production so that an objective analysis of health and production, including the costs of production, could be made.

The inclination to fill the program with every known preventive measure—whether the disease was likely to occur or not, whether the particular technique was highly effective or not, and often with more than one technique to prevent one disease—was one of the false steps made in the early stages of this new expansion into herd and flock health programs. Such programs could, and often did, cost more than the wastage they set out to eliminate. Subsequently, the analysis of these programs in terms of cost-effectiveness has put them on a sounder financial footing and made them more generally acceptable. Modern financially viable herd health programs were the eventual outcome of this evolutionary process.

Phase 4 in the development is taking place in the 1980s. In this phase, practicing veterinarians make regularly scheduled visits to the herd, examine animals and records for evidence of subclinical disease, and collect and analyze data with the assistance of the computer. Both the farmer and veterinarian agree on targets of performance for the herd. The veterinarian regularly analyzes the animal health and production data, compares the *actual performance* with the *targets of performance*, and identifies the reasons for failure to achieve the desired targets of performance. With the assistance of agricultural advisors (nutritionists, geneticists, engineers, economists), the veterinarian will make recommendations for improvement in animal health and production using the whole farm approach. The ideal objective is to maximize the utilization of the resources available on the farm.

It is now generally agreed that subclinical disease or production inefficiencies, many of which cause no recognizable clinical signs, are the most important contributors to reduced productivity. These production inefficiencies, which result from factors that impair animal health, can be eliminated in the foreseeable future if present knowledge is applied, if animal health delivery systems are improved, and if new technology is developed through basic and applied research in areas where suitable measures are not presently available. There are good prospects for major breakthroughs in animal health in the next decade that will have implications for animal production in the 21st century (Anderson and Pritchard 1980). The development of a totally integrated animal health and management system is the most important need. Epidemiologic surveillance will become the "core" activity of public and private practice of preventive veterinary medicine (Schwabe 1982).

FACTORS AFFECTING THE DEVELOPMENT OF HERD HEALTH PROGRAMS

Several factors have prevented the widespread adoption of herd health veterinary services by farmers and veterinarians.

Some farmers have not fully appreciated the existence of subclinical disease and the economic returns that are possible by accurately monitoring animal health and production and taking positive action to improve performance. Farmers have traditionally been willing to pay for emergency veterinary service on individual clinically ill animals. However, they have been and often still are reluctant to pay for veterinary advice when the results are not immediately obvious. Interviews with large-scale dairy operators have indicated that they perceive veterinarians as primary providers of clinical services only (Goodger and Ruppanner 1982b). Large dairies require an integrated approach to herd management, but the operators do not look to veterinarians to provide this integrated approach; instead, they rely on feed representatives, nutritionists, accountants, and staff of dairy cooperatives. Because veterinarians have little conflict of interest or vested interest in giving advice about nutrition, proper facility design, and other general management issues, this perception of the veterinarian as a clinician only deprives the dairy operator of an objective appraisal of herd health, management, and production. Changing this perception will require a restructuring of many veterinary medical school curricula, with an emphasis on courses in epidemiology, preventive medicine, herd management, nutrition, and similar subjects. This has been a major stumbling block in the rate of development of herd health services. Much of the gain in preventive veterinary medicine in the recent past has been because of a change in the attitude of farmers toward a more financially conscious appraisal of their activities than they applied previously. Some of the change has been due to better education generally, but primarily it has been an appreciation of the need to maintain a sufficient margin between costs and income in order to enhance their standard of living or simply to service their very large financial commitments. Cost-effectiveness and benefit-cost analysis have become the important yardsticks rather than winning at cattle fairs and shows or topping the prices at fat stock shows or wool sales. When this attitude about economic viability is applied to health and productivity, there is a tendency for

technical services and advice to be used much more to the mutual advantage of the service and the farmer. The trend to greater use of advisory services has been followed by a significant improvement in the standards of animal management and farming generally. This trend has been assisted by the disappearance of many inefficient farms, brought about by the cost-efficiency squeeze. In some areas, the surviving farms absorb the others, and farm size has increased. In general, the larger the farms, the more demand there is for advice on prevention of loss and for encouragement of the development of planned health and production programs.

The goals and values of farmers may also have been responsible for the slow growth of herd health (Gasson 1973). An analysis of the goals and values of British farmers reveals that the smaller farmers place more stress on intrinsic aspects of work, particularly independence. Farmers with larger businesses, however, are more economically motivated and are more likely to seek and consider consultancy advice about health and production management (Winkler 1979).

A major factor affecting the rate of development and the success of herd health programs has been the lack of reliable animal health and production records that can be analyzed regularly. The success of a herd health program depends upon the competence and enthusiasm of the veterinarian, the management expertise of the farmer, and the ability of the program to demonstrate progress through improved performance. Only the records can document improved cost-effective performance. When reliable records are lacking or cannot be easily analyzed, the veterinarian cannot demonstrate to the farmer that progress has been made. With no clear evidence of progress, the farmer may become disinterested in the program.

The economic value of the animal can influence the development of herd health. As the value increases, the need to insure against loss of the individual increases. As the value of food-producing animals continues to increase, the need for diagnosis and treatment of individual sick animals increases. At the other extreme, when the economic value of animals is low, such as beef cattle and wool sheep, the treatment of individual animals is given low priority, and there is a tendency for animal husbandry and management to be considered more important than specific health maintenance programs. The emphasis is on nutrition and breeding practice. Disease control programs such as those for internal parasites, blowfly infestation, and footrot are developed for application to all farms in the area rather than adapted to suit the circumstances or resources of a particular farm. For these reasons, planned animal health and production programs for wool sheep, and to a lesser extent for range cattle, tend to be strong on management and light on disease control and therefore tend to be dominated by animal husbandry advisors rather than veterinarians. The reverse is true in dairy cattle herds, beef feedlots, beef breeding herds, swine herds, and intensively-farmed fat lambs and fat sheep enterprises. Maximum veterinary intervention and domination of the management of the farm by veterinary rather than nutritional or genetic advice is demanded by the high level of disease prevalence that is potentially possible in such units and by the capital value of the individual animals. The risks of disease losses and the need for veterinary supervision are even greater in the large "factory" type farming units that are common in most developed countries (Watson 1980).

Emergency veterinary medicine and the revenue from the sales of drugs and vaccines have occupied a large part of well-established rural veterinary practices and in part have contributed to the slow growth of herd health in some areas. As long as veterinarians were making a good living from emergency veterinary medicine, which is satisfying to the veterinarian and the farmer, there was little incentive to develop herd health programs. Some veterinarians also lacked the confidence necessary to provide a comprehensive animal health service that included investigations of the nutritional status of the herd, housing requirements, reproductive performance, and other production-oriented aspects of the herds. However, there is ample evidence that veterinarians who give high priority to herd health will quickly develop a reputation as herd health specialists who can provide an integrated production-oriented preventive veterinary service. A busy veterinary practice can also schedule herd health work during those periods of the year when there is insufficient emergency work to financially support the practice staff. In this way, the work can be balanced throughout the year.

Other factors that can affect planned herd health programs include the availability of feed supplies, the market value of livestock, the prevalence of disease in the herd, and the diagnostic laboratory services available to the veterinarian. Large fluctuations in the supply of feed can cause major disruptions in reproductive performance. A marked decline in the market price of livestock will force farmers to invest scarce resources elsewhere on the farm. A sudden unexpected epidemic of an infectious disease can cause large economic losses, and the farmer may lose confidence in the veterinarian's ability to control disease.

THE REQUIREMENTS OF A HERD HEALTH PROGRAM

The three requirements for a successful herd health program are:
1. A willing farmer
2. An enthusiastic, competent veterinarian and
3. A system of record-keeping and animal identification

An even more fundamental requirement before a herd health program is begun is the establishment or growth of a satisfactory farmer-veterinarian relationship. Through experience with the veterinarian, the farmer must reach the point where he has confidence that the veterinarian can provide the service.

The Willing Farmer

The characteristics that identify farmers as being likely to be receptive to a herd health program and that will set an example for the rest of the community include the following:

□ Leaders in the community. These are the progressive farmers whose opinions are accepted by other farmers.

□ Successful businessmen. Business acumen is a highly desirable characteristic, especially if the farmer has a good farm. These farmers are aware of the principle of cost-effectiveness.

□ Stable, efficient farmers who have good judgment and who are recognized as "early innovators" in the community (Fig. 1–1).

□ Knowledgeable farmers. These are farmers who keep up to date with the farm literature and who are interested in learning more about the modern aspects of animal health and production.

□ Farmers who have not overextended their limit of resources, in terms of finance and of labor or land area, are most likely to be able to make changes in management and scale of operations.

□ Farmers whose inclination is to avoid taking risks are natural enlisters in herd health programs. There are significant differences between them and gamblers in farming performance (Camm 1980).

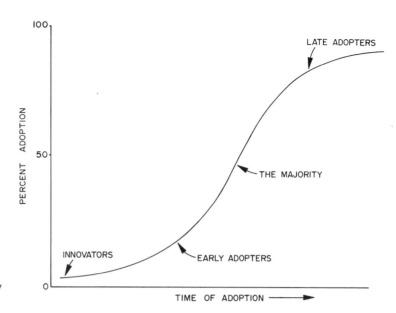

Figure 1-1. The community adoption curve.

To develop a situation in which farmers are committed to a herd health program requires two stages. The first is to convince them to begin by establishing a bond of confidence between the farmer and the veterinarian; by determining that there is a problem in the herd that is likely to be responsive to a cost-effective control program; and, if necessary, by beginning the program as a partial one, for example by improving reproductive performance and delaying action on other problems until obvious results are obtained.

Herd health management programs need to be viewed from the perspective of the livestock producer's decision-making framework. The farmer's goals and objectives must be considered. The producer's resource situation may be a primary determinant of feasible herd health alternatives. The role, nature, and size of livestock enterprises impose limitations on the type and scope of herd health management program that is (1) economically feasible, (2) workable in practice, and (3) acceptable to the livestock producer (Huffman 1979).

Having established the program and being aware that the bigger task is to maintain it, it is necessary to set the second phase in motion. This is most likely to be successful if the program has the following characteristics:

□ The simplest data recording system possible. A farmer's natural inclination is to avoid paper work, especially large sheets of it showing many columns and many figures. Data that have already been provided, e.g., herd and milk testing data and artificial breeding data, should be used where possible. The farmer's own observations should be restricted in scope if possible (e.g., limited to disease and reproduction and culling data) and it should be transcribed, collected, and entered into tables by professional data handlers.

□ The quickest possible turnaround time for analysis of data and reporting back to the farmer. Instant turnaround by computer printout or visual display is most satisfying. Reporting back in numerical terms is usual, but if the results can be expressed in financial terms they have more impact.

□ A data analysis system that gives early warning of impending deviations of production performance or disease prevalence from set targets.

□ The introduction into the production and disease control systems of the most up-to-date technical information as soon as it becomes available.

□ The creation of a data base of information accumulated from the cooperating farms to serve as a realistic guide to performance targets.

□ The conducting of interherd comparisons anonymously to indicate to each farmer where he stands with respect to performance in a variety of parameters and in contrast with his peers.

□ The promotion of exchange of information between farmers about modifications of techniques, problems with existing techniques, and developing needs by conducting group meetings at intervals of six months to one year.

☐ Visiting the herd regularly, punctually, and for a sufficient time period to allow discussion of all problems. In beef cattle or sheep operations where visitation is less frequent, the maintenance of surveillance must be less personal but can be complemented by written reports at intervals between physical visits.

☐ Ensuring that farm staff, especially managers and share-farmers, are included in the competitive atmosphere of the program. They are critical because they are responsible for putting the recommended procedures into practice (Henderson 1980). These parts of a total program are displayed graphically in Table 1–2. They all encourage a degree of psychological dependence by the farmer on the system. They also impose an acceptance of responsibility by the veterinarian to provide the necessary input, to keep on providing this input, and to be financially responsible if he provides the wrong advice.

The Enthusiasm and Competence of the Veterinarian

Veterinarians have traditionally been viewed as healers of the sick, but they are situated in the advisory support system of farmers in a way that makes them strategically the best person to ensure that there is integration of the various components of management (Goodger and Ruppanner 1982b). These include health maintenance, genetic input through artificial breeding, advice on nutrition and calving pat-

terns, and in the northern hemisphere, housing. All these advisory and management aid services must be integrated so as to have maximum beneficial effect on the total farm program. The veterinarian is the person closest to the interface between the support systems and the farm itself. He is one of the most frequent visitors and is often the most familiar with the farm's objectives and resources, especially its management skills. Also, much of what the veterinarian does can significantly affect the influence of the other advisory input. It is not intended to suggest that the veterinarian will necessarily proceed to encompass all areas of advice to animal farmers, but for the reasons stated he is a logical selection from the team of management advisors who could act as the coordinator of all of the sources of advice. If veterinarians had the proper training and interest to adopt such a role, they would be in a much better position than they are now to work with other specialist advisors. This would include a better appreciation of when such a specialist could help and should be called on to do so, and also how their advice should be incorporated into the overall plan of management. It would be a much better service of advice to farmers if it resulted in a reciprocal development of understanding and constructive criticism between veterinarians and agriculturalists rather than the interprofessional competition that tends to be the order of the day.

It is also desirable that the professional veterinarian be convinced that the conventional stance of the physician, with the treatment and control of clinical disease as the sole objective, is inappropriate to agricultural prac-

Table 1–2. CONVERTING FARMERS TO A HERD HEALTH SERVICE

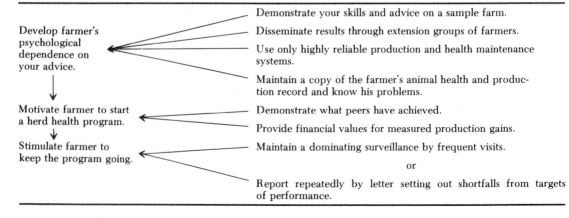

tice. This attitude fails to recognize the strong relationship between management and disease, especially the effect of disease on management, and the need to consider benefit-cost relationships in veterinary professional advice. There is ample evidence that veterinarians can play an important role in improving the profitability of farming because of the economic importance of disease and the large returns that have been shown to be attainable by investment in disease control programs.

To participate properly in planned animal health and production programs, a veterinarian has to make certain commitments. However, participation can be at a number of levels so that its intensity varies. It is important to make regular visits, punctually and at the specified times, and to complete the visits without interruption. This virtually creates a requirement for a practice employing more than one veterinarian. The veterinarian should maintain the necessary expertise in such things as pregnancy diagnosis in cattle, and semen examination in rams. He should check the analyses on every report that comes out of the data analysis system and advise the farmer of the implications of these results for that particular herd. The veterinarian should give first priority to being available for consultation on management matters to participating farmers. He should also keep up with technical and scientific advances and feed them into the information extension system. It is necessary for him to be aware of political, sociological, and financial pressures on the relevant industry that are likely to affect its financial status.

Participation of the veterinarian may be at one of several levels. The common ones are as a herd health veterinarian and as a species specialist. In the former, the veterinarian limits his expertise to the prevention, control, and treatment of disease and is aware of the implications of production matters but is not skilled in handling them. When questions related to nutrition and breeding program arise, the veterinarian consults with colleagues in the allied professions and arranges for their advice to be provided to the farmer (Lesch et al. 1980). The species specialist is skilled in all facets of knowledge and manipulation of the particular industry and deals with all of these matters. Whether or not the work is done by a private practitioner or a government-salaried officer seems to be irrelevant except where both are available. In those circumstances, the private practitioner would seem to be the logical person because of his greater familiarity with and preoccupation with individual herds or flocks. However, it is a common experience to find a private practitioner who is not skilled in the necessary techniques or who is not interested in participating in the program, and there is no reason why a veterinarian of another genre should not take over its direction.

The Records System and Animal Identification

A simple, reliable system of recording animal health events and production performance is a fundamental requirement for a successful herd health program. Without recording, the control of productivity is guesswork. The records system involves all of the components from the records containing the raw data through to the summaries of animal health and performance. Many different systems are available, but the fundamental requirements include the following:

□ Positive identification of the individual animal or groups of animals is a necessity.
□ The system must be simple to use and understand.
□ Only animal health and production data that are considered necessary to assess herd performance are collected and analyzed. The types of data collected will vary between species and classes of livestock, but clearly established terminology should be used to avoid confusion and to allow comparisons to be made between cooperating farms.
□ The system must be structured so that the data is easily collected, gathered, analyzed, summarized, and reported to the farmer within a few days of the herd health visit.
□ The veterinarian should maintain a file of each summary report that was sent to the farmer.

In the simplest form of record keeping, the data from individual animal cards or from groups of animals is collected and analyzed regularly, and summaries of herd performance are reported. In small cattle and swine herds, the manual handling of records is satisfactory but still time consuming. As the size of herds has increased, it has become necessary to consider the use of a computer.

The introduction of computer-based data recording systems has revolutionized the handling and analysis of animal health and production data. The computer is able to store a large amount of data about a large number of individuals. It has the capacity to analyze and integrate current data with historical data and provide a summary of up-to-date performance. It can be programmed to compare actual performance with preset targets of performance.

The computer can prepare action lists, which advise when certain events will occur or when certain procedures should be performed. It is now possible for the computer to take over the entire chore of record-keeping and to provide summaries of performance as frequently as necessary. Only the most elementary records of observations need to be made by the farmer.

Additional Requirements

Some additional requirements include adequate physical facilities on the farm for the handling of animals, particularly cattle, during the farm visit. Adequate facilities are required for performing rectal examinations on cattle. Pens for separating groups of animals near the examining point so that examinations and treatments can be completed with a minimum loss of time are necessary.

A veterinary diagnostic laboratory is also necessary for assistance in making a definitive etiologic diagnosis in the case of herd problems.

THE COMPONENTS OF A HERD HEALTH PROGRAM

The components of a herd health program include regularly scheduled farm visits by the veterinarian; good animal farming by the farmer; the recording and analysis of animal health and production data; and the provision and coordination of advice by the veterinarian.

The success of a herd health program will depend on the competence of the veterinarian, the level of management by the farmer, the reliability and adequacy of the records, and the competence with which the veterinarian provides advice and follows up the results of that advice.

The veterinarian should identify the objectives of the farmer before beginning a program. A clear picture of the production objectives compared with actual performance will often identify the presence of problems that have interfered with performance.

The initial stages of any program should concentrate on solving obvious disease or production problems for which there are simple and reliable solutions. When these problems are solved, attention can then be given to evaluating the health and production status of the herd and to the identification of other

economically significant problems. Gradually, over a period of two to five years, the veterinarian will become acquainted with the herd, its characteristics, and areas where additional effort should be directed to improve health and production. It is a gradual evolutionary process.

Frequency of Visits to the Herd

The most common aspect of any herd health program is the regularly scheduled visit to the herd. The frequency of each visit will depend on the class of livestock, the size of the herd, the incidence of disease, and the length of time the herd has been on a program. Twelve monthly visits are common for year-round dairy herds with less than 100 cows. Weekly visits become necessary for herds of 300 to 500 cows, and more frequent visits may be necessary for larger herds. Four visits per year are common for commercial beef herds, and weekly visits are usually necessary for beef feedlots with a total capacity of 5000 head. For 100-sow farrow-finish swine herds, monthly visits are common.

Activities During the Farm Visit

The veterinary activities conducted during each visit are similar for each species or class of livestock, but the specific activities will vary according to the class of livestock, the season of the year, and the length of time the herd has been on the program.

The primary purpose of the farm visit is to organize and concentrate the veterinary activities into a regular schedule to ensure that they get done. There are several animal health and production activities that occur during the production cycle of each animal. The primary objective of the farm visit is to determine the *actual performance* of animal health and production and to compare it with *targets of performance*. In other words, the regularly scheduled farm visit is a surveillance system designed to detect or predict animal health and production problems before they become economically significant and to indicate the necessary corrective action. Under ideal conditions, each visit should provide a summary of the animal health and production status, the reasons for failure to achieve certain targets of performance and, recommendations for corrective action. For some parameters of performance, the data will be available directly from the records or the computer print-out. Examples include milk production, number of pigs born alive, number of pigs weaned per litter, average daily gain in feedlot steers, and the somatic cell count of milk. For other parameters, the veterinarian will have to carry out certain diagnostic skills, such as pregnancy diagnosis, in order to obtain the information.

Some examples of specific activities follow.

Reproductive Performance

In breeding herds, the emphasis is on surveillance of reproductive performance. For example, in dairy herds, which calve year round, at each monthly visit all cows bred more than 40 days are examined for pregnancy by rectal examination. The cows to be examined are identified by examination of the individual cow records or by the use of a computer. Regular pregnancy examinations will identify nonpregnant cows as soon as possible so that early corrective action can be taken. In beef breeding herds, the bulls are examined for breeding soundness before the breeding season ends. Pregnancy examinations are done only once annually, usually following the breeding season. In swine herds, reproductive performance may be monitored regularly by pregnancy examination using an ultrasound pregnancy tester, monitoring of the number of sows that return to heat three weeks after breeding, and the number of pigs born alive per litter.

Production Performance

The production of livestock and livestock products can be monitored on a regular basis and can be used as indicators of performance. These include average daily milk production, butterfat test, average daily body weight gain in feedlot cattle, days to reach market weight in pigs, feed efficiency in feedlot cattle and finishing pigs, and grades of carcasses at slaughter.

Nutritional Status

The feeds and feeding program have a major influence on reproductive performance, growth rate, and milk production and must be monitored regularly. The veterinarian must be aware of any changes in the feeding program that have occurred since the last farm visit or that are intended in the near future. On breeding farms, there are several different age groups of animals at different levels of growth and production. This requires close surveillance to avoid under- or overnutrition.

Clinical and Pathologic Examination of Animals

On a herd basis, there are usually some animals affected with clinical disease that the farmer has identified. They should be examined, and the necessary laboratory samples should be taken to obtain a definitive etiologic diagnosis. In beef feedlots and swine herds, necropsy examinations of animals that have died naturally or of selected clinical cases is a common practice in order to obtain an etiologic diagnosis.

Disease Incidence

The records of all clinical diseases that have occurred since the last visit should be examined. If possible, the veterinarian should attempt to determine the etiology retrospectively from the evidence available and prescribe advice on the treatment and control of future cases.

Routine Elective Activities

In some programs, veterinarians perform certain routine activities at strategic times. These include vaccination, administration of anthelmintics, dehorning, castration, foot trimming, and other minor surgical procedures such as spaying beef heifers. While it may be argued that these procedures are too technical for a veterinarian, the veterinarian should be aware of when and how these things are being done if he is not doing them. However, many farmers prefer to employ their veterinarian for these tasks, which provide an excellent opportunity for him to get on the farm on a regular basis.

Examination and Discussion of Records and Reports

There are always some problems with the accuracy of completeness of the records and these should be corrected each month. All production and disease reports should be interpreted and recommendations made for corrective action if necessary. The results of the previous herd health visit should be discussed with the farmer. The results of recommendations made on previous visits should be assessed and changes made if necessary. This will require that the veterinarian bring with him to the farm a current client file that contains the results of herd health visits, necropsy reports, feed analysis reports, and recommendations that were made for the previous few months.

Emergency Farm Visits

The emergency farm visits are independent of the programmed visits. However, the nature and amount of emergency veterinary medicine necessary in the herd will be relevant to the overall herd health program. Every disease incident treated by the farmer or the veterinarian must be recorded. At each farm visit, the diagnosis, treatment, and control of the diseases encountered are discussed.

Investigation of Outbreaks of Disease

Unexpected outbreaks of disease should be investigated as soon as possible by means of a carefully planned clinical and epidemiologic examination of the herd (Kahrs 1978, 1980). The investigation will include clinical examination of affected animals and the submission of appropriate laboratory samples. Detailed recommendations for treatment and control should be reported in writing to the farmer and a copy of the report retained by the veterinarian for future reference.

Consultation by Telephone

A significant amount of consultation can occur by telephone and may consume a large amount of the veterinarian's time. Recommendations for the treatment and control of herd problems may be given over the telephone provided the veterinarian is confident that he has sufficient knowledge about the particular problem from previous visits to the farm. However, all major recommendations should be recorded and followed by a written report to the farmer. This is particularly important when prescriptions for mass medication of feed and water are given by telephone.

Meeting with Participating Farmers

A valuable aspect of any herd health service is the convening of regular meetings of participating farmers to discuss the results of performance of the herds. The results may be presented anonymously, and individual farmers can compare their performance indices with others in the anonymous group. The high levels of performance can be used as targets of performance that are possible under the conditions of the local area.

Provision of Drugs and Vaccines

Drugs and vaccines to be used in the herd can be supplied by the veterinarian at reduced cost. This will encourage the farmer to purchase these supplies from the veterinarian, who will provide recommendations for their use. The veterinarian will also then be aware of the drugs and vaccines being used in the herd.

RESPONSIBILITY OF THE FARMER

The success of a herd health program depends heavily on the level of management and the desire and ability of the farmer to carry out the recommendations of the veterinarian and any other agricultural advisors involved.

The principal mechanism in these programs is to encourage farmers to compete against each other for ranking and also against approved standards. The standards are presented as targets, which are arrived at by estimation of what should be possible in an ideal situation as created by experimental research, tempered with what appear to be attainable results in a particular environment, as disclosed by a data base developed in it. This does not appear to have been too difficult, but many of the targets in use have not been submitted to extensive field testing. What is difficult is selecting the individual criteria—the indices in which the targets are to be set. There is no rule for selecting the indices. They are peculiar to each species and are presented in each of the programs in later chapters.

The target concept assumes that the only objective is maximum financial profitability. That is often not so, and other objectives, as presented in the introduction to this chapter, are often included in a farmer's objectives. To ensure that the herd health program for a particular herd keeps these objectives in sight, it is recommended that they be recorded in a farm profile created for the purpose. The profile should include:

□ Details of other enterprises on the farm. This may be important, because they may compete with each other for available labor, land, and financial resources.

□ Details of physical resources, land area, water availability, and soil type and fertility. These are factors that are often responsible for variations in performance between apparently comparable farms.

□ The farmer's objectives. These might well include a guaranteed two-month vacation each year or a desire to win an agricultural contest that does not include economic profitability.

□ The management systems used, such as all-grass pasture, biological manures only, dry lot farming, and type of housing.

□ Classes and breeds of livestock, especially changes in them.

Each year when the performance of the farm is reviewed, the opportunity should be taken to update the farm profile and compare the achievement with the objective rather than just the target.

Farmers receive advice from a number of sources that often present different or conflicting opinions. The progressive farmer would prefer to have all of these channels of advice integrated through a common program. Planned herd health and production programs set out to do this, but the objective—admirable though it is in every way—is not easily attained. The problems encountered include the reluctance of the institutions that control production data to make it accessible and the difficulty created by different computer languages, different indices used in assessment, and different and incompatible computer programs.

The segments of information and attendant advice, which suggest themselves as potential facets of an inclusive data and advice program, include milk quality and volume in DHIA testing, artificial breeding records relative to reproductive efficiency, cow quality records in breed society catalogues, hard data from regional applied research on feeding programs and pasture utilization, and data from disease eradication programs, e.g., tuberculosis and brucellosis.

THE COLLECTION, ANALYSIS, AND USE OF ANIMAL HEALTH AND PRODUCTION DATA IN A HERD HEALTH PROGRAM

One of the most important components of a successful herd health program is the keeping of good records that can be used to monitor and evaluate the incidence of disease and production.

The kinds of records will vary considerably, depending on the class of livestock and the stage of the herd health program. In the simplest and most common form used in dairy herds, for example, there is an individual lifetime card for each cow. All events of the reproductive cycle and incidents of clinical disease are recorded on the card when they occur. At regular intervals, monthly or less frequently, the veterinarian analyzes the data and prepares a summary of the reproductive performance and disease incidence. This kind of an individual card manual analysis system has been successful for small 50- to 80-cow dairy herds. Some larger herds of up to 200 to 500 cows have maintained this manual system,

and various bookkeeping techniques have been used to make the analysis efficient. In dairy herds, the emphasis has been on assessment of reproductive performance, and the manual systems have been satisfactory. Similar manual systems have been used in beef breeding herds (Janzen 1983), swine herds (Pepper et al. 1977; Pepper and Taylor 1977), and beef feed lots (Church 1980) with success. However, as livestock herds become larger and more intensive, farmers become more cost conscious and require the rapid analysis of a wide spectrum of production data, which cannot be done manually. This has led to the use of the computer, which can store and analyze large amounts of data and provide useful performance statistics for decision making on a daily basis. The computer is "automating" the eyes of the herdsman (Puckett et al. 1981; Russell and Rowlands 1983).

The computer has already had a major impact on the development of efficient modern livestock production. Much of the progress in animal breeding programs in cattle and swine was made with the use of the computer. Initially, the information from the farm was mailed to the computer center, processed, and the report mailed out to the farm. One problem with this system was the long turnaround time, as long as two weeks or more, which often made the information too historical. The introduction of farm-located terminals linked to the central computer by telephone eliminated the turnaround problem. The recent development of microcomputers has now made it possible for farmers to own and operate a computer completely independent of any outside agency. However, there are two major problems with stand-alone on-the-farm microcomputers. The first is that the development of software programs has not kept pace with the development of computer machines. As a result, there is considerable worldwide activity in 1984 in the development of useful, reliable software programs for the different classes of livestock. The second problem or deficiency is the lack of access to central information for comparative purposes.

However, it appears that on-farm computers will be used extensively for analysis of farm accounting, crop production, and livestock performance on individual farms. Veterinarians providing a herd health service must use all the production information that is available from the farm programs or if unavailable, develop computer programs that are located and operated in the veterinarian's office (Sard 1981). The data is sent to the office on a regular basis, processed, and the results returned to the farm. In this way, both the farmer and the veterinarian maintain a record of the health and production of the herd.

The flow of data and information in a herd health program is represented diagrammatically in Figure 1-2. The data is collected from available sources on a regular basis and entered by codes into the computer, which analyzes the data and produces useful information. The veterinarian must then interpret the information and make recommendations for action to improve performance. The results of the action to improve performance are monitored over the next few farm visits, and the cycle is repeated. It is a *constant self-analyzing surveillance system*. For each action there is a measurement, and for each period of monitoring there is either more action or a decision that none is necessary. The targets of performance can be incorporated into the computer program and compared with actual performance. An examination of the computer print-out for the period will indicate the areas in which shortfalls have occurred.

As shown in the collection of data in Figure 1-3, data can come from several sources. In order to maintain the program's profile of economy and to use information efficiently and as inexpensively as possible, it is necessary to use data already accumulated for other purposes, e.g., herd testing, or the artificial insemination records from breeding cooperatives. Use of this material can effect considerable economy, especially if it is already computerized and is in a compatible language. Only data that is critical to the assessment being undertaken should be collected. It is easy to collect enormous amounts of data that are irrelevant or redundant. The sole purpose of the program is to perform every part of it with the greatest economic efficiency, and this applies to the data collection and analysis as much as it does to the veterinary part of the program.

The data provided by the participating herds

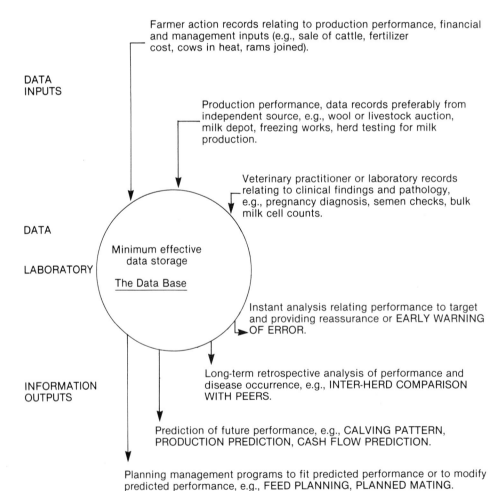

Farmer action records relating to production performance, financial and management inputs (e.g., sale of cattle, fertilizer cost, cows in heat, rams joined).

DATA INPUTS

Production performance, data records preferably from independent source, e.g., wool or livestock auction, milk depot, freezing works, herd testing for milk production.

Veterinary practitioner or laboratory records relating to clinical findings and pathology, e.g., pregnancy diagnosis, semen checks, bulk milk cell counts.

DATA

LABORATORY

Minimum effective data storage

The Data Base

Instant analysis relating performance to target and providing reassurance or EARLY WARNING OF ERROR.

INFORMATION OUTPUTS

Long-term retrospective analysis of performance and disease occurrence, e.g., INTER-HERD COMPARISON WITH PEERS.

Prediction of future performance, e.g., CALVING PATTERN, PRODUCTION PREDICTION, CASH FLOW PREDICTION.

Planning management programs to fit predicted performance or to modify predicted performance, e.g., FEED PLANNING, PLANNED MATING.

Figure 1-2. The flow of data and information in a herd health program.

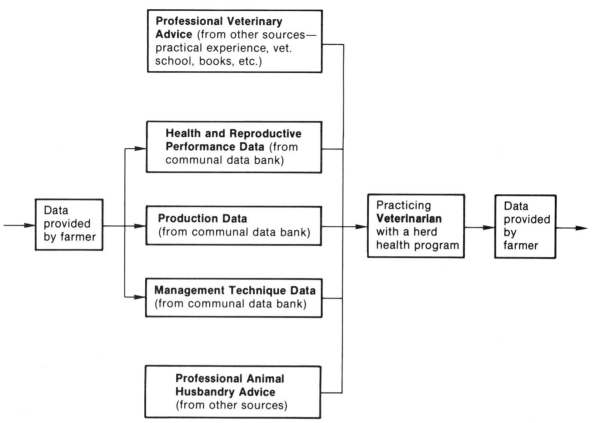

Figure 1-3. The flow of data and information in a herd health program.

and flocks can be accumulated into a data bank, and from this bank, performance levels can be estimated and targets set. This information usually comes to the data bank as a monthly return on a structured report form. It is desirable to accumulate as much basic and detailed information about the relevant animal species and industry as possible. For a practicing veterinarian, this may be limited to disease incidence and reproductive performance. For a species specialist, the expertise will extend over the fields of nutrition, breeding programs, and housing. A collaborative effort with an animal husbandry advisor would complement the service.

The pattern of flow of information was illustrated in Figure 1-3. A more detailed flow chart of an interactive program applicable to dairy herds at an advanced level is shown in Figure 1-4.

Analysis of Data

After the animal health and production data is collected from the farm, it must be transferred to and incorporated into the previously collected data and analyzed periodically. The data must be stored and retrieved easily and

economically. A variety of codes are used that simplify data handling. Manual systems are satisfactory for small herds, but as herds become larger the computer becomes necessary to minimize the number of errors and to obtain rapid analysis of the data.

The most important aspect of the analysis of the data is to select the most useful indices or parameters that are required to accurately monitor performance.

Following analysis of the data, reports containing useful information and recommendations are prepared and sent to the farmer.

Periodic Reports to the Farmer

Regular reports must be prepared and sent to the farmer. The reports are provided after each visit, and the number of reports depends on how frequently the veterinarian visits the herd as part of a herd health program. The reports contain the following kinds of information:

□ A list of clinical examinations and treatments carried out as a record of the events.
□ An updated list of the individual animals or groups of animals, depending on how they are handled in the particular program. This

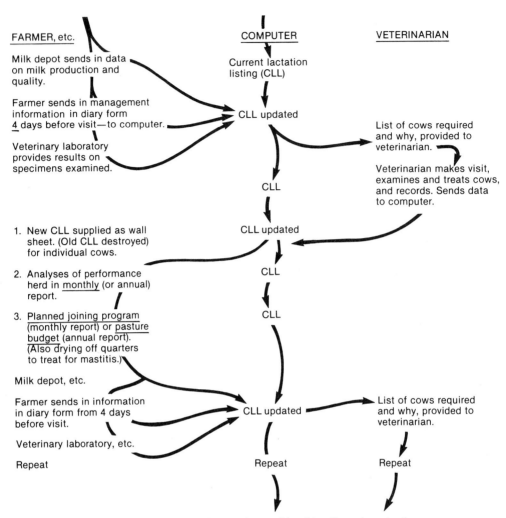

Figure 1-4. Pattern of information in an advanced herd health and production program.

includes all the data relating to disease, reproductive performance, and preventive procedures for the unit and enables each animal's (or group's) history for the immediate past to be reviewed. A lifetime history also is available on request for producers who require the information for decisions on culling and to provide a health and production record at the time of sale.

☐ An analysis of the parameters used to evaluate reproductive efficiency and the wastage caused by mastitis and other diseases. These are accompanied by the levels of performance proposed as targets and an opportunity for the veterinarian to comment on performance—good or bad. It is important that sufficient flexibility be retained when assessing changes in performance indices. For example, bulk milk cell counts fluctuate visibly from month to

month, and it is usual to wait until a three-month rolling average continues at a high level before raising an alarm.

☐ Recommended actions. These are recommendations arising from other programmed reminders for that particular time of the year or reproductive cycle or from the interactive part of the computer program. Based on the data that has already been provided to it, the computer identifies those cows that have had a poor reproductive performance, a poor production record, or serious disease incidents. These cows can be considered with a view to culling some of them. Similarly, the computer will identify the cows to be dried off and the dates on which this should be done, cows to be bred, and cows to be examined for pregnancy or for abnormal reproductive function.

□ Predicted production events. This is a developing and vital segment of the program. The farmer can preplan a calving or reproductive pattern for his herd or flock. Armed with a knowledge of the fertility index of the herd, the computer program can then advise when individual cows should be bred to conform with this pattern. Similarly, it is then possible, knowing the reproductive data, to predict what the milk production will be at particular times and to predict the feed requirements week by week. All of these functions are performed by modern programs. Farmers receiving this advice can plan their feed program six months in advance. This gives them time to plant a crop, boost pastures with nitrogen fertilizers, purchase more land, or cull more cows.

□ Cash flow predictions may also be included.

An annual report may be prepared that is a retrospective summation of the other reports that have already been provided for the year. This is the opportunity for a major review of the performance of the herd for the year and for an interherd comparison among a local group, with an annual meeting of participants to discuss progress and performance. The annual review of the herd needs to be done in conjunction with an updating of the herd profile. A copy of an annual interherd report is shown in Table 1-3.

General Advice in Output

This is advice that does not originate from the monitoring program. It relates mostly to those actions that the farmer must take regularly during the year. The action is generally directed at the prevention of specific diseases and the maintenance of production. Some of the actions are stimulated by events in the reproductive cycle. For example, it may be necessary to vaccinate cattle for vibrosis and other infectious diseases before breeding; ewes may need to be vaccinated for enterotoxemia in late pregnancy; cows that are susceptible to milk fever will need to be treated prophylactically close to the day of calving.

The range of the recommendations is not universal for every farm and will depend on the prevalence of disease in the individual herd and in the area. What the veterinarian recommends will depend on his knowledge of these matters and on his expectations of bad seasons or bad years for particular diseases, often depending on the climate and the availability of feed. Also, his recommendations will be affected by the need to remain cost-effective. For example, it may be financially more beneficial on some farms, in some years, to restrict the supplementary feeding of ewes, normally done to avoid pregnancy toxemia, because the expected prevalence may not warrant the additional expense.

This general advice can be sent by mail at strategic times of the year, without the necessity of visiting the farm. In addition, new information and techniques may be included and reported in the form of a newsletter to the veterinarian's clients.

BENEFITS OF A HERD HEALTH PROGRAM

Financial Gains

The economic benefits derived from a herd health program have been the subject of considerable debate. When progress has been made and performance has improved, it has been difficult to identify which factor or combination of factors was responsible. A successful comprehensive herd health program involves more effective management by the farmer, the introduction of specific disease prevention techniques, regular visits by the veterinarian, improved nutrition, improved breeding programs, and possibly some unidentified variables.

The veterinary costs of a herd health program are part of the variable or optional costs of farming such as those associated with feed, fertilizer, supplies, and services. The net return to the farmer of money spent on veterinary services directed toward a comprehensive

Table 1-3. ANNUAL INTERFARM COMPARISON OF TARGETS OF PERFORMANCE AND ACTUAL PERFORMANCE

Data	Target of Performance	District Average	Actual Performance
Average daily milk yield (liters)	15	13.2	14
Bulk milk cell count/ml	300,000	500,000	200,000
Per cent cows in heat last 30 days	100	85	75
Per cent cows pregnant at 90 days	100	80	70

herd health program has been calculated for some specific disease control techniques such as control of mastitis and improved reproductive performance in dairy herds. The net returns have been on the order of 200 to 500 per cent.

The technique of partial budgeting can be used to determine the gain or loss associated with the selection of certain strategies of disease control (Ellis and James 1979). The financial changes that occur are grouped according to extra costs, costs saved, revenue foregone, and extra revenue.

A herd health program will increase the costs of production, but the net return from improved performance must exceed the input costs or the program is inefficient. A detailed record of all input costs must be kept for an accurate assessment of the program.

The increased costs of a herd health program can be substantial and may include professional veterinary fees for the regular farm visits and for the analysis of problems and the preparation of reports; professional fees for consultants used by the veterinarian; records and computer costs; drugs, vaccines, anthelmintics, and other supplies; and the costs associated with changes in any aspect of the management of livestock such as nutrition, breeding, housing, additional labor, and new equipment.

Preventive veterinary medicine pays. Most of the documented evidence has been generated from dairy herd health programs in which comparisons in animal health and production performance were made on dairy farms before and after a herd health program was initiated and operated for up to three years (Jointex 1976; Sol 1982). In the Joint Exercise in Animal Health and Productivity (Jointex) in Britain, the effects of joint advice by veterinarians and agricultural advisors on productivity and profitability of 114 farms over a three-year period were examined and compared with farms not enrolled in the exercise. The combination of all the factors resulted in an improvement in total gross margins of 126 per cent on the exercise farms compared with 42 per cent on the farm management survey (Jointex 1976). Similar results were obtained in a three-year study of dairy farms in Holland (Sol 1982).

There is also some indication that as the level of performance improves, the health costs will decrease. The health costs are lowest in dairy herds with near annual calving intervals compared with much higher costs in herds with longer lactation lengths (Shanks et al. 1982).

Aids to Management

An established operative herd health program with a reliable records system will automatically result in the development of several useful aids to management. These have been most successful in dairy and swine herds and include action lists, which assist the farmer in identifying when certain events will occur or which actions must be taken in particular animals. These animals are highlighted by the records system, which prompts the farmer to perform the action when necessary. Some examples in a dairy herd include cows for reproductive tract examination (pregnancy diagnosis, postpartum examination, or infertility); cows to be dried off; cows due to calve; cows to be culled; cows for mastitis examination; and cows for examination because of history of clinical disease.

Other aids to management include predictions of calving pattern, feed requirements, milk production, and cash flow.

Continuous Assessment of the Farming Unit

The herd health program can be regarded as a recurring assessment of the farming unit as a functioning unit. The assessment can be used at any time as a check on the efficiency of a manager, herdsman, or partner (share-farmer). It can also be used by the manager or managing partner as justification for a change in shares in the proceeds. For a banker, investor, buyer, or seller, an annual report can provide evidence of biological managerial efficiency to supplement a financial statement of profit and loss. In extension exercises, field days, farmer's discussion groups, and meetings, the information provided in annual and monthly reports is most valuable because of the actuality and local origin of the data.

Efficient Utilization of Rural Veterinary Practitioners

Rural veterinary practices have participated in governmental disease regulatory work on a fee-for-service basis for many years. The government benefited by being able to extend its surveillance and eradication programs; and by using practitioners as part-time and casual employees, it was able to remain flexible and relatively uncommitted for a significant segment of its work. Veterinary practices benefited by an improvement in their financial viability, partly because of added income, but largely because the regulatory work could be programmed in parts of the year when emergency work was at a low level and practitioners tended to be underemployed. The success of eradication programs for brucellosis and tuberculosis, which provided most of this regulatory work for veterinarians, has resulted in a marked reduction in the volume of this work available to practitioners and in the regular income that it used to provide. In veterinary practices where work is seasonally distributed, with the peak at the time of calving, herd health programs are a suitable alternative to governmental regulatory work because the reproductive program on which they are based is busiest in the slow season for emergency work.

Encouragement for Veterinarians to Become Species Specialists

Good farmers are able to integrate the information and advice that they receive from various sources and make the appropriate decisions themselves. Many others are not capable of doing this, and this creates a vacancy in the ranks of advisors to food animal farmers—the professional advisor who can provide farmers with a list of alternative strategies and be able to recommend the best solution after making an objective evaluation of the herd, using all of the available information.

Veterinarians are situated in the advisory support system of animal farmers in such a way that they are the most strategically placed persons to ensure that there is integration, and not confrontation, between the components of management. However, veterinarians have traditionally been cast in the role of healers, and additional training and experience for them is required if they are to be involved in decisions on management. This is not to say that basic clinical skills will no longer be necessary. The entire preventive program depends on fast, accurate diagnosis and prompt action when problems arise, and this requires careful clinical examination and proper field and laboratory investigations. If a veterinarian in rural practice wishes to restrict his activities to traditional medicine, surgery, and theriogenology, he will find a need to consult animal husbandry advisors when necessary. A veterinarian who wishes to become fully involved in production management as well will need to develop his expertise as a species specialist (Blood 1978; Radostits 1974).

Increase in the Veterinarian's Involvement with Subclinical Disease

A large part of the impetus to the development of herd health programs has arisen from the realization that the most severe losses in productivity, especially in grazing animals, are caused by subclinical rather than clinically apparent disease. Subclinical disease may affect a large number of the herd and may require extensive epidemiologic and laboratory investigation if a diagnosis is to be made. Treatment and control procedures usually involve the whole herd, and economic considerations assume first priority. The treatment and control procedures for diseases such as parasitoses, nutritional deficiencies, metabolic diseases, and chronic staphylococcal mastitis in cattle and foot rot in sheep require not only herd treatments but need to be integrated with the grazing management of pastures and the management of technical procedures, such as shearing and milking, and the known epidemiology of pathogens, such as the seasonal appearance of fungi on pasture. Veterinarians have been increasingly involved with the diagnosis and management of subclinical diseases for some years, but the inclusion in our lists of diseases of such entities as "failure to meet mathematical targets" has increased involvement further.

Research and Development Opportunities

Field investigations into the effects of changes in management, the administration of anthelmintics, and vaccination schedules on the efficiency and volume of production are difficult and expensive to arrange. A well-managed herd health program provides data from a large number of cows whose health and production records are monitored for health maintenance purposes. However, it is relatively easy to insert a research protocol into such a system and to have access to many cows in a conventional, commercial situation and to determine the outcome of treatment in real-life circumstances.

SOME OTHER FEATURES OF ANIMAL HEALTH MANAGEMENT

Herd Health Programs and the Future of Rural Practice

There is a growing demand for veterinarians to participate in planned programs that set out to maintain health and production in dairy herds. If these programs are to be serviced properly, the number of veterinarians available would need to be modified. Their awareness of the industry and of animal management would need to be increased to the point where they could be involved in significant decisions in farm management. Formal postgraduate training as a species specialist would need to cross the traditional boundaries and provide an education in animal science, especially nutrition and genetics, agricultural economics and engineerin, agronomy, and veterinary science. The major objective is to train the veterinarian in these other fields and at a level that will provide an understanding of the problems and promote consultation and cooperation with the appropriate specialists with the goal of using a team approach to solving them. This should integrate knowledge from a number of disciplines and avoid confrontation between their spokesmen, an all too common occurrence.

The real need in farm management is to find compromises between the often conflicting requirements of the management tools, including health maintenance, nutrition, and breeding plans. The objective of planned health and production programs is to integrate the advice streams relating to these subjects and thus provide an overall whole-farm policy. Compromise between the conflicting demands to get the best whole-farm answer requires a sufficient understanding of all the needs, all the resources and their availability, and all the principles of feeding, reproductive management, and so on. Basically, it is the farmer who should have this broad understanding and be capable of putting advice from all of his advisors into its proper perspective. Some farmers do, but many do not, and it is these who require the coordinated advisory service that a properly educated veterinarian is capable of providing.

Alternatives to Herd Health Programs Provided by Veterinarians

The responsibility of coordinating animal production and health advice for farmers has been unclear for a long time, and the veterinary profession and animal scientists have not appeared anxious to assume the role. Veterinarians have seemed such an obvious choice because they are on most farms frequently, and if they provide herd health programs they are already making the periodic visits that are required for this kind of work.

Of the possible alternatives, the obvious one is to establish animal husbandry advisors in this role and have them use veterinarians as consultants in matters where etiologically specific disease is concerned. There are combinations of people and circumstances now where such an arrangement is producing satisfactory results. However, it is not possible to produce a species specialist in this way. A fully qualified veterinarian who develops a species specialty can provide a major component of a herd health service.

There are differences between the species in the balance between health and production problems as causes of economic loss. In dairy cattle, disease is probably the greater of the two or at least is so great that it requires a veterinarian in constant attendance. In beef cattle and pigs, the veterinarian and the animal scientist can probably make equal contributions, with the possible exception of beef feedlots and intensive pig units, which require more veterinary input. Sheep are probably a species in which planned animal health and production programs could logically be supplied by the animal husbandry profession, with the veterinary profession providing additional consulting services.

In most countries at the present time these programs are developing, and the opportunity is there to lead them and participate in them. The veterinary profession has not fully grasped the opportunity and may find itself in a secondary role as the leadership is taken up by others. For the veterinarian to retain or gain a firm hold on this role in agriculture, he will need to participate actively by ensuring that much of the information stored in the data bank is provided by veterinarians. This may be in the form of reproductive examination records for beef cattle, mastitis examination data in dairy cattle, or necropsy and clinical pathology data in feedlot and sheep enterprises. The greater challenge to the veterinary profession is to create ways of making even bigger contributions by devising new but cost-effective reasons for maintaining their involvement in planned herd health and production programs.

Payment for Services Provided

The service provided is strictly tailored to provide the best financial climate for the farmer, and it is logical that the farmer should pay for it. However, in the initial stages, when a program is beginning or in circumstances where the farmer's financial returns are poor, the question of subsidization or other forms of support may be raised. It is apparent that there are fringe benefits for units other than the farmer, and it is logical that they might contribute to initial or continuing costs if their involvement is great. Some of the receiving organizations are government departments of agriculture, which could have access to data on disease occurrence at all levels, including diseases recognized and treated by farmers; the pharmaceutical industry, which could have use for similar information relevant to potential demand for their products; dairy product processing units, which would be better able to rationalize their purchasing and storage data if accurate production prediction was possible; and university or other research organizations, which need access to source material for research.

Implementation of a Herd Health Program

There is considerable information available about animal health and production that is not being utilized by livestock producers. Failure to apply this information is a major cause of economic loss in livestock production. There is a need for a *Herd Health Alert* campaign directed toward livestock producers that will emphasize that an integrated animal health and production program on the farm can improve animal production and economic returns to the producer. There has been considerable research done on individual diseases and many aspects of animal production. However, there has been almost no research done on the implementation of animal health and production practices using the whole-farm approach, which will yield the best economic return to the producer. Educational efforts have been effective in implementing mastitis control producers in commercial dairy herds (Crist et al. 1982).

A Herd Health Alert Campaign

A campaign of this type would make producers more aware of the large economic gains that are possible by the application of an integrated animal health and production program. There is a need for veterinarians and agricultural advisors to put together, using the printed word and the mass media, the principles of the program that will change the attitudes of producers and motivate them to improve animal health and production. An important research objective is to address the issue of the education of livestock producers to apply the information that is already available

on the control and prevention of animal disease.

A major challenge of the 21st century is the efficient production of wholesome meat and milk using a completely integrated animal health and production system.

There is also an urgent need for a restructuring of veterinary curricula to meet the needs of veterinary students who desire to become food animal practitioners (Goodger and Ruppanner 1982b). There should be a continuum of courses and experiences throughout the veterinary curriculum that give proper emphasis to the herd health concept (Hagstad 1979; Hagstad and Hubbert 1979). Courses offered should include: (1) financial management; (2) farm management; (3) animal production; (4) animal nutrition; (5) experimental design; (6) data processing; (7) economic decision making; (8) statistics; and (9) business administration. Continuing education programs should also provide subjects with a new emphasis to update the skills of those currently in food animal practice.

On a more immediate level, practicing veterinarians must reorient themselves and make a commitment to provide an integrated animal health and production service.

The challenge of the 1980s for veterinarians in large animal practice will be to fill the scientific veterinary journals and textbooks with examples of how applications of preventive medicine have increased profit at the herd level (Hubbert 1979). This information is vital to the development of practitioners of preventive medicine who have confidence in their capability as consultants to management.

References

Anderson, D.P. and Pritchard, W.R. Animal Health. *In* Animal Agriculture, Research to Meet Human Needs in the 21st Century. Pond, W.G. et al. (eds.). Proc. of a meeting held at Boyne Mountain, MI, May 4–9, 1980, pp. 129–151.

Bailey, D.E. Preventive medicine in sheep and goat medicine, J. Am. Vet. Assoc., *174*:388–389, 1979.

Barfoot, L.W., Cote, J.F., Stone, J.B. et al. An economic appraisal of a preventative medicine program for dairy herd health management. Can. Vet. J., *12*:2–10, 1971.

Becker, H.N. Preventative medicine in swine practice. J. Am. Vet. Med. Assoc., *174*:389–393, 1979.

Blaxter, K.L. The limits to animal production. Vet. Rec., *105*:5–9, 1979.

Blood, D.C. The veterinarian in planned animal health and production. Can. Vet. J., *20*:341–347, 1979.

Blood, D.C., Williamson, N.B. and Morris, R.S. The future of large animal practice. Vet. Rec., *103*:246, 1978.

Camm, R.M. Animal health today: The problems of large livestock units. Economics of disease control. Br. Vet. J., *136*:313–320, 1980.

Church, T.L. Preventive medicine and management in beef feedlots. Can. Vet. J., 21:214–218, 1980.

Cope, G.E. Preventive medicine in feedlot practice. J. Am. Vet. Med. Assoc., 174:394–395, 1979.

Crist, W.L., Heider, L.E., Sears, P.M. et al. Effectiveness of educational efforts in implementing mastitis control procedures in commercial dairy herds. J. Dairy Sci., 65:828–834, 1982.

Ellis, P.R. and James, A.D. The economics of animal health. 2. Economics in farm practice. Vet. Rec., 105:523–526, 1979.

Gasson, Ruth. Goals and values of farmers. J. Agric. Economics 24:521–542, 1973.

Goodger, W.J. and Ruppanner, R. Historical perspective on the development of dairy practice. J. Am. Vet. Med. Assoc., 180:1294–1297, 1982a.

Goodger, W.J. and Ruppanner, R. Why the dairy industry does not make greater use of veterinarians. J. Am. Vet. Med. Assoc., 181:706–710, 1982b.

Hagstad, H.V. Preventive medicine in today's curriculum. J. Am. Vet. Med. Assoc., 174:384–386, 1979.

Hagstad, H.V. and Hubbert, W.T. Interfacing professional training in health maintenance and preventive medicine. J. Am. Vet. Med. Assoc., 175:210–211, 1979.

Haines, J.M. Preventive medicine in equine practice. J. Am. Vet. Med. Assoc., 174:396–398, 1979.

Harrington, B.D. Preventive medicine in dairy practice. J. Am. Vet. Med. Assoc., 174:398–400, 1979.

Heider, L.E., Galton, D.M. and Barr, H.L. Dairy herd reproductive health programs compared with traditional practices. J. Am. Vet. Med. Assoc., 176:743–746, 1980.

Henderson, D.C. Animal health today. The problems of large livestock units. The role of the farm staff. Br. Vet. J., 136:203–205, 1980.

Henderson, J.A. The prospect before us. Can. Vet. J., 1:3–9, 1960.

Hubbert, W.T. Perspective on veterinary preventive medicine in the United States. J. Am. Vet. Med. Assoc., 174:378–379, 1979.

Huffman, D.C. Economic decision making by livestock producers. J. Am. Vet. Med. Assoc., 174:381–384, 1979.

Janzen, E. Health and production records for the beef herd. Vet. Clin. North Am., Vol.. 5, No. 1. March 1983. pp. 15–28. Symposium on Herd Health Management—Cow Calf and Feedlot. O.M. Radostits (Ed.).

Jointex: Preventive medicine in practice. News and Reports. Vet. Rec., 98:349–350, 371, 1976.

Kahrs, R.F. Techniques for investigating outbreaks of livestock disease. J. Am. Vet. Med. Assoc., 173:101–103, 1978.

Kahrs, R.F. Teaching the techniques for investigating animal disease outbreaks. J. Am. Vet. Med. Assoc., 173:387–388, 1980.

Lesch, T.E., Troutt, H.F. and Jones, G.M. Expanding food-animal veterinary services through nutritional consultation. J. Am. Vet. Med. Assoc., 176:734–737, 1980.

Muirhead, M.R. The pig advisory visit in preventive medicine. Vet. Rec., 106:170–173, 1980.

Pepper, T.A., and Taylor, D.J. Breeding record analysis in pig herds and its veterinary application. 2. Experience with a large commercial unit. Vet. Rec., 101:196–199, 1977.

Pepper, T.A., Boyd, H.W. and Rosenberg, P. Breeding record analysis in pig herds and its veterinary application. 1. Development of a program to monitor reproductive efficiency and weaner production. Vet. Rec., 101:177–180, 1977.

Puckett, H.B., Olver, E.F., Harshbarger, K.E. et al. Automating the eyes of the herdsman. J. Anim. Sci., 53:516–523, 1981.

Radostits, O.M. Specialization in large animal practice. Can. Vet. J., 15:339–344, 1974.

Report of the Committee of Inquiry into the Veterinary Profession. Vol. I. Chairman, Sir Michael Swan. July 1975. pp. 1–238.

Russell, A.M. and Rowlands, G.F. COSREEL: Computerized recording system for herd health information management. Vet. Rec., 112:189–193, 1983.

Sard, D.M. Computer systems in veterinary medicine. Practice experience. Vet. Rec., 109:262–265, 1981.

Schnurrenberger, P.R. Defining preventive medicine in veterinary practice. J. Am. Vet. Med. Assoc., 174:373–380, 1979.

Schwabe, C. The current epidemiological revolution in veterinary medicine. Part 1. Prev. Vet. Med., 1:5–15, 1982.

Shanks, R.D., Berger, P.J., Freeman, A.E. et al. Projecting health cost from research herds. J. Dairy Sci., 65:644–652, 1982.

Sol, J. Economic and veterinary results of a herd health program during three years on 30 Dutch dairy farms. Proc. XII World Congress on Diseases of Cattle. The Netherlands. Sept. 7–10, 1982. Vol. I. pp. 697–701, 1982.

Watson, W.A. Large livestock units and notifiable disease. Br. Vet. J., 136:1–17, 1980..

Winkler, J.K. Prevention for profit. J. Am. Vet. Med. Assoc., 174:401–403, 1979.

Dairy Cattle—The Interaction Between Health and Production

2

INTRODUCTION

Before we begin a description of actual programs in use and projected for the individual species of farm animals, it is necessary to provide some discussion on the ways in which health and production interact in a farming enterprise. The discussion is provided here about the subject of dairy cattle, because that is the one with which we are most familiar. We have dealt with the subject by dividing farm profitability, maximization of which is the broad objective of the programs that we espouse, into its components of individual cow profitability—both annual and lifetime—and profitability of the herd as a whole. Within each of these sections, the principal health and management factors that affect these profitabilities are discussed.

The purpose of this chapter is to remind veterinarians that there is more to profitability than curing a disease, and to remind animal husbandmen that feeding well is not a sufficient solution. What we have to say would be of a great deal more value if we could put a monetary figure on what we do and achieve. Table 2–1 gives some indication of our views of the relative importance of the factors that affect productivity and profitability. The literature on the subject is sparse, but some data have been provided (Martin et al. 1982).

FACTORS AFFECTING THE PRODUCTIVITY AND PROFITABILITY OF DAIRY HERDS

One of the most difficult tasks in maintaining a health and production program is that of keeping in mind a picture of the total events and influences in a herd that affect productivity and eventually profitability. It would then be possible to say, for example, that if sufficient feed energy is not available, then milk production will be reduced. Fertility will also be reduced, so that there will be a further consequent lack of production nine months hence, requiring a purchase of lactating cows with a potential of 5% of introduction of disease, which would limit production, plus a preva-

Table 2-1. ESTIMATED RELATIVE IMPORTANCE OF FACTORS AFFECTING DAIRY HERD PROFITABILITY

Factor Affecting Productivity	National Estimates of Average Shortfall in Production Caused by Each Factor	
	Australian or Pastoral-type industry	Canadian or Intensive-type industry
Inheritance	*Nil effect.* Artificial breeders maintain adequate status quo	Major effect because of high economic value of individual cows
Age	*Nil effect.* Cows culled too young because of disease for age pinpointed as cause	Major effect because of high economic value of individual cows
Innate productivity	*Nil effect.* Farmers select strongly for productivity	
Body condition score	*10-20% loss.* Cows generally badly underfed and too light at sale for beef	Minor effect because of good nutritional state of cows. Major effect if cows are overfat
Length of lactation	*15% loss.* In year-round herds too many cows are kept milking far too long because of reproductive inefficiency. In seasonal herds induction of early parturition and heavy culling have similar effect	Similar losses of 15% because length of lactation too long owing to reproductive inefficiency
Nutritional sufficiency	*15% loss.* Nutrition often deficient when seasonal growth poor. Causes loss of milk production and nutritional infertility	A major effect in some herds because do not feed adequate nutrient intake to meet needs of high-producing cow
Reproductive inefficiency	*10% loss.* Average intercalving interval 30 days too long. Mostly poor estrus detection and undernutrition	Similar losses, intercalving internal too long because of poor estrus detection
Mastitis	*6% loss.* Average quarter infection rate 25%, 50% cows affected	Economic losses from 10 to 20%
Other diseases	*< 1% loss* overall, but individual farms suffer bad losses	Losses from 2 to 5% of adult cows per year

lence of acetonemia now, and so on and so on. The productivity of the herd is a very complex system consisting of a large number of events and factors all reacting with each other in a very complicated way. It is not usually possible for a farmer or an advisor to be able to correlate all of the relevant influences and produce an accurate answer to the farmer's big question of today—"BUT WHAT IF . . . ?" The question goes something like this: "If I buy that cheap feed now, I think that I can maintain my milk yield in the autumn, *but what if* my fertility efficiency jumps up 10% because of this program you have introduced? And that depends a bit on how much meadow hay I make. I assume my usual yield of X tons, *but what if* there's a drought? And so on and so on."

One of the main objectives of a health and production management program is to be able to answer questions by dairy farmers about the effects of some disease control or management techniques that have been recommended to be introduced into other subsystems in the total herd structure. For example, the introduction of a mastitis control program affects not only the mastitis status of the herd. It also requires an additional input of labor. The increase in labor force might then require the herd size to be increased to fully utilize the additional labor, and these additional cows might have an effect on procedures in the milking parlor, which could have a further effect on the mastitis problem.

The complex relationships that exist between disease, nutrition, mating management, stocking rate, culling policy, and other variables that influence productivity create difficulty in computing the output of the herd as a system. The difficulties are multiplied by the degree of variability of each of these factors, which can be applied at different pressures for periods as short as one day. These variations are measurable, and much of the measurement, e.g., milk yields and meteorological data, is on permanent record. All that is needed is a computational system that can deal with the data and produce the output. A computer simulation model provides an appropriate solution.

Some computer simulation models are available (James 1977; Fick 1980; Oltenacu et al. 1980; Bywater et al. 1981; France et al. 1982), but they are generally in the developmental stage and have, for the most part, only limited local application. There do not appear to be any that are universally applicable and that contain a full roster of disease and management factors. It is easy to construct a flow chart on which a suitable model could be based. The difficulty is in obtaining suitable mathematical data with which to invest each factor. These mathematical statements must have hard data backing them up, and this requires adaptive research of the type usually carried out by governmental research stations in the region. A guesswork figure can be used but leads to the inevitable question by the farmer, "That's OK, provided our estimate of calf mortality in the first three weeks of life is accurate, *but what if* the real figure here is twice that?" The whole purpose of the exercise that we are undertaking is to be able to tell an individual farmer on an individual farm, in a particular region and with his own set of intellectual, financial, geographical, climatic, and marketing constraints what is his best management and health strategy to extract maximum profitability from his enterprise. Therefore, the advice must be accurate, and for it to be accurate, a computer simulation model must contain very accurate information on which to perform its computations.

Some typical questions that are currently posed by progressive dairy herd owners, to which there can only be guesswork answers at present, and that an efficient health and production management program should be able to answer accurately are:

☐ At what percentage induction-of-calving rate does the induction of calving become uneconomic?

☐ What is the break-even price of irrigation water?

☐ What percentage of an annual heifer crop can be sold as surplus stock not required as herd replacement in two years' time, while still maintaining herd size and productivity?

☐ What is the optimum carrying capacity (stocking rate) on a particular farm, taking into account its area, soil fertility, fertilizer history, rainfall, and irrigation resource?

☐ Taking into account pasture growth and milk prices, what is the optimum calving pattern for a particular herd?

Although it is not possible to reproduce a flow chart for a usable computer simulation model here, we do present a scheme that includes very simply and briefly the factors that significantly affect cow and herd productivity (Figs. 2–1 and 2–2) (Bywater and Dent 1976; Bywater 1976). There are factors that exert their influence only on the individual cow

and those that operate only at the herd level. A combination of these two groups of factors produces an estimate of herd productivity. A cost-benefit analysis applied at this point, assuming that accurate data is available from the farmer on the costs of production, permits the estimation of financial profitability of the herd. Return on the investment can then be calculated so that a comparison can be made between the investment of money in modifying conduct of the herd's affairs and the investment of a similar amount in some other enterprise.

The farmer, having received this estimate, is faced with a number of unenviable tasks beyond the one that has confronted the veterinary adviser. It is important that these be kept in mind in order that the possibility of their occurrence can influence proposed changes. They are:

1. The significant alteration of the objectives of the enterprise in which the herd is involved, e.g., changing from a seasonal to a year-round pattern of calving. It is vital that the objective be kept in clear sight at all times and preferably reviewed constantly, at least at yearly intervals. The question to be raised is whether the farmer's objectives are the same as last year. It is not unusual to have a gradual shift away from maximum profitability and toward the inclusion of a softening life-style.

2. Modification of the relative importance of the enterprises on the farm, e.g., reducing the dairy herd and increasing the potato or other cash-cropping enterprise.

3. The degree of risk that the farmer is prepared to carry, e.g., continuing a dry-farming exercise rather than installing irrigation at greater cost but for increased security.

In order to make these decisions, all that the farmer needs is a total farm, as distinct from a herd, computer simulation model. It is probable that models of this sort will be installed in phone-in computerized video systems within the next few years.

ANNUAL PRODUCTIVITY OF INDIVIDUAL COWS

The productivity of a herd is the sum of the productivity of the individual cows in a herd. The profitability of a herd is not quite the same thing, because there are factors arising out of management, such as a decision on a routine of pasture management, that affect only the profitability of the herd as a whole. It is appropriate, therefore, to discuss the variables that affect individual cow productivity, which may be expressed as productivity at the time, as in the yield of milk per cow per year, this year.

One of the important factors affecting each cow's productivity is its age, with a rising production level to the sixth lactation, with milk volume 25% greater at that time than in the first lactation. There is a slight decrease in butterfat percentage of about 0.2% due to age during this period and an obvious increase in yield of butterfat for the older cow.

Stage of lactation is important also. Milk production increases to three to six weeks after calving and then declines by about 5% per

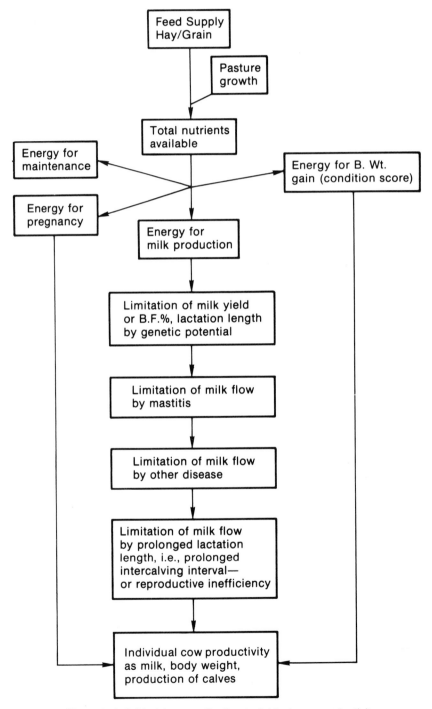

Figure 2-1. Critical factors affecting individual cow productivity.

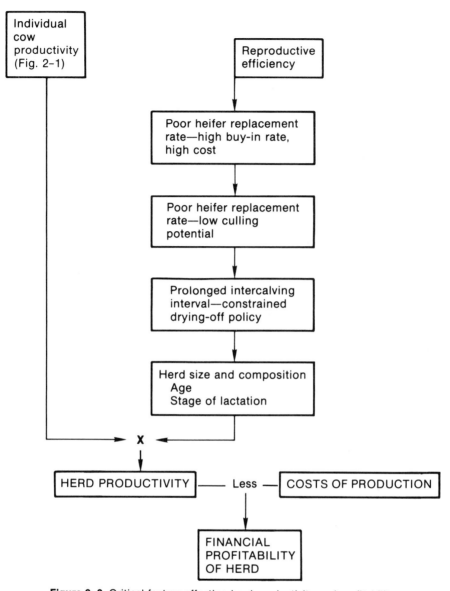

Figure 2-2. Critical factors affecting herd productivity and profitability.

month, the decline being slightly less in non-pregnant cows. There is also a strong relationship between size of cow and yield. This explains some of the difference between breeds, but there is the additional difference between breeds of an inherited butterfat content of the milk. Much use is made of this in commercial herds where cross-breeding to take advantage of hybrid vigor is practiced.

Although there are almost no data on the volumetric effect of sporadic disease incidents on milk production, this is an obvious limiter of production. However, constraints such as an attack of acute coliform mastitis may be ap-plied at a high level of intensity but for a very limited period of time. The effect on the individual cow's record is great, but the effect on the herd's performance may be hardly recognizable.

Nutrition is the most limiting factor in nearly all circumstances. In purely pastoral systems such as that in Australia, the limitation is mostly one of quantity of feed, although protein content may be very low in pastures on dry farms. Clover-grass pastures are generally used on irrigation farms where the capital value of the land warrants further investment in pasture seeding and fertilizer application. On pasture farms, it is still usual to provide supplementary feed in the season of poorest pasture growth, usually the winter months.

In housed and dry-lotted herds, the emphasis is quite different. Because of the capital investment involved, it is essential to keep numbers down and to extract maximum productivity and profitability from each cow. Thus, ration formulation with particular attention to digestibility, protein content, and mineral and vitamin composition in a total daily ration becomes the important factor.

Nutrition is important in a number of ways in growing the heifers quickly so that (1) the first pregnancy is begun at 15 months of age and subsequent pregnancies are at 365-day intervals; (2) the cow's genetic potential for milk production is realized without the cow developing a production disease such as milk fever, acetonemia, or osteoarthritis; and (3) she maintains sufficient body condition to survive seven or eight lactations and still retire at a body condition score that will mean a reasonable price at her cull sale. A cow's body condition score at calving is also an important factor influencing milk production in the subsequent lactation. There is an inevitable loss of body condition during the first three to six weeks after calving while the cow is in a negative energy balance. Cows starting a lactation in less than optimal condition have little reserve to counteract this drain, and production will fall short of potential. There is a concurrent reduction in reproductive efficiency.

Freedom from disease is always an important factor in avoiding production wastage. Management-induced diseases include inherited defects that should be avoided by a good cow quality control program and production diseases caused by failure to make good any nutrients being heavily used at particular stages of the lactation cycle. Infectious diseases are avoided by hygienic practices—especially the maintenance of a closed herd, the practice of prophylactic vaccination, and the careful selection of purchased feed. Within-herd infectious diseases may be completely eradicated, controlled to a financially bearable level, or treated early in their course.

Mastitis and reproductive inefficiency are universally recognized as the major causes of wastage among the common diseases. Mastitis is important because of its occurrence in almost every herd and at a quarter infection rate averaging about 25% and causing a significant decline in milk production in affected cows— about 50% in average herds practicing no effec-

tive control program. Reproductive inefficiency is expressed as a prolongation of the intercalving interval and averages 8 to 10% less than optimum in herds with moderately good management.

Inherited milking capacity is a factor of varying importance. In intensively farmed herds, where feeding is provided up to the maximum quality and energy density that the cow can accommodate, her genetic potential to produce milk or butterfat may be a limiting factor. However, in a pastoral economy, where the food intake is inevitably less rich in energy than is possible, the cows are often not fed to the limit of their inherited potential, so that cow quality or inherited milking capacity may be much less important.

In a dairy-farming system in which cows are bred only to ensure that lactation occurs, in which all bull calves and 50% of heifer calves are in surplus for use as herd replacements, and in which there is no veal-producing industry, the sale of surplus stock as cull calves adds little to a cow's total productivity. The position is different in stud herds, where calves may be very valuable. The cow's own value as a meat animal does affect her profitability, so that the maintenance of a reasonable body condition makes a contribution to the value of each cow.

The culling policy in a herd can have a marked influence on per cow profitability, early culling reducing the production of milk but enhancing the meat value of the cull. Early culling also reduces the wastage due to mastitis and reproductive inefficiency. These matters are set out under the heading of culling policy.

LIFETIME PRODUCTIVITY OF INDIVIDUAL COWS

As described in the previous section, a herd of three-year-old cows has a much lower level of production and profitability, all other things being equal, than a herd of six-year-old cows. The longevity of cows, but not just age alone, is a most important factor affecting profitability. It is a matter of age multiplied by annual productivity. A flow chart of factors affecting lifetime productivity is shown in Figure 2–3.

The total productivity of each cow will be the value of its total milk production, plus the value of its progeny kept as herd replacements or sold as culls, plus its own value when it is eventually sold as a culled-for-age cow. Some of these values will be high in stud herds, where most surplus stock are sold as producing animals rather than for meat.

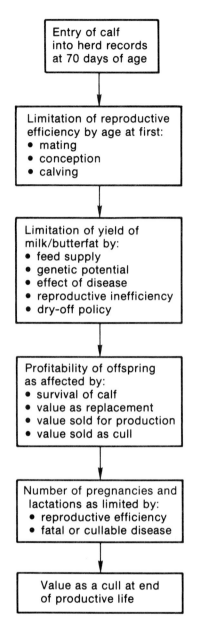

Figure 2-3. Factors affecting individual cow's lifetime productivity.

Understandably, there are a number of factors that affect the longevity of, or more particularly the number of lactations experienced by, each cow. However, the important ones are likely to be:

□ Disease control efficiency to avoid lethal disease. Many of them appear to be bad-luck diseases, unrelated to any lack of resistance in the cow or enhancement of virulence by the environment.

□ Reproductive inefficiency.

□ Poor production, usually in terms of milk yield, possibly in terms of poor butterfat percentage.

□ Genetic longevity. This often appears to be greatest in cows with a lesser annual production. Longevity has low heritability and is not usually a criterion for selection.

PRODUCTIVITY OF THE DAIRY HERD AS A WHOLE

Those factors that exert their influence on herd productivity by their influence on each cow in the herd have been discussed in the previous section, and the relationship between the two was shown in Figures 2-1 and 2-2. There are additional factors, and these follow.

Breeding strategies and techniques have an effect on profitability in some of the following ways: Artificial insemination by the owner/operator of the farm can be a highly profitable exercise if technique and conception rate are good. Insemination is carried out at the optimum time, and the semen used can be the cheapest available if genetic gain is not a principal objective. It is cheaper still to carry out an insemination program in a seasonally calving herd and then to turn in a nondescript but virgin—and therefore free of venereal disease—bull to mate with the late-conceiving cows. The conception rate is higher, the dams are potential culls for infertility, and the calves will not be kept as herd replacements and are therefore dispensable. Similarly, calves from heifers are not kept because the dams do not have production records as yet. The breeding program for heifers, therefore, is commonly one of running them with similar virgin bulls. For practical purposes, the alternative is insemination after synchronization, an expensive procedure. The technique of estrus detection, as discussed in the chapter on reproductive efficiency, is a factor of the greatest importance in determining the level of productivity of a herd as a whole. Prevention or eradication of infectious diseases that directly affect reproductive efficiency, the fertility of the sire, and the management decision to use a hormonal technique for widespread induction of parturition are similar factors.

Calf-rearing programs are described in Chapter 6. They contribute to herd profitability in several ways. The most important is their ability to keep the mortality rate low. Additionally, they influence the growth rate that they promote. Height and weight of young growing stock are closely related, and both of these characteristics therefore influence the age at which first estrus and mating occur. This is important because departure from the optimum of 15 months for these events and 24 months for their first calving represents lost income. The growth rate is critical during the period from weaning at 10 weeks of age until first breeding. During this time, the calves are pen-fed, often indifferent roughage, in intensive systems or are pasture-fed in dry paddocks in pasture systems. The two important influences are nutrition, both quality and quantity, and in the pastured animals, the control of internal parasites.

Pasture management can play an important part in herd productivity if there is almost complete dependence on pasture as a source of energy. This is expressed most dramatically where seasonal dairying is practiced. The objective is to have all the cows in the herd calve at approximately the same time to take advantage of the strong spring flush of growth. In many areas, there are two peaks of pasture growth, the second one being in the autumn, and the difficulties of a single massive calving can at least be halved. The obvious difficulty of having the human population milkless for two months of each year is avoided by staggering the calving season over a wide area, depending on the earliness or lateness of the spring flush in each small area. This system of pasture management creates another difficulty requiring the institution of yet another system of management. The problem arises because, in spite of the staggering of calving seasons from one area to another, there will always be a natural deficiency of milk production in the winter months at pasture. In order to maintain the flow of milk to the human population, the milk industry provides incentive prices for milk produced at these times. For farmers seeking these incentive prices, the profitability of the herd depends on a fine balancing of costs of feed against the price of milk.

The energy and other constituents of ingested feed are digested and metabolized and then partitioned to the various functions that the cow performs. There are, undoubtedly, differences between cows in their capacity to digest and metabolize, but for all practical purposes the digestibility of a particular feed and the metabolic fate of the absorbed nutrients are the same for all cows. However, the partitioning of the important classes of nutrients, especially energy, between milk production, growth or weight maintenance, walking or similar activity, and pregnancy is not readily identifiable and does appear to vary widely between cows. It is usually expressed, together with digestive and metabolic activity, as feed conversion efficiency.

The provision of suitable and cost-effective rations to intensively farmed cows on stored feeds is described in Chapter 7. In such diets it is possible to increase the energy intake, when the cow's dry matter intake limit has been reached, by reducing the fiber and increasing the energy content of the ration. When cows are grazing pasture, this is much more difficult because the energy and fiber content of the grazing plants can change dramatically over a very short time, and all of the pasture on the farm is likely to suffer the same fate at about the same time. Cows on summer pasture are likely to be seriously disadvantaged unless high-energy, high-density feeds, especially grains, are fed.

Estimation of the nutritional value of pasture is hazardous (Bywater 1976; Bywater and Dent 1976; Fick 1980) and is, in any case, of limited value because of variation in what the cow does with the absorbed nutrients at various levels of intake. This partitioning of energy into the several body functions can only be measured by using the cow as the measuring device. Some of the factors that affect the nutritional value of pasture are shown in Figure 2–4 and include:

□ the proportion of green or dry material with good feed value to old dead grass of almost no value. Each material will have its own digestibility, and the digestibility of the pasture as a whole will be the sum of them.

□ the proportion of the ground surface covered or occupied by pasture plants, i.e., the density of the pasture.

□ the proportions of clover and grasses and, among the grasses, those of high palatability and nutritional value compared with lesser grasses.

□ the duration of growth, flowering, seeding, and decay stages in the constituent plants.

□ responsivity of the pasture to climate and soil moisture as determined by its composition and the state and type of the soil on which the pasture is growing.

□ the application or cessation of application of artificial fertilizers, especially nitrogenous ones.

□ amount of trampling by livestock, especially when the soil is wet.

Although the cow's maximum voluntary feed intake (dry matter capacity) has been well identified as varying from 2.25 to 3.5% of the cow's body weight, with poorly digestible

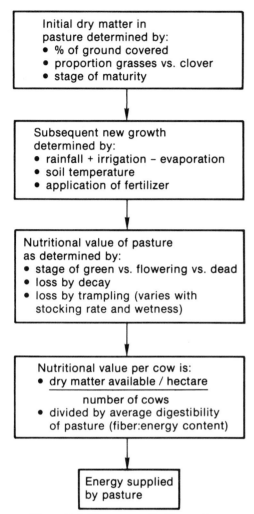

Figure 2-4. Energy supplied by pasture.

milking parlor. This assumes bulk tank milk collection and delivery. On most farms, a labor force of 1.3 to 1.5 persons per farm is usual, with the farmer's spouse being about a third of a full-time worker. This leads to a common herd size of 120 to 130 cows in milk for a one-man farm unit. With less cows, the worker's full potential is not realized, and the cost-effectiveness of the farm is less than optimum. With more cows than that, the efficiency of the herd's management is likely to be reduced in proportion to the reduced surveillance and care taken. In Canadian herds of dairy cows housed indoors for seven months of the year, a comparable figure is 40 to 60 cows.

Notwithstanding the general applicability of these estimates, it is still necessary to take into account other factors that affect the efficiency of labor. These include the design and efficiency of the milking shed; the use of automated milking and feeding machinery; the layout of the farm and the adequacy of fixed improvements, especially irrigation equipment and land-forming, fencing, and gates; the need or desirability of supplying supplementary feed from home-grown crops; the making of hay and ensilage and its distribution; the availability of hay-making and ensiling equipment; and, as much as any other factor, the distance from the farm to the nearest town and service center.

For pasture-farm dairying, as in Australia, the size of the herd is dictated by the size of the labor force available. If the original farm is not sufficiently large, the usual procedure is to buy more pasture land—often some distance away—and to run the heifers and dry cows on it. In spite of this apparent flexibility, there is still a great deal of room for error in deciding just how big a farm is before deciding to enlarge it, or in some cases decrease it, in size. The problem arises out of the difficulty in evaluating the individual classes of land with respect to productivity. Thus, it is important to know what proportion of the farm is irrigated, has improved pasture, is under crop, and so on.

Alternatively, the farm is managed more intensively by all possible means. In some circumstances, e.g., in Canada, such flexibility may not always be possible, especially because of the size and design of the barn, although there are a number of ingenious plans for adding new lounging pens and milking parlors to old-style housing. It is much more important, in these circumstances and with such expensive overhead, to feed more intensively and to concentrate on genetic quality and on develop-

roughage having the lower intake, there are other factors affecting food intake, especially the availability of grain and, to a much less extent, late pregnancy, which physically diminishes the rumen. These influences on the energy intake and partitioning from the diet are shown diagrammatically in Figure 2-5.

Herd Size

The size of a dairy herd, especially in relation to the amount of labor available, can be one of the most important factors influencing the profitability of the herd. There is no simple way of expressing this value or of measuring the value's validity in all circumstances. In Australian pasture farming, a single full-time worker can look after a 100-cow dairy herd and do all the chores including farm work, irrigation, feeding, harvesting meadow hay, calf rearing, milking the cows, and cleaning the

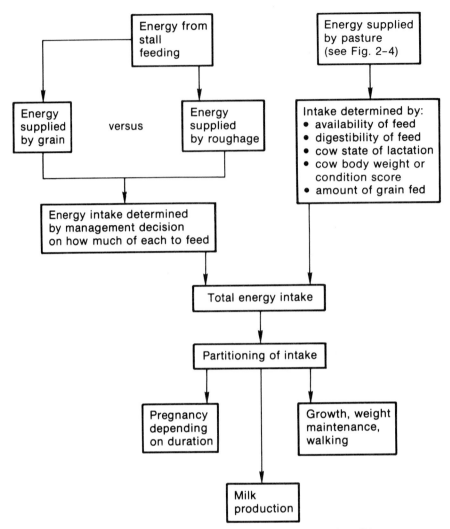

Figure 2-5. Factors affecting energy intake and partitioning in milking cows.

ment of sales of stud or at least on producing cattle when there is an excess of cattle over requirements.

Composition of the Herd

A number of qualities are important in the composition of the herd, because they influence the productivity of the herd as a whole at any particular time. They are the mix of milking cows versus calves, heifers, nurse cows, and bulls; the mix of milk and dry cows in the milking group; the average age of the milking cows, i.e, the mix of the various age groups; the average length of lactation (or dry period); and the quality of the cows. Each cow's potential to produce milk or butterfat is critical whether it be inherited or not, especially in intensive farming units of housed cattle.

The management practices that govern these all-important characteristics are shown diagrammatically in Figure 2–6. Largely, it is a matter of manipulating culling and drying-off to ensure a proper balance between producing and nonproducing cows and a willingness to breed (select) for high milk yield. This usually means using particular bulls for artificial insemination, but it may mean the purchase of quality females to make up numbers.

Stage of Lactation. In seasonal dairy herds, especially those with high reproductive efficiency, all of the cows will be at about the same stage of lactation at the same time. Hence all the cows will be in early lactation, or at their peak, or in decline, or stale, or dry together. In less well managed herds, there is a greater spread of each category. In year-round herds, a much greater mix is usual, with an objective of

17% of milking cows being dry at all times. In practice, there are usually one or more peaks of cows in milk related to the abundance of pasture feed at particular times of the year.

Age. The distribution of age groups within the herd is a very important indicator of its management efficiency. In herds where disease control is poor, the average herd age is lowered because of the higher prevalence of mastitis and reproductive inefficiency, especially in older age groups (Allaire et al. 1977), and the need to cull heavily for these diseases. Similarly, in herds where the genetic standard (cow quality) is poor and there is an opportunity to breed to high-quality bulls, the selection against the dams may be so high that, again, the herd average age will be lower than is desirable.

There are two obvious circumstances in which the average herd age will be higher than normal. Herds in which culling for disease is low because the diseases are controlled may have an average herd age that is two years older than normal, the profitability of each lactation may be 20% higher than in normal herds. The other circumstance in which average herd age is raised is where the herd is being increased in size, and the cows are retained for longer life spans than would ordinarily be the case.

Drying-off Policy

The type of drying-off policy used depends largely on the amount of attention that can be given to each cow. The choice is usually between drying off at the 300th day of lactation or the 222nd day of pregnancy, both of which can be determined by consulting herd records or by inserting an appropriate command in the herd's computer program. A decline in milk production to less than 4 liters per day or a decline in body condition score to below 3.5 (on a scale of 8) can also be used. The latter technique requires more detailed acquaintance with the cow's performance, health, age, and

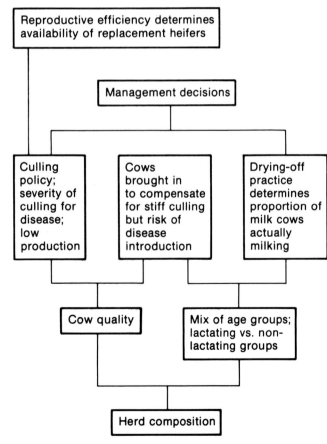

Figure 2-6. Factors affecting herd composition.

so on. In seasonal herds, the decision is usually more arbitrary—all the cows are dried off together on the day on which milking the herd ceases to be cost-effective. Some difficulties may be encountered with this procedure because already-infected quarters may develop clinical mastitis, and glands still secreting heavily may become painfully distended. The alternatives shown in Figure 2-7 have the virtue of being easily included in a computer program. Each method would be likely to select a slightly different group of cows.

Culling Program

An important and rather neglected part of a dairy herd management plan is the system of culling cows. In general terms, cows are culled because of poor production; susceptibility to or occurrence rate of disease, especially reproductive inefficiency and mastitis; and poor genetic quality including both productivity and breed type parameters. The guidelines for culling are presented in Chapter 8.

Quality of Labor

Given the same farm and the same herd, a good manager can improve the productivity and profitability by as much as 50%. The same types of differences are likely if a farm is run by an owner-manager rather than by hired help. There are exceptions to the rule, but the lack of personal financial involvement of the relief milker adds to the lack of familiarity of the help with the cows. Some of the factors that appear to affect the quality of dairy labor are:

□ innate managerial skill and capacity to make decisions.
□ numeracy and an appreciation of a cost-benefit relationship.
□ intelligence and some spirit of inquiry, i.e., a willingness to learn exemplified by attendance at discussion groups, short courses, field days; by joining a health and production management program; or by employing a farm management advisor.
□ motivation and consideration for animal welfare.
□ aversion to taking risks, which may mean a lack of enthusiasm for applying new technology or a willingness, for example, to risk the lives of cows in a bloating pasture.
□ amenity inclination, i.e., the farmer's enthusiasm to embrace a more comfortable lifestyle, gracious living, and quality of life.
□ experience.

Poor quality management, whatever the cause, is likely to depress the efficiency of estrus detection, of mastitis control by attention to teat dipping, and of the monitoring of pasture fields so that irrigation water can be applied and cows can be moved at the most advantageous times. Similarly, the proper

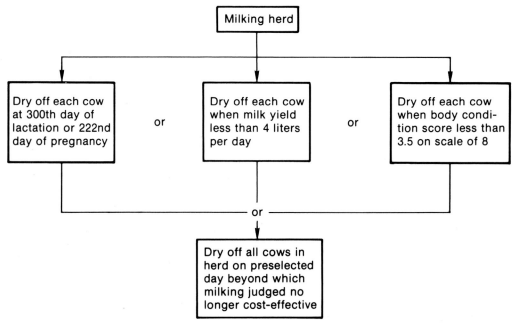

Figure 2-7. An outline of drying-off programs.

maintenance of floors, yards, lanes, and gateways may be neglected, resulting in a greater tendency for injury to occur.

ANNUAL SCHEDULE OF DISEASE OCCURRENCE RELATIVE TO MANAGEMENT PROCEDURES AND AGE GROUP

The occurrence of diseases and causes of suboptimal performance in dairy cattle other than reproductive inefficiency and mastitis are outlined here according to the age of the animal or stage of production. It is intended to be a reminder guide for the veterinarian in planning an integrated health and production management program on an annual basis. Certain diseases occur more commonly in certain age groups or during a specific part of the lactation-pregnancy cycle. Almost all of the infectious diseases can occur in animals of any age, but certain ones are age-related. At each herd health visit, the veterinarian should prepare an *action list* for each group of animals that outlines the routine procedures that are necessary and the diseases that are most likely to occur. Some of the diseases occur only sporadically, and a control program may not be practical or economical. Several diseases, for example salmonellosis, can occur in epidemic form and cause large economic losses due to death and costs of treatment. Other diseases like brucellosis may cause persistent problems because of the identification of new cases of serologically positive animals and the possible need for quarantine of the herd. Besides suboptimal reproductive performance and subclinical mastitis, inadequate nutrition—as presented in the chapter on nutrition—is a major cause of suboptimal performance in the dairy herd.

The successful control and prevention of these diseases and causes of suboptimal performance are dependent on an understanding of their etiology and epidemiology, the details of which are available in textbooks such as *Veterinary Medicine* by Blood, Radostits, and Henderson, 1983. Although the sporadic diseases such as salmonellosis may cause crippling damage on a farm, their overall impact on the dairy industry is quite small. For this reason, the importance of all diseases other than mastitis goes largely unchallenged. In developed countries it seems likely that all of them put together are likely to be less important than either bovine mastitis or infertility (Williamson et al. 1978).

In most of these sporadic diseases, recovery is common, and it is only the loss of production during the course of the disease that can be regarded as wastage. Thus, in a recovered case of indigestion there would be a loss of 70% of milk yield for three days, that is, a loss of two days of production, or 0.67% of the year's production. The additional cost of treatment would also be very small. The accumulation of data that will make losses due to disease measurable with some accuracy is one of the remaining largely unexplored areas of agricultural veterinary medicine.

Pregnant Cow or Heifer (During dry period for cow)
Examination of quarter milk samples one month or less before drying off
Dry cow therapy for mastitis control. Vaccinate pregnant dam for control of acute diarrhea due to enterotoxigenic K99$^+$ *E. coli*, rotavirus, and coronavirus and sometimes *Salmonella* sp.
Regular surveillance for summer mastitis
Avoid excess energy intake to prevent fat cow syndrome
Feed low-calcium diet or administer vitamin D_3 to minimize parturient paresis
Ensure adequate vitamin A/carotene intake
Place pregnant animal in calving box stall or calving paddock several days prior to parturition

Periparturient Cow (One week before and immediately after calving)
Increase surveillance for the following:
Peracute mastitis due to *E. coli* and *Staphylococcus* sp.
Udder edema
Dystocia, retained fetal membranes, and septic metritis
Parturient paresis and downer cow syndrome
Reduction in appetite due to simple indigestion associated with a change in diet
Left-side displacement of the abomasum
Abomasal ulceration

Early Lactating Cow (Fresh cow—calving to one month afterwards)
Primary acetonemia
Hypomagnesemia
Postparturient hemoglobinuria
Right-side displacement of abomasum
Cecal dilatation
Delayed onset of estrus
Repeat breeder
Mastitis (clinical and subclinical) control program

Middle and Late Lactating Cow (After first month of lactation)

Pregnancy diagnosis

Delayed onset of estrus/repeat breeder

Mastitis (clinical and subclinical) control program

Abnormalities of udder and teats

Suboptimal milk yield due to insufficient dietary intake of energy, protein, or minerals

Drop in butter fat test

Newborn Calf from Birth to Weaning

Provide necessary obstetrical assistance

Assess level of immunoglobulin in colostrum using hydrometer

Ensure adequate intake of colostrum and leave with dam for 48 hours; regularly examine serum immunoglobulins subsequently

Examine for evidence of congenital defects

Individual pen for first three weeks

Avoid lead paint in environment

Milk, stored colostrum, or milk replacer from colostral feeding period (first three days) to weaning

Offer hay and calf starter at two weeks of age; wean at six to eight weeks or when eating dry feed

Ensure adequate vitamin D intake

Major problems: acute diarrhea due to *E. coli*, rotavirus, coronavirus, *Cryptosporidia* sp. and others; omphalophlebitis and infectious arthritis

Calf from Weaning to Six Months of Age

Identification by tattoo or double ear tag

Adequate diet and housing to achieve optimum growth rate and prevention of specific vitamin and mineral deficiencies

Vaccination for:

Infectious bovine rhinotracheitis

Enzootic pneumonia

Bovine virus diarrhea

Brucellosis (where legislation permits)

Leptospirosis

Clostridial diseases

Salmonellosis

Ringworm control

Control of internal and external parasites

Avoid rubbish dumps (lead poisoning)

Weigh or tape calf monthly to measure if optimal growth achieved

Major problems: enzootic pneumonia of calves; infectious enteritides

Heifer from Six Months to 15 Months of Age

Selection for breeding

Removal of supernumerary teats

Adequate diet to ensure optimal growth and prevention of specific mineral and vitamin deficiencies

Administration of reticular magnet at 12 months of age for prevention of traumatic reticuloperitonitis

Adequate housing and stocking density to control infectious diseases such as coccidiosis and intestinal helminthiasis

Diseases that are likely to occur include:

Bovine virus diarrhea

Coccidiosis

Pneumonia

Ostertagiasis and other helminthiases

Papular stomatitis

Calf diphtheria (necrotic stomatitis)

Ringworm

Clostridial diseases

Hemophilus meningoencephalitis

DISEASES OF DAIRY CATTLE NOT NECESSARILY RELATED TO THE PRODUCTION CYCLE

Diseases Controllable by Vaccination

Leptospirosis

Clostridial diseases

Anthrax

Brucellosis (where legislation permits)

Infectious bovine rhinotracheitis

Infectious keratoconjunctivitis

Hemophilus meningoencephalitis

Rabies

Diseases Controllable by Nutritional Supplementation

Copper deficiency

Vitamin E and selenium deficiency

Polioencephalomalacia

Calcium, phosphorus, and vitamin D deficiencies

Several other mineral deficiencies, e.g., salt, magnesium, zinc

Simple indigestion

Rumen overload

Ruminal tympany

Traumatic reticuloperitonitis and allied syndromes

Low milk fat

Fat cow syndrome

Primary acetonemia

Diseases Controllable by Test and Slaughter

Leucosis

Brucellosis

Tuberculosis

Johne's disease

Diseases Controllable by Medication

Coccidiosis

Intestinal helminthiasis

Fascioliasis

External parasites (lice, chorioptic mange)

Anaplasmosis

Ringworm

Diseases too Sporadic to Warrant Prevention

Listeriosis
Contagious bovine pyelonephritis
Hemophilus meningoencephalitis
Actinobacillosis
Actinomycosis
Bovine papular stomatitis
Bovine malignant catarrh
Spondylosis in dairy bulls

Diseases Not Controllable by Other Than Usual Hygienic Precautions and Improved Animal Husbandry

Foot rot
Lameness due to diseases of the feet other than foot rot
Pneumonic pasteurellosis
Winter dysentery
Salmonellosis
Pseudocowpox
Bovine ulcerative mammillitis
Ringworm
Dermatophilus infection (mycotic dermatitis)
Diseases caused by chemical agents (lead, arsenic, fluorine, molybdenum, sodium chloride, hydrocyanic acid, nitrate, insecticides, urea, mycotoxins, dicumarol)

Diseases Controllable by Prevention of Introduction of Infection

Foot and mouth disease
Bluetongue
Brucellosis
Anaplasmosis
Tuberculosis
Johne's disease
Leptospirosis
Salmonellosis

Diseases Controllable by Genetic Surveillance

Congenital defects in newborn calves recognized and pedigree analyses carried out to identify and remove carrier animals

TECHNIQUES USED IN HEALTH AND PRODUCTION MANAGEMENT IN DAIRY HERDS

The techniques that are commonly used in animal health and production management programs in dairy herds and in which dairy species specialists are expected to be competent follow:

1. Nutritional surveillance; feed analysis; measurement of nutrient intake relative to needs, body condition score, milk production per cow, metabolic profile, tissue analysis for mineral content
2. Reproduction performance evaluation
3. Mastitis control; regular monitoring of somatic cell counts, dry cow therapy; evaluation of milking machine
4. Vaccination for certain infectious diseases; includes calfhood vaccination and annual revaccination of cows for endemic diseases (infectious bovine rhinotracheitis, leptospirosis)
5. Control of infectious disease without vaccination. Many infectious diseases must be controlled by one or more of the following:
   a. Adequate housing and ventilation; optimum stocking density; sanitation and hygiene; fly control
   b. Chemotherapeutic control; anthelminthic administration; foot bath for control of lameness caused by infections
   c. Isolation of infected animals; quarantine and testing of imported animals
6. Regular surgical procedures: foot trimming, dehorning, removal of supernumerary teats, castration of males
7. Specific infectious disease surveillance:
   Serological
      Brucellosis
      Leucosis
      Bovine virus diarrhea
      Leptospirosis
   Cutaneous testing
      Tuberculosis
      Johne's disease
   Fecal egg counts
      Helminthiasis
      Fascioliasis
8. Regular evaluation of production performance of individual cows and cull as necessary, using records from D.H.I.A. or R.O.P. Decision based on milk and butterfat yields. Selection of breeding stock, based on: production (milk volume and butterfat), reproductive efficiency, longevity, freedom from inherited defects
9. Regular analysis of health and production data of all age groups and classes of animals in the herd and comparison of actual performance with targets of performance
10. Regular calculation of the cost of milk production
11. Maintenance of a high level of animal husbandry

A summary of the disease control techniques and routine production procedures required in dairy herds according to age of animals or stage of production is presented in Table 2–2.

Text continued on page 47

Table 2–2. SUMMARY OF DISEASE CONTROL TECHNIQUES AND ROUTINE PRODUCTION PROCEDURES REQUIRED IN DAIRY HERDS ACCORDING TO AGE OF ANIMALS OR STAGE OF PRODUCTION (MASTITIS AND REPRODUCTIVE EFFICIENCY ARE PRESENTED SEPARATELY)

Disease or Production Procedure	Monitoring Technique(s)	Prophylactic Techniques			
		Management	Vaccination	Medication	Other
		1. Pregnant Heifer or Cow			
Fat cow syndrome	Body condition score	Feed dry cows separately and according to needs	—	May need to provide supplemental propylene glycol or glycerine	—
Parturient paresis	Previous episodes suggest close surveillance. Familial and breed predisposition do too. Pastured cows in high rainfall, heavy pasture growth seasons predisposed	Feed low-calcium diet (less than 100 g per day) during dry period up to 2 weeks prepartum	—	Administration of vitamin D_3 or analogues few days prepartum	Selection against susceptibility
		2. Periparturient Cow (1 week before and after calving)			
Parturient paresis	Look for staggering, muscle tremor, recumbency in cows every few hours for first 48 hours	Do not milk out completely	—	Treat with calcium salt in first stage of milk fever	Keep susceptible cows close to observation point
Retained fetal membranes and septic metritis	Placenta and/or malodorous discharge visible, straining in some	Adequate dietary intake of selenium and phosphorus	—	Treat with antibiotics for toxemia	Ensure brucellosis control not compromised
Udder edema	Edema along belly and up escutcheon. Udder swollen, very hard, milk normal	Premilking before parturition only if necessary to relieve pressure	—	Treat with diuretics	Consider terminating pregnancy with corticosteroids
Left-side displacement of abomasum	Clinical evidence of inappetence, ketonuria, and decreased milk production	Reduce heavy feeding finely ground grain, especially late in pregnancy	—	—	—
Simple indigestion	Clinical evidence of inappetence and rumen hypomotility	Avoid all dietary indiscretions (frozen, moldy, unusually high in carbohydrate or protein, or too high in fiber)	—	Ensure energy intake to avoid ketosis	—

3. Early Lactating Cow (1 to 8 weeks)

Problem	Monitoring	Prevention	Treatment	Medication/Supplement	Comments
Primary acetonemia	Clinical or periodic examination of urine for ketones. Depression of milk yield and food intake	Improve energy intake of high-yielding cows in late pregnancy and early lactation	—	May supplement diet with propylene glycol or glycerine	—
Hypomagnesemia	Compton metabolic profile or periodic examination of urine for magnesium	Avoid low energy intake, high grass intake. Supplement diet with magnesium	—	Magnesium-rich reticular implant bullets effective but inconvenient	Worst in cold, wet, windy weather. Provide tree or shed shelter
Postparturient hemoglobinuria	Compton metabolic profile, checking phosphorus status	Ensure adequate dietary phosphorus	—	Add sodium dihydrogen phosphate to ration or via dispenser	Avoid rape, cabbage, other cruciferous plants
Right-side displacement of abomasum and cecal dilation	Early detection of illness	No reliable preventive technique	—	—	—
Early lactation drop in milk yield	Milk production per day	Ensure adequate dry matter and energy intake	—	—	—
Delayed onset of estrus	Develop reliable system of daily heat detection	Ensure optimum body weight or body condition score at time of mating—nutritional needs supplied	—	No prophylactic medication	—

4. Newborn Calf (birth to weaning)

Problem	Monitoring	Prevention	Treatment	Medication/Supplement	Comments
Acute diarrhea due to *E. coli*, rotavirus, coronavirus, *Cryptosporidia sp*	Daily observation for clinical disease. Serum immunoglobulins at 24 to 48 hours of age	Ensure adequate obstetrical assistance at birth if necessary. Ensure adequate intake of colostrum	Vaccinate against all agents 6 and 2 weeks prepartum	Prophylactic antibiotics when situation very bad	—
Unthriftiness and suboptimal growth rate	Weekly body weight gains	Feed adequate levels of milk or milk replacer; offer hay and calf starter at 2 weeks of age; wean at 6 to 8 weeks of age when eating sufficient dry feed	—	—	Reduce environmental and nutritional stress

Table continued on following page

Table 2–2. SUMMARY OF DISEASE CONTROL TECHNIQUES AND ROUTINE PRODUCTION PROCEDURES REQUIRED IN DAIRY HERDS ACCORDING TO AGE OF ANIMALS OR STAGE OF PRODUCTION (MASTITIS AND REPRODUCTIVE EFFICIENCY ARE PRESENTED SEPARATELY) (Continued)

Disease or Production Procedure	Monitoring Technique(s)	Prophylactic Techniques		
		MANAGEMENT	VACCINATION	MEDICATION	OTHER
		5. Calf (weaning to 6 months of age)			
Unthriftiness and suboptimal growth rate	Monthly body weight gains, tape measure of height at withers. Fecal egg and oocyst counts	Feed adequate diet to support optimum growth rate. Pasture rotation to avoid massive larval infection	—	Anthelmintic at 3 and 6 months. Coccidiostat as required	—
Enzootic calf pneumonia	Observations for paroxysmal harsh upper respiratory tract coughing and tachypnea	Ensure adequate ventilation. Supplemental heat in calf barn. Use calf hutches	May consider vaccination	Medicate feed with tetracycline for few weeks during period of convalescence	—
Infectious bovine rhinotracheitis, clostridial diseases, leptospirosis, brucellosis, bovine virus diarrhea	Observation of fever, dyspnea, cough; sudden death, myositis; red urine, mastitis, abortion; diarrhea and mucosal erosions	Avoid introductions from herds with unknown health status	Vaccinate calves at 6 months of age for infectious bovine rhinotracheitis, clostridial diseases, leptospirosis if endemic in area. Vaccinate for brucellosis if best policy. Vaccination for bovine virus diarrhea of doubtful value	—	—
		6. Heifer (6 to 15 months of age)			
Intestinal helminthiasis and external parasites	Observation of diarrhea, weight loss, fecal egg counts	Helminth control by pasture rotation	—	Strategic administration of anthelmintics when necessary	—
Supernumerary teats	Inspection at 6 months of age	Remove all supernumerary teats surgically	—	—	—
Traumatic reticuloperitonitis	—	Feed hay from string-tied bales only. All concentrates should be passed over a magnet	—	Administer reticular magnet to all heifers nominated as herd replacements	—

Suboptimal growth rate	Monthly body weight gains or measure height at withers and compare with standards	Ensure adequate nutritional intake or delay mating heifers until optimum mating weight achieved	—	—	Watch for area-wide problem due to nutritional deficiency, e.g., copper, cobalt
Coccidiosis	Observe diarrhea, dysentery, poor growth	Avoid overstocking	—	Add monensin to feed	—
Bovine virus diarrhea	Observe diarrhea (sporadic cases—most die)	—	Consider use of vaccine	—	—
Clostridial disease	Observe sudden deaths and typical lesions	Special techniques for some diseases, like controlling liver fluke for black disease; clean castrations	Vaccinate with 8-way vaccine if not done earlier	Heavy doses of antibiotics in at-risk group	—
Intestinal helminthiasis	Regular observation of performance especially if on pasture; fecal examination for worm eggs	Pasture management to avoid heavy larval infestations	—	Strategic dosing with anthelmintics	—

7. Diseases of Dairy Cattle Not Necessarily Related to the Production Cycle

INFECTIOUS					
1. Respiratory					
Pneumonic pasteurellosis	Sudden onset of fever, cough, dyspnea	Adequate ventilation, avoid stresses of handling and transportation to cattle shows, quarantine herd imports	Efficacy of available vaccines which are used widely, has not been established	Medication with sulfonamides and antibiotics used to be widespread, not much used now	Wide scope of preconditioning program expensive and not shown to be cost-effective yet
Infectious bovine rhinotracheitis	Sudden onset of fever, cough, dyspnea	Same as for pneumonic pasteurellosis	Vaccinate calves at 6 months of age and cows annually	—	Major economic concern in abortion form of the disease
Lungworm	Observe chronic coughing in calves	Manage pastures to minimize larval contamination	Irradiated larval vaccine available. Expensive Experimental	Strategic treatment with appropriate anthelmintics	—
Atypical interstitial pneumonia	Not possible. Put pilot one or two cattle on suspect pasture	Restrict dust in barn	None available and technique not applicable	—	—
2. Enteric					
Winter dysentery	Explosive herd outbreak, severe diarrhea; brief non-fatal illness	Sanitation and hygiene, effective manure disposal	—	—	Probably cannot be prevented. Will occur under best management

Table continued on following page

41

Table 2–2. SUMMARY OF DISEASE CONTROL TECHNIQUES AND ROUTINE PRODUCTION PROCEDURES REQUIRED IN DAIRY HERDS ACCORDING TO AGE OF ANIMALS OR STAGE OF PRODUCTION (MASTITIS AND REPRODUCTIVE EFFICIENCY ARE PRESENTED SEPARATELY) (Continued)

Disease or Production Procedure	Monitoring Technique(s)	Prophylactic Techniques			
		MANAGEMENT	VACCINATION	MEDICATION	OTHER
Salmonellosis	Diarrhea and toxemia. Fecal culture in problem herd	Sanitation and hygiene, prevent introduction of carrier animals	Autogenous bacterin in problem herds	Mass medication of feed and water	Isolate and quarantine infected animals
Coccidiosis	Diarrhea, dysentery	Sanitation and hygiene, avoid crowding and fecal contamination of feed	—	Mass medication of feed and water for large herds raising many herd replacements	—
Bovine virus diarrhea	Acute diarrhea. Infection is ubiquitous	No management technique is feasible	Vaccination available but is unreliable	—	Isolate affected animals
Johne's disease	Chronic diarrhea	Eradication by identification and culling of infected animals attempted but often not effective	Vaccine available to control disease but not infection	—	Sheep and goats are susceptible. Complete removal of all livestock may be necessary
Intestinal helminthiasis	Diarrhea, wasting egg counts	Pasture management, improved husbandry	—	Strategic administration of anthelmintics if economical	—
Bovine papular stomatitis	Lesions visible in mouth. Disease is insignificant	Nil	Virus identified but vaccine not warranted	Nil	—
Bovine malignant catarrh	Fatal illness with profuse mucopurulent ocular and nasal discharge, ophthalmitis, oral mucosal erosions, terminal encephalitis, lymphadenopathy	Avoid contact with lambing ewes	None available	—	A very sporadic disease. No control program warranted.
Foot and mouth disease	Herd affected, lameness, sore mouth, milk yield drop	Prevent introduction of carrier animals into countries where disease does not occur	Vaccination in countries where disease endemic	Nil	Eradication by slaughter of herd and contact herds in free countries
Bluetongue	A very rare disease in cattle clinically identical with chronic bovine virus	Avoid introduction of infected animals. Insect control	Effective vaccines available for sheep. Not used but could be in cattle	Nil	Cattle are significant carriers for sheep

3. Skin and Feet

Disease	Clinical signs	Control/Prevention	Immunization	Treatment	Remarks
Warble; fly infestation	Lumps under skin	—	—	Regular strategic use of insecticides	—
Pediculosis	Itching, dandruff, hair rubbed. Lice visible. Some blood loss. Seasonal	Thin cattle most susceptible	—	Regular use of insecticides	—
Papillomatosis	Observe appearance of warts	Isolate infected animals	Autogenous or proprietary vaccines usually used as treatment	—	—
Pseudocowpox; mammillitis	Observe characteristic lesions on teats	Strict hygiene in milking parlor	Experimental mammillitis vaccine being tested	Iodophor teat disinfection preferred	—
Ringworm	Obvious skin lesions of scabs and alopecia	Sanitation, hygiene, avoid overcrowding	Extensively used in Europe	Griseofulvin	—
Dermatophilus infection (mycotic dermatitis)	Tenacious, widespread scabs; hair loss	Treat or remove affected animals	Nil	Individual medication of each affected animal with antibiotics to remove source of infection	An uncontrollable disease in developing high-rainfall countries
Foot rot	Lameness, crack in foot cleft, swelling	Provide well-drained stone-free alleyways. Daily formalin foot bath	—	May mass medicate feed if outbreak occurs	—
Lameness due to diseases of the feet other than foot rot	Regular clinical examination of feet	Regular foot trimming, foot bath, non-traumatic floor surface	—	Walk animals through foot baths on regular basis	—

4. Sudden Death Diseases

Disease	Clinical signs	Control/Prevention	Immunization	Treatment	Remarks
Clostridial diseases	Sudden death. May be swollen leg (blackleg, malignant edema), hemoglobinuria (bacillary hemoglobinuria)	Proper disposal of infected carcasses	Vaccinate all animals for clostridial diseases endemic in areas	Only in treatment of infected animals	—
Anthrax	Sudden death	Proper disposal of infected carcasses	Vaccinate for anthrax in endemic areas	Only in treatment of infected animals	—

5. Nervous System

Disease	Clinical signs	Control/Prevention	Immunization	Treatment	Remarks
Hemophilus	Number of cattle affected with somnolence, recumbency, blindness. Synovitis, pneumonia, pleurisy, endometritis	Constant surveillance, early treatment. Avoid stress	Vaccinate in outbreak. Annual vaccination of calves before weaning	Mass medication in face of an outbreak	—

Table continued on following page

43

Table 2–2. SUMMARY OF DISEASE CONTROL TECHNIQUES AND ROUTINE PRODUCTION PROCEDURES REQUIRED IN DAIRY HERDS ACCORDING TO AGE OF ANIMALS OR STAGE OF PRODUCTION (MASTITIS AND REPRODUCTIVE EFFICIENCY ARE PRESENTED SEPARATELY) (Continued)

Disease or Production Procedure	Monitoring Technique(s)	Management	Prophylactic Techniques Vaccination	Medication	Other
Listeriosis	May be number affected. Observe for neurological signs, especially circling	Cease feeding ensilage. May be source of infection	Vaccines used but results poor	In high-risk situation in feedlot feed tetracyclines all the time	Control not really feasible
Rabies	Posterior paralysis, slack jaw, dribbling saliva, choking. Occasionally maniacal	Avoid contact with wildlife	Vaccination in endemic area	Nil	—
6. Other Infectious keratoconjunctivitis	Lacrimation, photophobia, keratitis	Avoid overcrowding, control flies. Close surveillance, early treatment	Vaccine available but results indifferent	Treat affected eyes to reduce spread of infection. Twice weekly treatment of eyes is effective	—
Brucellosis	Monitor abortion rate. Greater than 2% check cows serologically with agglutination test for brucellosis. Cull positives	Eradication by test and slaughter	Vaccinate calves in initial stage of eradication program. Adult vaccination permissible in some countries	Nil	—
Leucosis	Serological	Eradication by test and slaughter. Maintenance of a closed herd	—	—	—
Leptospirosis	Abortion storms, mastitis, hemoglobinuria in calves. Can monitor for seroconversions	Avoid contact with carrier animals. Hygiene and water control	Vaccinate in endemic herd	To reduce carrier state, treat with streptomycin	Rodent control desirable
Tuberculosis	Regular herd or area testing	Cull reactors. Quarantine until clear tests. Prevent introduction of infected animals	—	—	Many nonspecific reactors to tests from infections with atypical mycobacteria. Badgers and other wildlife may be carriers
Actinomycosis	Observe osteomyelitis of bones of jaw	Cull affected animals quickly. Disinfect feed troughs	—	—	—

Condition	Clinical signs / Diagnosis	Control / Management	Comments	Treatment / Prophylaxis	Remarks
Actinobacillosis	Observe myositis of tongue	Treat or cull quickly. Disinfect feed troughs	—	Treat affected animals urgently	Ensure no abrasive material in ration
Contagious bovine pyelonephritis	Red urine, fatal subacute illness	Cease natural breeding. Isolate affected animals. Hygienic disposal of contaminated bedding	—	Prophylactic treatment with penicillin in high-risk situation	—
Anaplasmosis	Wasting disease with fever peaks. Monitor by complement fixation test	Insect control. Prevent infection through careful disinfection of instruments	Vaccines widely used and good value. Still some uncertainty about best procedure	Long-acting oxytetracycline to eliminate carriers	Introduce animals to endemic area only in winter and when younger than 2 years
Babesiosis	Acute febrile hemoglobinuric disease. Serological and hematological tests both used	Insect vector control	Vaccination effective. Best technique not yet identified	Chemoprophylaxis with long-acting drugs as a practicable technique	Eradication by tick eradication
7. Nutrition					
Carbohydrate engorgement	History of access, depression, ruminal stasis. Foul-smelling feces	Avoid access to unlimited supply of fermentable carbohydrate	—	Consider use of buffers added to diet	—
Simple indigestion	Anorexia, ruminal stasis	Avoid sudden changes in diet or damaged feeds e.g., frozen or moldy feeds	—	Consider use of buffers added to diet	—
Ruminal tympany	Ruminal and abdominal distention. Peracute, highly fatal	Pasture management, use nonbloating forages	—	Add surfactants to pasture, prepared diets, licks, or blocks	—
Polioencephalomalacia	May be several affected with blindness, nystagmus. Recumbency, tetanic convulsions	Ensure adequate intake of good quality roughage. Avoid periods of water intake reduction	—	Supplement diet with thiamine if necessary	—
Mineral deficiencies	Poor production and growth. Regular feed analysis. Plus:	Ensure adequate dietary intake of required minerals	—	Prophylactic administration of element (cobalt—intrareticular implants, bullets; copper—depot injections of copper salts; selenium—retention bullets, injection; phosphorus—medicated water supply	—
Cobalt	Urine MMA or FIGLU levels				
Copper	Serum ceruloplasmin levels	required minerals			
Selenium	Glutathione peroxidase levels				
Phosphorus	Clinical signs of poor growth and rickets in young animals				

Table continued on following page

Table 2-2. SUMMARY OF DISEASE CONTROL TECHNIQUES AND ROUTINE PRODUCTION PROCEDURES REQUIRED IN DAIRY HERDS ACCORDING TO AGE OF ANIMALS OR STAGE OF PRODUCTION (MASTITIS AND REPRODUCTIVE EFFICIENCY ARE PRESENTED SEPARATELY) (Continued)

Disease or Production Procedure	Monitoring Technique(s)	Management	Prophylactic Techniques		
			Vaccination	Medication	Other
8. *Genetic Defects*	Clinical recognition at birth. Pedigree analysis	Regular surveillance of pedigrees. Cull heterozygotes	—	—	—
9. *Diseases of Dairy Bulls*					
Lameness due to diseases of feet	Observe for lameness	Frequent examination and trimming of feet	—	—	—
Spondylosis	Posterior ataxia, paresis, recumbency	Electro-ejaculate old bulls in danger age group	—	—	—
Degenerative joint disease	Lameness in hind legs in young bulls 6 months old and older	Avoid growing calves too fast. Keep grain rations low	—	—	Select against animals with disease
10. *Chemical Agents*					
Too many are possible to list them all. Lead and arsenic are the most common	Signs relevant to suspect poison	Prevent access to toxic chemicals. Judicious use of others like urea and insecticides	—	—	—
Lead poisoning	Urine and blood levels	Don't pasture near rubbish dumps	—	—	—
Arsenic poisoning	Abdominal pain, severe diarrhea, die quickly	Dispose of all arsenic residues	—	—	Avoid arsenic dips and sprays for insect control

References

Allaire, F.R., Sterwerf, H.E. and Ludwick, T.M. Variations in removal reasons and culling rates for dairy females. J. Dairy Sci., *60*:254–267, 1977.

Blood, D.C., Radostits, O.M. and Henderson, J.A. Veterinary Medicine. A Textbook of the Diseases of Cattle, Sheep, Pigs, Goats and Horses. 6th Edition. Baillière Tindall, London, 1983.

Bywater, A.C. Development of integrated management information systems for dairy producers. J. Dairy Sci., *64*:2113–2124, 1981.

Bywater, A.C. and Dent, J.B. Simulation of the intake and partition of nutrients by the dairy cow. Part I—Management control in the dairy enterprise; philosophy and general model construction. Agricultural Systems, *1*:245–260, 1976.

Bywater, A.C. Simulation of the intake and partition of nutrients by the dairy cow. Part II. The yield and composition of milk. Agricultural Systems, *1*:261–279, 1976.

Fick, G.W. A pasture production model for use in a whole-farm simulator. Agricultural Systems, *5*:137–163, 1980.

France, J., Neal, St. C. and Marsden, S. A dairy herd cash flow. Agricultural Systems, *8*:129–142, 1982.

James, A.D. Models of animal health problems. Agricultural Systems, *2*:183–187, 1977.

Martin, S.W., Aziz, S.A., Sandals, W.C.D. et al. The association between clinical disease, production and culling of Holstein-Friesian cows. Can. J. Anim. Sci., *62*:633–638, 1982.

Oltenacu, P.A., Rounsaville, T.R., Milligan, R.A. et al. Systems analysis for designing reproductive management programs to increase production and profit in dairy herds. J. Dairy Sci., *64*:2096–2104, 1981.

Williamson, N.B., Cannon, R.M., Blood, D.C. et al. A health program for commercial dairy herds (5). The occurrence of specific disease entities. Aust. Vet. J., *54*:252–256, 1978.

3 Dairy Cattle—General Approach to a Program

INTRODUCTION

Changing Pressures in the Dairying Industry

The dairy industry has undergone dramatic changes during the past 20 years. Most of the changes have been the result of economic pressures produced by the high cost of hired labor, the rapid increase in interest rates on capital invested in a dairy farm, and the increasing costs of energy. The industry's response to these pressures has been to attempt to reduce costs by increasing automation, especially in feeding systems and the handling of cattle in such functions as milking. As a result there has been a large increase in capitalization on dairy farms, but the heavy interest payments on borrowed capital have exerted the next pressure—to reduce capital expenditure by increasing the efficiency of the individual cow. Genetic gain in productivity has therefore become a very important management technique (Young 1981). A need has been created by this trend to counter the increased rate of disease occurrence in these "super cows" that are bred, and then fed, to extract the highest possible yield in a lactation. These production diseases are created by an inability of input of food to match output of milk and the resulting negative metabolic balance. As a result, there is now a place for veterinarians who are also knowledgeable in balancing the nutritional requirements of very heavy–producing cows so that they can produce heavily, without wastage caused by production disease.

These influences are most noticeable in countries where animals are housed during the winter months. In herds that are always at pasture, for example in Australia, New Zealand and South Africa, the same pressures have been applied, but the responses have been different. It has been, for the most part, a response by way of reduced labor intensity, usually in the form of increased herd size and more highly automated milking parlors. Feeding programs have not been greatly changed, at least not by supplementary feeding, but there has been a marked trend toward seasonal dairying, with all the cows calving at the same time and at a time when pasture production is very high, that is, when feed is cheapest (Moller 1978). A variation of that policy is the one in which the cows are calved at the time when the profitability is greatest (when the price × yield of milk minus the costs of feed and other variables is greatest). Both of these influences—greater numbers of cows per man (1:120) and seasonal dairying—create a need for a management aid that keeps herd records, plans a mating program, predicts milk yield and feed requirements, and maintains reproductive efficiency and control of subclinical mastitis. Herd health programs and planned herd health and production programs are a natural consequence of such needs.

It is because dairy cattle are the most efficient of all farm livestock in converting feed protein and energy to human food (Hodgson 1979) that there is more concern about the financial solidarity of this industry than most others. It is apparent that high fossil energy costs and reduced supplies may precipitate sharp changes in the systems of livestock production in the world, particularly those that are energy-intensive. It would be counterproductive if these changes made dairy products too expensive for the consumer, because there is still plenty of opportunity to expand the industry. For example, the potential for world forage production and for milk production from forages is several times current production. One of the ways in which costs can be kept down is an increase in the efficiency of milk production through a planned animal health and production program provided by veterinarians. This chapter and this book are dedicated to that objective.

Not all warm climates are suited to extensive grazing of large, moderately producing herds. Where land is expensive and much supplementary feed is available at low prices, there has been another development, the confinement of cows in corrals or dry-lots. Provided the feeding and cattle handling can be automated, labor costs can be minimized. The system is capital-intensive, and the pressure is on keeping cows that are individually very efficient by virtue of their heavy milk production. Accordingly, the prevention of production diseases rates high as a priority. Another problem that arises—it has always existed with housed animals—is the disposal of effluent. The grazing of cattle has the advantage that the pasture sward and natural processes dispose of animal wastes, but doing it mechanically encounters problems of energy consumption and environmental pollution.

In all countries and with all systems of dairying, there has developed another highly significant influence that regulates the industry's activities at a more basic level—that of financial support from the public purse, i.e., from governmental aid. This may be by way of overt subsidy of the price of milk, dairy products, and beef or by less apparent means through lower interest rates from agricultural banks, costs of irrigation and land reclamation projects, government advisors, scientific diagnostic laboratories, and research into industry problems. In an era when government spending is being heavily reduced, the financial support to agriculture, including animal husbandry, is being closely reviewed (Thompson 1980). Part of this potential reduction in funding has to be credited to the growing power of consumers as a group. There is a disinclination to have particular segments of the community receive more than others, and the dairy industry—together with the other agricultural industries—is likely to be under pressure to be more cost-effective.

All of these influences have a general direction. It is to encourage farming to move more into the sector of business, with all the appurtenances that go with a commercial enterprise—cost-benefit analysis, adequate returns on investment, predictions of cash flow, evidence of collateral when borrowing money, and the use of commerce-oriented statistics rather than the classic statistics of scientific experimentation. Computerization is a logical answer to all of the problems created for the dairy farmer and for his veterinarian, and for all the other technical and financial advisors who work in the area that services the dairying industry.

Causes of Economic Loss in Dairy Herds

The relative importance of either disease or production problems to the wastage in commercial dairy herds helps to decide the orientation of the dairy farmer's thinking in terms of what advice he will seek first and where he will invest his available financial resources in an attempt to reduce costs. Although the consensus of opinion is that disease causes at least as much wastage as does management error, there is little supporting evidence on which to base that opinion. Some reports are available concerning the relative importance of illness (Keyser 1977) and the causes of disposal, including culling and death (Renkema and Stelwagen 1977; Williamson et al. 1978; Renkema and Stelwagen 1979), but the data, for the most part, refer to limited populations of cows. An East German survey (Eschenbach and Witt 1971) showed that 55 to 75% of all cows in a herd required treatment for mastitis, infertility, and foot injury, and mastitis accounted for 61% of all cows culled. Another large-scale survey in the United Kingdom (Beynon 1976) indicated that infertility and mastitis together accounted for 45% of losses, whereas poor production and similar problems accounted for 35%. In Canada, a survey (Burnside et al. 1971) showed that suboptimal reproduction was about equally important as a cause of culling. There were differences between breeds in the reasons for culling, udder disease being most important in Holsteins. In younger cows, low production was the more common cause, and in older cows, disease was more important. In the U.S., mastitis and suboptimal reproduction are estimated to account for 55% of the total costs incurred because of disease (Shanks et al. 1981). A similar large-scale survey in the U.S. (Allaire et al. 1977) showed that about one third of the cows culled were culled for low productivity, the other two thirds because of disease, mostly reproductive inefficiency and mastitis, which together were responsible for two thirds of the losses caused by disease. Figures from Zimbabwe suggest that similar conditions prevail

there. Reproductive inefficiency (39% of the culls) and mastitis (21%) were the principal reasons for culling cows (Higgins 1981). In some herds the culling rate may be as high as 25%, and this increases with the age of the cow (Cobo-Abreu et al. 1979a). The median survival time of cows after entry into the herd is approximately three years, which accounts for a major economic loss because of failure to achieve production potential. There is an association of mastitis, metritis, retained placenta, and pneumonia with culling (Cobo-Abreu et al. 1979b), and both disease occurrence and culling increase with age. Mastitis is associated with a drop in milk production, and metritis and retained placenta are associated with longer than optimum calving intervals. The diseases reduce milk production and number of calves and therefore lead to premature disposal. Identifying the causes of these diseases and instituting effective control procedures is a major goal in a herd health program.

Diseases associated with parturition such as dystocia, uterine prolapse, retained placenta and metritis may account for up to 8% of all diseases in dairy cows (Roine and Saloniemi 1978). Herds with a high incidence of retained placenta may also have more mastitis, ketosis, and parturient paresis.

There are notable differences between diseases in their contribution to wastage. These differences occur between breeds of cattle (Grommers et al. 1971), between different age groups, and between seasons of the year (Hansen et al. 1979), although much of this variation is related to the seasons of the year when particular events in the reproductive cycle occur. For example, in housed cattle there is no marked seasonality of disease occurrence other than that associated with calving and the onset of lactation, and as these events are concentrated into the housing period, there is a tendency for an increase in total disease occurrence in the months when cattle are housed (Erb and Martin 1978). Disease incidence is also much higher in the 50 days immediately after calving and increases severalfold with increasing age, owing largely to increments of damage to the mammary gland and an increasing incidence of the production diseases, milk fever, and acetonemia (Hansen et al. 1979). Another factor that causes great variation in the prevalence of disease in individual herds is the type and quality of housing used (Grommers et al. 1971), which is dealt with later.

Most of the data that are available relate to clinically recognizable disease, but there are other forms of loss that are equally important. Subclinical disease, for example in mastitis and reproductive inefficiency, causes suboptimal performance in a production parameter without identifiable lesions. Other factors, e.g., low fat content of milk on low-fiber diets, can also cause incidental related losses due to loss of reputation, or opportunity loss due to inability to supply a particular product in the appropriate quality or quantity.

Total losses due to disease cannot even be estimated, and until there is some system of national disease recording in a country, it is difficult to see how cost-effective disease control programs can be promoted with authority. Widespread planned health and production programs could provide more of this type of data than most other sources.

Some studies done in Canada indicate that the amount of concentrate fed to lactating dairy cattle accounted for the largest amount of variation in production and income per cow (Bowman et al. 1980). To optimize the level of production and income on these dairy farms, the level of nutrition must be improved. Management factors concerned with the milking procedure, calf rearing, calf nutrition and herd breeding practices were of tertiary importance in their effect on average herd production and income. Comparisons of the management in high-and-low-production herds showed that there was lower total feed intake and lower crude protein intake as a per cent of requirement in the low-production herds compared with the high-production herds (Martin et al. 1978). This illustrates the potential economic losses associated with undernutrition.

One of the effects of reducing wastage by disease in a herd is to move a problem to, or create a gain for, the management area and to alter the balance between the two. Two examples follow: First, the effect of a good health and management program is to produce milk more efficiently in a financial sense. This usually happens as a result of more milk being produced by the same resources. In most circumstances, the market for milk is limited, and its production in excess of a specific quota will be uneconomic. This places farmers in a position where they have to dispose of resources to gain the full rewards of the program. Farms are not usually readily divisible, so that if the size of the dairy herd is reduced, it is necessary to substitute an alternative enterprise.

Second, a reduction in the culling rate for disease can be expected within a relatively short time after a program commences. This moves cattle from the category of being culled as rejects to the category of surplus cattle sold for production purposes, with a resulting respectable increase in income. There is the more obvious effect of improved health and the reduction in the obligatory culling rate. The resulting increase in annual profitability in a herd with an average life increase of 3.5 lactations up to 5.5 lactations may be as much as 20% (Renkema and Stelwagen 1979).

One of the biggest problems encountered when assessing the gains made when a preventive program is introduced is that of appraising the financial gain when part of a farm is sold or when hired help is no longer employed. The only satisfactory method of attempting that task is to create a computer simulation model of a herd, with those factors included among the variables.

The Role of the Dairy Herd Health Program

The attention of the dairy farmer and the dairying industry has been attracted by the need to limit wastage caused by disease and to coordinate the control programs arising out of this policy with the production management programs. There is no clearly defined pattern for this interrelationship, because much depends on the individual enthusiasm, interest, and expertise of the persons involved in each situation. In one district or on one farm it is the animal husbandryman who is the focus of advice; on another, it is the veterinarian. In some circumstances, it is the farmer himself who is the innovator and the driving force. A schematic representation of the area of work to be covered in the advisory service to a dairy farm is shown in Figure 3-1. The veterinarian's contribution can be limited to the parts of the program that deal with health (heavily outlined) or, if he cares to develop sufficient extra expertise to qualify as a "species specialist," may extend to cover the management areas of nutrition, housing, genetics, and general management. There seems little doubt that the average farmer would be best served by having all sources of advice coordinated so that the effects of managerial change recommended in one area are accompanied by a description of the consequential effects in other areas. He also needs someone to maintain

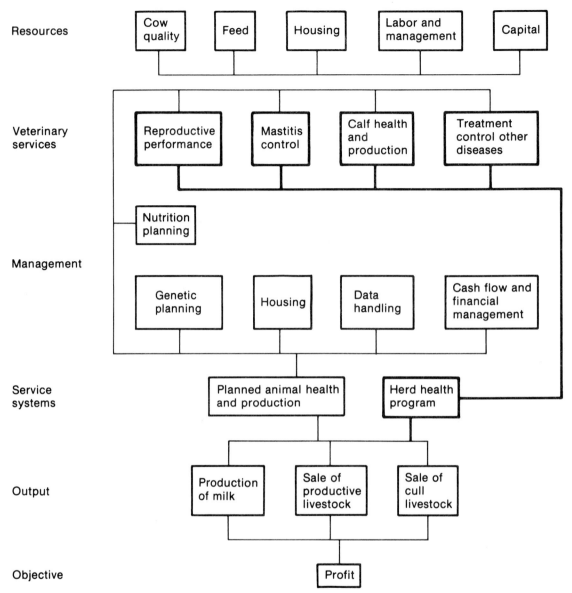

Figure 3-1. Schematic representation of the resources and management required in a planned animal health and production program and in a herd health program in a dairy herd.

his records and to originate recommendations emanating from routine and regular analyses of the data. The intensification of management processes also has created a special need for veterinary service and advice at a highly specialized level. A planned health and production program is now the standard method of countering these problems. This has added a new dimension to the work of veterinarians in food animal medicine. The opportunities for development of these programs are greater in the dairy industry than in any other because of the need to monitor production and health on a

daily basis and in a number of ways. Such a mass of data needs expert selection, storage, and analysis, and a computerized system provides the best answer.

Interviews with large-scale dairy operators in California indicate that as large-scale dairies have replaced smaller dairies, the operator's reliance on the veterinarian as a primary source of advice about a wide range of dairy health management issues has declined (Goodger and Ruppanner 1982). Large-scale dairies require a totally integrated approach to health management, which includes herd health, herd management, and production. Dairy operators do not look to veterinarians to provide this integrated approach, instead relying on feed representatives, nutritionists, accountants, and staff of dairy cooperatives. Operators perceive veterinarians as primary providers of clinical services only. Since veterinarians have little conflict of interest or vested interest in giving advice about nutrition, proper facility design, and other general management issues, this perception of the veterinarian as a clinician only deprives the dairy operator of an objective appraisal of herd health, management, and production. Changing this perception will require a restructuring of many veterinary medical college curricula, with an emphasis on courses in epidemiology, preventive medicine, herd management, nutrition, and similar subjects. Clearly, the future of large-scale dairy practice will depend on the development of a production-oriented system of veterinary service, which will require changes in the attitudes of veterinarians and in their education at veterinary colleges (Goodger and Kushman 1983).

A proposal for the integration of dairy cattle breeding management and herd health services for dairy farmers into a single computer-based data base has been described in Australia (Alexander 1978).

Objective of a Herd Health Program— Profitability

The primary justification for initiation of a health program is that productivity of dairy cattle differs substantially from the level regarded as economically optimal, owing to factors that a veterinarian can influence, such as diseases, nutritional disorders, and animal management problems. The primary objective of a dairy herd health program is to manage the herd in such a way as to achieve predetermined performance targets (Blood et al. 1978). The assumption must be made that achieving the biological target is synonymous with achieving the economic target, and an essential procedure in developing a herd health program is to produce evidence that this association is a valid one. At the present time, the achievement of these objectives is being attempted almost universally by a combination of regularly scheduled visits to the farm, by the dairyman managing the herd effectively, and by the use of a simple, reliable data system that records performance continuously.

It is generally accepted that these programs are highly profitable, with the common figure of 600% return quoted on the farmer's investment in the program (Barfoot et al. 1971; Williamson 1980). However, there is a great deal of difficulty in carrying out an accurate cost-benefit analysis of the programs and there is controversy about the conclusions (Williamson 1981; Alston and Ryan 1981).

TARGETS OF PERFORMANCE AND DATA HANDLING IN THE DAIRY HERD

Targets of Performance

A target of performance expresses what is thought to be a desirable level of production or incidence of disease that can be achieved economically given the resources available to the producer. In a dairy herd health program, the actual performance is regularly compared with present targets of performance. The differences between the two levels are calculated, and the causes of failure to achieve the targets must then be determined. This requires a continuous recording system that is simple, reliable, and preferably self-analyzing and that indicates clearly the shortfalls in performance or the increase in incidence of disease.

The targets of performance and disease incidence for dairy cattle are realistic and can be achieved economically. They have been established through the analysis of the lifetime production records of many cows over many years. The targets for reproductive performance and subclinical mastitis, which will yield the most milk over the lifetime of a cow, are particularly reliable. The targets presented in Table 3–1 are based on recorded material in the literature modified by our own experience in our own environments. They are probably applicable only in similar environments and are provided as examples into which dairy farmers and veterinarians can insert values applicable to their own circumstances. Performance targets for dairy herds on pasture in Australia and New Zealand and for housed cattle in North America and the U.K. are included in the table. The figures apply to commercial herds milking 100 to 400 cows year-round on improved pasture, either irrigated (Australia) or with good rainfall (New Zealand), or to housed cattle in herds of about 50 head.

Table 3-1. TARGETS OF PERFORMANCE AND DISEASE INCIDENCE FOR DAIRY CATTLE

	Australia and New Zealand	North America and the U.K.
REPRODUCTIVE PERFORMANCE		
Mean age at first calving (months)	24	24
Mean intercalving interval (days)	365	365–400
Mean interval calving to first estrus (days)	60	60
Mean interval calving to conception (days)	83	83–115
Mean length of lactation (days)	280	305
Mean length of dry period (days)	65	65
Culling rate for reproductive inefficiency (% per annum)	<10	<10
Abortion rate (% per annum)	<3	<2
MASTITIS PREVALENCE		
Quarter infection rate (%):		
Mid-lactation sample of herd	<7	<10
Each cow at drying-off	<10	<10
Bulk milk somatic cell count (monthly)	$<0.5 \times 10^6$ ml.	$<0.4 \times 10^6$/ml.
Individual cow milk somatic cell count (monthly)	$<0.3 \times 10^6$ ml.	$<0.15 \times 10^6$/ml.
No. of clinical cases per 100 cows per month	<2	<5
CALF HEALTH AND SURVIVAL		
Calf mortality (% under 28 days of age)	<5	<5
Total Disease Wastage		
Annual culling rate all diseases (% of total herd over 1 year of age)	<5	<5
Annual death rate (% of adult cows)	<2	<2
Average expected lifetime of each lactating cow (years)	10	8
Average number of lactations expected from each cow (years)	7	5
MILK PRODUCTION		
Average daily milk production of 4% F.C.M.* per cow (kg.)	15–20	30–45
Average annual milk production of 4% F.C.M.* per cow (kg.)	4500	6000–8000
Average annual production of butterfat per cow (kg.)	160–180	250–400
BODY CONDITION SCORE		
Of females at time of breeding (expressed as body condition score as described by Victorian Department of Agriculture or similar system)	5 out of 8	3 out of 5

*F.C.M. = fat-corrected milk.

Identification of Dairy Cattle

Accurate identification of individual animals and a system of keeping valid records are major prerequisites in the effective management of large dairy herds. The ideal method of marking animals for identification should provide permanent identity, be legible at a distance, be inexpensive and easy to apply, cause a minimum of pain or discomfort to the animal, conform to coding for data retrieval, and not be altered, destroyed, or lost (Hooven 1978). Permanent methods of marking include tattoos, color sketches, and hot and freeze branding. Nonpermanent methods include ear tags, neck straps and chains, and ankle straps. Electronic identification of animals using a transponder implanted in the animal, which emits signals to a receiver unit, is in the developmental stages (Holm 1981).

Data Handling Systems

Manual Card Systems

In a dairy herd health program, the basic recording unit is the individual dairy cow. In the simplest recording system, an individual cow card is assigned to each positively identified animal when it becomes a herd replacement. Using a simple code system, all events are recorded chronologically as they occur. These include the events of the reproductive cycle, pregnancy diagnosis by the veterinarian, diseases that occur, and the treatments given. Monthly milk somatic cell counts may also be recorded. Each individual cow card can hold the data for up to eight lactations. The data can be analyzed regularly using a manual system and the reproductive performance indices summarized and reported to the farmer. For small herds of up to 50 to 60 lactating cows, the individual cow card system is satisfactory. The major disadvantage is that the cow cards constitute the only record, and these must usually be taken back to the veterinarian's office for analysis, thus creating delays and periods of time in which the record book is not on the farm. This may result in loss of valuable data.

In addition to these health data, there is an equally strong demand for data relating to each cow's production status; this is acknowledged by dairy scientists in their selection and specification of least-cost diets, by geneticists in their selection of breeding stock, and by veterinarians in their monitoring of animal health and production (Puckett et al. 1981).

The amount of information that a dairy herdsman can record personally is limited. As the number of the cows in the herd increases, the detail of information collected and used decreases. In very large herds managed as a single unit, a bare minimum of data on individual animals is recorded. The resulting lack of individual animal management is reflected in lower than optimal milk production and an increase in intercalving interval, both of which lead to a decrease in lifetime production.

Computer Systems

The large amount of data that must be collected and analyzed on a dairy farm has led to the use of computers as an aid to the farmer in decision making and management of the herd (Speicher 1981). The potential use of the computer on a dairy farm includes dairy herd management, monitored crop production, financial accounting systems, decision aids, and communication systems. A computer-assisted dairy herd management system is one in which the herd is monitored and pertinent information on individual animals is entered into storage for retrieval at appropriate times and in a form designed to facilitate decision making. The computerized data acquisition system becomes an extension of the manager's memory, and it can rapidly sort and arrange information to be of the greatest value to the manager. The ultimate goal is for the computerized data acquisition system to be fully informed about the production, nutrition, reproduction, health, and economic status of all animals at all times and to initiate and carry out or notify the manager of any appropriate action to be taken (Ellis et al. 1983).

Production Management Systems

The Dairy Herd Improvement (DHI) program was the original computer-assisted dairy herd management system and has been one of the major factors contributing to the increase in milk production levels in the dairy industry. Input for the system is animal identification, performance status, and various measures of resource input, all of which are collected monthly by the DHI supervisor and mailed to the DHI center for computation with the assistance of a large, main frame computer.

The return report, received through the mail by the dairy manager, is a summary of individual animal status, overall performance, and some of the costs of production. These reports provide the manager with an organized summary of management information important to the decision-making process.

A typical DHI report would include the following information (Stout 1978):

Sample Day and Lactation Report
Kilograms of milk
Per cent butterfat
Grain mix fed on sample day
Total days of current lactation for each cow and totals of milk butterfat calculated for those days based on the sample-day production
Income over feed cost

Annual Projections
Each month the milk production accumulated for lactation-to-date is projected to a 305-2X-ME basis. This standardizes each cow's record to a 305-day lactation length, milked twice daily and the same age, mature equivalent (ME). By projecting all records to a standard level, valid comparison can be made between cows.

Management Data
Lactation number of each cow
Days dry for previous dry period
Last calving date
Intercalving interval
Results of pregnancy examination
Persistency (how well the animal is holding up in production)

Action Needed
Cows for drying-off
Begin feeding grain to cows before calving
Cows for pregnancy examination

Herd Summary—Reproductive Performance
Cows diagnosed pregnant
Cows possibly pregnant
Number of animals open
Intercalving interval
Calving-to-conception interval
Services per conception

Summary of Animals to be Milking, Dry or Due to Calve
Feeding Summary
Cost and Return Summary
Lactation Summary
Dry Days Summary
Production Summary

Programs of this type do not need the participation of the veterinarian—although that is usually provided for pregnancy diagnosis. It is highly desirable that reports to the farmer be channeled through an adviser of some sort who can provide information about the errors and potentialities that arise out of the herd's history.

Animal Health and Production Systems

Currently there are several herd programs that have attempted to build on the original management programs, such as the D.H.I. program, and to add health data and analysis. Some go further and add cash flow and mating selection programs. Each type has a major emphasis on one or another of the major inputs, and one of the large tasks still to be done in this area is the coordination of preexisting separate information from herd improvement, artificial breeding, and health sources into a single stream.

The principal programs in this category are from the University of Melbourne (Blood et al. 1978; Cannon et al. 1978) and the Daisy program (Stephens et al. 1979; Russell and Rowlands 1983; Martin et al. 1982). These programs were designed to serve veterinarians rather than the farmer. They feature simple minimal records, fast turn-around, and the production of reports that are most likely to reveal the best picture of the production and health status of the herd as a whole with respect to each of the diseases and to the production parameters. Then a suitable combination of skillfully selected indexes and a knowledgeable veterinarian who is familiar with each farm's management practice results in a monthly report to each farmer by a skilled adviser.

Data Input and Output

A properly designed program of this sort will collect only minimal data but will then dissect it in a multiplicity of ways and produce reports as shown below.

Data Collection

Until data loggers and hand-held computers reach practical prices, it is still necessary to record observations and actions with pen and paper. The requirement is for a diary in which the farmer can enter a record of those items of information about breeding and disease that are required by the program. The diary needs to be with the farmer at all times and be capable of producing a detachable record but leaving a copy. The shirt-pocket diary is most satisfactory with a guide to entries in the cover and self-carboned duplicate pages to facilitate copy production. Every two to four weeks, depending on the frequency of veterinary visits, the farmer is requested to forward the current diary pages (Cannon et al. 1978), and the information on them is immediately transferred to the Current Lactation Listing. The ultimate recording instrument is the hand-held data logger, into which data are entered as events occur. The data are transferred electronically into the office computer at the end of the day.

Notification of Visit and List of Cows Required

The updated Current Lactation Listing is searched by the computer for the identity of those cows that fall into the categories, such as no visible estrus, failure to conceive, pregnancy diagnosis, and drying-off examination for mastitis, that are needed for veterinary examination. A list of these cows is sent to the farmer together with a note advising of the date and time of the visit to examine the cows. The veterinarian is also advised if he is not initiating the action.

Examination Record

The list of cows required is presented as a report form so that the veterinarian can record his findings on it. There is also room to record treatments, recommended cullings, or treatment by the farmer. At the completion of the veterinarian's visit, the report is returned to the computer operator, who adds the information to the Current Lactation Listing.

Monthly Report

When the Current Lactation Listing has been updated it is sent to the farmer, with a copy to the veterinarian, as part of a monthly report that includes the sections listed below. The report provides an analysis of the performance of the herd in a variety of production parameters and a record of performance of individual cows.

Current Lactation Listing

Each lactation is dealt with as a separate record, and a cow may accumulate seven or eight such records on her lifetime chart. The Current Lactation Listing includes the current lactation record of each cow in the milking herd during that month. As each cow calves, aborts, or is purchased, she opens a new record on the Current Lactation Listing, and as she is dried off, dies, or is sold, the record is deleted from the Current Lactation Listing and is entered into the lifetime listing. The Current Lactation Listing includes all the data of the events in the cow's life during this lactation. Because it contains all the cows in the herd at the time, it can be used and is designed to be used as a catalogue of the herd. Each month it is updated, and a new listing is produced. In this way the farmer receives a new catalogue, and the previous one is discarded, every month. All entries in the listing are in an easily read code constructed especially for this purpose.

Reproductive Efficiency Status

This is indicated by average periods of calving to first estrus, to first service, to conception, and of calving to calving. In addition, as a guide to the possible causes of reproductive inefficiency, there may be included the percentage of cows submitted for pregnancy that are pregnant; the average interestral period; and lists of cows to be examined for problems, including no visible estrus, failure to conceive, repeated short estral cycles, and pregnancy rechecks for cows originally diagnosed as pregnant that have been observed to return to estrus.

Mastitis Status

This is indicated by the number of clinical cases per 30 days per 100 cows, the average bulk milk cell count for the past three months, the average individual milk cell count of each cow for the lactation so far, or the average quarter infection rate at drying-off for the past three months.

Milk Production

In herds that participate in a dairy herd improvement program, the record is personal to each cow and is essential if a selection program based on productivity is to be used. The alternative is a record of milk production provided by the milk reception depot at the retail outlet or processing plant. Divided by the number of cows milking at the time a computer program is required to keep this figure accurate on a daily basis, it is a valuable indicator of nutritional status in pastured cows, which are otherwise out of surveillance in this regard.

Other Disease Incidents

Only a limited number of codes is maintained in order to avoid the keeping of unnecessarily detailed records. The diseases likely to occur in significant numbers are listed.

The rest are in an omnibus group of "other diseases not listed above."

Assist Lists

These include lists of cows to calve arranged numerically and in order of expected date of calving, cows to be dried off, cows to treat at drying-off for mastitis, cows to receive prophylactic treatment for milk fever, and so on. The lists are provided by further dissection of the already accumulated data. Additional lists include those specifying which cows were examined, treated, recommended for culling, and so on. These are used to record what has in fact been done by the veterinarian and are essential for billing purposes.

Distribution of the Report

Two copies of the report go to the veterinarian, one for the owner and one for the veterinarian. The veterinarian comments on the performance of the herd, makes recommendations for its improvement where this is relevant, and sends one copy to the farmer. The report is discussed at the next regular visit or earlier if the situation requires it.

Annual Report

This report is provided annually and summarizes data for the preceding 12 months on reproduction performance, mastitis incidence, occurrence of other diseases, and causes of death and disposal. It is intended to be a retrospective analysis, whereas the monthly report deals with information that is sufficiently recent to provide some guidance on what to do now.

Accompanying the annual report are two tables, the *Anticipated Calving List* and the *Feed Planning Table*. These are management aids to help the farmer prepare for individual animals to calve and to help him determine the feed requirements for each week, based on the number of cows calving and the number being withdrawn from the herd. A further refinement of this system is to insert in the program a limit on the amount of milk production required. This may help to avoid a penalty for overproduction or, conversely, to fill a quota. In response, the program will advise, for example, that some cows should be deferred or advanced in their mating. This is in effect a planned breeding program. It can also be arranged that cows that do not attain specific disease or production levels are recommended to be culled.

Computerized Programs—Availability

The types of records, analyses of performance, and advisory tables described previously are really only possible at a reasonable cost by using a computer. There are three ways in which a computer resource can be used for this purpose, and they are discussed in detail in Chapter 13. They are:

□ The data is mailed in from the farm to a data laboratory that has access to a computer.
□ The veterinarian or other adviser maintains a microcomputer or has a terminal to a distant main-frame computer. This system has the advantage that a stand-alone micro could handle herd health programs for 50 to 100 herds and also carry out all the administrative work of the practice.
□ The farmer could have his own micro or main-frame link. A machine small enough to economically handle the preventive medicine and other records of 500 cows would be too small to carry out some tasks quickly enough. If it was large enough to do those tasks, it would be overcapacitated.

The well-developed computer software systems used in dairy cattle medicine have versions adapted to both mainframes and microcomputers. The University of Melbourne and the Daisy program were originally designed for mainframes linked to distant and dumb terminals, but both are now available in microcomputer versions. The way in which these systems will develop further and the likelihood that they will pass into the hands of farmers, veterinarians, or others is unclear. It seems likely that in some places it will be one system, and that, in other places—because another group of people is more active and enthusiastic—the alternative system will be used.

The following factors need to be taken into account when making a policy decision about which way the development of a computer system should go.

The major advantages of the computer are that the data can be stored cumulatively, can then be resorted, and an up-to-date retrospective analysis of the performance of each cow and of the herd can be made available immediately following the entry of the last item of data. This allows for instant analysis of the current performance, which is necessary in order to make intelligent decisions on management matters. The larger the memory of the computer, the better and faster the analyses.

Farmers joining a computer-based system will need to provide retrospective data for each cow for at least the previous 12 months in order to establish a baseline of data. This would be a daunting task to a farmer-operator, but is a small piece of business to an experienced person.

Whereas the use of microcomputers on individual farms will improve the speed and accuracy of handling data and of making decisions, there are some limitations. When they operate in isolation, they lose the considerable advantage that a cooperative of farmers achieves in being able to make anonymous interfarm comparisons. The development of a large common data base in an area in which data from thousands of cows are stored and analyzed provides valuable information on the levels of reproduction and production that are possible. This allows for the development of targets of performance that are related to the real practical farm situation (Crandall et al. 1979).

Progressive dairy farmers also need access to production and performance testing information, which is provided by central breeding agencies and dairy herd improvement associations. The evaluation of dairy bulls requires the participation of many dairy farms in a computerized official monthly milk recording system.

In addition to the data from individual cows, there is other information that must be recorded and reported to the farmer periodically. This includes information on all aspects of management, feeds and feed analyses, the results of necropsies, regular evaluation of the milking machine, specific disease incidence, and recommendations for control. All of this information can be stored chronologically in a veterinarian's office by the owner's name file and is used, along with the data collected from monthly farm visits, for the preparation of monthly and annual reports. This information is vital when there is a retrospective inquiry into the causes of a decline in production or a sudden increase in the incidence of disease.

Interaction with a Herd Health Computer Program

An effective herd health program is one in which the farmer reacts to advice about his performance by trying to improve it, often in a particular area of his work. An effective computerized program is designed to interact with the farmer. That is, the computer produces analyses of performance, the farmer reacts to them, and then feeds more data into the program, which reacts by producing new analyses, and the cycle is repeated over and over again, usually at monthly intervals.

In an effective dairy herd health program, the sequence is designed to serve the following functions:

- The computer generates a list of cows that have not matched targets and that need to be examined or to have their continued future in the herd decided. It is known that when farmers generate such lists they are much less rigid in their selectivity, and correspondingly, the program is less effective.

- The computer list goes to the veterinarian and the farmer. The veterinarian has the benefit of an exact list of what he has to do on his visit, the scope of the work, the treatment materials needed, the amount of time he will need, and an indication of developing herd problems, for example, a higher than normal proportion of cows failing to conceive. The farmer knows exactly which cows he should keep in for the veterinarian to examine and why he should keep them in.

- The veterinarian reacts by examining the cows, treating some, and recommending some for culling. A good program provides a list that invites a reaction because it not only specifies why the cow has been selected for examination but also recounts the cow's immediate past history on which the decision to examine was based and indicates gaps in which the veterinarian records his findings.

- The computer reacts when this information is entered into the program by discharging a report that analyzes the performance of each cow and of the herd as defined by the veterinarian's findings, the observations of the farmer, and information—such as volume of milk production—from still other sources.

- The veterinarian reacts in turn by viewing the analyses in the report and looking for early warning signs of impending herd problems such as a continuing rise in average milk cell counts. The response will be to advise the farmer on production management and disease control to counter the threat. The advice must be prompt, accurate, and up-to-date.

Besides this interaction there are obvious end-products of this data analysis, the principal one being the accumulation of a data bank that provides a reliable benchmark of what the herds are actually achieving, thus allowing targets to be more realistically determined. Further uses of the data are the production of interherd comparisons to encourage competition and the supplying of raw data to extension programs to give them some realistic, local, relevant information. Also, the information available about each herd can be used to provide the additional features of predicting cash flow, milk production, and feed planning.

THE COMPONENTS OF A DAIRY HERD HEALTH PROGRAM

Introduction

Dairy herd health programs vary, depending on the goals, values, and motivation of the producer and on the desire of the veterinarian to offer the service.

In the simplest form, a farmer deliberately sets out to improve his herd's performance by improving his management, especially in milking parlor hygiene and breeding techniques. The veterinarian is used only for emergency service.

In the next stage, the veterinarian is used on a selective basis. The farmer keeps all the records and selects the cows to be examined and treated by the veterinarian. A number of cows are treated at each of a number of visits, but there is no regular visitation, and no attempt is made to analyze the performance and status of the herd as a whole. There is no herd program.

A *herd health program* consists of regularly scheduled visits by a veterinarian in which all matters of health maintenance—especially the means of keeping reproductive efficiency high and mastitis and calf mortality low—are discussed, and individual animals and groups of animals are examined and treated in order to achieve these ends (Cote 1980).

A *planned herd health and production program* is one that combines a herd health program with one designed to incorporate advice and assistance about production management. This serves to relate the management advice aimed at reducing the prevalence of disease with that concerned with feeding and breeding plans and general management policies designed to promote production, either in volume or in economic efficiency.

The Basic Herd Health Program

In a basic dairy herd health program, the veterinarian makes regularly scheduled visits to the farm to examine animals, assess all aspects of health and performance, and make recommendations for improvement in those areas. The major theme is *constant surveillance* of health and production and the identification of reasons for failure to meet certain production objectives or targets.

Regularly Scheduled Farm Visits

In herds that milk all year round and have some cows calving every month, the usual schedule includes one visit from the veterinarian each month. This is satisfactory for average commercial herds of from 50 to 200 cows (Donovan 1981). In larger herds, more frequent visits are necessary, and these are usually conducted at two-week intervals. When cows are farmed intensively and strong emphasis is placed, for example, on reducing the calving-conception interval, more frequent visits than one each month are needed. As a result, farmers with intensively farmed herds of about 200 cows frequently request weekly visits. One of the effects of such numerous visits is that more frequent reports are required, and costs rise quickly. It is not only the costs of veterinary visits and services that increase but also the office work of recording, storing, analyzing, and reporting data and information. These costs are readily borne in herds where production and capitalization are high, the latter because of the high value of cows and buildings. In commercial herds farmed less intensively, but in which there is regularly more work than can be accomplished in a day, it can be advantageous to make visits on successive days and report only once each month. Herds of 300 to 500 cows are in this category.

In herds that milk only during a limited season, for example in New Zealand and Australia—where much of the milk is used for the manufacture of processed dairy products and where milking the cows can be arranged to take advantage of high seasonal pasture growth—the program is quite different. The entire herd is going through its lactation cycle at the same time, so that the functions of the veterinarian are different at each visit, in contrast to the activities in a year-round herd, which is calving some cows every month, and where the activities at each monthly visit are identical (Moller 1978).

Activities at Scheduled Visits. The standard practice in a herd health program is to monitor performance with the target and to make recommendations about management of the herd when performance falls behind that required for economic health. Translated into terms applicable to dairy herds this means periodic—usually monthly—visits to each farm by a veterinarian in order to:

- examine cows for evidence of one or more of the diseases against which a control program has been set up
- evaluate the results of these examinations and the data provided by farmer observations during the past month in order to assess the herd's situation with respect to fertility, mastitis prevalence, and other diseases
- discuss with the farmer why the performance in each of the health indices is good or bad in the light of the resources available, discuss his individual objectives, and make recommendations about variations in the application of existing measures or the introduction of new ones

The choice of which cows are to be examined is sometimes left to the farmer, and there is no reason why—provided he has access to the recommended targets and to the analysis of performance and, most importantly, is prepared to apply the criteria already selected—the farmer cannot select his own cows. However, it is a tedious task and is subject to many errors. The computer performs the task quickly and with no errors. In those circumstances in which the farmer has his own computer, he may elect to purchase the software program that enables him to nominate cows for examination.

All of his work is pointless unless the veterinarian is prepared to study the output of the program, relate errors in management to shortfalls in performance, and make recommendations about appropriate changes. This must also be followed by subsequent assessment of improvements or declines in the areas that are listed here. Before work can reasonably begin in a herd, the following minimal facilities should be arranged. The costs of the program are greatly increased if the veterinarian's visit time is doubled because of poor timing or inadequate facilities.

- Yards, stanchions, and milking parlors to permit easy and quick performance of rectal examinations, examinations for mastitis and other diseases, and the collection of samples
- Accurate and distinctive identification of every animal; freeze branding or large ear tags in both ears are best
- An accurate but very simple event diary must be maintained by the farmer, who must also report each month on any changes in management that are likely to have any effect on the prevalence of disease

□ A resource of some sort that will store, retrieve, and analyze data very quickly and without error. This may be a centrally located data bureau or a peripherally located computer equipped with an appropriate software package

Selection of Cows for Examination

The cows selected for examination at each monthly visit are determined by an inspection of the individual cow cards or by the use of a computer program that is provided with the information on each cow by the use of a pocket-sized diary. The daily events would have been recorded in the diary, which would have been sent to the computer center a few days before the scheduled farm visit. Cows are selected for examination of reproductive performance and mastitis and other diseases. The criteria for selection are presented in the sections on reproductive performance and mastitis and other diseases. Cows due to calve may also be vaccinated to increase the level of colostral immunity for the control and prevention of diseases of newborn calves.

Advice and Assistance Given

The following areas of activity are common to most programs:

Reproductive Performance. Cows that have not achieved the present targets of returning to estrus after calving by 60 days; had succeeding heat periods at intervals of 21 days, conceived by 83 days post partum, and then calved again at 365 days; and have not calved for the first time at 24 months are examined and, where necessary, treated. More important is the herd data, which may lead to a herd diagnosis, e.g., undernutrition, requiring a herd treatment such as a lift in energy intake. Individual cows with unsatisfactory performance may be marked for culling, induction, or parturition.

Mastitis. Individual cows will be marked for drying off, for treatment during the dry period, or culling on the basis of a drying-off examination by CMT and culture or more commonly on the basis of a summation of individual cow milk cell counts during the lactation. The overall level of infection or incidence of clinical cases will act as a guide to the necessity or otherwise of additional preventive hygienic measures.

Calf Health and Management. During each visit the health and management of the calves should be examined. The number of sick calves and the diagnoses and treatment should be recorded; the number of calves that have died and the necropsy findings should be evaluated. Calves that are selected as herd replacements may warrant special attention such as vaccination, dehorning, and removal of supernumerary teats.

Herd replacement calves should be vaccinated against the infectious diseases that are expected to occur in the herd or in the area. A calfhood vaccination program would give consideration to the bacterial and viral diseases of the respiratory and digestive tracts (Smith 1977).

Nutrition. The feeds and feeding programs used are reviewed each month in order to monitor major changes that may affect production or cause digestive diseases. Depending on the size of the herd and the availability of feeds, the composition of the diets fed to the different classes of dairy cattle in the herd will vary considerably and must be monitored. This may require an analysis of the feeds and adjustments in the formulation of the diet. Any change in the quality or quantity of feeds used should be recorded and filed for future reference. Feeding and management practices can account for major differences in milk yield between herds (Waheed et al. 1977).

Housing. In areas where dairy cattle are housed for several months of the year, particular attention must be paid to the diseases that are associated with the effects of housing. Infectious diseases of the respiratory tract precipitated by inadequate ventilation, infectious diseases of the digestive tract associated with a build-up of bacteria and viruses, outbreaks of peracute coliform mastitis due to poor sanitation, and injuries of the feet and musculoskeletal system associated with poor floor surfaces are examples of housing-related diseases.

Dairy Cow Quality. The provision of regular veterinary advice on the selection of bulls and cows for the breeding program is an option available to the veterinarian who expands the basic herd health program into a planned animal health and production program. Selection is a major tool in establishing a breeding program to meet national production requirements of milk products. At present the number of cows that are bred artificially in herds that are herd-tested by milk recording is inadequate if maximum genetic progress is to be made by selection of young bulls. Expanded levels of herd recording of milk production and of artificial breeding could greatly increase the potential for even further genetic improvement (McAllister 1980).

Discussion of Performance

During each monthly visit, the veterinarian should discuss with the farmer the quality of performance and how it can be improved. In a well-managed program there are usually many disease and production problems that will have occurred since the last monthly visit. The discussion can begin with an examination of the last monthly report which will invariably identify problems and some action. The farmer will usually indicate the problems that have arisen since the last veterinary visit. However, a checklist of analyses for a review of the major aspects of management and disease control will often reveal changes that have not been observed by the farmer.

Preparation of Reports to the Farmer

Following each monthly visit, a report should be prepared and submitted to the farmer within a few days. The report will contain a summary of animal health and production performance and the details of any recommendations for treatment and control of specific diseases. The report should be complete, comprehensive, and simple and should contain the results of all clinical and laboratory examinations performed on the farm and in the laboratory. Often it is necessary for the veterinarian to consult other specialists or reference textbooks or manuals to obtain information about particular problems. This follow-up is a vital part of a program, and failure to do so is a major cause of failure of these programs. It is the responsibility of the veterinarian to provide a complete analysis of the health and production of the herd and to make recommendations on paper and monitor the effects of those recommendations. A copy of the report is filed in the veterinarian's office, and the most recent monthly reports may be taken out to the farm on subsequent visits. Reference can then be made to recommendations made on previous monthly visits. Such a practice will illustrate to the farmer that the veterinarian is concerned about the state of health and production in the herd.

A major problem in the submission of monthly reports to the farmer is the delay that often occurs in the postal service. To overcome this difficulty, the use of on-farm computers, electronic mail, and telex systems may become more widespread in the future.

"When performance is recorded, performance increases; when performance is reported, performance accelerates."

Problems Involved in the Maintenance of a Herd Health Program

The maintenance and growth of a dairy herd health program requires the continued motivation and interest of both the farmer and the veterinarian. The causes of failure include the following:

1. Lack of psychological stimulation of the farmer. This may be due to the failure of the veterinarian to submit monthly reports on time.

2. Failure of the veterinarian to adhere to a regular schedule and to arrive at the farm on time for the herd health visit.

3. The introduction of too many disease prevention and management techniques, which may be too expensive or impractical for the particular herd.

4. Failure of the program to show progress in animal health and production. This requires diligence in the preparation and submission of regular reports.

Financial Aspects

Financial Budgeting

The farmer's principal interests are the financial outcome of his operation and the cost-effectiveness of any management changes that are recommended. Provided an accurate record of all the management inputs is kept, the cost of a management change is usually determinable. In a properly run herd health program, the benefits will be measured by weight or volume. Some relatively simple arithmetic in a partial budget then makes it possible to estimate the financial gain. Partial budgeting is a satisfactory technique for this assessment that can only profitably be done once each year. It is purely a bookkeeping exercise (Ellis and James 1979).

Financial Management

Once financial budgeting becomes part of the health and production program, it is a short step to financial management. This is the advisory response to the financial data accumulated in the budgeting exercise. It should provide the farmer with information on when cash will become available for investment and, alternatively, when an additional source of financial support will be necessary to maintain feed or other supplies over a particular period of time. A computerized financial management module added to a standard planned health and production program would make this possible.

No financial management system is described because none is generally available. As a general rule, however, it is the regularly occurring milk sales that are committed to providing day-to-day running costs, including veterinary services. On the other hand, it is the value of calves and cows sold as surplus that provides funds required for capital purchases and new ventures, including purchase of cows. For this reason, cash flow for regular supplies and services is generally applicable, although care is needed in seasonal herds to ensure that cash is available during the two months when no cows are being milked. Whether or not cash will be available for new enterprises may depend on how many excess stock are sold for production purposes instead of being sold as reject or cull cows. The purpose of the program is to ensure that the potential usefulness of the veterinarian in bringing this about is fully realized.

Profitability

A number of studies have been reported of the profitability of these programs. The programs themselves are very similar, being based on maintenance of reproductive efficiency and a low quarter infection rate of mastitis-producing bacteria. In spite of the difference in the methods used to assess profitability, the results are very much the same. They are of the order of 300% return on the total funds, including disinfectants and extra feed invested in the program (Barfoot et al. 1971; Blood et al. 1978; Ellis and James 1979). It might be expected that programs in herds where the earned income is much less because of the product's low value at sale point could be less profitable. However, the investment in the program, by virtue of the larger amount of work done, appears to proportionately offset the additional income.

Most studies have confined themselves to the direct effect of the program on the value of milk produced, although, of course, there are other less easily measured gains. The farmer who produces the same amount of milk with less cows needs less land and less labor. If the milk is improved in quality and produced at a time of the year when the price is inflated with incentives, the gains can be a great deal higher than those cited above. An Australian analysis of a full program (Williamson 1979) returned up to $90 per hectare in the third year of its

operation. This represented about 800 to 900% return on the investment.

Other reports relate the gains reported by simpler programs consisting of a segment of a total program. For example, an American study (Galton 1977) has shown a gain of $58 per cow per year over untreated controls in a reproductivity management trial. One analysis in the U.S. of the profitability of standard veterinary services to dairy farmers concluded that a return of 196% to the investment was achieved (McCauley 1974). A Dutch program (Sol 1982) reports annual gains over feed costs of $70 per cow, $184 per hectare of farm land, and $5000 per worker on the farm. The charges made for these services vary with the value of the gains that are made, i.e., they are proportional to the price of milk per liter. Australian figures (Tranter 1982) are $2 for computer work and $5 for veterinary work per cow per year. North American figures would be about twice as much as these.

One of the factors that need to be considered when comparing results reported from different workers is the enthusiasm and the expertise used by the workers themselves. Thus clinicians in university veterinary clinics might be expected to spend more time on the job and to charge less than their practitioner colleagues.

No reports appear to be available on the profitability of herd health programs that have had a production management system added. Because these programs utilize a lot of information that is already available in other systems, it is to be expected that the profitability could be much greater than that in the purely health sector.

Review Literature

Blood, D.C., Morris, R.S., Williamson, N.B. et al. A health program for dairy herds. 1. Objectives and methods. Aust. Vet. J., 54:207-215, 1978.

Blood, D.C. The veterinarian in planned animal health and production. Can. Vet. J., 20:341-347, 1979.

Gartner, J. Replacement policy in dairy herds on farms where heifers compete with the cows for grassland. Part 1. Model construction and validation. Agricultural Systems, 7:298-318, 1981.

Gartner, J. Replacement policy in dairy herds on farms where heifers compete with the cows for grassland. Part 2. Experimentation. Agricultural Systems, 8:163-191, 1982.

Goodger, W.J. and Kushman, J.E. The future of large-scale dairy practice: Toward a production-oriented system for veterinary services. J. Am. Vet. Med. Assoc., 183:50-54, 1983.

Goodger, W.J. and Ruppanner, R. Historical perspective on the development of dairy practice. J. Am. Vet. Med. Assoc., 180:1294-1297, 1982.

Goodger, W.J. and Ruppanner, R. Why the dairy industry does not make greater use of veterinarians. J. Am. Vet. Med. Assoc., 181:706-710, 1982.

Gould, C.M. Dairy husbandry. Vet. Rec, 81:657, 1967.

Harrington, B.D. Preventive medicine in dairy practice. J. Am. Vet. Med. Assoc., 174:398, 1979.

Nott, S.B., Kauffman, D.E. and Speicher, J.A. Trends in the management of dairy farms since 1956. J. Dairy Sci., 64:1330-1343, 1981.

Williamson, N.B., Cannon, R.M., Blood, D.C. et al.: A health program for dairy herds. 5. The occurrence of specific disease entities. Aust. Vet. J. 54:252-256, 1978.

Williamson, N.B. The economic efficiency of a veterinary preventive medicine and management program in Victorian dairy herds. Aust. Vet. J., 56:1-9, 1979.

Wilcox, C.J. and van Horn, Large dairy herd management. Univ. Presses of Florida, Gainesville, FL, 1976.

References

Alexander, G.I. An integrated approach to improvement of dairy cattle production. Bovine Pract., 13:14-18, 1978.

Allaire, F.R., Sterwerf, H.E. and Pudwick, T.M. Variations in removal reasons and culling rates with age for dairy females. J. Dairy Sci., 60:254-267, 1977.

Alston, J.M. and Ryan, T.J. The economic efficiency of a veterinary preventive medicine and management program in Victorian dairy herds: An alternative viewpoint. Aust. Vet. J., 57:572-573, 1981.

Barfoot, L.W., Cote, J.F., Stone, J.B. et al. An economic appraisal of a preventative medicine program for dairy herd health management. Can. Vet. J., 12:2-10, 1971.

Beynon, V.H. The disposal of dairy cows in England and Wales. Vet. Ann., 16:1-6, 1976.

Blood, D.C., Morris, R.S., Williamson, N.B. et al. A health program for commercial dairy herds. 1. Objectives and methods. Aust. Vet. J., 54:207-215, 1978.

Bowman, J.S.T., Moxley, J.E., Kennedy, B.W. et al. The dairy herd management system and farm productivity. Can. J. Anim. Sci., 60:495-502, 1980.

Burnside, E.B., Kowalchuk, S.B., Lambroughton, D.B. et al. Canadian dairy cow disposals. Can. J. Anim. Sci., 51:75-83, 1971.

Cannon, R.M., Morris, R.S., Williamson, N.B. et al. A health program for commercial dairy herds. 2. Data processing. Aust. Vet. J., 54:216-230, 1978.

Cobo-Abreu, R., Martin, S.W., Stone, J.B. et al. The rates and patterns of survivorship and disease in a university dairy herd. Can. Vet. J., 20:177-183, 1979.

Cobo-Abreu, R., Martin, S.W., Willoughby, R.A. et al. The association between disease, production and culling in a university dairy herd. Can. Vet. J., 20:191-195, 1979.

Cote, J.F. Twenty years of experience with dairy herd health in Ontario. Can. Vet. J., 21:340-342, 1980.

Crandall, B.H., Crandall, L.N. and Crandall, B.L. On-line use of DHI computers for large herd management. J. Dairy Sci., 62 (Suppl. 1):95, 1979.

Donovan, L.A. Dairy herd health in New Brunswick. Can. Vet. J., 22:103-106, 1981.

Ellis, P.R., and James, A.D. The economics of animal health. 2. Economics in farm practice. Vet. Rec. 105:523-526, 1979.

Ellis, P.R., Esslemont, R.J. and Stephens, A.J. COSREEL. Vet. Rec., 112:285, 1983.

Erb, H.N. and Martin, S.W. Age, breed and seasonal patterns in the occurrence of ten dairy cow diseases: a case control study. Can. J. Comp. Med., 42:1-9, 1978.

Eschenbach, E. and Witt, W. Analysis of disease prevalence in intensive dairy cattle units. Monatsh. Vet. Med., 26:561-563, 1971.

Galton, D.M., Bar, H.L. and Heider, L.E. Effects of a herd health program on reproductive performance of dairy cows. J. Dairy Sci., 60:1117-1124, 1977.

Goodger, W.J. and Kushman, J.E. The future of large-scale dairy practice: Toward a production-oriented system for veterinary services. J. Am. Vet. Med. Assoc., 183: 50-54, 1983.

Goodger, W.J. and Ruppanner, R. Why the dairy industry does not make greater use of veterinarians. J. Am. Vet. Med. Assoc., 181:706-710, 1982.

Grommers, F.J., Van De Braak, A.E. and Antonisse, H.W. Direct trauma of the mammary glands in dairy cattle. 1. Variations in incidence due to animal variables. Br. Vet. J., 127:271-282, 1971.

Hansen, L.B., Touchberry, R.W., Young, C.W. et al. Health care requirements of dairy cattle. 2. Nongenetic effects. J. Dairy Sci., 62:1932-1940, 1979.

Higgins, C.W. Survey of dairy cow wastage, 1978/79. Zimbabwe Agric., 78:71-74, 1981.

Hodgson, H.J. Role of the dairy cow in world food production. J. Dairy Sci., 62:343-351, 1979.

Holm, D.M. Development of a national electronic identification system for livestock. J. Anim. Sci., 53:524-530, 1981.

Hooven, N.W. Cow identification and recording systems. J. Dairy Sci., 61:1167-1180, 1978.

Keyser, H. De. Survey of cattle diseases in a practice area (Belgium). Vlaams Diergeneeskunding Tijdschrift, 46:94-112, 1977.

Martin, B., Mainland, D.D. and Green, M.A. Virus: A computer program for herd health and productivity. Vet. Rec., 110:446-448, 1982.

Martin, L.J.F., Christensen, D.A. and Armstrong, K.A. Feeding and management in Saskatchewan dairy herds classified according to milk production levels. Can. Vet. J., 19:331-334, 1978.

McAllister, A.J. Are today's dairy cattle breeding programs suitable for tomorrow's production requirements? Can. J. Anim. Sci., 60:253-264, 1980.

McCauley, E.H. The contribution of veterinary service to the dairy enterprise income of Minnesota farmers: Production function analysis. J. Am. Vet. Med. Assoc., 165:1094-1098, 1974.

Moller, K. Planned animal health and production service (PAHAPS) in New Zealand dairy herds. Bovine Pract., 13:26-30, 1978.

Puckett, H.B., Olver, E.F., Harshbarger, K.E. et al. Automating the eyes of the herdsman. J. Anim. Sci., 53:516-523, 1981.

Renkema, J.A. and Stelwagen, J. Productive life-span of dairy cows and its economic significance. 1. Disposal of dairy cows: The current situation. Tijdschrift voor Diergeneeskunde, 102:603-637, 1977.

Renkema, J.A. and Stelwagen, J. Economic evaluation of replacement rates in dairy herds. 1. Reduction of replacement rates through improved health. Livestock Prod. Sci., 6:15-27, 1979.

Roine, K. and Saloniemi, H. Incidence of some diseases in connection with parturition in dairy cattle. Acta Vet. Scand., 19:341-353, 1978.

Russell, A.M. and Rowlands, G.J. COSREEL: computerised recording system of herd health information management. Vet. Rec., 112:189-193, 1983.

Shanks, B.D., Freeman, A.E. and Dickinson, F.N. Post partum distribution of costs and disorders of health. J. Dairy Sci., 64:683–688, 1981.

Smith, P.C. Proposed calfhood immunization program for the commercial diary herd. J. Dairy Sci., 60:294–299, 1977.

Sol, J. and Renkema, J.A. Economic and veterinary results of a herd health program during 3 years on 30 Dutch dairy farms. 12th World Conf. Diseases of Cattle, Amsterdam, pp. 697–701, 1982.

Speicher, J.A. Computerized data acquisition systems for dairy herd management. J. Anim. Sci., 53:531–536, 1981.

Stephens, A.J., Esslemont, R.J. and Ellis, P.R. The Daisy dairy herd health program. Proceedings 2nd Int. Symp. Vet. Epidemiol. Econ., Canberra, pp. 53–59, 1979.

Stout, J.D. The role of DHI records in herd health programs. Bovine Pract., 13:31–38, 1978.

Thompson, S.C. The economics of dairy farming in Canada. Can. Vet. J., 21:113–118, 1980.

Tranter, W.P. Computerized herd health programs in tropical Australia. 12th World Conf. Diseases of Cattle, Amsterdam, pp. 701–711, 1982.

Waheed, M.A., Lee, A.J. and Harpedstad, G.W. Feeding and management effects on herd differences in milk yield. J. Dairy Sci., 60:773–782, 1977.

Williamson, N.B. The economic efficiency of a veterinary preventive medicine and management program in Victorian dairy herds. Aust. Vet. J., 55:1–9, 1979.

Williamson, N.B. The economic efficiency of veterinary preventive medicine and management programs in Victorian dairy herds. Aust. Vet. J., 56:1–9, 474–476, 1980.

Williamson, N.B. The economic efficiency of a veterinary preventive medicine and management program in Victorian dairy herds. Analytical methods defended. Aust. Vet. J., 57:573–576, 1981.

Williamson, N.B., Morris, R.S. and Anderson, G.A. Pregnancy rates and non-return rates following artificial and natural breeding in dairy herds. Aust. Vet. J., 54:111–114, 1978.

Young, G.B. Livestock improvement and disease in dairy cattle Br. Vet. J., 137:209–216, 1981.

Dairy Cattle—Maintenance of Reproductive Efficiency

INTRODUCTION

In most countries, the primary objective of a reproductive control program in a dairy herd is to have each cow calve and produce a live calf every 12 months. A secondary objective, especially in pastoral countries, is to have the cows calve at the time of the year best suited to the needs of the particular herd to meet milk quotas, or when feed supplies are at their most plentiful and best able to supply the nutrient demands of pregnancy and lactation. The more appropriate criterion is when the value of milk less the cost of feed is at its highest.

Although an intercalving interval of 12 months will yield the optimal amount of milk and number of calves over the lifetime of the cow in most circumstances (deKruif and Brand 1978; Britt et al. 1981; Britt 1977), it is generally

agreed that, for very high–producing herds, the optimum interval may be longer than 12 months. There is an interesting coincidental, and probably related, relationship between reproductive efficiency and low total expenditures on health matters (Shanks et al. 1982). The minimal total health cost has been shown to be least in those cows that first calve at 20 to 24 months and at near annual intervals subsequently.

The current level of reproductive performance in dairy herds is well below the optimum in most countries. The average intercalving interval is 400 to 420 days instead of 365 days, and the average conception rate is 45% to 50% instead of 65%. For example, in a Canadian study, the reproductive efficiency of artificially bred Holstein cows was as follows: mean services per conception—1.97; per cent conception on first service—47%; days from calving to first service—88; and days from calving to conception—121 (Tong et al. 1979). In this study, the reproductive efficiency was highest in small herds with 35 or fewer cows, and dairymen who managed their labor efficiently for the production of milk also managed their herd well for reproductive performance. The level of reproductive performance in dairy herds in the United States is also below the optimum (Spalding et al. 1975); the calving interval for dairy cows averages at least 13 months in most areas and longer in many states (Hawk 1979).

This suboptimal level of reproductive performance in dairy herds is matched by the knowledge that it can be substantially improved by a combination of routine genital examinations, the early treatment of abnormalities detected in these examinations, improved heat detection and breeding at the proper time, and an increased preoccupation by the herdsman with the reproductive status of the herd. Reproductive efficiency can also be improved by increasing the conception rate and by early culling for reproductive failure. Both of these strategies will reduce costs by decreasing the average number of services required for a herd as a whole (Rounsaville et al. 1979). There is a great deal of field evidence that this improved reproductive performance is economical (Morris et al. 1978; Whitaker 1980; Galton et al. 1977). An additional example is the evidence from computer simulation models that increasing the efficiency of estrus detection will shorten the mean interval from calving to first service, and the calving to conception interval.

THE CAUSES OF REPRODUCTIVE INEFFICIENCY

The reasons for failure to attain a 365-day intercalving interval can be divided into managerial errors in which the cow is not mated and reproductive failure in which the cow is mated but conception or the birth of a live calf does not result. The modes of reproductive inefficiency are shown in Table 4–1, and the causes of reproductive failure are shown in Table 4–2.

The relative importance of each of these causes varies widely from place to place and even from time to time on one farm, depending

Table 4–1. MODES OF REPRODUCTIVE INEFFICIENCY IN DAIRY CATTLE

| | Diagnosis | |
Modes°	By History	By Physical and Laboratory Examination
1. ANESTRUS		
a. Failure to observe heat	No visible estrus recorded	Not pregnant. Follicle or corpus luteum on ovaries. No other abnormalities
b. True anestrus	No visible estrus recorded	Not pregnant. No palpable structures on ovaries and no other abnormalities
2. FAILURE TO BREED Management decision	Heat observed, recorded, but not bred	Not pregnant. Follicle or corpus luteum on ovaries. No other abnormalities
3. FAILURE TO CONCEIVE		
a. Fertilization failure (female side)	Fails to conceive when bred. Interestral intervals 18–24 days	Not pregnant. Endometritis may or not be detectable on rectal or vaginal-cervical examination. Semen quality good
b. Fertilization failure (male side)	Fails to conceive when bred. Interestral intervals 18–24 days	Not pregnant. No clinical evidence of endometritis. Semen quality or serving capacity inferior
c. Technique of inseminator	Conception rate at first service compared with performance of other inseminators. Interestral intervals 18–24 days	Not pregnant. No clinical abnormalities detectable. Semen quality good
4. EARLY EMBRYONIC DEATH	Interestral intervals longer than 18–24 days	Not pregnant after previous positive pregnancy, returned to heat. No abnormalities on palpation
5. ABORTION	Abortion rate more than 2% per annum	Involuting uterus may be palpable
6. STILLBIRTH/ DYSTOCIA	History of difficult birth	Gross pathology of swollen calf head, edema and laceration of vulva

°Each mode represents a stage in the reproductive process, and all cases of reproductive inefficiency can usually be categorized into one of these modes based on the history and clinical findings.

Table 4-2. SOURCES OF REPRODUCTIVE FAILURE IN DAIRY CATTLE

Causes of Failure	Approximate Percentage of 100 First Services
Anatomical abnormalities	2
Ovulation failure	2
Loss of ruptured ova	5
Fertilization failure	13
Embryonic mortality	15
Fetal mortality	3
Total	40

(From Hawk, H.W. Infertility in dairy cattle. *In:* Beltsville Symposia in Agricultural Research. 3. Animal Reproduction, New York, John Wiley and Sons, Inc., 1979, pp. 19–29).

on the level of preoccupation of the farmer with the problem of getting his cows in calf. When farmers do not give high priority to reproduction, too little labor, time, and attention is given to such things as detecting estrus, inseminating cows at the best time, diagnosing pregnancy, and actively undertaking the correction of the identifiable causes of poor reproductive performance. Instead, inaccurate estrus detection results in the insemination of many cows that are not in estrus or even near ovulation. These cows have no chance to conceive.

Among defects of ovarian function and structure, as shown in Table 4-2, the important ones are anestrus, subestrus, and cystic ovaries, which account for 70% of treated infertility cases (Roine and Saloniemi 1978). Fertilization failure and embryonic mortality are preeminent as causes of reproductive failure. Factors that are known to decrease ovum fertilization rates include low-fertility bulls, insemination within the first several weeks post partum, insemination after ovulation, and several infertile services. Embryonic mortality may be associated with several previous infertile services and the fertilization of aged ova, but the real causes of most embryonic deaths are unknown (Sreenan and Diskin 1983). There is also a close relationship between fatty liver, fat cow syndrome, and ketosis, and poor fertility, and this emphasizes the importance of the need to reduce nutritional and lactational stress in early lactation.

Reproductive performance can be improved in each of the two major problem areas—estrus detection and fertility—by applying existing knowledge. For example, accurate detection of estrus would shorten calving intervals by providing more frequent opportunities to insem-

inate cows and by improving fertility through better timing of insemination relative to ovulation.

In cows with no diagnosable disease problem, the rate of embryonic mortality is probably quite stable and subject to decrease, mostly by reducing the mortality caused by poorly timed insemination and that caused by such identifiable factors as high environmental temperature and humidity and the use of semen from low-fertility bulls. The ovum fertilization rate can almost certainly be improved—to a marked degree in some dairy herds—by inseminating only estrous cows, by improving the timing of insemination during estrus, and by inseminating cows with semen from bulls of proven quality.

Other managerial decisions that are critical to high reproductive efficiency include positive action to prevent the introduction of brucellosis, vibriosis, leptospirosis, and trichomoniasis; selection against bulls, and possibly cow families, that have a bad record of stillbirths due to dystocia; and early insemination of cows after calving. During the past 30 years, the policy on early insemination has varied widely. Originally, the policy was that cows should not be bred until 60 days after parturition, by which time the cows were thought to have regained an effective level of fertility. Fifteen years ago, the pendulum swung in the other direction when it became apparent that delaying the first service to the period from 60 to 81 days after calving was increasing the intercalving interval unnecessarily. This change of view was more readily acceptable if a decline in conception rate at first service from 65% to 50% was acceptable. It was acceptable, because the cost of an additional 0.5 services per conception was more than offset by an additional income arising out of a 10-day reduction in intercalving interval. Now that there is an appreciation that an increased rate of infertile services may further increase the rate of failing to conceive, there is a renewal of interest in avoiding mating cows until the success rate is likely to be optimum for financial efficiency. The commonest recommendation is to breed cows at the first estrus after the 50th postpartum day.

The other management decision that has a very important effect on reproductive efficiency is the culling policy. If all cows that do not exactly match reproductive targets are immediately culled, the reproductive efficiency of the herd at any one time is considerably enhanced. The total effect on the herd's economy may be disastrous because of the young average age of the herd and the almost certain result of a lowering of the herd's milk yield. This conundrum highlights the need for a simulation model so that the effects of varying individual variables on the whole herd function can be properly assessed. If, on the other hand, the culling policy is directed toward improving milk yield, there may be a tendency to keep old or infertile cows because of their genetic worth. Again, only a simulation model will be able to compare the two strategies and come up with a whole-farm answer.

MEASUREMENT OF REPRODUCTIVE PERFORMANCE

The basic objective is a calving interval of 12 months, with the first calf born at 24 months of age. How this is achieved biologically is the same irrespective of the breeding plan used in the herd. The breeding plan may be year-round, with some cows calving every month, or seasonal or block mating, which may be one mating a year, e.g., in spring, or more commonly two matings, one in spring to catch the flush of feed and one in autumn to have milk available when winter incentive prices operate.

The measurement of reproductive efficiency is done differently for the two management systems. In a year-round herd it is possible to observe performance from month to month and recognize trends early. This enables the veterinarian to recommend changes in management and hygiene and then observe the effects of the changes over the next month or two.

In seasonal or block-mated herds, the emphasis in management is on concentrating the mating, and therefore the calving, into as short a season as possible. This may be as short as six weeks. It is not possible in these circumstances to watch trends, correct management, and observe results. Everything happens too quickly. In high-producing herds it can be worthwhile to make weekly visits and be on the watch for early warnings, but trends do not really become evident over such short time spans. What is done is to concentrate farmers' activity into the breeding period with a view to getting as many cows as possible in calf and using the veterinarian in the periods immediately before and at the end of the breeding period. In the early session, the veterinarian is required to intervene if the degree of estral activity in the herd is insufficient to suggest that all cows will be in heat during the first three

weeks of the breeding period. If the prebreeding estral cycling rate is adequate but the rate of submitting cows for insemination (the submission rate) is insufficient during the first three weeks of the breeding period, then it is necessary for the veterinarian to take urgent action to repair the situation quickly. At the end of the breeding period, it may be necessary for the veterinarian to intervene in the management of those cows that have not conceived. This usually requires synchronization of estrus and double insemination in the bulk of the cows that have no obvious structural lesions. There will be a few cows that need treatment for endometritis or cystic ovaries.

Measurement of Reproductive Efficiency in a Year-Round Herd

A calving interval of 12 months is optimal to maximize milk and calf production during the productive life of a cow. However, the measurement of the calving interval is too historical to be of real value in the regular assessment of reproductive performance if corrective action is to be taken quickly. To obtain a mean figure for the herd, all cows must calve twice so that the calving index will include events that, for some cows, will be 1.5 to 2 years old. Alternatively, the calving to conception interval can be calculated at the end of a breeding season before the subsequent calving season begins in seasonal calving herds and at the end of each monthly visit in herds calving year-round. Provided the pregnancy diagnosis technique and breeding history are accurate, it is usually possible to pinpoint the day of conception, calculate the calving to conception interval, and predict the calving date and the intercalving interval (Fig. 4-1). There are two sources of error: (1) a return to standing estrus, even though the cow is still in early pregnancy, occurs in a surprisingly large proportion of cows, i.e., about 13% in southern Australia; and (2) resorption occurs in a further 1%.

Seasonal or Block-Calving Herds

In a seasonal calving herd, those cows that do not conceive quickly provide a major problem. It is customary in these herds to look for an indicator that is even earlier than the calving-conception interval. The calving to first heat interval is the average period in the herd between calving and first heat and is the one usually used. It is about the earliest available indicator of the degree of reproductive activity, but because the effect of efficiency of

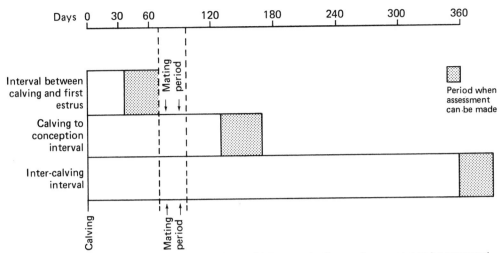

Figure 4-1. Times during reproductive cycle at which reproductive performance can be assessed.

conception is not included, it is not highly accurate as a predictor of overall reproductive efficiency. It is also subject to the error introduced by poor heat detection. As a herd measurement in seasonal calving herds, the degree of reproductive activity is commonly expressed as the percentage of open cows that are on heat in the 30 days before the breeding season commences. One step further in the breeding cycle in these herds is the submission rate, i.e., the percentage of open cows submitted for breeding in the 30 days after the breeding season commences.

In all of these estimations, it is important that the mean figure for the herd be quoted together with the standard deviation. It is the latter that indicates when there are cows in the group that have very long calving to conception, or to first heat, or to calving intervals. These cows can give a distorted view of the reproductive performance of the group as a whole.

Assuming a gestation period of 280 days, the target figure for the optimal calving to conception interval is 85 days (i.e., 365 less 280 days). The components of the calving to conception interval and the factors that affect them are shown in Figure 4-2.

The length of the interval from calving to first service is affected by farm policy, postpartum uterine involution, and the occurrence and detection of estrus. Farm policy regarding timing of first service varies considerably. In some herds, first service is not carried out until the first estrus after 70 days post partum. To achieve a mean interval of 65 days to first service, it is essential that all cows receive their first service at the first estrus after a 50-day interval post partum. This advice alone will

frequently shorten a calving to conception interval.

Rapid involution of the uterus post partum and return to normal ovarian cyclicity are prerequisites of good fertility. Dystocia, retained placenta, and endometritis will cause delays in the interval to first estrus and subsequent fertility.

Estrus detection is a major factor in breeding efficiency in dairy cattle. Only 40% to 60% of heats are detected on many farms, although 80% can be achieved by the use of heat mount detection aids or by observing cows for 30-minute periods before and after milking, at midday, and during the late evening. If farm policy is to serve cows at the first estrus after 50 days post partum, in seasonal calving herds it is possible to expect 50% of cows to have been served by 65 days post partum if estrus detection rates are 80% or more.

A summary of the fertility indices that can be monitored regularly is presented in Table 4-3. The targets or goals are considered to be optimal. The interference levels are those levels at which an investigation should be undertaken to determine the cause of failure to meet the targets.

The non-return rate is the non-palpatory method of pregnancy diagnosis. Cows that are bred and do not return to heat between 30 and 60 days are considered pregnant. This method has been used by the Dairy Herd Improvement Association. It is not as accurate as the palpation method (Williamson et al. 1978) because it depends so much on the accuracy of estrus detection on the farm and does not take into account those cows that develop a retained corpus luteum or that suffer early embryonic death. The method falls into disuse when

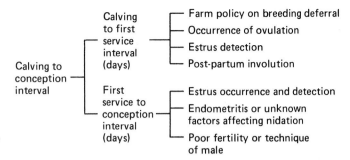

Figure 4-2. The components of the calving to conception interval.

inseminators employed by the artificial breeding organization, which could then estimate which cows are not returning to service, are replaced by farmers doing their own inseminations themselves. The insemination center then has no information on returns to service. The farmer may, of course, keep his own records. The method has always been useless on pastured herds where a make-up bull is put in when sufficient cows have been inseminated. This is a common policy in commercial herds and is aimed at not keeping the calves of cows that are late breeders, so that the sire used is immaterial. It is assumed that the fertility of the herd will improve as a result. For obvious practical reasons, the policy is really only applicable on farms where the cows are pastured and where seasonal or block breeding is practiced.

The interval from calving to first service and the interval from first service to conception are both affected by the conception rate and by the estrus detection rate (Esslemont and Ellis 1974). If, for example, a herd's interval to first service is averaging 80 days and the average conception rate is 50%, the calving to conception interval will range from 106 days, with an 80% estrus detection rate, to 122 days,

with a 50% rate. Obviously, the highest possible detection rate must be achieved. Herd management policy often dictates that insemination shall not take place until a certain number of days post partum and in certain months of the year. When insemination is allowed, the detection rate and the length of the normal estrus cycle will mean that, on average, it takes some 15 to 20 days from the start day for all cows to be inseminated for the first time. The combination of these factors means that in many seasonal calving herds, the mean interval to first insemination is 80 days. Consequently, an average calving to conception interval of 96 days is the lowest that can be achieved, and this level is only possible if a 60% conception rate is coupled with an 80% detection rate.

The indices recommended for use in assessing reproductive efficiency are shown in Table 4-3. All of them require:

□ accuracy of observation, especially in estrus detection. To be good enough, the farmer must be motivated not to miss anything. He can be helped by concentrating the times and the groups of animals that have to be watched.

□ accurate, easily understood recording. This

Table 4-3. FERTILITY INDICES TO BE CALCULATED WITH TARGET AND INTERFERENCE LEVELS°

	Targets	Interference Level
1. Calving interval (days)	365	375
2. Calving to conception interval (days)	85	>95
3. Mean calving to first service (days)	65	>70
4. Cows showing heat by 60 days post partum (%)	>85	<70
5. Conception rate to first service (%)	70	<50
6. Conception rate to all services (%)	58	<50
7. Services per conception	<1.5	>2
8. Average age at first calving (months)	24	>28
9. Culling rate for reproductive (per cent of breeding animals per annum)	<10	>12
10. Average number of lactations in lifetime (years)	>7	<5
11. Abortion rate (per cent of pregnant animals that abort per annum)	<3	>5

°The interference levels are the suggested levels of unsatisfactory performance at which investigative action should be taken.

can be facilitated by ensuring that the farmer always has the recording apparatus with him, which means that the recorder must be light in weight and simple to use.

□ a system of analyzing the data that is quick and efficient, reports areas of inadequacy, and makes recommendations about how cows are to be culled.

There is, in addition, a need for veterinary participation by way of pregnancy diagnosis, if this is done manually. In today's dairy industry, there is no room for the inaccuracies inherent in pregnancy diagnosis by non-return to estrus or by milk progesterone estimations. A further major input by veterinarians is the avoidance of loss by abortion, infectious infertility, and dystocia. Their participation in this sort of work generates data that are invaluable in measuring performance and supplying back-up data, which is usually critical when making an etiological diagnosis.

METHODS OF ACHIEVING A HIGH LEVEL OF REPRODUCTIVE EFFICIENCY IN A DAIRY HERD

Although the individual cow is an important factor in the management of the herd, and the summation of the performances of all the cows provides the data of the herd's performance, it is essential that the management of the herd as a whole be kept under constant surveillance. It is easy enough to treat each anestrous cow for that condition without appreciating that there are more cases with the problem than there should be and that the nutritional status of the herd as a whole might be bad enough to explain why the prevalence is high. Therefore, individual cows that do not match targets should be dealt with as individuals, but when that is done, the herd performance is assessed and, if necessary, a herd strategy of prevention is instituted. This is likely to be a managerial or nutritional problem, now that the infectious causes of infertility and abortion are under control in most countries. A protocol for conducting an examination of a herd for a reproductive inefficiency problem is illustrated at the end of this section (p. 79).

In order to achieve optimum herd reproductive performance, it is necessary to extract optimum performance from each cow. This requires that each cow calve every 12 months, beginning at 24 months of age, and the achievement of that objective is dependent upon detecting estrus in cows, beginning at about 40 days after calving, and breeding them

to conceive by an average of 85 days after calving. Two important points of procedure are involved:

□ concentration of reproductive management activity in the period right after parturition and up to three months later

□ frequent periodic physical examination of the cow's genital tract. There is no substitute for the perceptive fingers of a veterinarian in determining reproductive status

Concentration of Management Activity in the Early Postpartum Period

The achievement of a mean calving to conception interval of 85 days requires concentrated management activity during the first 90 days following calving. Ideally, cows should be bred on the first heat after 50 days, which usually occurs between 60 and 69 days. Under good management conditions, allowing for some cows that will repeat, breeding cows on that heat will result in a calving to conception interval of 85 days.

Early postpartum breeding in dairy cows results in more calves and higher milk yield per day of herd life, but early-bred cows require more inseminations per conception. Breeding can normally begin at about 40 days post partum with an acceptable rate of reproductive performance, and with current management practices, a calving interval of 12 months or less can be achieved by shortening the interval to first insemination to an average of about 50 to 60 days post partum (Britt 1975). Each day of delay beyond the optimum calving to conception interval of 85 days reduces the farmer's profit margin (Olds et al. 1979). The gestation period cannot be changed significantly by management practices and, therefore, attention must be focused on the period beginning approximately 40 days post partum when fertilizable heats begin.

The management activities that need to be actively pursued during this period are included in the following list.

Encouragement of Early, Active, Repeating Estrus Cycles. The simple monitoring of reproductive status, especially postpartum estrus cycles, will not of itself encourage greater reproductive efficiency (Munro et al. 1982). There must be interaction by the farmer or his veterinary advisor to the point that the recognition of an impending problem must be countered by some preventive reaction. Principal among these are management techniques, and of those, an adequate nutritional level to meet the needs of early lactation and conception is the most commonly invoked strategy.

Cows should be challenge-fed during early lactation to avoid the negative energy balance that is so detrimental to the return of the estrus cycle. The feeding program should avoid excessive weight gain in dry cows but should be a high-density energy diet after calving. The relationship between fertility and roughage, rather than concentrates, has been demonstrated (Bogin et al. 1982). For energy deprivation to have a significant effect on fertility, the degree of deprivation usually has to be severe; the effects of less extreme deficiencies (10% to 20% below recommendations) have not been clearly demonstrated. For example, feeding primiparous heifers at an energy level of 85% of the total recommended by NRC for the period from parturition to 84 days after calving did not affect their reproductive performance compared with animals that received 135% of the NRC recommended ration (Carstairs et al. 1980).

Heavy feeding to the point of causing the development of a fatty liver has a significant adverse effect on fertility by increasing the intercalving interval (Reid et al. 1979). Similarly, high-level feeding also increases the services per conception rate but at the same time increases the ovulation rate (Maree 1980). Nutritional deficiencies of phosphorus and trace elements are often purported to be causes of reproductive inefficiency, but, with the exception of manganese and zinc, there appears to be no direct association (Hidiroglou 1979). Nutritional deficiencies that lead to loss of body condition, including copper, cobalt, iodine, iron, and selenium, may reduce reproductive efficiency indirectly.

Of equal importance to a high level of feeding in early lactation is the need to have cows in good body condition, e.g., moderately heavy body weight or condition score of 5 out of 8, at calving. Thin cows do not return so quickly to estrus nor are their estral periods as fertile as in heavier cows (Grainger et al. 1982). Fat cows are at a similar disadvantage, as discussed later. The principal problem with body weight is in the heifers. Recommended weights at 15 months are 320 kg. for Holsteins and 220 kg. for Jerseys.

The most favored biologic treatment to restore resumption of estral cycling after parturition is the maintenance of good condition at calving and the provision of a high-energy diet, that will not produce a fatty liver, in early lactation. However, there is also a current trend toward the use of hormonal remedies. Gonadotropin-releasing hormone (Gn-RH) or prostaglandins are used to initiate and synchronize estrus in cows, beginning at about 40 days after calving. (Garverick et al. 1980) A regimen of two injections of prostaglandin 11 to 12 days apart, followed by one or two inseminations at 72 to 80 hours or 72 to 96 hours, respectively, following the second injection results in acceptable conception rates (Young and Henderson 1981; Bosu et al. 1981; Lamming et al. 1979; Drew and Gould 1980), as does the use of a progesterone-retaining intravaginal device (PRIDs).

A great deal of information is lacking about these hormonal techniques, both in results achieved and in the long-term undesirable effects on reproductive efficiency that may follow. The results with prostaglandin appear to be better in heifers than in adult cows when synchronization is matched with fixed-time double insemination (Dawson 1980). In general, the effectiveness of the hormonal treatments is much less than that produced by good husbandry. They will continue to be used because husbandry will continue to be poor on some farms.

Accurate Detection of Estrus. Simple observation of the herd for 30 minutes in the morning before and after milking, at midday, and late in the evening allows accurate detection of estrus, but few farmers can afford the time to do the task properly. For large herds of cows at pasture, steers injected with testosterone, and tail paint and heat mount detectors applied to cows are preferred to observation. Although each is successful and preferred in a particular environment (Fulkerson et al, 1983), tail paint is preferred in most cases because of its cheapness and ease of application (Williamson 1980b). The thick paint is applied to the skin over the dorsal spines of the sacral and first coccygeal vertebrae. It can be applied with a roller and brush and sits up on the hairs in the area. When a cow stands and is mounted more than momentarily, the paint is rubbed off. The accuracy of tail painting has been shown to be high and is superior, in most situations, to human observation of estrus behavior (Ball et al. 1983). Both of the above techniques are good enough to obviate the use of penis deviations created surgically in entire bulls, that is, in dairy herds where the tail paint or heat mount detectors can be adjusted twice daily. Vasectomy and partial epididymectomy are less distressing alternatives to the more multilative preparations but still have serious disadvantages including actual vaginal entry of cows and introduction of the possible transmission of venereal disease (McCaughey and Martin 1980).

Another tactic that also helps in estrus detection is grouping of the early lactation cows (10 to 12 weeks post partum) together both for observation of estrus and for supplementary feeding.

Early Treatment of Endometritis. Postpartum infection of the uterus has been considered to be the predominant cause of bovine infertility for a long time (Erb et al. 1981a; Erb et al. 1981b). However, its importance seems to vary greatly. For example, endometritis caused by *Corynebacterium pyogenes*, the principal bacterial cause of the disease, occurs in up to 10% of housed cattle but in less than 1% of many pastured herds. A recent observation of a high incidence of endometritis in some dairy herds has been attributed to uterine infection with *Hemophilus somnus.*

Whatever the cause, it is customary to recommend that endometritis be treated as early and as intensively as possible if the calving to conception interval is to be kept short (Studer and Morrow, 1978). This is probably a correct view within a cattle population that is adequately fed. However, there is a strongly supported view that heavily fed cows have more metritis but a higher conception rate than poorly fed cows, which have less endometritis but a poorer fertility rate (Francos 1979). There is also evidence that a single treatment of endometritis in a cow on about the 14th day after parturition is unlikely to have effect on the subsequent health of the uterus (deKruif et al. 1982).

Retained placenta and twinning are both conducive to the development of traumatic vaginitis and metritis. Both diseases have a deleterious effect on subsequent fertility (Kay 1978). Selection against twinning is advantageous from this and other points of view. Early and thorough treatment of retained placenta should be followed by a postnatal checkup at the next herd health visit.

Intensive Treatment of Postparturient Debilitating Diseases. The effects of milk fever, acetonemia, hypomagnesemia, and postparturient hemoglobinuria on the reproductive efficiency of affected cows is commonly discussed but not well identified. It is logical that postparturient debilitation due to any of these diseases causes an interruption of estrus cycling. For example, acetonemia is reported to have prolonged the calving to conception interval of affected cows by 51 days and increased the services per conception rate by 0.73 (Nenadovic et al. 1979).

Early Breeding After Calving. Early breeding after calving encourages a reduction in the intercalving interval, but this is at the expense of a lower conception rate. This does not appear (Whitmore et al, 1974; Williamson 1980c) to have any apparent deleterious effect on long-term fertility. If cost-effectiveness is the objective, there seems to be little argument with the view that the profitability is greatest when the first service falls in the period from 46 to 60 days postpartum (Fielden et al. 1980).

Correct Timing of Insemination. Inaccurate detection can lead to incorrect timing of insemination, even to insemination of cows that are not on heat at all. Using progesterone assay of plasma (Appleyard and Cook 1976) or milk (McCaughey and Cooper 1980) as an indication of true estrus, surveys have shown that from 7% to 22% of cows had abnormal levels of progesterone when they were inseminated. These cows failed to conceive because they were inseminated at the wrong time. For best results, the cow should be inseminated about 18 hours after estrus is first observable. If there is doubt or the cow is difficult to get in calf, a series of two inseminations, one early in the estrus cycle and one at the end, is recommended.

Pregnancy Diagnosis by Hormonal Means. The diagnosis by the assay of progesterone in milk (Heap and Holdsworth 1981; Laing et al. 1979) is still beset with problems, chiefly inaccuracy, which improves as the period between the test and insemination is lengthened. Progesterone levels in milk reach a peak 10 to 15 days after estrus and are maintained if the cow conceives but fall away sharply after 19 days if pregnancy does not result. Milk samples collected 20 to 24 days after insemination can be used to discriminate between pregnant and nonpregnant animals. The accuracy, when the sample is collected at the recommended time of 24 days after insemination, is only 85% for positive diagnosis, much of the error probably being due to early embryonic mortality. The accuracy of negative tests is much better but still less than 100% (Dawson 1980). The accuracy of the test can be improved by taking a series of three tests, but this is unlikely to be a practicable procedure (Laing et al. 1980). As a test for pregnancy, it is having little impact on the total number of pregnancy diagnoses made in the U.K., where the test has achieved its greatest prominence. Of the herds in the U.K. in which pregnancy diagnosis is carried out, 98% use the manual technique conducted by a veterinarian. Less than 2% rely solely on progesterone assay (Newton et al. 1982).

Regular Physical Examination of the Reproductive Tracts. The reproductive performance of the herd can be evaluated monthly, or more frequently in large herds, by the physical examination of the reproductive tracts of cows. The emphasis is on the examination of cows for pregnancy, cows that fail to demonstrate estrus by a certain time after calving, and cows that do not conceive following breeding. The list of cows selected for examination at each visit is determined by examination of the recent reproductive history of each cow. This can be obtained by examination of the individual cow cards or, in a computerized system, the cows will be selected on the basis of information provided by a daily diary in which all events are recorded.

Regular visits by a veterinarian to examine the reproductive tracts of cows for evidence of pregnancy or reasons for non-pregnancy are the basis for all modern herd health programs. The cows selected for examination, and the reasons for the examination, are as follows.

Pregnancy Diagnosis. Cows bred for at least 35 days are examined for pregnancy by palpation of the uterus per rectum. This is the cornerstone of an effective reproductive herd health program. The breeding dates should be available. Palpation of fluids in an enlarged uterine horn, slipping of the chorioallantoic membrane, or palpation of an amniotic vesicle is generally accepted as positive evidence of pregnancy in cows bred less than 70 days earlier. Palpation for fluctuation alone in cows pregnant 35 to 70 days is an accurate and safe method of pregnancy diagnosis, but palpation by membrane slip and, to a lesser degree, palpation of the amniotic vesicle may cause some fetal loss (Abbitt et al. 1978).

No Visible Estrus. All cows that have not shown a heat within 49 days after either calving or the last reproductive event should be examined. No visible estrus may be due to failure to observe the cow in heat or may be due to a true anestrus, which may be a result of uterine or ovarian pathology or undernutrition. In a computerized program, the computer will identify cows for which a heat has not been recorded by the herdsman over the 49-day period.

The examination of cows that have not shown heat for 50 days since calving will usually reveal evidence of ovarian activity (palpable follicles or corpora lutea), which indicates that the anestrus is due to failure to observe heat or failure to record an observed heat.

In herds where the cows are kept in good condition, the greater proportion of cows showing "no visible estrus" will be ones in which estrus has occurred but not been detected. In herds where the cows are kept in thin body condition, there will usually be about equal numbers of anestral cows and cows that were in estrus but were not observed. The former have very small ovaries, without apparent luteal activity, and a small uterus that is lacking in tone. Heifers and young cows are the group most likely to be affected (Fielden et al. 1976). The most common causes of anestrus are immaturity and a relative lack of dietary energy intake. Cows that were in too light condition at calving and that are short of feed at mating time are the most common group to be affected. Ostertagiasis is also a precipitating cause, especially in young females. Nutritional deficiencies of copper, cobalt, selenium, and phosphorus have the same nonspecific effect. Sporadic cases of anestrus are due to ovarian abnormality or pyometra.

The methods for detection of estrus in cattle running at pasture (Williamson et al. 1972) and in housed cattle (Esslemont and Bryant 1976) have been described. Because of the importance of this managerial feature, large herds are now being divided into smaller groups, which allows the herdsman to concentrate surveillance for heat detection on the recently calved group (Britt 1977).

The management of cows that have not demonstrated estrus is dependent on the cause. When failure to observe estrus is the cause, an improvement in the surveillance for heat detection is necessary. Heat mount detectors and tail paint (Williamson 1980b) are indispensable aids to heat detection in pastured cattle. However, increasing the frequency of observation of the animals will usually improve the rate of heat detection in housed cattle.

Failure to Conceive or "Repeat Breeders." Cows that fail to conceive following three successive breedings are classified as repeat breeders and should be examined for clinical evidence of disease of the reproductive tract. The timing of the insemination, the expertise of the inseminator, and the quality of the semen must also be considered. The cause of a repeat breeder is not always obvious but may include endometritis, lactational stress, poor quality semen, and failure to ovulate. A special category within this group is the cow that returns to estrus at intervals longer than the normal 19 to 24 days but not at multiples of 21 days, which implies faulty estrus detection. The long interestral group may consist of cows that have had early fetal deaths (embryonic mortality, see Table 4-1).

Postnatal Examination. Examination of all cows during the period three to seven weeks after parturition is designed to detect abnormalities that are likely to interfere with subsequent reproductive performance. In many commercial herds, the procedure is uneconomic because of the rarity of any positive findings. This applies particularly to cows that run at pasture all year round. In housed animals, the incidence of endometritis and slow uterine involution is thought to be higher, but there is no concrete evidence of this. However, repeated examinations and treatment during this period are credited with making major improvements in reproductive efficiency (Bostedt et al. 1976). There is no hard evidence on the effect of reduced physical activity on fertility in cows confined in corals as opposed to those confined in barns, but it is commonly thought to be an influential factor.

A postnatal examination and treatment is recommended in all cows reported to have experienced dystocia or postparturient problems such as retained placenta or uterine prolapse. The record of complications in cows in which parturition has been induced by the administration of corticosteroids indicates that they should also be included in the group requiring a postnatal examination. In cows that have metritis prior to the breeding season, there is a high probability that conception will be impaired, but retention of the placenta appears to exert little effect on the subsequent conception (Sandals et al. 1979).

Retained placenta, metritis, cystic follicle, and luteal cyst can directly increase the intercalving interval by up to 20 to 27 days (Erb et al. 1981a; Erb et al. 1981b) and should be recognized and treated as soon as possible. (Whitmore et al. 1979).

Abnormally Short Interestral Intervals. Cows with abnormally short interestral intervals are those that have been on heat three or more times in a 35-day period. Large follicular cysts are palpable on some ovaries in these cows.

Recheck for Pregnancy. The computer is programmed to identify cows whose records indicate that they were previously diagnosed as pregnant and are now recorded as having returned to estrus. This is a relatively common occurrence in cows that are still pregnant and suffer no ill effects from the occurrence. However, any attempt to inseminate these cows may result in an abortion. Those cows that are not pregnant are presumed to have resorbed an early fetal death if death occurs before the 4th month of pregnancy or to have aborted unobserved if death occurs after that time. Those that have aborted should be dealt with as presented under that heading.

Early Embryonic Mortality. This form of wastage is estimated to represent 75% of all reproductive wastage (Sreenan and Diskin 1983). The conceptus dies within 20 days of fertilization, and the cow returns to estrus with a longer than normal interestral interval. Little is known about the specific causes of the problem, but chromosomal abnormalities (King and Linares 1983), *Campylobacter fetus*, and prolongation of the ovulation to fertilization interval are likely.

Abortion and Fetal Resorption. Cows that are found to be not pregnant after a prior diagnosis of pregnancy should be submitted to the same examination as cows that have been seen to abort or show evidence of having done so. A protocol for the examination of such a cow is presented later, but an extensive discussion of the causes is not undertaken. However, most authors agree that in the presence of brucellosis and with a very low incidence of infection with *Campylobacter* spp. or trichomonads, the proportion of abortions that remain undiagnosed after laboratory examination is of the order of 66%. A survey in the U.S. (Rowe and Smithies 1978) showed 62% of bovine abortions to be undiagnosed, and of those that were diagnosed, 38% were caused by infectious bovine rhinotracheitis virus, 12.7% by mycotic infections, and lesser percentages by *Campylobacter* spp., *Corynebacterium pyogenes*, listeriosis, brucellosis, leptospirosis, and chlamydia. The diagnosis of abortion in cattle may be improved by the use of immunofluorescent examination of the fetal tissues (Miller and Quinn 1957).

Prolonged Gestation. Cows that have not calved within three weeks after the anticipated calving are immediately selected for examination. Cases of prolonged gestation (either giantism or with an immature fetus) may have inherited the relevant genes or may have been exposed to toxic substances. Most cases submitted for examination turn out to be pregnant cows in which the service date and the stage of pregnancy have been recorded wrongly.

No Events. A small percentage of cows annually will emerge on the record system because of no events. The cow may have been culled and the record not removed, or she may still be in the herd and may not have been examined for several months. She should be examined at the earliest opportunity.

Additional Means of Promoting Fertility. Although intensification of breeding management during the first 90 days of lactation, including repeated physical examination of female genitalia, is the principal means of improving reproductive efficiency, there are other ancillary measures that should be invoked.

Control of Specific Diseases That Cause Abortion and Infertility. In most developed countries, the control of bovine brucellosis by vaccination of calves with *Brucella abortus* strain 19 has been discontinued because the prevalence of the disease has been reduced to almost zero. Further reduction in prevalence is likely to be achieved only by continuing active vaccination. Leptospirosis is still a serious cause of abortion and is controllable only by vaccination twice yearly, usually with a bivalent vaccine containing killed *Leptospira interrogans* var. *pomona* and *Li.* var. *hardjo.* Vibriosis is almost a forgotten disease because it is controllable by artificial insemination. Where natural breeding is practiced, vaccination of the bull before the breeding period is an effective counter to the spread of this venereal disease. Trichomoniasis is rarely if ever seen and is effectively controllable by artificial insemination.

Virus abortion due to the bovine virus diarrhea virus (B.V.D.) and to the herpesvirus of infectious bovine rhinotracheitis are both dealt with by vaccination with an attenuated virus. An inactivated B.V.D. vaccine is now available. The desirability of the procedure is open to doubt, and in many countries the high prevalence of the infection, as manifested by serology rather than clinical illness, is used as justification for taking no prophylactic measures.

Maintenance of Optimum Fertility of the Bulls. Bulls are still used in some commercial herds, especially in a makeup capacity in seasonal herds. When the majority of the herd have conceived by artificial breeding and the remainder are principally cows of marginal fertility, there is some merit in mating them with a bull allowed to run with a herd. However, because of the bull's minor role, he is often neglected and can be of low fertility. To avoid this, it is recommended that he be treated for lice, worms, and liver fluke on three occasions; that he be vaccinated against vibriosis and leptospirosis; and that his feet be examined and trimmed as necessary. These activities should begin at least two months before it is anticipated that he will be used (O'Conner, 1981). It is also desirable to conduct both a physical examination of the bull and a serving capacity test near mating time. The bull should be excluded from the cows as they come into milk, and for large bulls a serving crate should be provided for use with small cows that may need to be hand-mated.

Termination of Pregnancy. This has become a very important technique in areas where seasonal calving is the prevailing strategy. Cows that did not conceive must be sold at the end of their lactation. Those that conceive late in the season will be dried off while still milking heavily. If they are to be retained in the herd, they need to be brought back to the normal conception date. The only way to arrange this is by inducing parturition. When the loss of the calf, as commonly happens, is not important but precipitation of lactation is, this is a relatively safe and cheap method of bringing it about (Weich et al. 1979). It should not be attempted before the appropriate stage of pregnancy—26 weeks—as indicated by presence of fetus, cotyledons, and fremitus on rectal examination, and farmers should be warned of the possible unfavorable outcomes including death of the calf, retention of the placenta, and photosensitive dermatitis, which are known untoward sequels of the use of corticosteroids for this purpose. A recent addition to the pharmaceutery surrounding the induction of parturition is the injection of 300 μg of clenbuterol, which delays parturition for up to 12 hours when that time is more appropriate than the expected one (Dawson 1983).

Pharmaceutical Control of Breeding. When husbandry techniques fail to bring the reproductive efficiency of a herd up to the desired standard, it may be necessary to attempt to manipulate the breeding cycle by pharmaceutical means. The usual technique is to synchronize estrus by the use of a prostaglandin, then to diagnose pregnancy by a progesterone assay on milk, and finally to terminate pregnancy at a time most appropriate to the management of the herd, usually by means of a corticosteroid. The technique is effective but expensive (Eddy 1983). A cost-benefit analysis of the program shows a significant gain but not as great a gain as when husbandry techniques—especially good detection of estrus—are implemented. In terms of reproductive efficiency, good detection of estrus is as effective as controlled estrus by cloprostenol, either by observing estrus after a single injection or by blind insemination after two (King et al. 1983).

Induction of Lactation in Nonpregnant Cows. From one point of view, this practice is the ultimate answer to the problem of reproductive inefficiency because it dispenses with the need for pregnancy and proceeds directly to the real objective by inducing lactation. At present the outcome falls far short of the aspiration and it seems unlikely, using present technology, that the technique will be adopted commercially. A combination of estradiol and progesterone is effective in inducing lactation, but the milk yield is low and there are undesirable side effects (Tervit et al. 1980).

Monitoring of Inseminator Efficiency. The act of artificial insemination is such a simple and positive one that the only common problem encountered is in the early stages of training, when failure to penetrate the cervix and palpate the end of the catheter in the uterus causes low conception rates. Some trainees never do learn how to do it properly, but their conception rates are so low that they are excluded at the training level. Once trained and working, either as an inseminator employed by an artificial breeding service or as a do-it-yourself farmer, it is unusual to have a significant decline in efficiency.

As in other situations that require constant monitoring of performance, a small computer program written to extract the relevant data from a large data base collected for other reasons serves this purpose. The large data base provided by a herd health program is ideal for the purpose and is another justification for the development of these programs. They are particularly advantageous when data are not available from an artificial breeder service because it sells straws to farmers, who are under no obligation to inform the artificial breeder organization of the results achieved with the semen.

Avoidance of Stillbirths/Dystocias. There is nothing new or exciting in this area. The staple recommendations from past years still pertain. They include careful surveillance at calving, selection against cow families that encounter

problems of maternal-fetal disproportion and resulting dystocia, and avoidance of mating with bulls with the same predisposition.

Surveillance at calving has two objectives. One is to avoid the loss of the present calf by intervening early enough to save it but not so early as to make things difficult for an as yet undilated dam. The other is to avoid trauma and infection of the tract, which is more likely to occur in cows where dystocia is present for more than a few hours.

In females, the pelvic diameter, as measured by an instrument or as judged by the distance between the tuber coxae (Ben-David 1980), is used as a guide to selection. Absolute targets are not set, but in a herd with a problem, it will be necessary to cull about the bottom 20% of the pelvic sizes to exert any significant effect on its prevalence. Although the above recommendations are generally agreed upon, the evidence of any significant heritability of the physical size of the pelvis is lacking. Most of the observations in beef cattle (e.g., Brinks et al. 1973) indicate that heritability of freedom from dystocia in the dam is low and that calf size is the principal determinant (Lasater et al. 1973).

Mating the herd to bulls with a history of offspring that encountered no problems is a favored policy. The effect of the bull is probably manifested through the size of the calf—calves with large birthweights being more likely to encounter difficulty. It is not uncommon for beef farmers to appreciate that they are going to encounter calving difficulties when feed supplies are good. The cows will have too much pelvic fat, and the calves will be too big. Realization of the impending problem late in the breeding season and a reaction by the farmer to reduce food intake may result in an outbreak of pregnancy toxemia, with heavy death losses as a result. This would be a most unlikely event in a dairy herd.

Much of the work on selection against families for freedom from dystocia has been done on beef cattle. It seems likely that the same conditions would operate for dairy cattle. An exception to this is twinning, which is inherited and can often be the cause of dystocia and subsequent infertility.

Selection of Cows for Examination, Treatment, and Culling. In any program directed at improvement of reproductive activity, it is necessary to periodically review the data about each cow and decide whether she is achieving the target set by the farmer. Those cows that do not should be called in for examination and treatment or culling. There are a number of inherent weaknesses in the system, and it is often unsuccessful because of these weaknesses. They are:

1. The criteria are too lax. This can only be overcome by having the farmer develop tough targets.

2. The records are inadequately maintained. In many cases this has been due to lack of expertise, but this is no longer true. A computer program that collects, stores, retrieves, and analyzes data and prints out information is accessible to any farmer. It is still possible to wreck the recording, but this is seldom done.

3. The person comparing each cow's record with the approved target may be too flexible in the decisions made about each cow. A computer will select 15% to 20% more cows using the same information, because it can be programmed to operate without flexibility.

4. The regularity of the reviews often suffers when there are other pressures on the farm. A call by an external agency often produces a more active response.

5. A reminder that examinations of cows are due at farm X is more likely to meet a positive response if it is accompanied by a list of cows, their histories, and the reason for the examinations.

CLINICAL INVESTIGATION OF REPRODUCTIVE INEFFICIENCY IN A DAIRY HERD

General Procedure

The recommended procedure for examination of a fertility problem in a dairy herd is the same whether the problem appears in a herd managed by a herd health program or whether a farmer calls for help with a herd that is not under constant veterinary surveillance. In herds on a computerized herd health program, a decline in reproductive performance will become obvious early if the responsible veterinarian is paying close attention to the reproductive indices produced at monthly intervals by the program. In other herds, the problem is often much further advanced. It is a great advantage in these herds, if they have sufficient good data—and they usually do not—to run the data from a year or two through the herd health computer program and produce an analysis of the reproductive performance. This procedure has the dual advantage of giving a ready estimate of the size of the problem and, at the same time, helping to indicate in what general area the problem is likely to lie. The herds in which it is possible to do this are usually limited to those that keep an individual cow card record system. A barn sheet can be used as a data base provided the farmer has been meticulous in recording every reproductive event, but the labor input required at the computer is higher. The procedure is to construct a series of current lactation records and analyze them through the computer in terms of calving to conception interval, calving to first estrus, interestral interval, and so on.

A general recommendation is to carry out a complete examination of reproductive functions in any herd in which a problem is thought to be present. The examination should be a complete one, even in those herds in which the farmer or referring veterinarian requests a specific investigation of a particular function, e.g., repeat breeders. In most herds where there is a problem caused by a management error, there will be departures from normal in a number of areas rather than in just one. For example, a herd that is having a problem with so-called anestrus often also has a problem of repeat breeders, and correction of, for example, the poor detection of estrus often solves both problems. On the contrary, herds that encounter a specific abortive agent, e.g., *Brucella abortus*, are likely to have a specific problem in a specific area and if they have another problem, it will be in an unassociated area.

A protocol for the examination of a herd with a fertility problem follows.

Protocol for Examination of a Herd with a Problem of Reproductive Inefficiency

History

The essential part of the history is the breeding history of each cow, including heats not served, breedings, pregnancy diagnoses, examination and treatments for breeding aberrations, and calvings, cullings, and sales. After consideration of some of the analyses of this data, it may be fairly obvious what particular avenues of evidence should be explored. At the beginning, it is worthwhile to obtain a general history about breeding practices, artificial or natural breeding, timing of mating, techniques employed, method of estrus detection, status of nutrition and body score, introduction of new breeding animals, accidental incursions from outside the farm, and so on.

Reproductive Status of Each Cow

Using a combination of each cow's reproductive record for the past year and the findings on physical examination of the genital tract, it is usually possible to define the cow's reproductive status. It is much easier to do this if the breeding history of the herd has been submitted beforehand, the data has been computerized and then analyzed, and a request-for-examination form has been produced. This will indicate those cows that need examination and also outline their immediate past histories and the reasons for nominating them for examination.

The common findings on examination of the genital tracts of infertile cows are:
□ pregnancy
□ very small ovaries containing no structures, which occur commonly in nutritionally stressed females, especially heifers after their first calf is born
□ apparently normal ovaries with a large corpus luteum in one and no structures or a follicle in the other. This is the classic finding in a so-called anestrus cow that is cycling normally but is unobserved. The situation in the ovaries is changed at the next monthly examination
□ a single large corpus luteum in one ovary that is unchanged at subsequent monthly examinations, the so-called retained corpus luteum
□ large cystic ovaries in cows that have nymphomaniac behavior or anestrus
□ the thick-walled, hard-feeling, double-normal-sized uterus of chronic endometritis, not to be mistaken for the turgid-feeling estral uterus. The vaginal contents are purulent-viscid in endometritis, crystal clear and tenacious in estrus
□ on visual examination of the vagina with an endoscope, congestion/inflammation of the cervix is accompanied by a discharge of purulent or viscid-cloudy exudate

A summary of the way in which the analyses should be interpreted in order to arrive at a patho-anatomic diagnosis is included in Table 4-1.

Comparison of Fertility Indices of the Herd with Optimal Targets of Performance

Having completed the examination of the reproductively inefficient individual cows, it is now necessary to compare the herd's performance with the targets used to identify normality.

For Herds Calving All Year Round	Optimal Target
Calving interval (months)	12
Calving to first heat interval (days)	35
Calving to conception interval (days)	85
Calving to first service (days)	65
Per cent showing heat by 60 days	>85
Conception rate to first service (%)	70
Conception rate all services (%)	58
Services per conception	<1.5

The optimal distribution of cows according to the stage of production and reproduction (Spalding et al. 1975) for herds calving year round is as follows:

Pregnant and dry	17%
Pregnant and milking	42%
Not pregnant and milking	41%

The frequency distribution of the length of interestral intervals can be used to determine the efficiency of estrus detection. If estrus detection is reliable and accurate, the ratio of interestral intervals of 18 to 21 days to interestral intervals of 36 to 42 days is 6:1. A ratio of less than 6:1 indicates that the herdsman is missing some cows in heat but is detecting these same cows later in the next heat, which increases the frequency of interestral intervals 36 to 42 days in duration.

Seasonal or Block Mating Herds. The targets used in dairy herds or beef herds that mate all cows at a particular time each year are added to those listed previously (Malmo 1982). They are:

Per cent of cows on heat by 60 days after calving	95
If estral activity and detection are good, the herd should match the target of:	
Submission rate for first 30 days of breeding season (60 to 90 days after calving) (%)	>95
Per cent conception on first (and on each subsequent) service	>65
Per cent cows pregnant by end of first 60 days of breeding	>85
Per cent cows not pregnant by end of first 5 months of breeding	<5

Define the Modes of Reproductive Inefficiency and Determine the Cause

Comparison of the actual performance with optimal targets will identify the stages of the reproductive cycle in which there is a shortfall in performance. Using a decision tree as a guideline (Fig. 4-3), the modes of reproductive inefficiency can be identified and an indication of the cause of the infertility deduced. A summary of the more common

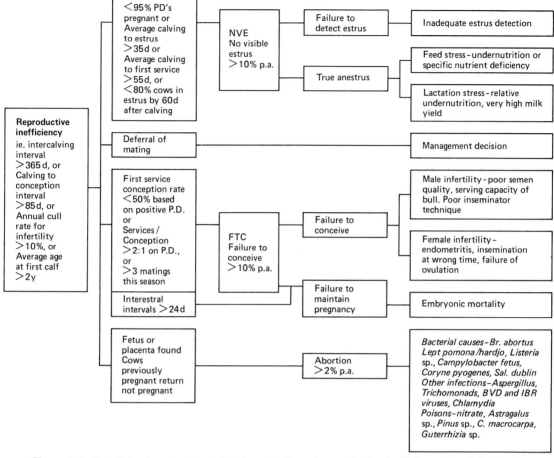

Figure 4-3. A decision tree for the clinical investigation of reproductive inefficiency in a dairy herd.

causes of infertility (Table 4–4) and abortion (Table 4–5) is provided.

The step of passing from a definition of the mode of the infertility to the specific cause requires some knowledge of the relative frequency of the common causes. This knowledge will ensure that, when an investigation is undertaken to determine the cause, the most likely one is not left until the end of the investigation before it is considered. The most common causes of reproductive inefficiency are, in order of descending frequency:

1. *Inadequate estrus detection.* As herds have increased in size and labor input per cow has been reduced, management generally has declined. Detection of estrus is the most sensitive activity in breeding management, and failure to breed cows is the result. This commonly leads to an erroneous snap diagnosis of "anestrus." The diagnostic exercise required is not a laboratory one, although whether a cow has been in estrus or not can be deduced from blood or milk levels of progesterone. What is

required is a careful clinical examination of ovaries of so-called anestrus cows to demonstrate that they are, in fact, cycling; and, as a subset of this group, a careful watch for a high proportion of nonpregnant cows among those presented for pregnancy diagnosis is also required.

2. *Breeding nonestral cows.* When cows are not observed to be in estrus at the level that probability demands, the average herdsman will commence breeding cows that might be in season. This is one of the disadvantages of the artificial breeding program; natural service would avoid the error. There is the other small facet of this group in which cows have gone off season by the time they are bred. This error is not identifiable by any physical or laboratory examination.

3. *Nutritional stress.* Inadequate nutrition, mostly by way of an insufficient supply of energy, is a common cause of reproductive inefficiency. This may be because of an absolute shortage of feed or because of a shortage

Text continued on page 86

Table 4-4. DIAGNOSTIC SUMMARY OF CAUSES OF INFERTILITY IN DAIRY CATTLE*

Initial Clinical Classification	History—The Problem Presented	General Clinical Findings	Clinical Findings of Genitalia	Lab Findings	Patho-anatomic Diagnoses
NVE (No visible estrus)	*Individual cow:* No estrus observed in 49 d after calving or 35 d after mating or other reproductive event *Herd:* 1. <95% pregnancy diagnoses pregnant at examination, or 2. average calving to first service >55 d, or 3. <80% cows on heat by 60 d after calving, or 4. average calving to first estrus >35 d 5. >10% no visible estrus (per annum) *Herd seasonal or block mating:* Additional problems: 6. Cycling rate 30 d preceding mating start 95% 7. Submission rate 30 d after mating start 95% 8. Late calves requiring induction of parturition 10%	1. Body condition score <3.5. Evidence of undernutrition or parasitism in heifers 2. Intercurrent disease, e.g., acetonemia, metritis, fat cow syndrome, LDA 3. Body condition normal. No other signs 4. Body condition normal. No other signs	Small ovaries, no structures; small, delicate uterus Ditto, except metritis obvious on rectal palpation Corpora lutea in ovary, uterus normal size and tone. Same findings on same ovary one mo later Corpora lutea and/or follicles in different ovaries at serial examinations 1 mo apart	— Of intercurrent disease — —	Undernutrition anestrus Secondary anestrus Retained corpus luteum Defective estrus detection

Condition	History / Criteria	Other findings	Clinical findings	Laboratory / herd action	Diagnosis
Nymphomania	*Individual cow:* Abnormally long estral cycle. Short intercycle intervals. Intense estral activity	Tail head may be raised or trauma to pelvis	Large follicular cysts one or both ovaries	—	Cystic follicles
FTC (Failure to conceive)	*Individual cow:* More than 3 matings this breeding season. *Herd:* 1. 1st service conception rate 50% on pregnancy diagnosis 2. Services/conception >2.0 on pregnancy diagnosis 3. >10 FTC's per yr	May be heavy producer. Insemination time may be too late. Inseminator may be inefficient. Semen fertility may be poor. Cow may have vaginal discharge	Normal uterus and ovaries or enlarged, thick-walled doughy uterus. Vaginal exam—inflamed cervix; pus from os	Bacteriological exam of vaginal pus. Biopsy of uterine wall	Endometritis; not on heat when bred; fault in male; unspecified
PDR (Pregnancy diagnosis recheck)	*Individual cow:* Cow diagnosed pregnant, returns to estrus. Interestral intervals >28 d. Large S.D. about mean	Nil —	Not pregnant. Uterus may be involuting Not pregnant No abnormality	Check for *Campylobacter* sp. in herd Check for *Campylobacter*	Fetal resorption or abortion Embryonic mortality within 20 d of conception
Abortion (problem >3% p.a.)	*Individual cow:* Aborted fetus or retained placenta found. Cow previously diagnosed pregnant >x mos. *Herd:* Intercalving interval >365 d. Calving to conception interval >85 d. Animal cull rate for infertility >10%. Average age at first calf >2 yrs	Involuting uterus, metritis, fetal dystocia	Not pregnant, uterus may still be involuting	Microbiological and serological search Serological cause	Abortion 33% with specific cause

*Abortion is dealt with separately.

Table 4–5. DIAGNOSTIC SUMMARY OF CAUSES OF ABORTION IN CATTLE

Disease	Epidemiology			Field Examination		Laboratory Diagnosis	
	Clinical Features	Abortion Rate	Time of Abortion	Placenta	Fetus	Isolation of Agent	Serology
Brucellosis (Br. abortus)	Abortion	High, up to 90% in susceptible	6 mos +	Necrosis of cotyledons. Leathery, opaque placenta with edema	May be pneumonia	Culture of fetal stomach, placenta, uterine fluid, milk, and semen	Serum and blood agglutination test, milk ring test, whole milk plate agglutination test. Whey plate agglutination, semen plasma, and vaginal mucous agglutination test
Trichomoniasis (Tr. fetus)	Infertility—return to heat at 4–5 mos, abortion and pyometra	Moderate, 5–30%	2–4 mos	Flocculent material and clear serous fluid in uterine exudate	Fetal maceration and pyometra common	Hanging drop or culture examination of fetal stomach and uterine exudate within 24 hrs of abortion	Cervical mucous agglutination test
Vibriosis (Campylobacter fetus)	Infertility, irregular moderately prolonged diestrus	Low, up to 5% (may be up to 20%)	5–6 mos	Semi-opaque, little thickening. Petechia, localized avascularity and edema	Flakes of pus on visceral peritoneum	Culture of fetal stomach, placenta, and uterine exudate	Blood agglutination after abortion (at 3 wks). Cervical mucous agglutination test at 40 d after infected service
Leptospirosis (Li. pomona and Li. hardjo)	Abortion may occur at acute febrile stage, later, or unassociated with illness	25–30%	Late, 6 mos +	Avascular placenta, atonic yellow-brown cotyledons, brown gelatinous edema between allantois and amnion	Fetal death common	Isolation from pleural fluid, kidney, and liver of fetus. Direct examination of urine of cow is best	Positive serum agglutination test 14–21 d after febrile illness
Listeriosis (L. monocytogenes)	May be an associated septicemia	Low	About 7 mos	—	No abnormality	Organisms in fetal stomach, placenta, and uterine fluid	Agglutination titers higher than 1:400 in contact animals classed as positive

Agent	Season / Occurrence	Incidence	Time of abortion	Placenta	Fetus	Culture	Serologic test
Infectious bovine rhinotracheitis	Uneventful	25–50%	Late, 6 mos	—	Autolyzed	Culture of placenta and fetus	Acute and convalescent sera —
Mycoses (*Aspergillus, Absidia*)	—	Unknown 6–7% of all abortions encountered	3–7 mos	Necrosis of maternal cotyledon, adherence of necrotic material to chorionic cotyledon causes soft, yellow, cushion-like structure. Small, yellow, raised, leathery lesions on intercotyledonary areas	May be small, raised, gray-buff, soft lesions or diffuse white areas on skin. Resemble ringworm	Direct examination of cotyledon and fetal stomach for hyphae, suitable cultural examination	—
Epizootic bovine abortion	Mainly winter. Herd immunity develops	High (30–40%)	6–8 mos	Negative	Subcutis edema, ascites, esophageal and tracheal petechia, degenerative lesions in liver	Cause not identified	No accurate test

Miscellaneous bacterial infections that cause a large number of bovine abortions are *Corynebacterium pyogenes* and *Salmonella dublin*.

Poisonings: The following poisonous agents are credited with causing abortion in cattle: preformed estrogens, perennial broomweed (*Gutierrezia* sp.), *Astragalus* sp., *Pinus ponderosa, P. radiata, P. cubensis, Cupressus macrocarpa*, nitrate in high concentrations.

Isoimmunization of pregnancy. Has not been observed to occur naturally in cattle. It has been produced experimentally by repeated intravenous injections of blood from the one bull. Intravascular hemolysis occurs in the calves.

Unknown. From 30 to 75% of most series of abortions examined are undiagnosed. The ingestion of large quantities of pine needles is suspected as a cause of abortion in range cattle in the United States. Infection with the virus of mucosal disease and *Mycoplasma* spp. are other causes of undetermined importance.

relative to a high milk yield. For example, a heavily producing cow may receive a diet high in fiber and deficient in starch density. An analysis of feed is not required to provide this answer. The cow's body condition and milk yield are both good indicators of the cow's nutritional status. It is only when these appear normal that an evaluation of specific nutritional elements by laboratory techniques is required. It is recommended that cows have a body condition score of 5 (out of 8; 1 = emaciation, 8 = obese) at calving to still have a condition score of 3.5 at mating.

4. *Inadequate male input.* Artificial insemination provides a guarantee against poor semen, or at least warns the farmer if the reproductive efficiency of the semen is poor. It does, however, have the disadvantage of allowing error by an incompetent inseminator, although in our experience of examining herd infertility problems, we have never encountered the circumstance in which the inseminator was the cause of a major infertility problem, except in the early training period.

5. *Infectious agents.* Brucellosis, vibriosis, and trichomoniasis have almost completely disappeared as significant causes of infertility. Brucellosis survives to plague individual herds and should not be forgotten in investigations of herds with abortion problems. The other infections listed in Figure 4–3 and Table 4–5 are probably of more importance, with no single one of them always dominating the others. These are the diseases that lend themselves to diagnosis by serological examination; by bacteriological examination of uterine discharge, placenta, or fetus; by pathological examination of tissues; by uterine biopsy; or by examination of tissues from necropsied animals or animals slaughtered for meat.

Although the infectious agents usually account for very few of the infertility problems and for only 30% of the abortions, they are still a significant cause of loss in individual scattered herds. For this reason, a complete examination is always necessary.

Laboratory Investigations

A complete laboratory examination includes the following:

1. *Metabolic profile test.* Blood glucose, total serum protein, serum copper, glutathione peroxidase for selenium deficiency, serum calcium, and phosphorus estimations will provide a guide to the cow's nutritional status with respect to each of these dietary ingredients.

2. *Feed analysis.* A complete analysis of the feed for digestible energy, crude protein, and minerals may rarely be indicated. This needs to be accompanied by an accurate estimate of total feed intake per cow per day. When a dietary deficiency of energy, protein, or macroelements such as calcium and phosphorus is suspected, it is more usual to consult a feed component table in a textbook than to do an analysis.

3. *Tissues.* Analysis of liver and other body tissues for minerals such as copper may be indicated and is a common exercise when examining herds with reproductive problems.

4. *Abortions.* Aborted fetuses and placenta must be submitted for laboratory evaluation. Acute and convalescent sera from the dam must also be examined serologically.

5. *Semen evaluation.* The quality of a batch of semen can usually be assessed by the conception rates in other herds using the same semen. A sudden, unexpected decrease in the conception rate should prompt a laboratory evaluation of the semen.

6. *Abattoir specimens.* The reproductive tracts of cows culled for infertility may be available from the abattoir and should be examined when possible.

7. *Genital discharges.* Samples of abnormal genital discharges should be taken for microbiological culture. Special transport media may be necessary when genital mycoplasmosis is suspected.

Corrective Action and Monitoring the Results

Having made a definitive diagnosis, it is now customary to introduce corrective measures and to monitor the effects. The corrective action may include improvement in the surveillance of heat detection, the use of heat detection aids, improvement in nutrition, the specific treatment of cows affected with endometritis, the use of different semen, insemination at a more optimal time, or response trials. The specific nature of the corrective action should be documented for future reference, and the results should be monitored and recorded. Failure to achieve the desired results may necessitate a reinvestigation of the problem in greater depth.

FINANCIAL IMPLICATIONS OF REPRODUCTIVE INEFFICIENCY

It is not possible to be very specific when describing the financial gain that results from improving reproductive efficiency in dairy herds. The value of dairy products varies so widely between countries that gains in dollars and cents mean little. There are also very great variations in the costs of feed and housing between countries where cattle are housed and countries where the industry is entirely pastoral. Capital investment in livestock also varies widely between these two and other groups of countries. It is therefore necessary to express gains in terms of increases proportional to the investment in making the change—the percentage return to investment (Williamson 1980a).

What estimates of profitability there are, are suspect unless they emanate from a simulation model of a dairy herd. To say that such and such an additional management technique has so and so an effect by assessing the cost of the technique and the observed gain in isolation without taking into account the effects of the technique on other than reproduction functions, and without taking into account the effect of other factors that might have affected production, is to oversimplify the system.

In spite of these shortcomings, the usual means of expressing the profitability of improving reproductive efficiency is to quote the increased net profit that results by each day that the intercalving interval is shortened. This presupposes that the optimum intercalving interval is 365 days; that the value of milk is the same at all times of the year; and, because one of the large costs of reproductive inefficiency is the premature culling of cows, that the value of cull cows is the same at all times of the year. It also presupposes that the herd is calving all year round and that cows having difficulty conceiving can be carried on for a significant length of time in order to conceive. In those herds that practice the alternate strategy of seasonal or block calving (Bailie 1982), this is not possible, and cows with conceptual difficulties must be culled or bred late and have their pregnancies terminated by pharmacological means. Thus, any expression of profitability of a reproduction program must take into account the value of additional milk produced (less the additional cost of feed) plus the lowered depreciation per cow as a result of a lower culling rate. For example, an improvement in detection of estrus could have the effect shown below (after Bailie 1982).

The effects of terminating pregnancies in late calving cows instead of culling them would seem to have been a cheaper alternative.

Any estimates of financial gain relative to reduction in the calving interval will show great variation. This wide range of values in profitability is apparent at different times during the year when milk prices differ in order to provide incentives for better milk production.

The available computer simulation models of reproductive systems in dairy herds (Oltenacu 1980; Bailie 1982) take into account all the important factors affecting reproductive efficiency. The use of such a model to evaluate the profitability of changes in the management system or in the value of individual variables, e.g., estrus detection (Bailie 1982), has demonstrated their usefulness. The costs of the culling program and its attendant replacement program are available from a similar computer simulation model (Gartner 1981, 1982).

Review Literature

Britt, J.H., Cox, N.M. and Stevenson, J.S. Advances in reproduction in dairy cattle. J. Dairy Sci., 64: 1378–1402, 1981.

Dawson, F.L.M. Reproduction and infertility. Vet. Annual, 23:1–9, 1983.

Konermann, H. Fertility problems in cattle breeding, causes and possible counter-measures. Vet. Med. Rev., 1:32–38, 1974.

deKruif, A. and Brand, A. Factors influencing the reproductive capacity of a dairy herd. N.A. Vet. J., 26:178, 183–189, 1978.

Lamming, G.E., Foster, J.P. and Bulman, D.C. Pharmacological control of reproductive cycles. Vet. Rec., 104:156–160, 1979.

Mather, E.C. and Melancon, J.J. The periparturient cow—a pivotal entity in dairy production. J. Dairy Sci., 64:1422–1430, 1981.

Miller, P.D. Artificial insemination organizations. J. Dairy Sci., 64:1283–1287, 1981.

Morris, R.S., Williamson, N.B., Blood, D.C. et al. A health program for dairy herds. 3. Changes in reproductive performance. Aust. Vet. J., 54:231–246, 1978.

Oltenacu, P.A., Milligan, R.A., Rounsaville, T.R. et al. Modelling reproduction in a herd of dairy cattle. Agricultural Systems, 5:193–205, 1980.

Rumler, R.H. Dairy cattle breed organizations in the United States. J. Dairy Sci., 64:1278–1282, 1981.

Voelker, D.E. Dairy herd improvement association. J. Dairy Sci., 64:1269–1277, 1981.

Length of Breeding Season	Improvement in Estrus Detection Conception Rate 60%	Value of Improved Milk Production Resulting (January Calving)	Value of Improved Milk Production Plus Lowered Depreciation for Culling of Cows (January Calving)
274 days (year round)	50→80%	£11.8 per cow ($17.70)	£25.1 ($37.65)
130 days (seasonal or block)	50→80%	£4.7 per cow ($7.05)	£26.4 ($39.60)

References

Abbitt, B., Ball, L., Kitlo, G.P. et al. Effect of three methods of palpation for pregnancy diagnosis per rectum of embryonic and fetal attrition in cows. J. Am. Vet. Med. Assoc., 172:973–978, 1978.

Appleyard, W.T. and Cook, B. The detection of estrus in dairy cattle. Vet. Rec.., 99:253–256, 1975.

Bailie, J.H. Management and economic effects of different levels of estrus detection in the dairy herd. Vet. Rec., 110:218–221, 1982.

Ball, B.J.H., Cowpe, J.E.D. and Harker, D.B. Evaluation of tail paste as an estrus detection aid using serial progesterone analysis. Vet. Rec., 112:147–149, 1983.

Ben-David, B. The distance between tuber coxae of heifers as an aid in the prediction of difficulty of parturition. Refuah Vet., 37:12–14, 1980.

Bogin, E., Avidar, Y., Davidson, M. et al. Effect of nutrition on fertility and blood composition in the milk cow. J. Dairy Res., 49:13–23, 1982.

Bostedt, H., Reissinger, H. and Gunzler, D. Clinical findings on the course of the puerperal period in cows on farms with fertility problems. Berl. Münch. Tierarztl. Wochenschr., 89:24–28, 1976.

Bosu, W.T.K., Doig, P.A. and Barker, C.A.V. Pregnancy and peripheral plasma progesterone levels in cows inseminated after synchronization of estrus with prostaglandin F2α. Can. Vet. J., 22:59–61, 1981.

Brinks, J.S., Olson, J.E. and Carroll, E.J. Calving difficulty and its association with subsequent productivity. J. Anim. Sci., 36:11–17, 1973.

Britt, J.H. Early postpartum breeding in dairy cows. A review. J. Dairy Sci., 58:266–271, 1975.

Britt, J.H. Strategies for managing reproduction and controlling health problems in groups of cows. J. Dairy Sci., 60:1345–1353, 1977.

Britt, J.H., Cox, N.M. and Stevenson, J.S. Advances in reproduction in dairy cattle. J. Dairy Sci., 64:1378–1402, 1981.

Carstairs, J.A., Morrow, D.A. and Emery, R.S. Postpartum reproductive function of dairy cows as influenced by energy and phosphorus status. J. Anim. Sci., 51:1122–1130, 1980.

Dawson, F.L.M. Reproduction and infertility. Vet. Annual, 21:1, 1980.

Dawson, F.L.M. Reproduction and infertility. Vet. Annual, 23:1–9, 1983.

deKruif, A. and Brand, A. Factors influencing the reproductive capacity of a dairy herd. N.Z. Vet. J., 26:178, 183–189, 1978.

deKruif, A., Gunnink, J.W. and deBois, H.W. Examination and treatment of post-parturient endometritis in dairy cattle. Tijdschr. Diergeneeskd., 107:717–725, 1982.

Drew, S.B. and Gould, C.M. Fertility of cloprostenol treated dairy cows. Vet. Rec. 107:88–89, 1980.

Eddy, R.C. The use of the prostaglandin analogue, coprosterol and the milk progesterone test to control breeding policy in one herd. Br. Vet. J., 139:104–108, 1983.

Erb, H.N., Martin, S.W., Ison, N. et al. Interrelationships between production and reproductive disease in Holstein cows. Conditional relationships between production and disease. J. Dairy Sci., 64:272–281, 1981a.

Erb, H.N., Martin, S.W., Ison, N. et al. Interrelationships between production and reproductive disease in Holstein cows. Path. analysis. J. Dairy Sci., 64:282–289, 1981b.

Esslemont, R.J. and Bryant, M.J. Estrus behaviour in a herd of dairy cows. Vet. Rec., 99:472–475, 1976.

Esslemont, R.J. and Ellis, P.R. Components of herd calving interval. Vet. Rec., 95:319–324, 1974.

Fielden, E.D., Harris, R.E., Macmillan K.L. et al. Some aspects of reproductive performance in selected town-supply dairy herds. N.Z. Vet. J., 28:131–142, 1980.

Fielden, E.D., Macmillan, K.L. and Moller, K. The pre-service anestrus syndrome in New Zealand dairy cattle. Bovine Pract., 11:10–14, 1976.

Francos, G. The relationship between the incidence of endometritis and repeat breeders in dairy herds. Ref. Vet., 36:131–134, 1979.

Fulkerson, W.J., Sawyer, G.J. and Crothers, I. The accuracy of several aids in detecting estrus in dairy herds. Applied Anim. Ethol., 10:199–208, 1983.

Galton, D.M., Barr, H.L. and Heider, L.E. Effects of a herd health program on reproductive performance of dairy cows. J. Dairy Sci., 60:1117–1124, 1977.

Gartner, J.A. Replacement policy in dairy herds on farms where heifers compete with the cows for grassland. Part 1. Model construction and validation. Agricultural Systems, 7:289–318, 1981.

Gartner, J.A. Replacement policy in dairy herds in farms where heifers compete with the cows for grassland. Part 2. Experimentation. Agricultural Systems, 8:163–191, 1982.

Garverick, H.A., Elmore, R.G., Vaillancourt, D.H. et al. Ovarian response to gonadotrophin releasing hormone in postpartum dairy cows. Am. J. Vet. Res., 41:1582–1585, 1980.

Grainger, C., Wilhelms, G.D. and McGowan, A.A. Effect of body condition at calving and level of feeding in early lactation on milk production of dairy cows. Aust. J. Exp. Agric. Anim. Husb., 22:9, 1982.

Hawk, H.W. Infertility in dairy cattle. In: Beltsville Symposia in Agricultural Research. 3. Animal Reproduction, pp. 19–29, 1979.

Heap, R.B. and Holdsworth, R.J. Hormone assays in reproduction and fertility. Br. Vet. J., 137:561–571, 1981.

Hidiroglou, M. Trace element deficiencies and fertility in ruminants. A review. J. Dairy Sci., 62:1195–1206, 1979.

Kay, R.M. Changes in milk production, fertility and calf mortality associated with retained placenta or the birth of twins. Vet. Rec., 102:477–479, 1978.

King, G.J., Malo, D., Papageorges, M. et al. Controlled breeding of dairy cows with cloprostenol. Can. Vet. J., 24:105–107, 1983.

King, W.A. and Linares, T. Cytogenetic study of repeat breeder heifers and their embryos. Can. Vet. J., 27:112–115, 1983.

Konermann, H. Fertility problems in cattle breeding, causes and possible counter-measures. Vet. Med. Rev., 1:32–38, 1974.

Laing, J.A., Eastman, S.A.K. and Boutflower, J.C. The use of progesterone concentration in milk and plasma for pregnancy diagnosis in cattle. Br. Vet. J., 135:204–209, 1979.

Laing, J.A., Gibbs, H.A. and Eastman, S.A.K. A herd test for pregnancy in cattle, based on progesterone levels in milk. Br. Vet. J., 136:413–415, 1980.

Lamming, G.E., Foster, J.P. and Bulman, D.C. Pharmacological control of reproductive cycles. Vet. Rec., 104:156–160, 1979.

Lasater, D.B., Glimp, H.A., Cundiff, L.V. et al. Factors affecting dystocia and the effects of dystocia on subsequent reproduction in beef cattle. J. Anim. Sci., *36*:694–705, 1973.

Malmo, J. Planned animal health and production services for seasonally calving dairy herds. 12th World Conf., Diseases of Cattle, Amsterdam, pp. 670–677, 1982.

Maree, C. Observations on the influence of high level feeding on the ovarian activity and fertility in dairy cows. J. South Afr. Vet. Assoc., *51*:167–176, 1980.

McCaughey, W.J. and Cooper, R.J. An assessment by progesterone assay of the accuracy of estrus detection in dairy cows. Vet. Rec., *107*:508–510, 1980.

McCaughey, W.J. and Martin, J.B. Preparation and use of teaser bulls. Vet. Rec., *106*:119–121, 1980.

Miller, R.B. and Quinn, P.J. Observation on abortions in cattle. A comparison of pathological, microbiological and immunological findings in aborted fetuses and fetuses collected at abattoirs. Can. J. Comp. Med., *39*:270–290, 1975.

Morris, R.S., Williamson, N.B., Blood, D.C. et al. A health program for commercial dairy herds. 3. Changes in reproductive performance. Aust. Vet. J., *54*:231–246, 1978.

Munro, C.D., Boyd, H., Watson, E.D. et al. Monitoring pre-service reproductive status. Vet. Rec., *110*:77–81, 1982.

Nenadovic, M., Radakovic, N. and Karadzic, V. Relationship between the occurrence of acetonemia and endometritis and various production and breeding indices in Holstein Friesian first calves. Veterinarski Glasnik, *33*:555–562,1979.

Newton, J.M., Shaw, R.C. and Booth, J.M. Pregnancy diagnosis in dairy herds in England and Wales. Vet. Rec., *110*:123–125, 1982.

O'Connor, P. Care of the bull in a seasonal dairying practice. Vict. Vet. Proc., *39*:25, 1981.

Olds, D., Cooper, T. and Thrift, F.A. Effects of days open on economic aspects of current lactation. J. Dairy Sci., *62*:1167–1170, 1979.

Oltenacu, P.A., Milligan, R.A., Rounsaville, T.R. et al. Modelling reproduction in a herd of dairy cattle. Agricultural Systems, *5*:193–205, 1980.

Reid, I.M., Roberts, C.J. and Manston, R. Reduced fertility associated with fatty liver in high-yielding dairy cows. Vet. Res. Commun., *3*:231–236, 1979.

Roine, K. and Saloniemi, H. Incidence of infertility in dairy cows. Acta Vet. Scand., *19*:354–367, 1978.

Rounsaville, T.R., Oltenacu, P.A., Milligan, R.A. et al. Effects of heat detection, conception rate, and culling policy on reproductive performance in dairy herds. J. Dairy Sci., *62*:1435–1442, 1979.

Rowe, R.F. and Smithies, L.K. Causes of abortion in dairy cattle: A diagnostic survey. Bovine Pract., *13*: 102–103, 1978.

Sandals, W.C.D., Curtis, R.A., Cate, J.F. et al. The effect of retained placenta and metritis complex on repro-

ductive performance in dairy cattle—a case control study. Can. Vet. J., *20*:130–135, 1979.

Shanks, R.D., Berger, P.J., Freeman, A.E. et al. Projecting health cost from research herds. J. Dairy Sci., *65*:644–652, 1982.

Spalding, R.W., Everett, R.W. and Foote, R.H. Fertility in New York artificially inseminated Holstein herds in Dairy Herd Improvement. J. Dairy Sci., *55*:718–723, 1975.

Sreenan, J.M. and Diskin, M.G. Early embryonic mortality in the cow. Its relationship with progesterone concentration. Vet. Rec., *112*:517–521, 1983.

Studer, E. and Morrow, D.A. Postpartum evaluation of bovine reproductive potential. J. Am. Vet. Med. Assoc., *172*:489–494, 1978.

Tervit, H.R., Fairclough, R.J., McGowan, L.T. et al. Induction of lactation in dry dairy cattle. N.A. Vet. J., *28*:15–19, 1980.

Tong, A.K.W., Kennedy, B.W., Chicoine, R.L. et al. Reproductive efficiency of artificially bred Holsteins in Quebec. Can. J. Anim. Sci., *59*:419–425, 1979.

Welch, R.A.S., Day, A.M., Duganzich, D.M. et al. Induced calving, a comparison of treatment regimes. N.Z. Vet. J., *27*:190–198, 1979.

Whitaker, D. A fertility control programme in dairy cows in new South Wales. Br. Vet. J., *136*:214–221, 1980.

Whitmore, H.L., Hurtgen, J.P., Mather, E.C. et al. Clinical response of dairy cattle with ovarian cysts to single or repeated treatments of gonadotropin-releasing hormone. J. Am. Vet. Med. Assoc., *174*:1113–1115, 1979.

Whitmore, H.L., Tyler, W.J. and Casida, L.E. Effects of early postpartum breeding in dairy cattle. J. Anim. Sci., *38*:339–346, 1974.

Williamson, N.B. The economic efficiency of a veterinary preventive medicine and management program in Victorian dairy herds. Aust. Vet. J., *57*:1–9, 1980a.

Williamson, N.B. Tail painting as an aid to estrus detection in cattle. Aust. Vet. J., *56*:98–100, 1980b.

Williamson, N.B. The effect of variations in the interval between calving and first service on the reproductive performance of normal dairy cows. Aust. Vet. J., *56*:477–480, 1980c.

Williamson, N.B., Morris, R.S. and Anderson G.A. Pregnancy rates and non-return rates following artificial and natural breeding in dairy herds. Aust. Vet. J., *54*:111–114, 1978.

Williamson, N.B., Morris, R.S., Blood, D.C. et al. A study of the estrus behavior and estrus detection methods in a large commercial dairy herd. Vet. Rec., *91*: 58–62, 1972.

Young, I.M. and Henderson, D.C. Evaluation of single and double artificial insemination regimes as methods of shortening calving intervals in dairy cows treated with dinoprost. Vet. Rec., *109*:446–449, 1981.

5

Dairy Cattle—
Mastitis Control

INTRODUCTION

The control of mastitis in dairy herds has always consisted of surveillance, so that the mastitis status of the herd could be assessed, and the application of preventive techniques to reduce the quarter infection rate. Great strides have been made during the past 20 years, first in the development of preventive techniques and recently in the development of surveillance or monitoring methods. The first real control program (the NIRD program) did not include a surveillance segment because none was available at the time. This absence of monitoring meant that the small proportion of

herds that did not respond to the preventive techniques continued without being quickly recognized—to the serious disadvantage of the individual farmer. Also, the dramatic decrease in prevalence of the common forms of strepto-coccal and staphylococcal forms of the disease was followed by a significant increase in prevalence of opportunist infections, which required that a surveillance system be in place. These infections, largely gram-negative bac-teria commonly residing in the environment and bovine feces, have had a great deal of attention and still present a significant but surmountable problem.

The largest problem still extant is the failure

90

of farmers to take advantage of the available control programs. For this reason, new programs and modifications of them are taking their acceptability to the consumer into account. The principal barrier to adoption of programs in the past has been the additional labor involved. Most programs depend on extra activity at milking time when the farmer can least afford it—either out of his or her time or as an additional task for hired labor.

COST-EFFECTIVENESS

Eradication of mastitis has never been seriously considered, except where it is incidental in the course of a systemic disease such as tuberculosis. Mastitis control is almost entirely a matter of reducing the wastage of milk production and the premature culling of valuable cows. This overriding criterion of profitability makes it necessary to financially evaluate the control techniques to be used to ensure a profitable return on the investment. There are many levels of dairying in developed countries, and for this reason it is not possible to describe a mastitis control program in which the individual techniques are compatible with economic circumstances in all localities. What can be economical in a heavily capitalized complete housing enterprise could be quite unprofitable in a total pasture enterprise in which individual cows are worth only 20% and the price of milk is only 50% of the values in the housed environment.

It is not intended to expand on the detailed economic aspects of mastitis control programs in this discussion because of the infinite variations in the value of the product and the great variability in costs, especially of labor and land, in different countries. It is the responsibility of all persons who promote mastitis control to do their own partial budgeting of their own particular financial circumstances. Some guidelines are discussed in a later section (pp. 110–111).

LIMITATION OF PREVALENCE

If limitation of the prevalence of mastitis is to be the objective, the question that arises is the level of prevalence that is to be recommended as a reasonable target.

An analysis of the costs and benefits of any mastitis control problem will indicate the level of expenditure that is appropriate and thus the level to which the prevalence of the disease can be reduced. The initial gains are more easily

and cheaply accomplished than the later ones. There is also the question of whether reduction of the population of the resident major and minor pathogens increases susceptibility to the opportunist pathogens, the coliforms, the *Pseudomonas* sp., and so on.

It is therefore not unreasonable to propose an objective that is, e.g., 10% or 5% quarter infection rate, depending on the financial and epidemiologic circumstances of the herd.

THE CLASSES OF INFECTION

The Parasitic Versus the Opportunist Infections

The obligate parasites, *Streptococcus agalactiae*, *Str. uberis*, *Str. dysgalactiae*, and *Staphylococcus aureus*, are resident parasites of the skin of the teat and the tissues of the teat and mammary gland. As such they are controllable if the teat skin can be maintained in a disinfected state and the mammary tissue cleared of infection, i.e., the area that needs to be controlled is defined and can be physically dealt with. If the rate of new infections with these bacteria is to be reduced, their population numbers around the tip of the teat and the entrance to the teat canal must be reduced. Thus the critical line in the control program is disinfection of the end of the teat and the maintenance of the disinfected state for as long as possible.

Because disinfection of the end of the teat cannot be infallible, a second line of defense is necessary—one in the gland itself. The only suitable and available defense is the presence of abundant leucocytes. Their numbers must be large if they are to be effective, because they are relatively inefficient in milk, which has so many other particles to phagocytose. In fact, some bacteria—e.g., staphylococci—survive in leucocytes, which they might not do if they were exposed to the accompanying antibiotic treatment. Thus a reduction of the cell count of milk—e.g., below 400,000—may expose the quarter to infections of all sorts, and if the resident mastitis pathogens—the staphs and streps—are well under control, the predominant infections may be the gram-negative opportunists.

The opportunist invaders, typified by *Escherichia coli*, penetrate the teat sphincter and canal without first colonizing the teat skin. Disinfection is therefore of no avail. If the milking technique and the milking machine tend to leave the teat canal dilated and its keratin barrier rendered ineffective, and if the leucocytic defenses of the mammary tissues have been greatly reduced, the pathway is clear for opportunist bacteria. If the cow's environment is changed so that its contamination rate is multiplied several times, it is understandable why coliform mastitis could become a major problem.

The Major Pathogens Versus the Minor Pathogens

The major pathogens are the well-recognized obligate parasites of the udder, *Streptococcus agalactiae*, coagulase-positive *Staphylococcus aureus*, *Str. uberis*, and *Str. dysgalactiae*. The minor pathogens are *Corynebacterium bovis* and *Staphylococcus aureus*, which are nonpathogenic and coagulase negative. It is the latter that are credited with maintaining a higher than normal cell count and thus increasing the resistance of the infected quarter to invasion by a major pathogen. Correspondingly, eradication of these minor pathogens, as might occur in an intensive program of dry cow therapy, could significantly increase the susceptibility of the herd to opportunist pathogens.

The Opportunist Pathogens

These organisms invade when defenses are low and usually create very severe damage, even to the point of killing the host, but they do not stay in the host and do not provide a source of infection for other cows. They pose a threat because of the serious damage that they do and because the standard mastitis control programs do not restrain these infections. It has often been said that a too intensive conventional mastitis program will be followed by a surge of coliform mastitis. The case is still not proven, but there are incidental records that support the view (Marr 1978; Robinson et al. 1983).

PRINCIPLES OF PREVENTION

To be effective, a mastitis control program must first be adopted. This usually requires an extension program dedicated to promoting a state of mastitis awareness. This needs to be supported by a control program which is:
- known to be cost-effective
- within the scope of the average farmer's understanding
- adaptable to the current management system
- a visible success in that the number of clinical cases will be seen to diminish very rapidly

What is then required to complete the circle is a test that will show individual farmers whether or not *they* have a mastitis problem on *their* farm—the initial assessment.

Mastitis Awareness

There are many ways of creating an atmosphere in which lack of control of mastitis is a management disgrace. The most obvious but least used technique is to put an incentive price on to the value of mastitis-free milk. A number of European countries do this by placing a premium on milk with a low cell count. In some countries, sale of milk containing more than a sufficient number of cells is prohibited.

Dairy factories and manufacturing companies are in the best position to do this but are usually disinclined to disaffect their suppliers. What they can do as an alternative is provide a free cell-counting service. This may be a herd cell count or the average of individual cow cell counts. The farmer can be advised each month of his absolute count and also where he is in the merit list of local herds.

Assessing the Mastitis Status of the Herd

The details of these procedures are dealt with elsewhere (pp. 110–112). Briefly, the choice is between tests carried out by the farmer and those carried out at an external site, the obvious one being the milk reception depot. Tests conducted by farmers are divided into two groups: (1) keeping a running total of clinical cases occurring in lactating cows; and (2) cow-side tests, as they are called, especially the California Mastitis Test (CMT).

In most areas of do-it-yourself activities, farmer input is very variable. The principal difficulty is to get farmers to assiduously repeat the task each week or month and then to interact with the herd by comparing the herd's performance with a target and to introduce reparative measures when these are needed. This is especially true if the test is mathematical or biological and therefore quite outside the farmer's range of expertise and normal activity.

The alternative to farmer-conducted tests is the assessment of the herd by an external authority. The obvious test is on milk, and the obvious site is the milk collection depot. The first test used, which is still highly relevant as a means of drawing attention to a herd with a problem, is the bulk milk cell count. Because of the inaccuracies that characterize a test carried out on the combined milk of a hundred or more cows, there is much more interest now in the use of the mean of the herd's individual cow milk cell counts. The bulk milk count is carried out on a sample of the bulked milk at the milk receiving depot. The individual cow cell count is most economically carried out on samples forwarded to a herd milk testing laboratory. If the herd does not belong to a herd improvement organization, it is necessary for the farmer to collect individual cow composite samples. This can be time-consuming or expensive if the veterinarian is to collect a sample from each of four quarters from each cow on four occasions during each lactation.

The Availability of a Cost-Effective Mastitis Control Program

Until the NIRD program—devised by the National Institute for Research in Dairying at Reading in the U.K.—was released, the outlook for mastitis control was very grim. Then the atmosphere changed and has remained good since then, because the program satisfied the criteria set out previously. It requires very little additional labor, the farmer can readily understand why he is carrying out each technique, and each of them fits into the milking shed routine. In addition, it is very cheap, and the response is rapid and dramatic, provided the infection rate is moderately severe. The number of clinical cases subsides sharply, and the number and value of mastitis ointment tubes used provides even more tangible evidence of the beneficial effect of the program.

Most countries now employ a basic NIRD program but adapt it to suit their own circumstances. For example, it is universal now to add a monitoring segment to the control techniques, but it is not essential to do so in those countries where laboratory back-up is not available. In our experience, a reasonable evaluation of the program is that it can reduce the mastitis prevalence in a herd by two-thirds in one year and at a high cost-effectiveness, as indicated by a 300 to 500% return on the money invested in the program.

If veterinarians are involved in herd health programs and have constant access to sources of information about their clients' productivity, they are in a position to provide the ingredients that are essential in order to make this program run—to monitor the performance by way of cell count, to comment on the performance as shown by the graph of the herd average, and to advise on the most economical way in which the desired end result might be achieved.

The Epidemiologic Basis of the Control Program

The principal mastitides are those caused by the resident major pathogens, the obligate parasites that survive in the tissues of the host. Accordingly, the program devised to control them had to (1) *reduce the duration of the infection* in the donor host; and (2) reduce the rate at which the infection spread from the donor hosts while they were being eliminated. This reduction in spread is most simply expressed as *reducing the rate of new infections*.

Expressed in the simplest terms and at the least cost with the least disruption of the farmer's activities, this consisted of:

1. *Reducing the duration of the infection by:*
□ treating intensively during the dry period when the infections are most vulnerable and when most new infections begin
□ avoiding treatment during lactation because it is inefficient and because much loss of milk results from the prolonged withdrawal times. Only clinical cases should be treated during lactation, and a great deal of study needs to be given to selecting the treatment of choice
□ culling the chronic cases that do not eventually clear with repeated dry period treatments

2. *Reducing the new infection rate by:*
□ dipping all teats in an effective teat dip after each milking
□ backflushing teat cups and washing udder and teats before each cow is milked
□ ensuring that the milking machine is chosen, installed, and operated in such a way that least damage is done to mammary tissues and least infection is spread

METHODS OF MONITORING MASTITIS PREVALENCE

The purpose of the techniques that follow is to periodically assess the number of quarters affected by mastitis. This is not necessarily synonymous with knowing how many quarters have a specific infection. Infection is not necessarily equated with loss of milk production; however, the presence of inflammation, that is, mastitis, is accompanied by production wastage.

The objective may be to determine the existing state of mastitis in a hitherto unfamiliar herd or to repeat an assessment in a herd where prevalence is being monitored over a long period. In either case, the prime target of the investigation is subclinical mastitis, particularly that caused by *Staphylococcus aureus*, because of its insidious spread and irreversible damaging result.

The monitoring methods in significant use at present are (1) the individual cow somatic milk cell count; (2) the bulk milk cell count; (3) indirect chemical tests based on the cell content of the milk, such as the California Mastitis Test, with or without microbiological examination; (4) electrical conductivity; and (5) recording of clinical cases. There are many other indirect tests that have been largely discarded, mostly because they depended on a bacterial result. The emphasis at present is on detecting damage rather than infection. There are also a number of other tests currently being evaluated, but none appears to have the promise of those already in use.

Methods of surveillance set up to detect clinical mastitis are not to be neglected if an accurate record is to be maintained as part of a mastitis monitoring exercise.

Bulk Milk Cell Counts

Cell counts on bulked milk samples collected from storage vats at the farm and tested at the milk receiving depot have come to be recognized as a screening test for dairy herds. It is acknowledged that they are too inaccurate to be highly dependable as a diagnostic tool, but as a warning signal to indicate that a more intensive examination needs to be carried out, they are the first step in creating a state of awareness about mastitis in individual farmers. The use of automated cell counting machines brings these counts within the range of everyone, and the fact that they are being conducted is taken as the first sign that the farmer is ready to discuss a complete program.

The test is simple and requires only an automated cell counter such as a Coulter counter, which counts particles of a particular size, or a Fossomatic, which recognizes stained cell nuclei. The accuracy of the instruments used must always be a concern, and the instruments that count particles of a given size may mistakenly count aggregated casein micelles produced in milk that has been through a centrifugal pump on the farm (Hill et al. 1982; Hoare et al. 1982). The error can be avoided by prior heating of the sample to 55°C before fixing it. Fixing and staining of the samples must be done quickly. Fixation in formalin is preferred to fixation in glutaraldehyde. Fresh milk stored at 21°C is unsuitable for examina-

tion after 16 hours because of the disappearance of cells. The addition of dichromate keeps the milk suitable for testing for 14 days (Dohoo et al. 1981) and overcomes many of the logistic problems in the laboratory.

The bulk milk cell count used as a positive criterion is 300,000 cells per ml. in North America. A level of 500,000 is often used as a beginning standard. In some European countries levels of less than 300,000 are used. It is probably safest to interpret counts of less than 250,000/ml. as indications of good udder health and counts over 500,000 as indications of a serious mastitis problem. The problem in interpreting bulk milk cell counts is that the bulk milk represents a mixture of milks, all of which have been influenced by their own particular set of factors. These include:

□ infection, which exerts by far the greatest influence. But even within this category there are great variations. For example, *Streptococcus agalactiae* infections produce much higher cell counts than *Staphylococcus aureus* infections

□ the number of quarters infected, which will exert a large effect on the herd's cell count

□ cell counts that increase with age but are not due to age. The increase is due to the increasing prevalence of infection as the cow gets older

□ stage of lactation. It is only during the first week and the last few days of the lactation that the count is higher and then only by a factor of about two

□ a milk rise in summer months

□ diurnal and day-to-day variations without apparent reason

□ a diluting effect in herds that calve all year round. There will be only a few recently calved cows in the herd at one time. In seasonally calved herds, all the herd is likely to be recently calved or to be dried off at the same time

These sources of error limit the value of the bulk milk cell count. Attempts to improve its accuracy by combining a total cell count with an approximately differential cell count, based on cell size, have not been satisfactory (Meek and Barnum 1982). The use of a rolling three-month average is recommended to overcome the temporary changes that can occur for environmental reasons.

Although bulk milk cell counts—with or without differential bulk milk cell counts—are not sufficiently accurate to be used as a monitoring technique for mastitis status, they are useful as indicators of approximate pro-

Individual Quarters	**Cells/ml.**
Normal uninfected quarters	50,000–150,000
Quarters uninfected but with a history of previous infection	600,000
Composite Samples	
All quarters free of infection	100,000–250,000
Quarters harboring minor pathogens	200,000–500,000
Quarters harboring major pathogens	<600,000
Clinical cases	10 million

ductivity loss. Thus a 100,000 cell/ml. increase in bulk milk cell count has been equated with a loss of 13.26 liters milk/cow/month (Barnum and Meek 1982).

Individual Cow Milk Cell Counts

The availability of automatic cell counting equipment and the already collected milk samples for butterfat testing have been combined to create an enormous breakthrough in mastitis monitoring. There has been an extraordinary rapidity of acceptance of the technique, and the supporting evidence on which the choice should have been made is only now becoming available (Poutrel and Rainard 1982; Lindstrom et al. 1981; Geringer and Thierley 1982; Dohoo and Meek 1982).

Factors that affect somatic cell counts have been dealt with in the previous section, but the only significant factor at the level at which we are considering the counts—infection—need be considered. Suggested critical levels are shown at the top of this page.

The most suitable threshold level for normality is a composite sample with less than 250,000 cells/ml. Most common recommendations are for <500,000 cells/ml. For a single quarter, the normal threshold level is 300,000 cells/ml.

The cell count is interchangeable with the California Mastitis Test, and the conversion data are shown at the bottom of this page (Schneider and Jasper 1964).

Because knowledge about cell counts is still being collected, it is probably best to avoid being dogmatic about any of the figures quoted. The following generalizations are thought to be applicable:
- The relationship between cell count and infection status, based on a single count, is not strong and is best in herds and in cows that have a high level of infection with a major pathogen. The results are comparable within herds, but between herds there are large differences in what appear to be significant levels of cells (McDermott et al. 1982).
- Division of the cells on the basis of size into presumptive groups of leucocytes and tissue cells does not increase the accuracy of the test (Meek et al. 1980).
- The results are more accurate with quarter than with cow or herd samples (Lindstrom et al. 1982).
- Infections with minor pathogens cause cellular responses nearer to normal levels than to the responses caused by major pathogens.
- There is a strong relationship between high cell counts and lowered milk production, high CMT reaction, and a high prevalence of clinical cases (Gill and Holmes 1978), so that a culling program or the selection of cows for dry period therapy can be based on a cell count.
- The standard procedure is to test composite samples of all quarters from each cow. A positive result means that all quarters must be treated, which doubles the number that actually need treatment, assuming an average of two infected quarters per cow.
- Because milk samples for herd testing are collected four times in a lactation, four cell counts can be done. It is reasonable to make a decision on the basis of the mean of all counts, but the recommendation is to use the peak count of the four as the critical finding.
- For greatest accuracy, cows judged to be infected on the basis of composite samples and possibly by quarter cell counting or CMT plus culture should be examined for physical evidence of fibrosis, which warrants culling. The result of not doing any cultural examinations is the possibility of an unusual pathogen gaining a secure foothold in the herd.

CMT Score	**Individual Cow Cell Count** (Cells/ml.)	**Loss of Milk** Yield for Lactation (%)
Negative	0– 200,000	
Trace	150,000– 400,000	6.0
1	300,000–1,000,000	10.0
2	700,000–2,000,000	16.0
3	>2,000,000	25.0

Combined California Mastitis Test and Microbiological Examination

The California Mastitis Test is accurate in the hands of a skilled operator. Some farmers can handle it satisfactorily, but some won't because they have no confidence in their capacity to read the results consistently. Since it is based on the amount of cellular nuclear protein in the milk, it reflects the cell count accurately and has always been a reliable indication of the severity of the mastitis and the loss of potential milk yield. The relationship was shown in the table on page 95.

The test has the advantage that it can be used on a bulk milk sample or as an individual cow test. For individual cows, a trace is considered to be a positive test warranting further examination. For a herd test, the criteria are less severe, and for large herds, because of still further dilution, the criteria could be even less severe.

As a herd test, a grade 1 reaction should be interpreted as a positive indication of mastitis. About 18% of cows with mastitis in a herd will stimulate a grade 1 reaction. A grade 2 reaction suggests that a serious situation exists. The relationship between mean individual cell count and CMT is of the order of:

		Mean Individual Cell Count/ml.
CMT	negative	100,000
"	trace	300,000
"	1	900,000
"	2	2.7 million
"	3	8.1 million

A positive California Mastitis Test is a sufficiently accurate indicator that further examination can be dispensed with, except that recently calved and about-to-be-dried off cows are likely to give false-positives. For completeness, and to determine which bacteria is the causative agent, it is common practice to culture CMT positive samples and identify further the staphylococci as positive or negative coagulase producers, and the streptococci as being *Str. agalactiae* or *Str. nonagalactiae*. This sort of testing requires a bacteriology laboratory, costly human labor input, and a further delay of 48 hours. Also, a special sample must be collected and submitted. Although a composite sample may be used, it is worthwhile, having gone to this trouble, to base the tests on individual quarter samples.

A satisfactory report on a milk sample should include an assessment of the degree of inflammation (CMT or cell count), an identifi-cation of the bacteria, the number of colonies per loop, and an impression of its pathogenicity and sensitivity to antibiotics. A proportion (10 to 20%) of CMT positive samples will be bacteriologically sterile and should be recultured. They are interpreted as being infected but are negative on culture because the bacteria are intracellular in leucocytes.

Electrical Conductivity

Mastitic milk has a higher electrical conductivity than normal milk because of its higher electrolytic content, especially sodium and chloride ions. As a monitor of mastitis, the technique of measuring electrical conductivity is attractive, because a conductivity sensor could be introduced into the milk line and the normalcy of the milk from each cow, potentially each quarter, could be checked at each milking (Linzell and Peaker 1972). A further advantage is that a change in electrolytic content is the earliest change in the milk in mastitis, and electrical conductivity is therefore the earliest warning system. The lack of accuracy in the technique at present prevents its commercial use. Variations in sensitivity and specificity of the electrical conductivity (EC) between herds is the principal problem (Sheldrake and Hoare 1981), and predetermined thresholds of EC result in serious errors in some herds. Agreement between conductivity and cell counts is good (Mielke et al. 1981; Fernando, 1982), and there is no interference with the milking procedure. Conductivity above 6.9 m./cm.^{2} at 20 to 30° C is considered to be abnormal.

Hand-held conductivity meters are also available and are suitable for checking individual quarters, e.g., to determine response after treatment. They consist of a funnel into which the milk is squirted, a cell in which the milk to be tested is held, and a clockface indicator marked +, ?, and −.

Recording of Clinical Cases

This may seem simple enough, but farmers often need advice or a standard procedure to keep watch for clinical cases. Acceptable guidelines are:

- attention by observation or palpation of new asymmetry of the udder
- palpable hardness or soreness when washing or stripping the udder
- use of a strip cup with a black shiny top to detect watery milk before each milking when cows are milked in situ in a barn

- stripping of the foremilk onto the floor, preferably onto a black tile, in a milking parlor where the floor is constantly wet
- installation of stainless steel or plastic filters in the milk line on each handset. Clots are evident through the glass and, if they are heavy, the tube is blocked and the handset falls off.

MASTITIS CONTROL STRATEGIES

A mastitis control program should not be looked upon as a rigidly enforceable set of rules. There are a number of basic techniques, each of which can be enforced with varying degrees of strictness, and a number of additional techniques, each of which provides a small additional gain and which is usually applicable in a certain set of circumstances. For example, early and late dry period treatment may be applied in areas where summer mastitis is prevalent. In addition, there is a relatively large number of items, such as cleanliness and hygiene in the milking parlor, that have a supportive but probably immeasurable effect on mastitis control.

The program discussed in the following sections is basically the NIRD program adapted to an advanced dairy farming culture but set at varying levels depending on the economy of the local dairy industry. It is capable of still further fine tuning to fit the economic situation and the managerial expertise on a particular farm. It is the individual farm and its program that is the objective to keep in sight at all times. There is also a need to achieve the best financial gain for the least expenditure on that particular farm.

Area control is not a feasible objective, and national area programs have to be based essentially on an extension program that arouses enthusiasm for the introduction of mastitis control machinery and provides financial incentives to encourage farmers to participate. In most developed countries the adoption of effective programs lags far behind the potential level of adoption—usually the adoption rate is 25 to 35%.

There is another important feature of an effective program, which is that the war may be won in the milking parlor but the overall campaign is won or lost outside it. The golden rule for an area program is that there must be:
- a mastitis awareness program to sensitize the farmer group
- a herd test (e.g., the bulk milk count) to identify herds that have a problem
- an effective program

- a group of enthusiastic and knowledgeable veterinarians
- a monitoring system capable of marking progress

The most effective extension tool is the presence in the community of farmers who are pursuing mastitis control and who are acknowledged as early innovators and community leaders. Veterinarians in the community may need special attention if they are to be fully cooperative. One of the best encouragements is the incorporation of a mastitis control strategy into a planned herd health and management program. The teaming of mastitis control with maintenance of reproductive and productive efficiency and the control of other diseases tends to relieve the boredom of undiluted mastitis control.

The profitability of mastitis control programs is often discussed but seldom defined. Most arguments for the program are related to the dire effects of not using one or of withdrawing a herd from the program (Robinson et al. 1983). Computer programs (Kirk 1982) are available for calculating the cost-effectiveness of various mastitis control strategies. This subject is given some attention in a later section (Chapter 13).

The Basic Control Program

Much has been made of five-point programs to control mastitis because of the need to have farmers concentrate on the critical parts of the program. Listed here are the many other characteristics of a good mastitis program:
- If possible, select against families with a poor mastitis history and concentrate the breeding program away from them
- Do not feed mastitis milk to heifer calves, especially if they run together as groups
- Milk in a dairy that is easy to clean and disinfect
- Use only the most efficient milking machine, avoiding those features that predispose to mastitis
- *Maintain the milking machine properly* with 6-month checkups carried out by a qualified technician who also replaces worn parts
- Ensure a good, gentle, milking technique
- When examining the foremilk for clots, ensure that the Phillips method is used to prevent reflux from the perhaps transiently infected teat cistern back into the mammary gland itself. The base of the teat must be closed off before pressure is exerted on the teat to expel the milk. In herds with a high

quarter infection rate, failure to use this technique may lead to a further increase of infection.

□ Ensure that an adequate labor force is available for the number of cows to be milked

□ Avoid environmental conditions that result in coldness; wetness; muddiness of the udder; and chapping, cracking, and abrasions of the teats. In housed animals, ensure that the bedding is least likely to be a focus of infection

□ *Ensure early diagnosis of clinical cases and their prompt and efficient treatment*, e.g., use a strip cup

□ Give constant attention to maintenance of good health of teat skin

□ Constantly monitor for subclinical mastitis by individual somatic cell count or drying-off CM test

□ *Ensure effective teat dipping after each milking and after drying-off treatment*

□ *Provide dry period treatment* with a superior treatment in either the blanket mode or the selective treatment mode, depending on the quarter infection rate. In some circumstances this may need to be repeated

□ *Cull chronic subclinical* or repeating acute clinical cases of mastitis

□ Maintain accurate records on identification, clinical and laboratory findings, and treatment used

□ Ensure that the water supply is free from contamination by animal effluents

□ *Backflush teat cups after each cow* or provide chemical or heat disinfection if this is possible

□ Consider vaccination in circumstances in which results are not as good as might reasonably be expected

□ Avoid antibiotic residues in milk by limiting treatment in lactating cows to clinical cases

□ Avoid undertreatment with too small doses of antibiotic, which are likely to induce a state of antibiotic tolerance in pathogenic bacteria

□ If the herd is divided into groups based on stage of lactation, milk the freshest cows first.

However, for purposes of promotion through activities in the media or in talking to farmers, a simpler format is highly advantageous. What is shown below is a three-tiered program designed to be used at various levels in farms or areas of increasing enthusiasm or capacity to pay. Theoretically it would also be possible at the beginning of a campaign to start with the basic option and build on it gradually as the farmer developed enthusiasm for the program.

A three-level mastitis control program is as follows:

1. *The minimum level* is dry period treatment only and is capable of reducing the quarter infection rate to 15 to 18%.

2. *The medium level* program includes dry period treatment, teat dipping after milking, and special attention to milking machine function and use. This regularly reduces the quarter infection rate to 10%.

3. *The maximum level* includes teat dipping, dry period treatment, milking machine care and proper use, sanitation of teat cups and teats before each cow is milked, premilking stripping, and careful detection and treatment of subclinical cases in lactating cows. A quarter infection rate of 7% is not unusual with this strategy.

In all of the above it is assumed that lactating clinical cases will be dealt with adequately, chronic cases will be culled, and prevalence will be monitored. Dry period treatment will be blanket when the quarter infection rate is more than 15%, the bulk milk cell count is >500,000/ml., the average individual cow cell count is >250,000/ml., or there are four or more clinical cases/100 cows/30 days. Failure to carry out these tasks and observe these criteria could mean a serious deterioration in the level of control.

Individual Control Program Techniques

The following techniques are all basic to the control program but are capable of great flexibility and application at varying levels of intensity.

Dry Period Treatment

An awareness of the processes involved in drying off makes them more understandable. Milking is stopped, either because there is so little milk present that the labor of harvesting it is worth more than the milk or because the farm policy is to calve near a certain date, and all cows must have had a suitable 60-day rest period before that date. They may be dried off abruptly or by gradually dropping out milkings. The latter is particularly suited to cows that are still milking heavily, e.g., 10 kg./day or more.

New infections occur most commonly during the dry period, especially at the beginning and end of it (Smith and Todhunter 1982). At these times, the teats are distended, and there is often milk in the teat canal and a drip at the end. Infection passes easily through the dilated canal, and there is no flushing-out mechanism because the cow is not being milked. Although the method of drying off has no effect on subsequent milk yields, the abrupt technique can cause an increased rate of new infections, especially if there is a mastitis problem in the herd already.

The factors that increase the chances of new infection during the dry period are:
☐ distention of teat cistern and canal, which facilitates entry of infection
☐ lack of flushing action
☐ lowest cell count in milk when it is most dilute, favoring invasion
☐ level of infection of teat skin likely to be greatest in a herd in which mammary infection is commonest.

The obvious control measures at this time are to avoid overdistention of the udder, i.e., dry off slowly; infuse dry period treatment; infuse a teat sealer to block the teat canal; and disinfect teat skin frequently during the most dangerous periods.

The efficacy of dry period treatment in reducing the number of infected quarters and the number of new infections during the dry period is now well established. The two areas that are still being strongly debated are the wisdom of blanket treatment as opposed to selective dry period therapy and which is the most cost-effective preparation to be used.

Blanket Versus Selective Dry Period Therapy. The original recommendation was to treat all quarters and to avoid laboratory involvement. Since then it has become evident that the cost of treating uninfected quarters is high and that there might be disadvantages in removing all infections from the quarters. This latter argument has gained strength from recently acquired knowledge about the role of minor pathogens in encouraging greater resistance to other infection. Currently it is customary to advise that all quarters in the herd be treated if the bulk milk cell count is >500,000 cells/ml. for any single examination or if the quarter infection rate in the herd is more than 15%. Below this, selective treatment is recommended. This may take several forms:

1. If the quarters have been individually examined, then treat only the positive quarters. This will inevitably miss those quarters that become infected after the examination and the new infections that occur during the first four weeks of the dry period, the period during which the dry period treatment can be assumed to be effective.

2. The alternative to (1) is to treat all quarters in those cows in which one or more quarters have been found to be affected. This recommendation is based on the high probability that the next infected quarter will be in a cow that is already infected in another quarter.

3. A compromise program is to treat known infected quarters with a major agent such as benzathine cloxacillin and the remainder with a newer product such as procaine penicillin 100,000 units or streptomycin 0.5 g.

4. In cows found positive on a composite sample, treat all quarters. The alternative would be to examine these cows more closely to identify the individual infected quarters; this is not recommended because of the high additional cost.

All selective treatment programs have the drawback that they will miss new infections in the first month of the dry period. Proponents of the selective therapy approach feel that the saving in cost (up to 70% reduction) more than compensates for the loss incurred by the new infections. Real cost comparisons are shown in Table 5–1. There are no hard data on which to base an authoritative opinion. Nor are there data on which to base the commonly stated view that blanket dry cow therapy of all quarters makes a herd more susceptible to the opportunist coliforms (Marr 1978). The final statement on the subject is that none of the

Table 5–1. COMPARISON OF COSTS OF VARIOUS
DRY PERIOD TREATMENT STRATEGIES*

		Selective Treatment		
Item	Blanket	Special Visit	Herd Health Visit	Cell Count On Free Sample
Drug costs	$900.00	$135.00	$135.00	$270.00
Examination costs	Nil	250.00	200.00	100.00
Total	900.00	385.00	335.00	370.00

*Based on drug costs of $2.25 per tube, milk test in a herd health program of $2/cow, at a special visit $2.50 per cow, in herds of 100 cows.

selective treatment strategies have been shown to be more effective than the blanket treatment (Philpot 1977), which does not take into account the fringe benefits of having the results of the mastitis program under constant review.

Selection of Quarters for Dry Period Treatment. The subject of monitoring quarter infections for selective dry period treatment has not been examined in great detail. The two most common methods used, as described previously under mastitis monitoring techniques, are serial individual cow cell counts during lactation and application of the California Mastitis Test in the period just prior to drying off.

Individual cell counting has the disadvantage that when the quarter infection rate is low, a large number of quarters will be treated unnecessarily because the test only identifies the cow, and all the quarters must be treated on the infected cows. It would be possible to recheck each cow in order to find which quarter is infected, but this would be a costly exercise. Examination of each quarter with the California Mastitis Test avoids this difficulty but is probably not as accurate in its identification of cows. A single examination four weeks before drying off has an accuracy of 80%; two examinations four and eight weeks before drying off have an accuracy of 90% (Poutrel and Rainard 1981).

The recommended procedure in herds with a quarter infection rate of greater than 15% is to treat all quarters in all cows—blanket therapy. Where the infection rate is less than this, selective dry period therapy should be practiced. The method of selecting quarters to be treated in year-round herds where regular monthly visits are made and cows are dried off in approximately equal numbers each month is a CMT at the last visit, cultural examination of all quarters with a trace result, and treatment of all quarters showing a 1+ or a trace plus positive culture with a known pathogen. Unless the cultural examination is made, many quarters with minor pathogen infections will be treated unnecessarily. Alternative recommendations are to rely on the CMT alone carried out at eight and four weeks before drying off and to treat all quarters in cows that show one infected quarter.

In herds that calve all the cows as near as possible to the same date, the above monitoring procedure is not possible. The amount of laboratory work involved during a brief period of two months would present a logistic problem of the greatest magnitude. Individual cow cell counts are the prevailing technique. They are usually carried out on milk already collected for butterfat testing, but failing that, a special sample is usually collected as described previously at eight and four weeks before the expected drying-off date. Automatic counting equipment makes it possible to test enormous numbers of samples quickly.

The number of counts and thus the accuracy of the technique vary, but the greater the number of counts, the greater the accuracy. A New Zealand system based on five tests of milk for butterfat content during the lactation, followed by treatment of all cows with mean cell counts of greater than 300,000 cells/ml., has been highly successful in terms of milk yield gains (McMillan et al. 1980). This procedure of measuring success by improvement in productivity has an appearance of greater relevance than relating a positive finding to the presence or absence of a major pathogen. Australian workers (Nicholls et al. 1982) have also demonstrated this relationship. Their observed relationship between high cell counts (peak of four counts at 300,000 cells/ml.) and infection had an accuracy of 70 to 75%.

The original New Zealand work included a classification of cows into three groups on the basis of average milk cell count for the lactation: (1) very high cell counts—about 4% of the herd to be culled; (2) high cell count >300,000/ml.—treat at drying off and expect improved yield in early lactation; (3) low/normal cell counts—cows not given dry period treatment.

An innovative use of this cow cell count information is the development of a computer program that estimates the loss of potential milk yield caused by a particular cell content, and also the economic loss that will probably result (Kirk 1982).

Summary of Criteria. Cows to receive dry period treatment are:

Bulk milk cell count >500,000	
Four or more clinical cases/100 cows/ three days	Treat all quarters all cows
Q.I.R. >15%	
Individual cell count average all cows >250,000	

Individual cows with
 peak composite cell
 count >250,000
Cows that had clini-
 cal mastitis during
 lactation
Q.I.R <15%
CMT >trace plus posi-
 tive culture major
 pathogen (May opt to
 treat *only* the positive
 quarters)

Treat only
these cows

The thresholds quoted are notational only. At the present time, they are being lowered at frequent intervals. They are also capable of being adjusted upward or downward as a program progresses.

Timing of the Dry Period Treatment. This should be applied to each cow individually immediately after the last milking for the lactation and creates no problem in herds that milk cows year round. In seasonal herds, farmers would prefer to dry off their herd gradually over a period of two or three weeks and then treat them all. This is a dangerous procedure and not recommended because of the probability that new infections will be allowed to develop unchecked in this most dangerous segment of the dry period. It also provides a better chance for the udder infusion to cause a chemical mastitis. If the quarter is still full of milk, the treatment is diluted; if it has been dry for two weeks, there is much less dilution and some compounds, e.g., tetracyclines, are too irritant to be infused at this time.

When a year-round herd is on a herd health program, the usual procedure is for the veterinarian to examine the cows at the last visit before drying off and then to supply the treatment, usually 48 hours later. Another recommended program is to identify the quarters at an earlier meeting eight weeks before drying off (Poutrel and Rainard 1981).

If treatment is to be repeated during the dry period, this should be done about three weeks before calving and the milk kept out of the vat for the next four weeks.

Technique of Dry Period Treatment. The clean dry teats to be treated should have their ends defatted and swabbed clean with methyl or propyl alcohol, taking care to evert the tip end. Strip out enough milk to ensure that the quarters are not going to leak after the manipulation. Insert the tube or other medicament and dip the treated teat in a disinfectant teat dip such as 5% tincture of iodine after cleansing it with sodium hypochlorite. Repetition of the teat dipping on several occasions during the first week of the dry period effectively reduces the new infection rate of *Staphylococcus aureus*.

Choice of Dry Period Treatment. Benzathine cloxacillin in 500-mg. doses (Orbenin Dry Cow) has led the market for a long time and is undoubtedly an excellent product. It has a cure rate of about 85% for *Staphylococcus aureus* and over 90% for *Streptococcus agalactiae*. Spontaneous cure rates for these infections are about 30% (Pankey et al. 1982). Neopen D.C. White (neomycin sulfate 500 mg. and benzathine penicillin 325,000 units) has approximately the same result. A combination of procaine penicillin (1×10^6 units) and dihydrostreptomycin 1 g. is also effective at the same level. Smaller doses, e.g., procaine penicillin 100,000 units plus 100 mg. dihydrostreptomycin, or neomycin 500 mg., are much less effective—with the 50 to 60% cure rate range for staphylococci.

Post-treatment Monitoring. A good mastitis control program will include a system of keeping a check on the mastitis of a herd. This can be done by one of the following: (1) number of clinical cases recorded; (2) number of tubes of mastitis ointment used; (3) periodic weekly or monthly checks by the milk depot on the bulk milk cell counts or California Mastitis Tests on bulk samples; (4) monthly checks of cows about to be dried off.

Other Dry Period Techniques

Besides the standard programs outlined previously there are several additional innovative programs being tested.

Levamisole Treatment During Dry Period. The cows are injected at weekly intervals with 2.5 mg./k. BW weekly for six weeks, the last injection usually four weeks before calving and always at least two weeks before. A dramatic reduction in the number of clinical cases in the postparturient period is reported in one study (Flesh et al. 1982), but no effect was observed in another in which the cows also received standard dry period treatments with antibiotics (Ziv et al. 1981). Additional benefits have also been recorded in the reduction of number of fetal deaths and the occurrence of mastitis after similar levamisole treatment (Flesh et al. 1982).

The treatment is based on the known effect of levamisole of enhancing immunity at a time when blood levels of humoral antibody are at a very low level at parturition.

Intramammary Polyethylene Devices. The insertion of polyethylene loops or spirals into quarters of bovine udders causes a rise of somatic cell counts, especially in the foremilk and in the strippings. A similar rise in the midstream milk is of short duration. A significant reduction in susceptibility to experimentally induced infection results (Brooks and Barnum 1982; Paape 1982). The diminution in susceptibility appears to be related to the degree of somatic cell increase in the foremilk. Infection does not occur when the cell count exceeds 9×10^5/ml. (Paape et al. 1981), but not many counts reach this level, most being about 5 to 6×10^5/ml. (Jasper et al. 1982). There are varying reports about whether the devices reduce the volume of milk produced. There may be a decrease of 2.4 kg./day/cow (Jasper et al. 1982). The devices are approximately 2 mm. in diameter and 115 mm. long in a loop 25 mm. across.

Induced Mammary Involution. Involution can be hastened by the infusion of the quarter with a tissue-damaging agent such as colchicine or *E. coli* endotoxin at the end of the lactation. The procedure reduces the new infection rate in the early part of the dry period, but the rate returns to normal later in the same dry period (Oliver and Smith 1982).

The Milking Machine

Not all the mastitic ills of the past 50 years can be attributed to the milking machine, but there is no doubt that a poorly designed, badly constructed, and negligently used machine can wreak havoc in an otherwise well-run herd of dairy cows. A summary of recommendations for milking machine use follows. If these are adhered to carefully, it will be a reasonable expectation that mastitis will not be a problem, unless there are serious errors in hygiene.

In this section, the subject of milking machine construction, use, and maintenance is dealt with briefly. For those veterinarians who include milking machine surveillance in their herd health programs, more detailed discussions are available (Thompson 1977; Britt 1977; Noorlander and Heckman 1980, 1981, 1982; Williams and Mein 1982; McDonald 1971), but some knowledge of the milking machine is necessary for all veterinarians who work with dairy cattle.

The Role of the Milking Machine. The milking machine has relevance to mastitis in a number of ways:

□ It carries infection from cow to cow in the herd. This occurs principally by the physical removal of the cups contaminated with infected milk from one cow and applying them untreated to the teats of another cow. It is also possible that momentary reverse flow of milk during milking may do the same thing.

□ It aids the transfer of infection from quarter to quarter in the same cow during milking. This occurs because of circulation of milk within the cluster as a result of reverse flow due to vacuum fluctuation.

□ The milking machine encourages the penetration of the teat canal by particles of milk carrying bacteria derived from the colonized skin of the teat; the environment, e.g., dirty wash-water; or transfer from another teat. The vacuum pressure of the machine dilates the teat sphincter and canal and then jets the particles of milk at the sphincter as a result of abrupt removal of the cups or by liner slip.

□ It causes damage to the skin, especially at the teat end. These erosions are prime sites for colonization with major mastitis pathogens. The probability of mastitis developing from one of these sites is high because of the proximity of the lesion of the teat sphincter.

Desirable Standards for Machine Functioning. The desirable standards for good machine function (Schroder 1968) are shown at the bottom of this page.

Level of vacuum pressure at meter	50 kPa (or 15 in./37.5 cm. Hg)
Vacuum pressure at meter in high-line installation	43–50 kPa (12.5–13.5 in./31.3–38.8 cm. Hg)
High-line installation	48–50 kPa (14–15 in./35–37.5 cm. Hg)
Level of vacuum at teat cup under full load	40–42 kPa (11–12 in./27.5–30 cm. Hg)
Minimum vacuum residual for massage	20 kPa (6 in./15 cm. Hg)
Reserve capacity of vacuum pump	1 cfm. (28 l./min.)
Pulsation rate	40–60/min. (with preference for close to 40)
Ratio of vacuum to rest in cycle	50:67
Ratio of milk to rest in cycle	35:65 to 65:35
Claw-piece air bleed	7 l./min. (¼ cfm.) of free air per claw piece

Vacuum Pressure Errors. The vacuum pressure should not exceed the manufacturer's recommendations, which are available in the machine's service manual. When checking the machine's pressure, it is best to utilize an independent vacuum meter, which is periodically checked for accuracy, because the machine's meter may be inaccurate. It is surprising how few of them are not accurate when one considers the dusty, humid atmosphere in which they operate.

Standard pressure recommendations are 15 in. (37.5 cm.) Hg or 50 kPa. Higher pressures cause teat damage—especially at the end, encourage the entrance of mastitic organisms, and result in higher cell counts and C.M.T. readings (Langlois et al. 1981). Lower than normal pressures increase milking time and allow the cups to fall off but are not causes of mastitis.

Excessive pressure can be created very briefly if the cups are forcibly removed without releasing the vacuum. It is a fairly common problem when the milker is trying to cut corners and to milk too many cows. A similar effect results from not releasing the vacuum before pulling the cups off. Too much weight being exerted on the handpiece when carrying out machine stripping also has this effect. Excessive pressure may also develop in a part of a system, e.g., if the air vent in the claw is blocked or if there is a blockage in a long milk line that isolates the vacuum meter. In the latter case, the pressure in the unblocked part of the system may be elevated to 50% above normal. A particular local error is when the air vent at the end of the claw—which is essential for the onward passage of milk—becomes blocked, causing milk to accumulate in the liner and exert excessive pressure on the teat.

The increased pressure in the milking system is transferred to the end of the teat and, when the teat sinus is open, to the interior of the mammary gland. The effect on the teat end is to cause, in sequence, engorgement and chapping, eversion of the sphincter first presenting as a prominence and then as an obvious prolapse, erosion, the development of a sore, and then a scab and eventually "black spot" or "black pox." Mastitis due to mixed infection, especially gram-negative organisms, is a common sequela. These teats are very painful, and affected cows will interrupt the milking by kicking off the cups and will fail to let milk down properly and this will result in a decline in yield. Permanent obstruction of the teat canal may also be a sequela.

A side issue in the vacuum pressure discussion is the comparison between the low-line and high-line milking machines. The latter are the more modern design and are usually associated with heavily capitalized new installations. They are a great improvement on low-line machines in the matter of moving milk and in maintaining milk quality, and they also appear to have a beneficial effect on udder health (Gudding and Lorentzen 1982). The effect on mastitis occurrence is not due just to vacuum pressure, because although the general pressure in the line is lower than in a high-line, the pressure at the teat is slightly higher. However, it is more stable, and this lack of fluctuation in vacuum may be the important factor.

INADEQUATE VACUUM RESERVE. Large fluctuations in vacuum pressure are caused by an inadequate reserve of vacuum pressure in the pump and vacuum tank. These fluctuations are associated with an increase in the new infection rate, but the exact reason for this is not known. It might be the result of a reverse flow of milk when the pressure drops. Fluctuations exceeding 5 cm. Hg in a long-line bucket system and 7.5 cm. in a milking parlor milk line are thought to be excessive. The method of measurement is to stuff a vacuum gauge into a milking cup while all the other handsets are in use. If the fluctuations last for more than five seconds, the machine needs a technical inspection.

Reverse Flow of Milk. Reversal of flow of milk in a machine has serious consequences. It may cause a transfer of infective material from one cow and her set of cups to an adjoining clean cow. It may also cause a transfer of infectious material from one teat cup and its resident teat to another teat cup on the same cow. Reverse flow can occur when the milk line diameter is too small. This is most likely at peak flows and, for example, when Jersey cows are replaced by Holstein-Friesians or when the number of milking stands is increased without increasing the milk line diameter. It may also occur when the milk tube from the cluster or the liner tube is inadequate to take peak milk flow. Reverse flow is a characteristic of high-line milkers and is unlikely to occur in low-line machines.

Reverse flow can also occur at the end of milking if there is too little milk in the pipe system. This is avoided when automatic units are installed that remove the cups when milk flow falls below a certain rate (Philpot 1972).

Duration of Milking—Overmilking. Some

of the same effects occur with overmilking, i.e., leaving the cups on after milk flow has ceased, as occurs with excessive vacuum pressure. However, damage to the teat end is not as marked and under experimental conditions (Natzke et al. 1982) does not occur at all. There is a much greater transfer of infection from infected to uninfected quarters when overmilking is a problem, but the increase in mastitis may not be very great if the infection rate is very low. In herds where the infection rate is high to begin with, a serious exacerbation in subclinical mastitis is likely, and clinical cases will also be more frequent. This is partly due to the increased rate of spread of infection and also to injury to the lining of the teat canal and cistern caused by milking a dry teat, which tends to be crammed into the cup. When individual quarters are lighter than others on the same cow, removal of individual cups can be carried out if there are sight glasses in the milk lines from each cup.

The optimum time of milking per cow varies with the amount of milk flow and the size of the teat cistern and the diameter of the canal. However, four minutes is a good average milking time for a herd. Average times of more than six minutes are taken to indicate poor equipment or labor.

Too Rapid Removal of Milking Machine Cluster/Liner Slip. Abrupt removal of the cluster, especially if the vacuum pressure has not been released, is a potent means of increasing the new infection rate. The effect is to jet milk from the cup and the milk tube back up through the dilated teat canal, thus increasing the chance of infection from other infected quarters of the same cow. The same effect is achieved when the negative pressure in the udder is made greater than that in the teat cup by serious overmilking. Liner slip is another cause of excessive turbulence of milk within the liner and of jetting of milk toward the sphincter at the end of the teat.

Shields fitted in the base of the liners deflect the surge of milk that would otherwise jet up into the teat and udder cisterns. They are credited with controlling most of the new infections that would otherwise occur (Griffin et al. 1982). They are of major importance as a defense against the bacteria that do not colonize the teat skin—the opportunist invaders, especially *E. coli.*

Number of Stands per Milker. The number of machines, handsets, and milking stands that one person can handle efficiently varies. Because of the cost of labor there is always a

great pressure to increase the number of cattle, and contemporary milking parlors, e.g., the carousel, are very heavily capitalized with automatic machinery to reduce the need for human participation. Therefore, there is a tendency for overmilking to occur unless mechanical cup removers are installed. Even with their use, errors can still occur if they are not properly installed and maintained.

Pulsation Rate. Although the pulsation rate is more important to the efficiency of milking than to udder health, there is a connection. Recommended pulsation rates vary from 40 to 60/min., with most machines recommending 40. Slower rates mean slower milk harvesting and may cause discomfort due to the prolonged squeeze on the teats. Faster rates result in insufficient time for the teat to refill after emptying. As a result, the teat is gradually crumpled and crammed into the liner. It is assumed that this causes damage to the mucosa and the sphincter. It has also been observed that there is a greater infection rate of quarters when the inflation rate is too high and the period of liner closure is insufficient (Reitsma et al. 1981).

Teat Cup Liners (Inflations). Construction of the inflations is now realized to be an important factor in maintaining udder health. The bore and length of the liner are critical. At the present time all liners are small bore (2 cm.) with varying diameters and with additional length, because short liners pinch teat ends and cause injury, and wide-bore (2.5 to 3.0 cm.) liners also cause injury. A combination of short liners and overmilking is very damaging to the end of the teat. Long liners do not squeeze the end of the teat. It is also important that the mouth of the liner not damage the base of the teat or leave too much milk in the udder.

The composition of the liner is important. The original natural gum rubber inflations were relatively nonporous, which was good, but they were insufficiently firm. Synthetic rubbers, which have been used for many years, have firmness but may be too firm for teat comfort, and the material is relatively porous. Silastic (silicone rubber) is experiencing a wave of popularity because of the ease with which it can be cleaned. Other rubbers rapidly develop cracks, which become filled with fat and make disinfection increasingly inefficient (Noorlander and Hickman 1980, 1981, 1982).

When the liners are being placed in the cups, it should be obvious that they do not have to be stretched a great deal or distorted to fit them to the cups. They should also be long enough so that they can collapse completely below the teat and not pinch it as described previously. They should have an effective barrel length of 14 cm.

Care of liners has always been a prime concern in dairy management, and techniques for cleaning and sterilizing them after milking and disinfecting them between cows have undergone much scrutiny. Liners that are used for too long lose their shape and resilience. They are then slower at milking and likely to cause teat damage. Cracking can also be a problem, and cracked, misshapen and saggy liners should be discarded. It is bad policy to discard one of a set. The others milk less rapidly than the new ones, so that some teats are still being milked when milk has ceased to flow. These teats are then crammed into the cup, and damage is likely to occur.

The problems with teat cup liners stem from the fat in the milk, which clogs up the pores in the rubber liner, making it difficult to disinfect and leading to loss of resilience, to cracking, and to milk stone, a mineral deposit resulting from hard water and minerals in milk. Depending on the nature of the liner, there is a need to periodically clean the liners to remove these deposits and to prolong the efficient life of the equipment. There are many efficient milk line cleansers available.

Teat Dipping

Dipping of the teats of all cows immediately after each milking and dry period treatment are the backbone of the modern mastitis control program. The realization that dipping at this time, rather than the procedure of disinfecting the teat before milking, which had been the standard recommendation for many years, completely revolutionized mastitis control. It was based on the observation that bacterial colonization of the teat skin occurred during the period between milkings and that if the skin could be disinfected and kept disinfected between milkings, the new infection rate was much less. The technical achievement that made it all possible was the development of teat dips, which would have a residual effect on teat skin for a long period and would not be greatly affected by having the teats dragged through water or long grass and which would not damage the skin. One deficiency of the dips in use at present is that they are effective against streptococci and staphylococci but not against coliforms.

The sprays are much easier to apply and are preferred by farmers to the dips, but they are more wasteful, much of the fluid being lost in the air. They are also likely to be diluted beyond their effective concentration so that they will pass through the spray. The most effective means is to dip the teats in the liquid. A colored liquid such as an organic iodide, especially iodophors, is preferred because it discolors the skin and provides evidence that it is being used (Meek 1981).

Choice of Teat Dip. Only post-milking teat dipping is recommended, premilking disinfection having little discernible effect on the new infection rate (Sheldrake and Hoare 1983). Iodophor solutions containing 1% of available iodine, hypochlorite solutions containing 4% of free chlorine and very low levels of alkali, and chlorhexidine 0.5 to 1% in polyvinylpyrrolidone solution or as a 0.3% aqueous solution are well known to be effective. Clorox, a commercial bleach powder (U.S.), meets the requirements of a teat dip, but most other commercial hypochlorites are too irritant to teat skin and hands. The choice between these compounds can be decided on price because of their equal efficiency as teat dips (Natzke and Bray 1973; Schultze and Smith 1972). Other teat dips reported to reduce the new infection rate by more than the required 40% are chlorhexidine digluconate (0.5%) with glycerine (6%) (Hicks et al. 1981), quaternary ammonium compound (0.5%) (Stewart and Philpott 1982), and dodecyl benzene sulfonic acid (Barnum et al. 1982).

The biggest problem with teat dips is chapping of the teats that occurs in some herds. Glycerine is the best emollient, but care must be taken not to add too much because it does reduce the bactericidal efficiency of the dip (Sheldrake et al. 1980). Lanolin or mineral (paraffin) oil is also used, the latter being a favorite do-it-yourself mix with a bad record of reducing the efficiency of the dip. Soluble lanolin does not have this problem and is highly recommended. Another efficient emollient is a mixture of methylglucoside and urea.

A problem is reported with iodine residues in milk, purported to result from enthusiastic use of an iodophor teat dip. These dips are now prohibited in some areas under pure food legislation (Sheldrake et al. 1980). A teat sealant that creates a film of acrylic latex over the end of the teat has achieved some currency because of its efficiency against new coliform infections of the udder, but it appears to lack effectiveness against invasion by gram-positive organisms (Farnsworth 1980).

Premilking Techniques

Teat Cup Disinfection. The currently favored method of reducing the chances of spread of infection via the teat cups is to flush them with cold water after each cow. The milk line from the cluster is plugged into an automatically operated nipple, which flushes water back through the milk line and out through the cups, which are then immediately applied to the cow standing opposite in the parlor. A warm water method has been described (Box and Ellis 1978).

The alternative methods are boiling water pasteurization, which creates difficulties in herringbone parlors where speed of throughput is paramount, and chemical disinfection. The latter is so often misused that it is probably best not to contemplate it.

Where the lowest possible quarter infection rate is desired, this technique should be included. However, it does require more work in the parlor, the mechanical equipment installed to do the work automatically has a habit of breaking down, and the operation is commonly omitted. If the prevalence of mastitis is high, it should be included in the program.

Premilking Preparation of Teats and Udder. The usual premilking technique is to wash the teats and lower udder with running water, which should preferably be warmed. This has largely replaced chemical disinfection and relies on physical dilution of the existing skin contamination. Concurrent massage of the area promotes let-down of the milk and faster milking out. Chemical disinfection of the area is still practiced when water supplies are short, but care must be taken to avoid contaminating the disinfectant wash water and to use either paper towels or to boil cloth towels between single cow uses. The same chemicals used in teat dips are applicable here but in a much greater dilution. Hibitane, a diguamide disinfectant, is suitable at a concentration of 4 to 8 g./L.; quaternary ammonium compounds as 0.2%, iodophors at 100 ppm. of free iodine, or sodium hypochlorite at 800 to 1200 ppm. free chlorine are all suitable for the purpose if used in accordance with the manufacturer's directions.

Teat Stripping. It is a common practice to squirt out a few streams of milk while preparing the udder. Clots in the milk will be observed, and let-down will be stimulated. Care is needed with the procedure because when the infection rate in the herd is high, there are likely to be many transient infections in the milk in the teat cistern. If the teat is carelessly squeezed, some of the milk in the cistern will reflux back up into the udder and may carry the otherwise innocuous infection up with it to invade the mammary tissue. If care is taken to block off the teat at its base and then strip out the milk, this danger can be everted. This premilking stripping, preferably just before washing, combined with stripping at the very end of milking is thought to increase the new infection rate, but the effect is likely to be small unless there is already a high rate of infection.

Because infection can be spread by contaminated hands, care must be taken when premilking hand stripping is practiced. A bucket of disinfectant should be available for washing between cows, especially after known infected cows have been handled. In circumstances where the infection rate is high, the hands should be rubbed with antiseptic cream at the end of each milking. Colonization of human skin by major mastitis pathogens should be kept in mind as a potential source of infection.

Stripping at the end of milking should be avoided except by exerting light pressure on the handset.

Genetic Selection Against Mastitis

There are conflicting views about the genetic susceptibility of cows to mastitis (Gonyon et al. 1982), in most cases due to failure to identify the site of operation of any resistance or susceptibility mechanism. There does not appear to be any direct relationship between total milk yield and increased susceptibility (Miller et al. 1981), although there is conflicting evidence. Differences in susceptibility between breeds appear to be well established, also without the mechanism being identified (Grootenhuis et al. 1979; Grootenhuis 1981). For example, genetic variations in susceptibility to *Str. agalactiae* and high cell counts have been established, but it is unlikely that much selection pressure will be mounted against these or other susceptibilities. Much of the work is equivocal, and no indicator test has been developed (Miller and Schultze 1981).

Although the heritability of teat size and shape and udder size is not accurately identified, there are some minor relationships between these factors and mastitis prevalence. A difference is apparent in the susceptibility to *Staph. aureus* infection in cylindrical as contrasted to funnel-shaped teats, the latter being more susceptible (Bakken 1981). Teats with pointed ends also suffer from more teat-end erosions than others. Fast milking cows, which are likely to have easily dilated teat canals and are therefore likely to be more susceptible to mammary infection, are thought to have high susceptibility (Pearson and Mackie 1979), but it would seem to be unwise to select against fast milkers for this reason.

Other Miscellaneous Control Measures

Feeding Mastitis Milk to Calves. This has been a convenient way of disposing of an unwanted material but is not recommended if heifer calves are run together, for fear the infection may be introduced into the immature udders when the calves suck each other. Provided the calves are kept in separate pens, there is no apparent systemic infection in the calves and no increase in mastitis subsequently (Barto et al. 1982).

Segregation of the Herd and Order of Milking. Segregation of groups within a herd for the purposes of mastitis control would be an unusual strategy. Any partition of a herd these days is for the purpose of regulating feed supply to cows in early lactation and for purposes of concentrating the breeding group for best accuracy in estrus detection. If there is an opportunity to segregate into groups, the plan should be to milk the heifers first and the aged cows last. Further segregation could be on the basis of mastitis history or somatic cell count status. Determining which is the optimum milking order would be an excellent task for a computer program.

Bedding and Bed Stalls. The bedding may significantly affect the rate of infection with *E. coli*. Wet sawdust is the worst vehicle for the infection, shavings are next on the list, and straw is the least likely to initiate infection. Sand appears to be safe. Another factor in bedding is that it appears to be safest when it is left undisturbed. Fluffing it up to make it look nice may bring heavily contaminated material to the surface where it achieves close contact with the teat skin.

Special precautions must be taken if a control program is to be mounted against mastitis due to opportunist invaders such as *E. coli*, and these are discussed under the heading of special programs (p. 109).

Stall beds are an important risk area for mastitis in housed cattle (Klastrup 1981). Cubicles in loose housing have the lowest prevalence over tie stalls, which are better than loose housing, with the cows reclining unconstrained on a strawpack. If stalls or cubicles are too short, the risk is higher because of contamination of, and damage to, the udder by the curb.

Rearing Calves on Nurse Cows. Calves sucking nurse cows with mastitis may spread infection to other cows if allowed to suck them, or they may spread infection between quarters in the one cow. The heifer cows may then spread it to each other.

Disposal of Infected Milk. Hygienic disposal of the milk and cleaning of contaminated utensils are logical procedures.

Amputation of the Tail. This procedure has been touted as an aid to mastitis control, but no relationship exists. It has advantages of the comfort and perhaps the health of the person milking the cows.

Drying Off of Chronic Mastitic Quarters. Cows that have one or more functionless quarters that contain only pus tend to be culled. However, it may be desirable to retain a valuable breeding cow. In those animals, it is advisable to dry up the quarter by chemical means. An infusion with silver nitrate (30 to 60 ml. of a 3% solution) or copper sulfate (20 ml. of a 5% solution) or other chemical escharotic agent is the usual means. The infusion is left in the quarter for 10 to 14 days, but if a severe reaction with painful swelling occurs, the quarter is stripped out several times. Quarters containing a lot of pus may need to be treated on several occasions.

Health of Teat Skin. The importance of maintaining healthy teat skin is gravely underestimated by farmers. Sores and cracks on the teats provide excellent opportunities for colonization and then infection of the mammary gland by the gram-positive major pathogens. What is required is regular treatment with a teat dip containing an emollient such as soluble lanolin, or the vigorous use of an antibiotic ointment. Chlorhexidine or iodophor creams are most valued.

Culling of Chronic Cases. This is a very much neglected technique, especially in large herds where cows lose their identities. Problem cows tend to be missed unless there is a computerized herd health program in place that flags a cow that has more than a specified number (usually three) of attacks of clinical mastitis. These cows are then brought in for examination and consideration for disposal. The history and examination of the milk—physically on the strip cup and by cell count and culture in the laboratory—will be important, but a careful clinical examination of the teats and udder by palpation to detect serious fibrosis is a very illuminating procedure that can reveal irreparable damage to the quarter or quarters. Farmers are often reluctant to cull cows with a good productive and reproductive record. They really need access to a computer simulation model of mastitis in a dairy herd that will demonstrate the consequences of leaving an active spreader of infection in a loosely guarded, highly susceptible population of cows.

Infection-free Water Supply. The opportunist infections such as *E. coli* and especially *Pseudomonas* spp. can achieve very high populations in water if the supply is heavily contaminated by effluents containing animal fecal material. If the water is used for udder and teat washing, premilking preparation, and back-flushing of teat cups, large numbers of bacteria will be lodged in the environment immediately surrounding the teat sphincter. Any machine or milking error that then jets fluid up against a dilated teat canal can precipitate a new infection.

Avoidance of Developing Resistance in Bacteria. Extensive use of low levels of antibiotic in treatment, especially dry period treatment, can encourage the development of strains of bacteria that can tolerate the presence of high levels of the same antibiotic. Strains of these bacteria can then be produced that, because of their resistance to antibiotics, present large problems in mastitis control. Staphylococcal mastitis is an example of a mastitis that is much less susceptible to penicillin than it used to be, for this reason.

Avoidance of Creating Toxic Residues in Milk. It has become very important, for human public health reasons, to keep antibiotics out of the human food chain, in this instance milk. A withdrawal time of 72 hours of all milk from a lactating cow that has been treated intramammarily means that a lot of milk is lost from sale. This means that the treatment of lactating cows is less than popular. The intramammary infusion of large volumes of procaine penicillin suspension or the use of a long-acting dry period treatment in lactating cows, which used to prevail as a treatment, is no longer permissible. Penalties for not keeping contaminated milk out of the sale vat are now very heavy. A second dry period therapy must be at least one month before the first milk sale is proposed.

Actually, the program described here is directed away from unnecessary treatment of lactating cows and has a decided bias against the possibility of antibiotic residues occurring in the milk. Recommended withdrawal periods are:

Udder infusion in a lactating cow, quick release compound	72 hours
Udder infusion of slow release dry period treatment in dry cow	4 weeks
Parenteral injection, single injection, not long-acting bases	36 hours
Parenteral injection, series of injections, not long-acting bases	72 hours
Parenteral injection, in long-acting bases	13 days
Intrauterine tablet	72 hours

Vaccination. The only vaccination prospect in bovine mastitis is that aimed at *Staphylococcus aureus*. There was work done on *Str. agalactiae* at one time, but it appears to have lapsed completely. Commercial vaccines administered parenterally are available for staphylococcal mastitis, and they may reduce the severity of the disease sufficiently to warrant including it in a program for a problem herd in which the regular program is not achieving great success.

In cattle, humoral antibodies do appear in the serum after vaccination but do not pass into the milk. Much of the experimental work on these intramuscular and similar systemic vaccinations has been carried out on sheep, and the results may not be extrapolable to cattle. A rise in antibody titers in serum and an increased resistance to *Staph. aureus* is recorded in sheep after intramuscular injection of a live *Staph. aureus* vaccine (Watson and Kennedy 1981). Failure of systemic vaccination in cattle has led to an attempt to produce cellular antibodies against *Staph. aureus*. Thus the intramammary infusion of vaccines has been tried commercially, but the results claimed are at most a reduction in the severity of subsequent mastitis and in loss of milk yield (Groothuis and Grootenhuis 1981). The killed vaccines for intramammary use are often combined with an antibiotic and used as a dry period treatment.

Treatment of Lactating Quarters. An important part of a control program is the early recognition and treatment of cases of clinical mastitis. Recognition of their occurrence depends on:

- good observation while preparing the udder and teats for milking. The presence of swelling, pain, heat in acute cases, or scar tissue or atrophy in chronic cases is not hard to detect, although it may be more obvious at the end of milking. Clots in the milk or wateriness of it should also be noticeable if the premilking preparation is carried out properly
- clots present in the in-line filter or on filter paper in the filter at the holding tank

It is essential that the incident be recorded. A

sample taken for microbiological examination would be a great advantage. Treatment should begin at once. One infusion is usually sufficient to effect an apparent clinical cure, and this is what most farmers do to avoid having to reject too much milk. However, to have some chance of significantly reducing damage to the quarter and of gaining some return to normal function, there should be three infusions at 24-hour intervals of a quick-release preparation or a single infusion of a long-acting preparation. In both cases, all milk from the cow will have to be withdrawn from sale for six days. Because the penalty for antibiotic contamination of milk is so high, it is suggested that a dramatic means be used to advise that a cow's milk must be withheld and the date that it can be returned to the milk supply.

It is not proposed to discuss here the relative merits of individual treatments. There are many of them, and almost the only information about them is that provided by the manufacturers. The recovery rate of subclinical cases of mastitis is so poor that treatment of them is not generally recommended.

Sources of Error in Mastitis Control Programs

If a mastitis control program is in place and the results are not as good as expected, the following list can be used as a guide to the most common errors.

Problem of a High Bacterial Count in Milk. Milk receiving depots constantly monitor the bacterial count of milk as it is received as a part of their quality control. The threshold count is 100,000 bacteria/ml., and counts above this result in a refusal to accept further milk. The farmer's response is to call for help. Almost always, the problem arises because of faults in the cleaning system of the milking machine or containers used for transport. However, a very high incidence of mastitis, expecially that caused by *Str. agalactiae*, has been known to cause a high bacteria count, but the mastitis status of the herd would have to be calamitous, an unlikely occurrence in a herd with a control program. Most farmers are aware of the importance of keeping mastitic milk out of the tank, and this would prevent any possibility of such a high bacterial count. Examination of the milking equipment usually pinpoints the problem. In some cases, gross contamination of the wash water used in the dairy may be the cause.

Problem of High Incidence of Mastitis. This may be indicated by a high bulk milk cell count, a high herd average of individual cow cell counts, an increase in quarter infection rate, or an increase in the number of clinical cases. The procedure to be adopted is the same as that discussed for the examination of a mastitis problem herd in a later section (p. 110).

Special Programs for Particular Circumstances

What has been described in previous sections is a general all-purpose mastitis control program. It is now necessary to define special modifications of the program that are necessary to suit special circumstances.

Year-round Herds. Because of the relatively leisurely speed at which the herd recycles itself, it is possible to adopt a continuous surveillance program. This makes it practicable to have a three-month rolling average of cell counts, new infections, or clinical cases as a guide to status. It is then possible to impose new control techniques or to gently relax or increase existing ones, in response to a gradual change in the mastitis status of the herd. Because there are only a few cows drying off each month, careful assessments of each cow and of each quarter may be conducted. Physical palpation and cultural examination are possible.

Seasonal Herds. When almost all of the herd calves during a six-week period together with all the other herds in the area, there is little time to realize, for example, that the new infection rate has jumped dramatically, and there is little time to institute a major alteration in the program. Collection of samples at monthly visits for cell counting and cultural examination is not possible. In these circumstances, the examination must be done over a long period of the lactation, and the data must be made available for decision as to mastitis status and possibly as to which cows to treat in a selective dry period therapy program. Selective dry period therapy becomes a less attractive prospect in these herds than in year-round ones, but it can be done using cell counts during lactation as the guide.

Housed Cattle. Housed cattle are exposed to much greater contamination of their immediate environment than are pastured ones. Coliform and other opportunist mastitides are very serious threats. A number of corollaries follow:

□ Wash water used in the milking parlor must be pathogen-free
□ Use of the milking machine must avoid high vacuum pressure, heavy machine stripping, removal of the cups before the vacuum is

released, and abrupt removal of the cups—in short, anything that is likely to cause a rapid jet response of milk to the teat end

- Ensure that fecal contamination of the parlor is minimal and that the bedding area is clean and dry and has fresh straw. Shavings and sawdust are not acceptable as bedding. Sand is acceptable. Sawdust can be rendered innocuous for two to three days by a paraformaldehyde spray
- Stall beds must be just long enough to avoid contamination of the udder and damage to the teats
- Premilking hygiene MUST be at a very high level, with the udder and teats carefully washed with warm water and dried with an individual single-use paper towel
- Ensure careful attention to surveillance of a cell count and cultural examination just before drying off and again just before calving, if that is possible
- Although attention is often drawn to the greater susceptibility of quarters with a low cell count, it is not recommended that any positive attempts be made to maintain a high cell count during the dry period
- Dry cows should be kept away from the heavily contaminated environment, on pasture if possible. Their udders should be clipped free of long hairs. Two weeks before calving, an intensive program of udder washing and teat hygiene should begin. Cows with leaking teats should receive special attention. They may require a teat sealant
- Downer cows are likely to have massive coliform contamination of the teats and udder. Extreme care must be practiced to keep the udder clean and the chances of udder infection minimized.

Summer Mastitis Areas. Suppurative mastitis in dry cows at pasture in the summertime, caused by *Corynebacterium pyogenes* and unspecified staphylococci and streptococci, can be very difficult to prevent. Flies are thought to be one of the principal carriers of the infection, but there is little that can be done to control them. The recommended procedures to prevent summer mastitis are:

- infusion of all quarters with procaine penicillin 100,000 units in mineral oil twice during the dry period, at an interval of three weeks. Alternative procedures are monthly infusions of benzathine cloxacillin (500 mg.) or infusion every three weeks of ampicillin (250 mg.) plus cloxacillin (500 mg.) throughout the dry period (Edmonds and Welsh 1979)
- sealing the teat ends with collodion
- spraying the udder and cow's sides with insect repellent periodically
- maintaining a careful watch in summer and in pastures where flies abound
- close observation of the cows so that early treatment can be administered if cases occur

Assessment of Cost-Effectiveness of Mastitis Control

A realistic comparison of costs and benefits in a herd operating under a mastitis control program must take into account:

- expected additional income from greater milk production
- savings in costs of drugs used for treatment because of reduction in clinical cases
- costs of additional feed to produce the additional milk
- costs of dry cow therapy. The costs will be about the same for blanket therapy of all quarters and for selective treatment, because the costs of selecting the quarters to be treated will about offset the savings in treatment
- costs of teat dip. Careful buying will mean a great saving. Some teat dips are very expensive

Some partial budgets are provided in Table 5–2. The material is adapted from a monograph by Asby et al. 1975.

Examination of a Problem Herd

Basic Protocol for Examination of a Problem Herd

A problem level is defined as one in which one or more of the following findings apply:

1. An average bulk milk cell count for three months that exceeds 400,000 cells/ml.

2. An average individual cow milk cell count (the more counts the better) that exceeds 500,000/ml.

3. A quarter infection rate at drying off of 13% or more

4. A quarter infection rate in mid-lactation, random samples of more than 10%

5. A prevalence of clinical cases of more than 4 cases/100 cows/30 days

Death and cull rates would also be useful guides, but there are no criteria of any substance.

The following protocol is presented as a suitable procedure for the examination of a herd in which a mastitis control program does not achieve its targets and also for herds that come forward as primary accessions, i.e., the

Table 5-2. PARTIAL BUDGETS OF COSTS/BENEFITS
FOR A MASTITIS CONTROL PROGRAM

	Year 1	Year 3	Year 5
Benefits—Income from:			
Less mastitis treatment	$ 18.00	$ 57.00	$ 63.00
More milk produced	397.00	1411.00	1588.00
Total benefit	415.00	1468.00	1651.00
Costs—Expenditure on:			
Dry cow therapy	90.00	90.00	90.00
Iodophor teat dip	149.00	149.00	149.00
Milking machine test	7.00	7.00	7.00
Total basic program cost	246.00	246.00	246.00
Extra concentrate fed	77.00	280.00	316.50
Total costs	92.00	526.00	562.00
Margin benefits/costs	92.00	941.00	1088.00

farmer complains that there are too many clinical cases or that his bulk milk cell count or average individual cell count is too high. What is proposed is a practical procedure, designed to be cost-effective and completed in one visit.

Before the Visit

◻ Look for evidence that the problem is really one of mastitis and not one of poor milking technique. The best evidence is a high milk cell count

◻ Have a technician check the milking machine for proper vacuum pressure, adequate vacuum reserve, correct pulsation rate, squeeze-rest ratio, and especially free electricity

At the Visit (must include at least part of a milking)

The visit can be made at the afternoon milking but is better made in the morning so that milk samples collected can hopefully reach the laboratory the same day.

Before Milking

So that there might be some warning of what to look for during milking:

◻ examine bedding and stallbeds for size and cleanliness; also examine lanes and entrances for places where teats can be soiled or damaged

◻ Examine teat cups and liners for signs of wear, uncleanliness, cracks, or milk stone deposits

◻ check premilking udder wash liquid and cloths

During Milking

It is essential to actually observe the milking procedure but without alerting the milker to what is being done because he might correct faults for the occasion.

◻ Collect *aseptic* quarter samples for cell count or CMT and culture from at least 10% of cows, including some known chronic cases and some normals but avoiding recently treated cows. These samples are critical and

should be collected by a veterinarian or a technician with special training. A farmer can be trusted to collect them but only if he understands what he is doing and performs the task conscientiously. A laboratory report that classifies 20% of samples as contaminated is an indication that the entire task must be done again

◻ While collecting the sample, observe the teat skin for lesions likely to harbor infection, especially pseudo-cowpox, and examine teat ends for evidence of overmilking or high vacuum in the form of teat sphincter eversion or black spot

◻ Mark some cows to be segregated after milking if history, udder asymmetry, obvious fibrosis, or abnormal milk suggests severe udder disease. There is insufficient time to examine these cows properly during milking without delaying the milkers

◻ Observe the premilking udder preparation for effectiveness, especially if foremilk is examined, reflux from teat is prevented, and udder massage is performed. If towels are used, observe whether they are in fact single-use

◻ Observe milking procedure for normality of vacuum pressure on machine gauge, checked by your own gauge

◻ Observe that teat spray or dip gives complete cover to all teats of all cows but does not grossly waste teat dip; check for avoidance of overmilking and abrupt removal of cups without first releasing vacuum; note presence of liner slip and large fluctuations in vacuum pressure

After Milking

◻ Bring back the segregated cows for a more detailed examination, including palpation of mammary tissue and supramammary lymph nodes

◻ Check materials used for treatments and take samples for laboratory examination if bulk materials are used, if home sterilized syringes and cannulas are used, or if purchased materials are diluted or otherwise handled. It is best to suspect any medicament that is not in a single-dose disposable unit. Even those may be contaminated and should be sampled if that is suspected

☐ Before leaving the farm, make positive recommendations of a general sort and include the following:

Tighten up the hygiene, especially teat sanitization, before milking; use hypochlorite or iodophor udder wash

Reintroduce back-flushing or teat cup sterilization in disinfectant solution

Segregate and milk last the chronic cases and known clinical cases; also milk heifers last

Ensure teat dip is maximum strength; may have to change from spray to dip

Increase the dry period treatment intensivity by insisting on disinfection of teat before treatment and teat dipping afterwards, plus maximum strength intra-mammary treatment

☐ Correct obvious errors that may account for obvious errors, e.g., contaminated water that houses *Pseudomonas* sp.

After Farm Visit

It is important to move quickly to avoid too much further damage. There should be prompt action:

☐ submit milk and other samples for culture, specifying peculiar pathogens, e.g., mycoplasmas and yeasts if they are suspected. Request culture, sensitivity, number of colonies per loop, and pathogenicity tests, e.g., coagulase status of staphylococci

☐ comment on the lab report to the farmer with directions on what to do about specific findings, e.g., a high prevalence of *Str. agalactiae* that reinforces your clinical suggestion that teat dipping fluids are of inadequate concentration

Checklist of Common Causes of Failure in Mastitis Control Programs

1. Relaxation of teat dipping procedure by
☐ reducing the concentration, especially for spraying as distinct from dipping
☐ adding too much oil or glycerine to dip to prevent teat skin damage
☐ stopping altogether

2. Reduction in efficiency of dry period treatment by purchase of cheaper product containing much lower antibiotic content

3. Inadequate treatment of clinical cases in lactating cows usually by way of reducing number of infusions of short-acting product

4. Labor problem in milking parlor causing overmilking or abrupt teat cup removal

5. Inadequate culling pressure, especially in stud herds and when herd is trying to expand its size

6. Sudden appearance of an *exotic* infection e.g., *Leptospira hardjo* or *Mycoplasma* sp.; *Escherichia coli* in bedding or *Pseudomonas* in wash water.

Other Problems Masquerading as Mastitis

Other causes of reduced milk production in a dairy herd that may resemble a mastitis problem on superficial examination include situations in which there is apparently plenty of food and no obvious illness or loss of condition of the cows. Examples are free electricity and inherited poor milk production, an inadequate milking system, or an overlong intercalving interval (Bushnell 1982).

Free Electric Voltage. This is a not uncommon cause of a sudden reduction in milk flow. In most instances, the dairy is a new one, or new electrical work has been carried out. In old installations, it may be a matter of simple wear and tear with baring of wiring where vibration shakes rotted insulation loose. However, most cases are due not to faulty wiring but to the accumulation of low voltages because of faults in the grounding of the installation. They are therefore neutral to earth voltages. In new constructions the earth (or ground, or neutral) connection is not far enough into the ground, or there are insufficient grounding rods, or the ground is very dry, or the water table in the ground has fallen below the level of the rods. The observed problem may be intermittent and associated with periods of dry weather.

When there is a defect in the wiring installation, the problem is usually a continuous one and more serious than with a poor grounding. Many of the metal parts in the milking parlor, including construction materials and the milking machine, are connected to one another and radiate out from the electric motor and the vacuum tank so that cows come into contact with the free current from the stanchions and feeders. The milker often feels nothing because his contact is less, and rubber boots prevent any passage of current. The cows are very susceptible and make large surface contact with the metal conductor and the wet concrete. Because the amperage is often small, an electrician with an amp meter or volt meter should make the examination, and this while the machine is working.

Free electrical voltage may cause fatal electrocution in the milking parlor or may cause stunning, restlessness, frequent urination, bawling, refusal to enter the parlor, or simple failure to let down the milk. This retention of milk may lead to flare-ups of what has been subclinical mastitis; this may be interpreted as causing mastitis. Provisional guidelines for diagnoses are (Williams et al. 1981):

	Volts
Normal	<0.5
Suspicious	0.5 –0.75
Mild reactions	0.75–1.5
Strong reactions	1.5 –3.5
Critical reactions	3.5 –5.0
Life at risk	>5.0

Because of the often intermittent nature of the problem and the differences in the effects depending on the nature of the contact, any examination of suspected free voltage by a veterinarian should be carried out with extreme care. It is much safer to have a qualified electrician investigate the problem.

Moisture is the principal variable in determining the current flow. Wet conditions between the electrified object and the cow, between the cow and the concrete, and between the concrete and the ground facilitate the passage of current through the cow. There are also factors that govern the response of the animal to the passage of the current. For example, cracked teats are much more sensitive than uncracked teats, and worn or freshly trimmed feet are much more sensitive than others. A detailed description of electrical wiring systems on farms and their faults, together with examination techniques for these systems, is available (Gustafson et al. 1982).

Inherited Poor Milk Production. This is a very long-term problem. A farmer who has concentrated on breeding to one bull that has not been progeny-tested and is used for natural breeding—a very unlikely set of circumstances in these times—may find his herd producing much less milk than he anticipated. He may call for assistance because of his misunderstanding of the cause of the problem. There is usually only a preliminary difficulty in deciding that mastitis is not at the root of the matter.

PROMOTION OF MASTITIS CONTROL

Encouragement of farmers to use mastitis control programs is best done by a coordinated campaign which includes:

◻ an educational program in various media to publicize the availability of the program and the benefits of it

◻ reinforcement of the view that the benefit is by way of income

◻ demonstration on local peer farms, allowing farmers to observe the results in commercial circumstances. The quarter infection rate is reducible from the common beginning level of 30 to 10% in a year, and to 8% in two years. The return on investment in southern Australia will be of the order of 250 to 500%

◻ utilizing existing farmer discussion groups to have the program promoted by government veterinary officers, with accredited private practitioners available to do the veterinary work on the farms, with government laboratory back-up

◻ provision of government or industry support by way of laboratory and recording charges

◻ having a specific trouble-shooting system to look at those problem farms where the program does not work satisfactorily

◻ encouraging an interfarm comparison with explanation of good performance and examination of reasons why some farms perform poorly

Financial pressure is the argument best understood by all groups in the community, including farmers, and if an incentive scheme can be introduced by legislation or even by city ordinance or processing plant rule, the task of convincing farmers to improve their mastitis control program is greatly simplified. Some European countries have done this, and it does apply in some parts of South Africa, where penalties are imposed on milk containing higher than an approved cell count (Bryson and Hobbs 1981).

The keynotes in any extension campaign to promote mastitis control could include:

1. Don't wait until disaster strikes—have a control program that monitors the status quo

2. It is easy to reduce the prevalence in most herds that are without a program by two-thirds in one year (e.g., 30% to 10%).

3. It can be combined with a reproductive control program to constitute a total herd health program.

Review Literature

Dodd, F.H. and Griffin, T.K. The role of antibiotic treatment at drying off in the control of mastitis. Proc. IDF Seminar on Mastitis Control, Brussels. International Dairy Federation Annual Bulletin, Document 85, pp. 282–302, 1975.

Jackson, E.R. The control of bovine mastitis. Vet. Rec., 107:37–40, 1980.

McMillan, K.L. and Tauga, V.K. Dairy production from pasture. N.Z. and Aust. Soc. Anim. Prod. Conference Proceedings, February, 1982, Ruakura Animal Research Station, New Zealand.

Merrill, W.G. and Gorewit, R.C. Some restatements and further thoughts on milking management. Proc. 20th Ann. Mtg. U.S. Natl. Mastitis Council, Inc., pp. 93-107, 1981.

Morris, R.S. Criteria for the design and evaluation of bovine mastitis control systems. Proc. IDF Seminar on Mastitis Control, Brussels. International Dairy Federation Annual Bulletin, Document 85, pp. 395-409, 1975.

Morris, R.S., Blood, D.C., Williamson, N.B. et al. A health program for dairy herds. 4. Changes in mastitis prevalence. Aust. Vet. J., 54:247-251, 1975.

Natzke, R.P. Elements of mastitis control. J. Dairy Sci., 64:1431-1442, 1981.

Philpot, W.W. Control of mastitis by hygiene and therapy. J. Dairy Sci., 62:168-176, 1979.

References

Asby, C.B., Ellis, P.R., Griffin, T.K. et al. The benefits and costs of a system of mastitis control in individual herds. Study No. 17, University of Reading, Dept. of Agriculture & Horticulture, pp. 1-14, 1975.

Bakken, G. Relationships between udder and teat morphology, mastitis and milk production in Norwegian Red cattle. Acta Agric. Scand., 31:438-444, 1981.

Barnum, D.A. and Meek, A.H. Somatic cell counts, mastitis and milk production in selected Ontario dairy herds. Can. J. Comp. Med., 46:12-16, 1982.

Barnum, D.A., Johnson, R.E. and Brooks, B.W. Evaluation of a teat dip with dodecyl benzene sulfonic acid in preventing bovine mammary gland infection from experimental exposure to Streptococcus agalactiae and Staphylococcus aureus. Can. Vet. J., 23:50-54, 1982.

Barto, P.B., Bush, L.J. and Adams, G.D. Feeding milk containing Staphylococcus aureus to calves. J. Dairy Sci., 65:271-274, 1982.

Box, P.G. and Ellis, K.R. Apparatus for pasteurising teat cup liners between cows in a herringbone parlor. Vet. Rec., 102:35-38, 1978.

Britt, J.S. Mastitis problem herds. J. Am. Vet. Med. Assoc., 170:1239-1243, 1977.

Brooks, B.W. and Barnum, D.A. The use of polyethylene intramammary device in protection of the lactating bovine udder against experimental infection with Staphylococcus aureus or Streptococcus agalactiae. Can. J. Comp. Med., 46:267-269, 1982.

Bryson, R.W. and Hobbs, W.B. A successful herd mastitis control scheme in Natal. J. S. Afr. Vet. Assoc., 52:113-117, 1981.

Bushnell, R.B. Mastitis. Update on recent findings. Proc. 14th Ann. Conv. Amer. Assoc. Bovine Practitioners, pp. 73-77, 1982.

Dohoo, I. and Meek, A.H. Somatic cell counts in milk. Can. Vet. J., 23:119-125, 1982.

Dohoo, I.R., McMillan, I. and Meek, A.H. The effects of storage and method of fixation on somatic cell counts in milk. Can. J. Comp. Med., 45:335-338, 1981.

Edmonds, M.J. and Welsh, J.A. The prevention of summer mastitis in dry cows by intramammary infusions of ampicillin and cloxacillin. Vet. Rec., 104:554-555, 1979.

Farnsworth, R.J., Wyman, L. and Hawkinson, R. Use of a teat sealer for prevention of intramammary infections in lactating cows. J. Am. Vet. Med. Assoc., 177:441-444, 1980.

Fernando, R.S., Rindsig, R.B. and Spahr, S.L. Electrical conductivity of milk for detection of mastitis. J. Dairy Sci., 65:659-664, 1982.

Flesh, J., Harel, W. and Nebken, D. Immunopotentiating effect of levamisole in the prevention of bovine mastitis, fetal death and endometritis. Vet. Rec., 111:56-57, 1982.

Geringer, M. and Thierley, M. Relationship between bulk milk cell count, herd size, management and udder infection. Tierarztl. Umschau, 37:358-360, 1982.

Gill, M.S. and Holmes, W. Somatic cell counts, mastitis and milk production in dairy herds. N.Z. J. Dairy Sci. Technol., 13:157-161, 1978.

Gonyon, D.S., Everson, D.O. and Christian, R.E. Heritability of mastitis score in Pacific North West dairy herds. J. Dairy Sci., 65:1269-1276, 1982.

Griffin, T.K., Grindal, R.J., Williams, R.L. et al. Effect of the method of removal of the milking machine cluster on new udder infection. J. Dairy Res., 49:361-367, 1982.

Grootenhuis, G. Mastitis prevention by selection of sires. Vet. Rec., 108:258-260, 1981.

Grootenhuis, G.J.K., Oldenbrook, J.K.A. and Van Den Berg, J. Differences in mastitis susceptibility. Vet. Qtly., 1:37-46, 1979.

Groothuis, D.G. and Grootenhuis, G. Effect of intramammary vaccination on experimental staphylococcal infection in cows. Tijdschr. Diergeneeskd., 106:304-313, 1981.

Gudding, R. and Lorentzen, P. The influence of low-line and high-line milking plants on udder health and lipolysis. Nord. Vet. Med., 34:153-157, 1982.

Gustafson, R.J., Cloud, H.A. and Appleman, R.D. Understanding and dealing with stray voltage problems. Bovine Practitioner, 17:4-15, 1982.

Hicks, W.G., Kennedy, T.J., Keister, D.M. et al. Evaluation of a teat-dip of chlorhexidine digluconate (0.5%) with glycerin (6%). J. Dairy Sci., 64:2266-2269, 1981.

Hill, A.W., Hibbitt, K.G. and Davies, J. Particles in bulk milk capable of causing falsely high electronic cell counts. J. Dairy Res., 49:171-177, 1982.

Hoare, R.J.T., Nicholls, P.J. and Sheldrake, R.F. Investigations into falsely elevated somatic cell counts of bulked whole milk. J. Dairy Res., 49:559-565, 1982.

Jasper, E.H., Smith, A.R., McPherron, T.A. et al. Effect of an intramammary polyethylene device in primiparous dairy cows. Am. J. Vet. Res., 43:1587-1589, 1982.

Kirk, J.H. Application of programmable calculators to mastitis control programs. J. Dairy Sci., 64:2048-2058, 1981.

Kirk, J.H. T1/59 program based on somatic cell counts for estimating subclinical mastitis loss. Bovine Practitioner, 17:20-25, 1982.

Klastrup, O. Mastitis Control in Denmark. Proc. 20th Ann. Mtg. U.S. Natl. Mastitis Council, Inc., pp. 38-45, 1981.

Langlois, B.E., Cox, J.S., Hemken, R.H. et al. Milking vacuum influencing indicators of udder health. J. Dairy Sci., 64:1837-1842, 1981.

Lindstrom, U.B., Kenttamies, H., Arstila, J. et al. Usefulness of cell counts in predicting bovine mastitis. Acta Agric. Scand., 31:199-203, 1981.

Linzell, J.L. and Peaker, M. Day to day variations in milk composition in the goat and cow as a guide to the detection of subclinical mastitis. Br. Vet. J., 128:284-296, 1972.

Marr, A. Bovine Mastitis Control. (Corresp.) Vet. Rec., 102:132-134, 1978.

McDermott, M.P., Erb, H.N. and Natzke, R.P. Predictability by somatic cell counts related to prevalence of intramammary infection within herds. J. Dairy Sci., 65:1535-1543, 1982.

McDonald, J.S. Relationship of milking machine design and function to udder disease. J. Am. Vet. Med. Assoc., 158:184–196, 1971.

McMillan, K.L., Duirs, G.F. and Hook, I.S. Relationships between milk somatic cell counts, production index and dry cow therapy in seasonal dairy herds. Proc. N.Z. Soc. Anim. Prod., 40:180–188, 1980.

Meek, A.H. and Barnum, D.A. The application of bulk tank somatic cell counts to monitoring mastitis levels in dairy herds. Can. J. Comp. Med., 46:7–11, 1982.

Meek, A.H., Barnum, D.A. and Newbould, F.H.S. Use of total and differential somatic cell counts to differentiate potentially infected from potentially non-infected quarters and cows and between herds of various levels of infection. J. Food Protection, 43:10–14, 1980.

Meek, A.H., Goodhope, R.G. and Barnum, D.A. Bovine mastitis, a survey of Ontario dairy producers, 1978. Can. Vet. J., 22:46–48, 1981.

Mielke, H., Schulz, J., Beuche, W. et al. Monitoring udder health by measuring the electrical conductivity of first-milk samples from individual animals. Arch. Exp. Veterinarmed., 35:259–276, 1981.

Miller, R.H. and Schultze, W.D. Genetic resistance to mastitis. Proc. 20th Ann. Mtg. U.S. Natl. Mastitis Council Inc., pp. 51–78, 1981.

Miller, R.H., Pearson, R.E., Rothschild, M.F. et al. Comparison of single and multiple-trait selected sires. Response in mastitis traits. J. Dairy Sci., 64:832–837, 1981.

Natzke, R.P. and Bray, D.R. Teat dip comparisons. J. Dairy Sci., 56:148–150, 1973.

Natzke, R.P., Everett, R.W. and Bray, D.R. Effect of over-milking on udder health. J. Dairy Sci., 65:117–125, 1982.

Nicholls, T.J., Youl, B.S., Browning, J.W. et al. Individual cow cell counts, mastitis and production. Aust. Adv. Vet. Sci., pp. 158–159, 1982.

Noorlander, D.O., and Heckman, R. Scanning electron microscopy and etiological studies of teat cup inflations for mastitis control. J. Food Protection.43: 205–207, 1980.

Noorlander, D.O. and Heckman, R.A. Milk gases, mastitis and milking machines. Mod. Vet. Prac., 62:590–594, 1981.

Noorlander, D.O. and Heckman, R.A. Teat cup rubber design and mastitis. Mod. Vet. Prac., 63:655–659, 1982.

Oliver, S.P. and Smith, K.L. Nonantibiotic approach in control of bovine mastitis during dry period. J. Dairy Sci., 65:2119–2124, 1982.

Paape, M.J. Effectiveness of polyethylene intramammary device (IMD) in mastitis prevention. J. Dairy Sci., 65(Suppl. 1), 205–206, 1982.

Paape, M.J., Schultze, W.D., Guidry, A.J. et al. Effect of an intramammary polyethylene device on the concentration of leukocytes and immunoglobulins in milk and on the leukocyte response to Escherichia coli endotoxin and challenge exposure with Staphylococcus aureus. Am. J. Vet. Res., 42:774–783, 1981.

Pankey, J.W., Barker, R.M., Twomey, A. et al. Effectiveness of dry cow therapy in N.Z. dairy herds. N.Z. Vet. J., 30:50–52, 1982.

Pearson, J.K.L. and Mackie, D.P. Factors associated with the occurrence, cause and outcome of clinical mastitis. Vet. Rec., 105:456–463, 1979.

Philpot, W.N. Effect of milking machines equipped with automatic quarter take-off devices on milk quality and health of the udder. J. Milk Fd. Technol., 35:544–547, 1972.

Philpot, W.N. Comparative effectiveness of different dry cow treatment systems. Proc. 10th Ann. Conv. Amer. Assoc. Bov. Practitioners, pp. 55–64, 1977.

Poutrel, B. and Rainard, P. California Mastitis Test guide of selective dry cow therapy. J. Dairy Sci., 64:241–248, 1981.

Poutrel, B. and Rainard, P. Predicting the probability of quarter infection (by major pathogens) from somatic cell concentration. Am. J. Vet. Res., 43:1296–1299, 1982.

Reitsma, S.Y., Cant, E.J., Grindal, R.J. et al. Effect of duration of teat cup liner closure per pulsation cycle on bovine mastitis. J. Dairy Sci., 64:2240–2245, 1981.

Robinson, T.C., Jackson, E.R. and Marr, A. Within herd comparison of teat dipping and dry cow therapy with only selective dry cow therapy in six herds. Vet. Rec., 112:315–319, 1983.

Schneider, R. and Jasper, D.E. Standardization of the California Mastitis Test. Am. J. Vet. Res., 25:1635–1641, 1964.

Schroder, R.J., McIntyre, R.W., Delli Quadri, C.A. et al. How a large milk-producing county met the mastitis control challenge. J. Am. Vet. Med. Ass., 153:1676–1687, 1968.

Schultze, W.D. and Smith, J.W. Effectiveness of post-milking teat dips. J. Dairy Sci., 55:426–431, 1972.

Sheldrake, R.F. and Hoare, R.J.T. The detection of mastitis in individual quarters using electrical conductivity or somatic cell concentration. N.Z. Vet. J., 29:211–213, 1981.

Sheldrake, R.F. and Hoare, R.J.T. Role of pre-milking teat disinfection in preventing Staphylococcus aureus mastitis. J. Dairy Res., 50:101–105, 1983.

Sheldrake, R.F., Hoare, R.J.T. and Hutchinson, J.E. Post-milking iodine teat skin disinfectants. J. Dairy Res., 47:19–38, 1980.

Smith, K.L. and Todhunter, D.A. The physiology of mammary glands during the dry period and the relationship to infection. Proc. 21st Ann. Mtg. Natl. Mastitis Council, Inc., pp. 87–100, 1982.

Stewart, G.A. and Philpot, W.W. Efficacy of a quaternary ammonium teat dip for preventing intramammary infections. J. Dairy Sci., 65:878–880, 1982.

Thompson, P.D. Effects of physical characteristics of milking machines on teats and udders. J. Am. Vet. Med. Ass., 170:1150–1155, 1977.

Watson, D.L. and Kennedy, J.W. Immunization against experimental staphylococcal mastitis in sheep—effect of challenge with a heterologous strain of Staphylococcus aureus. Aust. Vet. J., 57:309–313, 1981.

Williams, D.M. and Mein, G.A. Physical and physiological factors affecting milk flow rate from the bovine teat during machine milking in dairy production from pasture. Proc. Aust. and N.Z. Soc. Ani. Prod. Conf. in N.Z., Feb. 1982.

Williams, G.F.H. Stray Electrical Current. Proc. 20th Ann. Mtg. U.S. Natl. Mastitis Council, Inc., pp. 13–17, 1981.

Ziv, G., Storper, M. and Saran, A. The effect of levamisole therapy during the dry period on clinical and subclinical bovine mastitis. Refauh Vet., 38:108–113, 1981.

6 Health Management of Dairy Calves

The successful rearing of dairy calves as herd replacements depends on a well-managed combination of early feeding of colostrum, adequate housing, and adequate nutrition following the colostral feeding period.

The infectious diseases of digestive and respiratory tracts are the most important diseases of calves from birth up to several months of age. Approximately 75% of the mortality of dairy animals under one year of age occurs during the first month of life. This serves to point out the necessity of giving high priority to a health management system for rearing newborn calves, especially during the first month of life.

Causes of Economic Loss in Dairy Calves. Economic loss in dairy calves from birth to six months of age is due to mortality and suboptimal performance caused by the following diseases or inadequacies in production management.

ABORTIONS, STILLBIRTHS, AND CONGENITAL DEFECTS. These account for approximately 2 to 3% of calf mortality and include brucellosis, leptospirosis, intrapartum hypoxemia due to prolonged parturition, and inherited and non-inherited congenital defects (see Table 6–1).

ACUTE DIARRHEA. This accounts for approximately 75% of the mortality of dairy calves under three weeks of age. Some causes are: enterotoxigenic *E. coli* in calves under three to five days of age; rotavirus in calves seven to 10 days of age; coronavirus in calves seven to 15 days of age; *Cryptosporidia* spp. in calves 15 to 35 days of age; *Salmonella* spp. usually in calves several weeks of age; and coccidiosis (*Eimeria* spp.) in calves older than three weeks of age.

CHRONIC DIARRHEA. Inferior milk replacers cause emaciation.

OMPHALOPHLEBITIS. This is due to *E. coli*, *Corynebacterium pyogens* and other mixed flora, which cause omphalitis and arthritis.

SEPTICEMIA. This is usually seen in calves under four days of age that are agammaglobulinemic and that have coliform septicemia due to serotypes of *E. coli*.

ENZOOTIC PNEUMONIA. This occurs primarily in housed calves over two months of age. It is due to infection with respiratory viruses and inadequate ventilation and accounts for about 15% of calf mortality from birth to six months of age.

NUTRITIONAL DISEASES. Suboptimal perfor-

116

mance due to inadequate nutrition of calves from birth to six months of age is common, but accurate data on the magnitude of the economic losses incurred are not available because dairy producers do not usually monitor calf performance during the first several months after birth. Enzootic muscular dystrophy due to vitamin E and selenium deficiency occurs in well-nourished calves two to four months of age raised indoors and then turned out to pasture. Inferior growth rate may be due to:

1. Inadequate dietary intake of energy, protein, vitamins, and minerals. This occurs in housed dairy calves fed roughage and grain and in young calves reared on pasture where the quality of the pasture does not meet the nutrient requirements for optimal growth.

2. Mineral deficiencies (copper, zinc, iron).

3. Post-weaning unthriftiness. This occurs in calves that have been weaned too early, before they have been consuming an adequate amount of dry feed. It also occurs in calves that have been weaned from cow's whole milk or milk replacer onto an inadequate diet. The diet may be inadequate because of poor quality roughage, low energy and protein content of the grains, or inadequate concentration of minerals and vitamins. In calves reared on the pasture, the nutrient content of the grass may be inadequate to meet the needs of optimal growth following weaning. The veterinary aspects of the nutrition of young calves are presented in Chapter 7.

PARASITIC GASTROENTERITIS. This occurs especially in calves from two months of age and older that are being reared on pasture. The common parasites include *Trichostrongylus* spp., *Ostertagia* spp., *Nematodirus* spp., *Bunostomum phlebotomum*, and *Haemonchus contortus*.

PARASITIC PNEUMONIA. This is due to *Dictyocaulus viviparus* in calves being reared on pasture after about four to five months of age.

ARTHROPODS. This category includes lice due to *Linognathus vituli*, *Hematopinus eurysternus*, and *Damalinia bovis;* ticks; and flies.

MISCELLANEOUS. This category includes abomasal ulcers and poisonings (lead).

EPIDEMIOLOGY OF CALF DISEASE

Mortality Statistics and Targets of Performance

In dairy herds, the population mortality rate of live-born calves under one month of age averages about 10% and varies from 3 to 30%

between individual herds. Even higher losses have been recorded in large dairy herds with 1000 to 2000 milking cows (Martin et al. 1975a, 1975b, 1975c). This represents a major cause of economic loss on an industry basis. On a herd basis, it has been estimated that a 20% postnatal population mortality rate in calves results in a 38% reduction in net profit. (Martin and Wiggins 1973).

Time studies have indicated that the extent of death losses increased during mid-summer (June, July, August) and mid-winter (November, December, January), with mortality rates being 20% higher than those in summer. The risk of death of calves is greatest in their first week of life on most farms. Of all deaths in calves less than five weeks of age, 55% occur during the first week of life and 25 to 30% during the second week. In general, the death loss in calves between five weeks and three months of age is less than 5%. In well-managed herds, the mortality rate of calves under 30 days of age can be controlled at a level of 5% of all calves born alive and normal.

In general, the problem of dairy calf mortality is best minimized by a comprehensive management program that is followed stringently (Kertz 1977). The published studies emphasize the relationship of a multitude of management factors to calf mortality.

The epidemiologic determinants of disease and suboptimal performance that are considered to be important in calves under one month of age include colostral immunoglobulins, the personnel caring for the calves, the quality of milk replacers, herd size, housing, and the season of the year. A brief description of the importance of each of these factors is presented here. Each factor is then reiterated and incorporated in the principles of control of infectious diseases of calves presented in a later section in this chapter.

Colostrum. The most important factor influencing health of the newborn calf is the ingestion of liberal quantities of colostrum within a few hours after birth and the subsequent absorption of the colostral immunoglobulins within 24 hours after birth.

The factors that affect the levels of serum immunoglobulins achieved in calves at 24 hours after birth include the concentration of immunoglobulins in colostrum, the amount of colostrum available, the time after birth of the first ingestion of colostrum, and the amount of colostrum ingested, which is a reflection of the maternal behavior of the dam and the vigor of the calf.

Personnel. The people feeding and caring for the calves have a marked influence on their health. In a field study, calf survival was highest when the owner's wife fed and cared for the calves, whereas survival was lower when hired labor was responsible for the feeding and care of the animals (Speicher and Hepp 1973; Oxender et al. 1973). In 16 large dairy farms in California where calf mortality rate over a period of at least two years on individual farms varied from 3 to 30%, the calf management personnel was the only factor significantly related to the mortality rate.

There were considerably fewer death losses on farms where the owner managed the calves than on farms where employees performed the duties. In general, other factors such as herd size, calving location, and calf housing were not related to calf deaths in the survey.

In conclusion, the investigators stated, "A relatively low calf mortality rate for owner-managed calf rearing systems suggests that owners may be motivated sufficiently to provide the care necessary to ensure a high survival rate in calves. Economic considerations are undoubtedly a part of the motivating force, and a profit-sharing scheme could possibly provide additional incentive for farm employees to improve their calf management practices. The majority of dairymen in the present study give high priority to the construction of calving pens and calf rearing barns. However, the results reported herein indicate that investment in personnel might yield a higher return in terms of a lower calf mortality rate" (Martin et al. 1975c).

In a study of Minnesota dairy herds, calf mortality was higher in herds owned by inexperienced managers than in herds owned by older and more experienced managers (Hird and Robinson 1982). In a survey of 140 dairy herds in South Carolina, calf survival was highest when the owner or his family rather than hired labor was responsible for the calves (Jenny et al. 1981). In Libya, calf mortality increased in dairy farms when the experienced animal attendants were replaced by less experienced workers (Gusbi et al. 1983).

All of this suggests that regardless of the herd size, housing pen construction, calving site, and many of the other factors that have been associated with calf mortality, the calf rearer and his motivation to raise healthy calves has the greatest influence on calf survival.

Milk Replacers. The use of inferior quality milk replacers containing heat-denatured skim milk powder and added indigestible nutrients in calves under three weeks of age can result in a high incidence of nutritional diarrhea that may predispose to infectious diarrhea and increased calf mortality (Roy 1969, 1980). This subject is presented in Chapter 7.

Herd Size. As herd size increases, mortality commonly increases (Speicher and Hepp 1973; Oxender et al. 1973). In an expansion program, the total number of cows and milking facilities might be enlarged without a parallel increase in calf-raising facilities and labor. A marked increase in population density commonly results in an increase in the incidence of infectious disease. Outbreaks of infectious disease in calves under four weeks of age occur more commonly in large herds (over 100 cows) than in smaller herds and can cause major economic losses due to death, the costs of treatment, and suboptimal calf performance.

Housing. The type of barn may influence calf mortality. Mortality is lower in smaller herds in stanchion barns than in larger herds in free stall housing. Three primary factors may account for this: (1) Stanchion environment is conducive to minimal calf mortality in that calving facilities and cow barns are commonly warm; (2) dairymen do not always provide adequate facilities for calving and for newborn calves as they enlarge their herds and move into free stall housing; and (3) management is spread over a greater number of cattle and consequently is less than optimal.

The type of pen construction used may influence calf mortality. Rearing calves in individual stalls elevated from the floor has generally been more successful than rearing them directly on the floor in groups (Simensen 1982). Elevated stalls are easier to keep clean than group pens and, therefore, may not allow pathogens to accumulate in bedding and manure packs in the large pens. Individual pens also enable the calf feeder to know how much feed the calf is eating, the feed intake can be controlled, and illnesses and performance are more easily and quickly recognized. Surveillance of each calf is necessary to help minimize mortality, especially during the first three weeks of life. Individual calf record cards may be posted above individual pens, and the health status and performance data are easily recorded and evaluated. This is difficult to do when calves are raised in groups. Calves may be raised successfully as groups in large pens with a less intensive surveillance system when they are older, because the incidence of infectious disease declines after one month of age.

Season of Year. The season of the year during which the calf barn is occupied by the largest number of calves has a major influence on calf mortality. Many studies have shown that calf mortality is significantly higher during the winter months in colder climates when all calves born may be housed from two to six months, depending on the length of the winter. This long period of occupation results in an increase in the infection pressure, discomfort because of wet bedding, and perhaps poor ventilation.

During the winter months, increases in calf mortality were associated with cold, wet, windy weather; in summer, greater death losses were associated with hot, dry weather. In general, the calf losses in winter were more closely related to the effects of extreme weather than those in summer.

THE RELATIONSHIP BETWEEN HOUSING AND DISEASE OF CALVES

Many cases of poor health in dairy calves have been traced to bad management and inadequate ventilation in the calf nursery (Anderson 1978). Calves reared indoors are commonly affected with pneumonia caused by viruses and bacteria, which may reach high concentrations in the air of poorly ventilated, damp, cold calf barns. Calf barns that are overcrowded, dark, and damp in the winter months and hot and poorly ventilated during the summer months commonly predispose to diseases of the respiratory tract. Unfortunately, in most dairy herds the emphasis is on the milking cow, and the calf barn traditionally has received low priority, resulting in uncomfortable rearing conditions that predispose to infectious diseases. Some producers have had so much difficulty raising calves indoors that they have resorted to rearing young calves in calf hutches outdoors. Whereas considerable research and effort have been expended in elucidating the infectious causes of respiratory diseases in calves raised indoors, only little research has been done to develop economical and practical methods of providing an optimum environment for calves raised indoors.

Some of the common environmental problems in calf barns include the following:

1. Overcrowding in situations where calves are grouped in pens and where calves of different sizes and age groups are raised in the same pens

2. High relative humidity due to overcrowding, low temperature of incoming air and lack of supplemental heat

3. Inadequate movement of air in and out of the building due to inadequate inlets or insufficient capacity or poor location of fans

4. Rearing calves in close proximity to adult cows

The important principles of calf housing include:

1. A calf rearing facility completely isolated from the adult herd

2. Periodic depopulation for cleaning and disinfection. An ideal system would be to rear calves in separate groups of stalls or pens that would allow serial depopulation, with some of the units being emptied, sanitized, and ready for the next batch of calves

3. An effective ventilation system that is flexible according to the seasonal changes of outside weather. This includes supplemental heat when necessary

4. Sufficient space for each calf according to its size

5. An effective feeding system

6. An adequate lighting system so that each calf can be seen daily

7. A system that will allow regular monitoring of calf performance such as body weight and height measurements

Optimal Environment for Housed Calves

The following descriptions of an optimal environment for housed calves are offered as guidelines for the veterinarian who may assist the producer in designing a calf barn or evaluating existing calf barns. The reader is encouraged to consult the review literature and the general references for excellent articles (Mitchell 1976; Turnbull 1980; Appleman and Owen 1975); and books that contain the necessary details (Anderson and Bates 1979; Bates and Anderson 1979).

Insulation. Adequate insulation of calf barns is essential if extreme temperature variations are to be avoided in winter and to keep the calf barn cool in summer. The main aim is to use construction materials with a low thermal conductivity in the walls and ceilings. Resistance values for the various insulating materials are available. Insulation of the roof is of utmost importance. It is essential to have a vapor barrier, such as a layer of plastic sheeting over the insulating material, to prevent moisture produced in the calf barn from penetrating the insulation and reducing its effectiveness.

Inside Temperature. One of the aims of a well-ventilated calf barn is to keep the calf's deep temperature normal within narrow limits. Newborn calves have a slightly reduced body temperature, rising to 38.7°C (101.6°F) on the first day of life and 38.9°C (102.1°F) on the second day. Thereafter, body temperatures remain at about 38.8° to 39°C (101.8° to 102.2° F) for the first three weeks of life. With high levels of feeding, there is an increase in body temperature, whereas low levels of feeding result in a reduction of temperature. The environmental comfort zone for calves ranges from 50° to 70°F (10°C to 21°C), and achievement of this will depend on the number of calves, their total heat and moisture production, the total surface area and volume of space available, the outside temperature, the insulation properties of the building materials, the type of bedding used if any, the ventilation rate, and whether or not supplemental heat is provided. If the environmental temperature of the calf barn goes above the upper limit of the comfort zone, productivity will fall progressively. On the other hand, the effect of a drop in temperature below the lower limit of the comfort zone may be slight at first except for the "wastage" of part of the calf's feed intake in increasing its metabolism to keep warm. The cost of feed intake used as internal fuel in this way is approximately four times the cost of external fuel sources, such as electricity or gas used to keep the calf barn at least at the lower critical temperatures.

Calves must be kept on clean dry bedding and free from cold drafts. The construction and ventilation system of the calf barn will depend on the geographical location of the calf barn and the mean maximum and minimum ambient temperatures experienced in that area. It is much more difficult to ventilate a calf barn during the winter months when the mean outside temperature is −15°F than during other seasons when the mean outside temperature may be 15°F. Veterinarians should seek the assistance of state or provincial departments of agriculture, which will usually provide the necessary assistance in designing calf barns and in modifying existing calf barns (Anderson and Bates 1979; Bates and Anderson 1979).

In some areas and under certain circumstances, it may not be economically justifiable to construct or maintain a controlled environment calf house. In the northeast of Scotland, calf house temperatures within the range of 1 to 20°C (with relative humidities from 64 to 96%) have no demonstrable effect on calf health and

performance (Mitchell and Broadbent 1973; Mitchell 1972). The extra capital cost involved in a controlled environment type of calf house does not appear to be justifiable in terms of calf health or performance of calves in a climatic house in the northeast of Scotland. The controlled house is insulated, of concrete block construction with an insulated roof, and has fan-assisted ventilation and provision for supplementary heat. The temperature and ventilation are controlled. In the climatic house, the salient features are its low-cost wooden-frame construction of exterior grade hardboard, without insulation and with no supplementary heat. Ventilation is by ridge outlet and perforated inlets in the upper half of the walls. In both types of calf houses the calves are straw-bedded.

Relative Humidity. The generally accepted ideal range of relative humidity for calf barns is 70 to 80%. The relative humidity and inside temperature are interdependent in that a high relative humidity and low temperature promote condensation on walls and ceilings and ultimately on calves, resulting in cooling, shivering, discomfort, and a high incidence of respiratory tract disease. Calves give off considerable sensible heat loss and moisture, but the heat production is not sufficient to lower the relative humidity and thus, under most conditions, supplemental heat is necessary to counteract the additive cooling effect of cold incoming air, which tends to decrease the inside temperature and increase the relative humidity. In Canada and the northern United States, where the mean daytime temperature during the winter months may be as low as −15°C, owners will usually close the air inlets in the calf barns because the incoming air is too cold. However, this is counterproductive because it effectively reduces the ventilation rate to almost nothing, which increases the concentration of aerosal infection. Under these circumstances, supplemental heat is a requirement.

If the relative humidity in the building is high at an abnormally high air temperature, the ability of the animal to dissipate heat by vaporization of water (by sweating or via the lungs) may be seriously impaired, whereas with a low temperature, high humidity will intensify the loss of heat from the animal. A high humidity (over 70 to 80%) at normal or subnormal temperatures almost invariably leads to condensation on the inside surfaces of the building and to damp floors and building, which may adversely affect the livestock and the building. The humidity is also closely connected with the ventilation of animal barns. The ventilation rate should be adjusted to remove all the moisture produced by the animals. This will ensure that the relative humidity of the air remains within the correct range and will prevent condensation; in addition, it will reduce the danger of cross-infection by respiratory droplets.

Air Intake, Air Circulation, and Air Outlets. The amount of air coming into a calf barn must equal that being exhausted. The air is extracted by fans vented through the roof or through the walls or gable ends. The incoming air is introduced through inlets high in the walls or in the ceilings. The movement of the air in the calf barn should function to remove excess moisture, dust particles, gases, and infectious agents without creating drafts that increase loss of heat from the calves and result in chilling. Drafts usually occur near inlets, doors, and fans.

Ventilation Rate and Heating Requirements of Calf Barns. In an inadequately ventilated calf barn, the stagnant air becomes humid, and there is a progressive increase in the concentration of dust, ammonia, and other gases. Bacteria and viruses adhere to dust particles, and the combination of these factors predisposes to a high incidence of both acute and respiratory disease and poor growth rates. In cold climates, these effects are most marked in the winter months and less so during the summer months.

If calves are housed during the summer months, the main aim of ventilation is to limit the temperature rise in the calf barn above the outside temperature. This is accomplished by providing sufficient fan capacity. The aim is to provide sufficient ventilation to keep the calf house at or below the upper limit in the optimum temperature range and also to provide a degree of air movement that allows sufficient dissipation of heat to keep the calf cool and comfortable. The ventilation required to meet these standards is based on empirical evidence, but for calves housed in temperate climates during the coldest weather, the minimum ventilation rate recommended is 8 cu. ft./min./calf and the maximum for the warmest weather is 50 cu. ft./min. and even higher in subtropical climates.

The supplemental heat requirements for housed calves will depend on the insulation value of the building, the population density of the calves, and the severity of the outside temperature, but 350 British Thermal Units (BTU) per hour per calf has been recommended (Sainsbury and Sainsbury 1979). During the cold winter months, the aims of ventilation are to provide an environment that is comfortable, to ensure that condensation does not occur on any of the materials in the building, and to remove noxious gases, dusts, and pathogens.

Population Density. The floor area requirement per calf depends on (a) whether the calves are to be penned individually or in groups and (b) on the decision of the producer as to what minimum area is acceptable as humane.

The smallest area, as used in veal calf crates, for calves up to 300 lb. (135 kg.) is 10 sq. ft. (0.92 m.^{2}), but this area will not allow such calves to turn around after they weigh more than 170 lb. (77 kg.). Some workers have suggested a minimum area of 17.5 sq. ft. (1.63 m.^{2}) at this weight. At three months of age a well-fed calf that is individually penned requires 18 sq. ft. (1.67 m.^{2}) of total area or a pen size of 6 ft. × 3 ft. × 5 ft. (180 cm. × 90 cm. × 150 cm.). Younger calves can be kept in 15-sq.-ft. (1.39 m.^{2}) pens (5 × 3 ft.) (150 cm. × 90 cm.), but an area of 12 sq. ft. (1.12 m.^{2}) should be considered the absolute minimum for newborn calves.

Pen Construction. Calves are housed in either individual or group pens. There are many different types of pen design and of materials used. Individual pens are usually constructed with raised slatted floors, and bedding is not required. The pens are narrow and long and do not allow the calf to turn around. Regardless of the design of the pen or of the materials used, individual pens should be large enough to allow the calf to lie down comfortably. Some slatted or expanded metal floors in individual pens will cause decubitus ulcers on the legs of calves, which may result in suppurative arthritis.

Individual calf pens made from metal are easiest to clean but are more expensive than those made from wood, which are pervious and often difficult to clean and sanitize.

Individual pens should be scraped down, washed with disinfectant, and left vacant for at least one week before placing a new calf in the pen. Some pens can be easily dismantled for cleaning and sanitizing, but the labor involved usually precludes this procedure.

Pens for groups of calves are usually large enough to hold six to 10 calves and must be bedded with straw, shavings, or sawdust. They should also be cleaned out, sanitized, and left vacant to dry after each batch of calves is removed. Only calves of uniform size and age should be mixed into groups.

Sanitation and Disinfection. When large numbers of calves are housed in a calf barn, there is a gradual increase in the population of infectious agents, which creates the potential for increasing the incidence of clinical and subclinical disease. The infection rate increases with the length of time over which the calf barn is occupied by calves. This build-up of infection can be minimized by depopulating the calf barn and by cleaning and disinfecting the calf pens. This principle is applied successfully in veal calf operations where the previously cleaned and disinfected barn is filled with newly purchased calves within a few days. The calves are fed as a unit for several weeks and then marketed as a unit. This has been called the *all-in all-out system* and is very effective.

Cleaning and disinfecting calf pens includes the removal of all bedding and manure, scraping the floors and walls of pens, washing them with a high-pressure sprayer (300 to 500 lb. per sq. in.), applying a suitable disinfectant, and leaving the pens dry and vacant for at least two weeks. The kind of disinfectant used is not critical provided that cleaning and washing are scrupulous. Many disinfectants are available, but some of the cheaper ones include: 2% sodium hydroxide (caustic soda or lye) and 5% sodium carbonate (washing soda). The reader is referred to a review article on disinfection in veterinary practice (Graham-Marr and Spreull 1969). Terminal disinfection of calf houses by formaldehyde fumigation is effective (Scarlett and Mathewson 1977). Efficient precleaning and sealing prior to fumigation are of paramount importance.

Calf Hutches. In some areas, calf hutches or "igloos" are used to raise calves during the first month of life. These consist of a three-sided covered pen, large enough for a calf to lie down and move around, and a small fenced exercise yard in front of the pen. These are erected outside and separate from the main barn and provide another method of removing the newborn calf from the main source of infection to a clean environment. When sufficient bedding is provided, they have proved to be very comfortable for newborn calves even when the ambient temperature is well below freezing. Calves raised in these hutches must be well fed with milk and some hay and grain to provide sufficient energy and protein intake to meet the increased requirements for maintenance and growth that are necessary when the outside temperature is below 0°C. However, it can be an excellent system for rearing calves with a minimal incidence of enteritis and pneumonia (McKnight 1978). The hutches do not, however, replace poor management. They are an excellent alternative for housing calves during the summer months when the calf barn can be depopulated, cleaned, disinfected, and left vacant for several months.

THE PRINCIPLES OF CONTROL AND PREVENTION OF INFECTIOUS DISEASES OF DAIRY CALVES

Most of the common diseases of dairy calves under one month of age cannot be totally prevented, and control at an economical level must be the major objective. With good management and disease control techniques, mortality can be maintained economically at a level of from 3 to 5% of live-born calves under one month of age. A prerequisite for effective economical control of disease of calves is to establish a simple recording system that the producer can understand and use. An effective monitoring system will record the following data on a regular basis:

1. Number of calves born alive and dates of birth
2. Number of calves born dead and dates of death
3. Number of sick and the diagnoses, treatments, and dates of treatment
4. Number of dead calves and the diagnoses
5. Growth rate and height of calf according to age and breed
6. Feed intake; the composition and the amount of feed intake should be monitored regularly

The most common diseases of calves under two months of age are the infectious diseases of the digestive and respiratory tracts (Radostits and Acres 1974). This provides a basis for a calf herd health program that should give high priority to the control of these infectious diseases using the details of the three principles outlined here.

Reduction of the Degree of Exposure of Calves to Infectious Agents

From birth to about six months of age, the calf is subjected to different infection pressures. In the first few days of life, the calf is very susceptible to enterotoxigenic *E. coli;* between five and 15 days and sometimes later, rotavirus and coronavirus infection are the most common causes of enteritis; salmonellosis may occur at any age but commonly occurs in calves from one to two months of age; and the respiratory infections occur most commonly between two and six months of age. Therefore, every economical management effort is made to reduce the infection pressure on the calf from birth to several months of age.

The reduction of the degree of exposure to infectious agents begins with the birth of the calf, which should take place in a clean environment. The perineum and udder of dirty cows should be washed shortly before calving. The umbilicus of the calf may be swabbed with a 2% tincture of iodine immediately after birth to control the entry of environmental pathogens, but there is no documented evidence that this practice will reduce the occurrence of disease. Calves affected with diarrhea should be removed from the main calf nursery and treated in isolation. Well-bedded calving barn stalls, calving corrals, and pastures provide the ideal environment for the newborn calf. The calf is usually left with the dam in the calving area and allowed to suck the dam for two to four days and then transferred to an individual stall for rearing up to weaning age. This is an ideal system of rearing calves, since it allows the herdsman to minimize exposure of the newborn calf to infectious agents and individual care and feeding can be provided during the first month, which is the most critical time in the calf's life. The individual stalls vary considerably in their construction, but the most important concerns are that they should be cleaned and disinfected between calves and be comfortable.

In large dairy herds in which the animals are confined during the winter months, diseases such as enterotoxigenic colibacillosis and enzootic pneumonia may be endemic because of the long occupation time of the barns in which adult cows and calves are housed closely together. Disease may become a major problem and may necessitate the construction of a separate calf barn detached from the main barn. The calf is born in a box stall in the main barn, allowed to nurse its dam for two or four days, and then transferred to the calf barn.

Regular sanitation and hygiene is of paramount importance in the calf nursery, especially during the first few weeks of age when the calf is most susceptible to infectious disease.

From two to six months of age, the major concern is the control of respiratory disease, which is dependent on the effectiveness of the ventilation system in maintaining a low level of aerosol infection. The optimal environmental condition for housed calves was presented in an earlier section.

Maintenance of High Level of Nonspecific Resistance

This is dependent on the ingestion of adequate quantities of colostrum within a few hours after birth and on the management and nutrition of the calves.

Fresh Colostrum. The ingestion of liberal amounts of colostrum containing high levels of immunoglobulins as early as possible after birth is the most important factor. At least 50 ml. per kg. body weight should be ingested within the first six hours after birth. The termination of absorption of colostral immunoglobulins in the calf occurs spontaneously with age at a progressively increased rate after 12 hours postpartum (Stott et al. 1979a). The rate and amount of absorption are a function of the concentration of immunoglobulins in the colostrum (Stott and Fellah 1983), the amount fed, and the age at first feeding (Stott et al. 1979b). Increasing amounts of colostrum fed (up to 2 L. to Holstein calves) increases the amount of absorption (Stott et al. 1979c). The rate of absorption and maximum absorption are superior in calves that suck their dams (Stott et al. 1979d). However, up to 42% of calves left with their dams for one day following birth either fail to suck or absorb immunoglobulins from colostrum and are hypo- or agammaglobulinemic (Brignole and Stott 1980). Forced bottle feeding of calves following sucking for one day will improve the serum levels of immunoglobulins. To overcome the problem of insufficient absorption of colostral immunoglobulins, it generally is advised to force-feed colostrum to calves as soon as possible after birth. Calves force-fed colostrum at a dose of 80 ml. per kg. body weight by stomach tube at six hours of age achieve high levels of serum immunoglobulins by 24 hours of age (Molla 1978, 1980). Higher levels are achieved in calves fed colostrum compared with those allowed to suck their dams (Logan et al. 1981).

To ensure that calves are fed colostrum containing the largest concentration of immunoglobulin, a practical field test is available. A colostrometer (a hydrometer calibrated for the purpose) will estimate the concentration of immunoglobulin in colostrum (Fleenor and Stott 1980). This should enable the dairyman to establish the quality of colostrum prior to feeding and to avoid a first-stage failure in passive transfer of immunity from inferior colostrum. It also allows pooled colostrum to be extended over a greater number of neonates by adjusting the amount fed to a minimum volume that delivers a fixed mass of immunoglobulin. Calves that are deficient in serum immunoglobulins after being left with their dams for the first 24 hours after birth either did not or could not suck their dams. The mothering instinct, shape, size, and placement of the udder and teats in the cow or the lack of vigor in the calf to seek, find, and suck the teat are all interrelated factors resulting in failure to ingest sufficient quantities of colostrum early enough (Brignole and Stott 1980).

Stored Colostrum. Colostrum is the product of the first six postpartum milkings from cows. Colostrum is unmarketable, and in dairy herds with high-producing cows a surplus is usually available in sufficient quantities to feed heifer replacement calves for up to 28 to 35 days of age (Foley and Otterby 1978). The feeding of colostrum to calves during the first month of life replaces the need for whole milk in calf-feeding programs and is thus highly economical. The continued presence of colostrum in the intestinal tract also exerts a local protective action against the infectious enteritides. The details of the availability, storage, treatment, composition, and feeding value of surplus colostrum are available (Foley and Otterby 1978).

Most healthy dairy cows will produce colostrum in excess of the calf's requirement during the three-day colostrum feeding period. With an average production of colostrum of approximately 44 kg. per cow during the first six postpartum milkings and an average consumption of 11 kg. per calf during the first three days postpartum, about 32 kg. of colostrum would be available per cow for feeding calves over three days of age. Calves have commonly been fed 1.8 to 3.2 kg. of undiluted colostrum daily from day four of life until weaning. If bull calves are sold after their colostral feeding period, there may be sufficient colostrum to feed heifer replacement calves for up to four to five weeks of age.

Colostrum can be stored economically at ambient temperatures in plastic-lined containers with minimum handling requirements. However, losses due to spoilage and undesirable fermentation can limit the shelf-life of fermented colostrum. Acceptability can also be a problem with storage at ambient temperatures. Acceptability of thawed colostrum by calves in excellent, warm temperatures may enhance putrefactive fermentations. When colostrum is stored at warm ambient temperatures, use of chemical preservatives is recommended. Whereas chemical additives have not decreased total numbers of microbes, some preservatives effectively decrease numbers of coliforms, molds, and yeasts while preserving a greater portion of the nutrient content of colostrum than is possible with natural fermentation. However, unavoidable nutrient losses occur during storage with and without chemical additives. As acidity increases total solids, protein and lactose concentrations decrease.

The generally recommended guideline is to feed colostrum at about 6% of body weight equivalent daily. It is commonly diluted with water at the rate of two parts colostrum to one part water to approximate the solid content of whole milk. When diluted with water at a rate of 2:1 it should be fed at 8 to 10% of body weight equivalent daily.

Calf feeding programs should make maximal use of available colostrum. When fed at recommended levels, it supplies an excellent economical diet for young calves.

Management of Newborn Dairy Calves. Keeping dairy calves alive and healthy starts with the maternity area. Herds that use well-bedded box stalls for calving and for the calf during the colostral feeding period have consistently lower calf mortality. Maternity pens should be well bedded and dry. A Michigan study showed a significant relationship between the dry matter content of the bedding and calf mortality. Calf mortality was significantly lower when the bedding in the maternity pen was dry when compared with maternity pen with wet bedding. Straw is considered the ideal bedding; sawdust is questionable because it will not absorb equivalent amounts of moisture. Also, calves tend to eat sawdust, which may precipitate digestive upsets and serve as a vehicle for the entrance of pathogenic organisms into the digestive tract.

The nonspecific resistance of the newborn calf is markedly influenced by the type of housing, the temperature of the calving facilities, the temperature of the calf barn, the person caring for the calves, and whether or not attendance and assistance are provided at birth. Calf mortality may be higher in herds housed in loose housing than in stanchion-type barns. Calf mortality is also lower in herds that provide heated calving facilities and when the calf house is provided with supplemental heat. It is also much less when the calves are cared for and fed by the owner than when managed by hired help. This is particularly important in large herds where hired help may be necessary.

The practice of collecting and transporting calves from farms to sale yards during their first week of life and especially during cold weather has contributed to high mortality from pneumonia and enteritis. Losses in young calves following transportation are highest in those under two weeks of age compared with older calves. This suggests that calves should be retained on the home farm for two to three weeks before being moved. Calves transported from one farm, through sale yards, and to their final destination during the first week of life are prone to disease because of the combined effects of inadequate intake of colostrum, the stress of transportation, starvation and overcrowding during transportation, and the type of starting feed used in the new premises. Mortality is usually higher in calves started on milk replacers than in those fed whole milk or skim milk.

One of the greatest needs in the calf industry is the development of an orderly marketing system for newborn calves that are sold from farms and transported to specialized calf-rearing units. The system must consider that during the first 10 days to two weeks of life, the calf is extremely susceptible to the effects of stress, irregular feeding practices, and rough handling, all of which predispose to infectious disease, high mortality, and major economic losses.

Increasing the Specific Resistance of the Newborn Calf by Vaccination of the Pregnant Dam

The passive immunization of calves against the infectious diarrheas caused by enterotoxigenic K99+ E. coli, rotavirus, and coronavirus by vaccination of the pregnant dam a few weeks before parturition has received considerable research attention in recent years, and the results are promising. The pregnant cow is vaccinated six to two weeks before parturition to stimulate the production of specific antibodies against the common enteropathogens; these antibodies are then transferred to the colostrum. The calf must ingest the colostrum and absorb the colostral immunoglobulins within 24 hours after birth for protection against systemic infection. The colostral immunoglobulins also provide local immunity in the intestine for the duration of their presence in the colostrum. This is known as lactogenic immunity and is contingent on the frequent ingestion of colostrum or milk containing adequate levels of protective antibodies. The serum antibodies may provide protection against enteric infection if present in high titers and are

transferred from the serum into the intestine.

It must be emphasized that vaccination is an aid to good management and not a replacement for inadequate management. The success of the vaccine is dependent upon several factors. The pregnant cow must be vaccinated at the optimum time before parturition to ensure maximum production and transfer of antibodies to the colostrum. The concentration of antibodies in the colostrum of vaccinated cows may vary widely, depending on the size of the cow, the amount of colostrum produced, the concentration of antigens in the vaccine, and the age of the animal. The calf must still ingest colostrum in sufficient quantities soon enough after birth to acquire the protection before invasion by the pathogens.

For the control of enteric colibacillosis, the pregnant cow is vaccinated six to two weeks before parturition with either purified E. coli K99+ pili or a whole-cell preparation containing sufficient K99 antigen (Acres et al. 1979). Good protection is also possible when dams are vaccinated with a four-strain E. coli whole-cell bacterin containing sufficient K99+ pili antigen and the polysaccharide capsular K antigen.

The levels of K99+ E. coli antibodies in the colostrum of vaccinated cows are very high for the first two days and then decline rapidly. These high levels of specific antibody protect the calf from enterotoxigenic colibacillosis during the first few days of life, which is the most susceptible period for the disease.

The passive immunization of calves by vaccination of the pregnant cow with rotavirus and coronavirus vaccines has also received considerable attention (Saif et al. 1983; Myers and Snodgrass 1982). The colostrum of the majority of cows contains antibodies against the rotavirus and coronavirus, which cause diarrhea in calves after about five days of age. However, the levels in the colostrum decline very rapidly in a few days and are at nonprotective levels in the milk at three to five days after parturition. This probably explains the occurrence of the disease in calves after five days of age. The colostral levels of rotavirus and coronavirus antibodies can be markedly increased by vaccination of the pregnant cow, but the increased levels are usually not more protective than the naturally occurring levels in unvaccinated cows. A mechanism for prolonging the level in milk for the first several days or few weeks would be highly advantageous.

One method of providing a daily source of viral antibody in the milk of calves for up to two to three weeks is to feed pooled stored colostrum containing the antibody. Another method is to supplement the daily milk supply with colostrum containing high rotavirus antibody titers from vaccinated cows (Saif et al. 1983). Experimentally, a simultaneous intramuscular and intramammary vaccination of pregnant cows with a modified live adjuvant bovine rotavirus greatly enhances the colostral rotavirus antibody titers (Saif et al. 1983). This colostrum protects calves against experimental challenge with rotavirus when fed as a 1% supplement of the daily intake of milk. On a practical basis, the feeding of one-half colostrum from vaccinated or unvaccinated cows with one-half whole milk will protect calves from rotavirus- and coronavirus-induced diarrhea from birth to two to three weeks of age, during which time they are most susceptible to these viral diarrheas.

VEAL CALF PRODUCTION

The raising of dairy calves for veal production has been a profitable opportunity when the economic conditions are right. A readily available supply of inexpensive healthy calves, good quality milk replacers at an economical price, reliable labor, inexpensive housing, and a market potential provide the opportunity to produce veal calves.

Consumers of veal prefer a well-fleshed calf of a "blocky" conformation with only a small cover of white fat. The meat must be pale pink, an index of youth to the packer that is found only in an anemic calf. The American market desires a live weight ranging from about 200 to 300 lbs. (90 to 135 kg.). The calves should grow at a rate of over 2 lb. (0.9 kg.) daily with a feed conversion of 1.4 to 1.5 kg. of milk replacer powder per kilogram of body weight gain. At the end of the feeding period, calves will often gain in excess of 3 lb. per day. A 100-lb. calf should be ready for market in 12 to 16 weeks.

The major causes of economic loss due to disease in veal calf operations are the infectious disease enteritides and pneumonias.

The enteritides are commonly associated with the low serum and intestinal levels of immunoglobulins in calves that are purchased from different, usually unknown, sources (Williams et al. 1980). Calf pneumonia may also be associated with low levels of protective immunoglobulins, but inadequate ventilation of the calf barn probably has a greater influence on the health of veal calves raised under intensive conditions.

An emerging problem in veal calf production is the welfare of the animals (Van Patten 1982). Veal calves may be housed in individual raised-floor stalls with no bedding, a restricted floor space for lying down, and no special contact with adjacent calves. These restrictions may encourage calves to reach each other at feeding times or to attempt to turn around in their stall to see each other. When veal calves are reared in groups, they suck each other's navels and penises. If straw is provided in group pens, they will eat the straw, which may exaggerate the incidence of abomasal ulcers. When they are housed in groups of 15 to 50, automatic milk replacer dispensers can be installed economically at the rate of one per 15 animals, which may overcome the sucking problem. However, it appears that a well-designed individual stall with slatted fronts for visibility and a sufficiently wide floor that allows the calf to stretch out is satisfactory and humane.

Health Management of Veal Calves

Purchase of Calves. Ideally all calves should be at least 45 kg. (100 lb.) in body weight and at least 10 days of age when delivered to the vealing unit. This will ensure obtaining calves of optimal physiological maturity and with adequate levels of serum immunoglobulins. In other words, a 100-lb. calf that has survived for 10 days has a better chance of living for a few months than a smaller calf that is only a few days of age. In the absence of an economical practical laboratory method of identifying calves that are a good risk, the probability is greater that the larger calf at 10 days of age possesses a greater degree of inherent or acquired resistance to infectious disease than the smaller calf at two days of age. An algorithm can be used to assist in deciding how to manage purchased calves with low serum levels of immunoglobulins and to determine what premium can be paid for calves with high immunoglobulin levels (White et al. 1983).

Within a few hours after arrival, all calves should be given a complete physical examination by the veterinarian. Calves with obvious abormalities such as navel ill, arthritis, diarrhea, or pneumonia should be isolated, treated if deemed necessary, or culled immediately. Each calf should be weighed on arrival and identified with a tag, and an individual calf card should be made out and clipped to its pen. All relevant information for that calf is recorded in chronological order: weight in and out, date in and out, diagnosis of illness, treatments, feed refusals, and nature and date of vaccinations given. These cards are then analyzed when the calves are shipped to market.

The vealing unit should be filled with calves within the shortest time possible, and almost all calves should be marketed within the shortest time possible. The *all-in all-out system* of intensified livestock production has been highly successful in the poultry industry and should be encouraged in the cattle industry for complete depopulation and an effective clean-out and disinfection. The system of introducing new calves and selling a few on a continuous basis does not allow for effective disease control.

Feeding. Veal calves are usually fed solely on a reconstituted liquid milk replacer containing 20 to 25% fat (D.M.). The digestive problems associated with these milk replacers occur during the first few days when the calves are adjusting to the ration and later in the feeding period when large amounts of the liquid are ingested at each feeding.

Nutritional diarrhea occurs in calves that consume too much milk replacer during the first few days. This can be controlled by feeding only one half of a total daily allowance to new calves on the first day, increasing up to three quarters on the second day, and finally a full allowance on the third to fifth day. The total daily allowance is increased each week as the calf grows older. The nutritional diarrhea associated with the feeding of milk replacers containing heat-denatured skim milk will be discussed in Chapter 7.

Abomasal bloat occurs during the finishing period in veal calves, which are by this time consuming large quantities (9 to 12 kg.) of liquid milk replacer per feeding. The disease is highly fatal. Affected calves will bloat and die within 15 minutes after first being noticed. The etiology and pathogenesis of the disease are unknown, but presumably it is related to the ingestion of large quantities of milk replacer, most of which enters directly into the abomasum. This sudden overloading of the abomasum may cause a reflex outpouring of fluids from the abomasal mucosa, which may further exaggerate the dilatation. Death results from peracute abdominal distention and acute heart failure due to failure of venous return.

The method of feeding—whether once or twice daily; the temperature of the milk replacer when fed; and the use of buckets, nipple pails, or automatic dispensers may affect the performance of the calves under certain management conditions, but in general almost any feeding system will be successful if properly used with good care, management, and sanitation.

Vaccination. Because veal calves commonly originate from many different sources, their immunological background also varies considerably, and it is difficult to plan an effective reliable immunization program.

Other than autogenous bacterins given to the dams during the latter part of pregnancy, there are no vaccines available for the control of enteric colibacillosis and salmonellosis. Control will depend on the purchase of healthy calves that have an adequate colostral status and on the minimization of the natural challenge by the calf's environment.

The use of modified live virus vaccines for the control of infectious bovine rhinotracheitis and enzootic pneumonia caused by parainfluenza-3 virus infection may be considered in veal calves. Most veal calves will be marketed by 16 weeks of age, and the use of viral vaccines at an early age, soon after the calves have arrived in the unit, is controversial. Colostral immunity begins to wane at four to six weeks of age, and vaccination with viral vaccines may be considered shortly after this time.

Housing. Veal calves are usually raised under intensified conditions in which many calves are housed in individual pens with raised floors. Because veal calves are fed large quantities of fluid, they give off large quantities of moisture in their urine and feces, and thus an effective ventilation system is necessary to remove excess moisture. Supplemental heat may be necessary during cold winter months to maintain a satisfactory minimum inside temperature of at least 50°F (10°C). In cold climates, the calf barn must be insulated with material having an R value of 15 in the walls and 20 to 25 in the ceiling. A continuous air exchange through the building at a minimum rate of four changes per hour is essential. For the winter months in cold climates, the most satisfactory method to bring in fresh air is over the heating unit. During the summer months, 30 air exchanges per hour are desirable. With any system, careful management and common sense in operation are essential to its success, regardless of its design. Veterinarians should consult their local state or provincial agricultural engineering extension service for assistance in evaluating the ventilation system of calf barns. When investigating a problem with respiratory tract disease in a group of housed calves, the ventilation system and its adequacy assume primary importance.

Surveillance System. Each calf should be

Table 6–1. CONGENITAL DEFECTS OF CATTLE (INHERITED AND NON-INHERITED)

Nature of Defect	Cause/Breed Affected	Name of Defect	Outcome
Dropsical swelling of legs, sometimes trunk	INH.° Ayrshire	Lymphatic obstruction	Not fatal, but not worth rearing
Edema, ascites, dyspnea	INH. Hereford	Ventricular septal defect	Death by 3 months
Dyspnea	Unknown	Diaphragmatic hernia	Not worth rearing
Bulging forehead, blindness, imbecility	INH. Friesian, Hereford	Hydrocephalus	Not fatal, but not worth rearing
Bulging forehead; short face, neck, and limbs; tongue protrusion; cleft plate	INH. Jersey, Guernsey, Friesian	Achondroplasia with hydrocephalus (bulldog calves)	Should be destroyed
Cleft palate and harelip	INH. Hereford, Angus, Charolais	Cleft palate and harelip	Difficult to rear
Small eyeballs, often accompanied by heart defect	Unknown	Microphthalmia	Can be fattened for veal
Short legs, short head, protruding tongue, difficult respiration, pot belly, bloat	INH. Angus, Hereford, possibly Friesian, Shorthorn	Achondroplastic dwarfism	Should be destroyed
Bulging forehead, blindness, imbecility	Unknown	Hydrocephalus	Should be destroyed
Resembles inherited achondroplastic dwarfism	Unspecified nutritional deficiency	Acorn calves	Should be destroyed
Small deformed calves, gestation period up to 15 months, absence of pituitary gland, cyclops	INH. Jersey, Guernsey	Prolonged gestation (cyclops type)	Dead at birth
Prolonged gestation and very large calves	INH. Friesian	Prolonged gestation (monster type)	Cesarean; nonviable
Impacted, abnormally positioned premolars; short lower jaw	INH. Breed not identified	Inherited displaced molar teeth	Not worth rearing
Short mandible, impacted molars, patent fontanelle, small body size	INH. Angus	Congenital osteopetrosis	Not worth rearing
Underdeveloped lower jaw	INH. Shorthorn, Jersey, Friesian, Ayrshire	Inherited mandibular prognathism	Fatten for slaughter as veal
Head looks like a sheep's; many other defects	INH. Limousin	Inherited probatocephaly (sheepshead)	Early death
Do not prosper; poor hair coat, hypersalivation, small tongue papillae	INH. Holstein Friesian	Smooth tongue	Do not prosper
Blindness, absence of iris, cataract, corneal opacity in some; often associated with albinism and may be accompanied by hydrocephalus and optic nerve hypoplasia	INH. Jersey, possibly Friesian, Shorthorn (especially whites) and Hereford	Inherited multiple eye defects	Fatten for slaughter as veal
Unable to stand, tetanic convulsions when started, can drink	INH. Polled Hereford	Inherited neuraxial edema	Fatal, permanent recumbency
May be blindness and inability to stand, extreme staggering	INH. Friesian, Guernsey, Hereford	Cerebellar hypoplasia	Calves that can stand may be fattened for veal
Tremor of limbs and neck	INH. Jersey	Congenital spasms	Should be destroyed
Posterior paralysis, tremor, rigid extension of legs	INH. Red Poll, Norwegian, Red Poll/Red Danish	Posterior paralysis—inherited, congenital	Should be destroyed

Clinical signs	INH / Cause	Condition	Recommendation
Abdominal distention and abortion in the cow, flexion and fixation of all limb joints	INH. Friesian	Multiple ankylosis	Should be destroyed
Limbs fixed rigidly, either flexed or extended; can be freed by cutting tendons	INH. Shorthorn	Multiple tendon contracture	Should be destroyed
Absence of bones below fetlocks, normal foot connected to leg by skin	INH. Breeds not defined	Inherited reduced phalanges	Should be destroyed
Complete absence of limbs or vestigial, front or hinds	Not inherited, cause unknown	Amputates	Should be destroyed
Fixation of joints in extension or flexed	Akabane virus infection	Arthrogryposis	Should be destroyed
Knuckling over at fetlock joints	Unknown	Contracted flexor tendons	May recover spontaneously, can be treated surgically
Imbecility, blindness, may be associated with fixed joints	Akabane virus infection	Hydranencephaly	Should be destroyed
Blindness, convulsions, paralysis of all legs	Any breed	Vitamin A deficiency	Early cases respond to treatment
Muscle weakness and paralysis	Unknown	Enzootic muscular dystrophy (white muscle disease)	Early cases respond to treatment
Thin skin, well-demarcated highly developed limb muscles, may cause dystocia to dams	INH. Charolais, Piedmont, South Devon, and many other European breeds	Inherited musclar hypertrophy (double muscle)	Highly sought after
Lack of hair, plates of horny skin over most of body surface	INH. Friesian	Inherited fish scale disease (congenital ichthyosis)	Not worth rearing
Hyperelastic skin due to excessive fragility of skin and connective tissue	INH. Belgian cattle	Dermatosparaxia	Not worth rearing
Absence of hair, except around eyes, mouth, and feet	INH. Guernsey, Jersey	Inherited congenital hypotrichosis	Fatten for slaughter
Streaks of hairless skin	INH. Friesian	Inherited congenital partial hypotrichosis	Fatten for slaughter
Short curly coat with some very coarse hair	INH. Hereford	Inherited congenital partial hypotrichosis	Fatten for slaughter
Absence of skin on lower legs and muzzle	INH. Friesian	Inherited congenital absence of skin (epitheliogenesis imperfecta)	Die within a few days
Gestation period up to 12 months, difficult calving, giant calves	INH. Friesian, Ayrshire	Prolonged gestation (giant type)	Die soon after birth
Swelling at navel	INH. Friesian	Umbilical hernia	Can be repaired surgically, do not keep for breeding
Distention of abdomen, may cause dystocia, no defecation	INH. Swedish Highland	Inherited alimentary tract atresia	Die unless surgically corrected
Difficult swallowing of solids, chronic bloat	Unknown	Persistent right aortic arch	Die unless surgically corrected
Urine dribbles from navel	Unknown	Pervious arachus	Can be fattened for veal or treated surgically
Poor immune defense mechanism, incomplete albinos	INH. Hereford	Chediak-Higashi syndrome	Die of septicemia
Stillborn or weak calves with enlarged thyroid glands	Iodine deficiency in diet	Goiter	Respond to treatment with iodine

INH = Inherited

Table 6–2. INHERITED NON-CONGENITAL DEFECTS OF CATTLE

Nature of Defect	Breeds Affected	Name of Defect	Outcome
Inflammation of skin on light-colored parts exposed to sun; brown-colored teeth	Friesian, Shorthorn	Inherited congenital porphyria	Can be reared indoors
Epilepsy	Brown Swiss	Inherited idiopathic epilepsy	May die accidentally
Recurrent convulsions followed by persistent ataxia, specific cerebellar cortical degeneration (dominant)	Angus	Familial convulsions and ataxia	Fatten for slaughter
Gross staggering of gait appearing 2 days to 2 weeks after birth	Jersey, Friesian, Shorthorn	Inherited neonatal	Mild cases can be fattened for veal
Normal till 2 days, then incoordination, deviation of head, recumbency, tetanic convulsions	Jersey, Hereford	Inherited neonatal spasticity	Fatal at 1 month
Extreme straightness with shortening of one or both hind legs	Friesian, Angus	Elso heel (inherited spastic paresis)	Fatten for slaughter
Rigidity of one or both hind legs on rising	Friesian, Guernsey	Inherited periodic spasticity (stall cramp)	No difficulty usually encountered
Protrusion and deviation of eyeballs, defective vision	Shorthorn, Jersey	Exophthalmos with strabismus	No difficulty usually encountered
Gradual loss of hair beginning at top of body	Friesian	Inherited symmetrical alopecia	Fatten for slaughter
Absence of horns; loss of hair on ears, knees, axillae, and flanks; long hooves; salivation	Friesian	Baldy calves	Always fatal
Normal to 4–8 weeks, then alopecia and thick crusts on head, neck, and legs; poor growth, hypoplasia of thymus	Black Pied Danish, other European breeds, including Friesian	Inherited parakeratosis	Die at 4 months, but can be maintained on daily intake of zinc
Stagging gait, failure to grow, complete paralysis	Angus, Galloway Murray Grey	Inherited mannosidosis (storage of mannose excessive due to deficiency of mannosidase; detected by mannosidase level in plasma)	Fatten for slaughter
Congestion of mucosa, dyspnea, high RBC count	Jersey	Familial polycythemia	Early death
Sudden death due to internal hemorrhage	Unnamed breed in Holland	Inherited aortic aneurysm	Sudden death
Osteoarthritis—particularly of stifle joint—develops slowly over 1–2 years	Holstein-Friesian, Jersey	Inherited osteoarthritis	Usually worth nursing but not to be used as a dam
At birth very curly coat, die suddenly at up to 6 months old; are very big calves; at necropsy have myocardial dystrophy	Polled Hereford	Inherited myocardiopathy	Always fatal
Hip lameness at 6 months and older, exacerbated by heavy feeding and fast growth rate	Hereford	Degenerative joint disease of young bulls	Useless for breeding
Curved claw—lateral digit narrow, curves inward, cracks in coronet, lame	Hereford, Holstein, Shorthorn	Curved claw	Permanently lame
Very mobile joints, no tooth dentine, pink teeth	Holstein	Collagen defect	Not viable
Very mobile joints, teeth normal	Jersey	Collagen defect	Not viable

examined twice daily for clinical evidence of disease. A nasal discharge, crusty nose, salivation, dyspnea, coughing, diarrhea, reluctance to get up, and refusal to feed are common clinical findings in sick veal calves. The diagnosis and treatment given should be recorded on the individual calf card, and on a regular basis a summary of diseases and mortality should be prepared, analyzed, and interpreted and the necessary control procedures instituted.

A decrease in appetite is one of the first and most reliable indicators of anemia in veal calves. A concentration of 25 to 30 mg. of soluble iron per kg. dietary dry matter will provide sufficient hemoglobin for normal appetite, growth, and oxygen transport, and also will result in carcasses light enough in color for the veal trade (Bremner et al. 1976).

Review Literature

Appleman, R.D. and Owen, F.G. Symposium: Recent advances in calf rearing, breeding, housing and feeding management. J. Dairy Sci., 58:447-464, 1975.

Foley, J.A. and Otterby, D.E. Availability, storage, treatment, composition, and feeding value of surplus colostrum: A review, J. Dairy Sci., 61:1033-1060, 1978.

Roe, C.P. A review of the environmental factors influencing calf respiratory disease. Agricultural Meteorology 26:127-144, 1982.

Roy, J.H.B. Symposium: Disease prevention in calves. Factors affecting susceptibility of calves to disease. J. Dairy Sci., 63:650-664, 1980.

References

Acres, S.D., Isaacson, R.E., Babiuk, L.A. et al. Immunization of calves against enterotoxigenic colibacillosis by vaccinating dams with purified K99 antigen and whole cell bacterins. Infect. Immun., 25:121-126, 1979.

Anderson, J.F. Medical factors relating to calf health as influenced by the environment. Bovine Pract., 13:3-5, 1978.

Anderson, J.F. and Bates, D.W. Influence of improved ventilation on health of confined cattle. J. Am. Vet. Med. Assoc., 174:577-580, 1979.

Appleman, R.D. and Owen, F.G. Symposium: Recent advances in calf rearing, breeding, housing and feeding management. J. Dairy Sci., 58:447-464, 1975.

Bates, D.W. and Anderson, J.F. Calculation of ventilation needs for confined cattle. J. Am. Vet. Med. Assoc., 174:581-589, 1979.

Bremner, I., Brockway, J.M., Donnelly, H.T. et al. Anaemia and veal calf production. Vet. Rec., 99:203-205, 1976.

Brignole, T.J. and Stott, G.H. Effect of sucking followed by bottle feeding colostrum in immunogloblin absorption and calf survival. J. Dairy Sci., 63:451-456, 1980.

Fleenor, W.A. and Stott, G.H. Hydrometer test for estimation of immunoglobulin concentration in bovine colostrum. J. Dairy Sci., 63:973-977, 1980.

Foley, J.A. and Otterby, D.E. Availability, storage, treatment, composition and feeding value of surplus colostrum: A review. J. Dairy Sci., 61:1033-1060, 1978.

Graham-Marr, T. and Spreull, J.S.A. Disinfection in veterinary practice. N.Z. Vet. J., 17:1-31, 1969.

Gusbi, A.M. and Hird, D.W. Calf mortality rates on five Libyan dairy stations, 1976-1980. Prev. Med., 1:205-214, 1983.

Hird, D.W. and Robinson, R.A. Dairy farm wells in southeastern Minnesota. I. The relation of water source to milk and milk fat production. II. The relation of water source to calf mortality rate. Prev. Vet. Med., 1:37-51, 53-64, 1982.

Jenny, B.F., Gramling, G.E. and Glaze, T.M. Management factors associated with calf mortality in South Carolina dairy herds. J. Dairy Sci., 64:2284-2289, 1981.

Kertz, A.F. Calf health, performance, and experimental results under a commercial research facility and program. J. Dairy Sci., 60:1006-1015, 1977.

Logan, E.F., Muskett, B.D. and Herron, R.J. Colostrum feeding of dairy calves. Vet. Rec., 108:283-284, 1981.

Martin, S.W. and Wiggins, A.D. A model of the economic costs of dairy calf mortality. Am. J. Vet. Res., 34:1027-1031, 1973.

Martin, S.W., Schwabe, C.W. and Franti, C.E. Dairy calf mortality rate: Characteristics of calf mortality rates in Tulare County, California. Am. J. Vet. Res., 36:1099-1104, 1975a.

Martin, S.W., Schwabe, C.W. and Franti, C.E. Dairy calf mortality rate: Influence of meteorologic factors on calf mortality rate in Tulare County, California. Am. J. Vet. Res., 36:1105-1109, 1975b.

Martin, S.W., Schwabe, C.W. and Franti, C.E. Dairy calf mortality rate: Influence of management and housing factors on calf mortality rate in Tulare County, California. Am. J. Vet. Res., 36:1111-1114, 1975c.

McKnight, D.R. Performance of newborn dairy calves in hutch housing. Can. J. Anim. Sci., 58:517-520, 1978.

Mitchell, C.D. Some environmental aspects of calf housing—a review. Farm Building R and D Studies, 02 January 1972, pp. 3-19.

Mitchell, C.D. Calf housing handbook. Scottish Farm Buildings Investigation Unit. Craibstone, Bucksburn, Aberdeen, U.K. 1976.

Mitchell, C.D. and Broadbent, P.J. The effect of level and method of feeding milk substitute and housing environment on the performance of calves. Anim. Prod., 17:245-256, 1973.

Molla, A. Immunoglobulin levels in calves fed colostrum by stomach tube. Vet. Rec., 103:377-380, 1978.

Molla, A. Estimation of bovine colostral immunoglobulins by refractometry. Vet. Rec., 107:35-36, 1980.

Myers, L.L. and Snodgrass, D.R. Colostral and milk antibody titers in cows vaccinated with a modified live rotavirus-coronavirus vaccine. J. Am. Vet. Med. Assoc., 181:486-488, 1982.

Oxender, W.D., Newman, L.E. and Morrow, D.A. Factors influencing dairy calf mortality in Michigan. J. Am. Vet. Med. Assoc., 162:458-460, 1973.

Radostits, O.M. and Acres, S.D. Diseases of calves admitted to a large animal clinic in Saskatchewan. Can. Vet. J., 15:82-87, 1974.

Roy, J.H.B. Diarrhea of nutritional origin. Proc. Nutr. Soc., 28:160-170, 1969.

Roy, J.H.B. Symposium: Disease prevention in calves. Factors affecting susceptibility of calves to disease. J. Dairy Sci., 63:650-664, 1980.

Saif, L.J., Redman, D.R., Smith, L.K. et al. Passive immunity to bovine rotavirus in newborn calves fed colostrum supplements from immunized or non-immunized cows. Infect. Immun., *41*:1118–1131, 1983.

Sainsbury, D.W.B. and Sainsbury, P. Livestock Health and Housing. Second Edition. London, Baillière Tindall, 1979.

Scarlett, C.M. and Mathewson, G.K. Terminal disinfection of calf houses by formaldehyde fumigation. Vet. Rec., *101*:7–10, 1977.

Simensen, E. An epidemiological study of calf health and performance in Norwegian dairy herds. II. Factors affecting mortality. Acta Agric. Scand., *32*:421–427, 1982.

Speicher, J.A. and Hepp, R.E. Factors associated with calf mortality in Michigan dairy herds. J. Am. Vet. Med. Assoc., *162*:463–466, 1973.

Stott, G.H. Immunoglobulin absorption in calf neonates with special considerations of stress. J. Dairy Sci., *63*: 681–688, 1980.

Stott, G.H. and Fellah, A. Colostral immunoglobulin absorption linearly related to concentration of calves. J. Dairy Sci., *66*:1319–1328, 1983.

Stott, G.H., Marx, D.B., Menefee, B.E. et al. Colostral im-

munoglobulin transfer in calves. I. Period of absorption. J. Dairy Sci., *62*:1632–1638, 1979a.

Stott, G.H., Marx, D.B., Menefee, B.E. et al. Colostral immunoglobulin transfer in calves. II. The rate of absorption. J. Dairy Sci., *62*:1766–1773, 1979b.

Stott, G.H., Marx, D.B., Menefee, B.E. et al. Colostral Immunoglobulin transfer in calves. III. Amount of absorption. J. Dairy Sci., *62*:1902–1907, 1979c.

Stott, G.H., Marx, D.B., Menefee, B.E. et al. Colostral immunoglobulin transfer in calves. IV. Effect of sucking. J. Dairy Sci., *62*:1908–1913, 1979d.

Turnbull, J.E. Housing and environment for dairy calves. Can. Vet. J., *21*:85–90, 1980.

Van Patten, G. Welfare in veal calf units. Vet. Rec., *111*: 437–440, 1982.

White, M.E., Pearson, E.G., Davidson, J.N. et al. An algorithm for minimizing financial losses due to immune deficiency in calves. Cornell Vet., *73*:76–81, 1983.

Williams, P.E.U., Wright, C.L. and Day, N. Mortality in groups of purchased Friesian cross calves. Br. Vet. J., *136*:561–566, 1980.

Veterinary Aspects of Dairy Cattle— Nutrition and Housing

Barn Environment
Heat Stress
Corral Systems
Veterinary Handling Facilities
Calf Housing

Periodic Depopulation
Manure Storage and Disposal,
   and Sanitation in Dairy Barns
Manure Handling Systems

Nutrition

INTRODUCTION

Feed is the largest cost in the production of milk by dairy cattle. Therefore, both the producer and the veterinarian must be concerned about using the most economical source of high-quality feed that will consistently yield the best level of production with a minimal incidence of nutritionally related disease. Thus regular surveillance and analysis of the nutritional program should be a major component of a totally integrated dairy herd health service provided by a veterinarian.

In a typical dairy herd that raises its own heifer replacements, there are several different classes of animals, each of which needs nutritional attention on a regular basis. They are as follows:

Calves from birth to weaning at about two months of age (or earlier in some cases)

Calves from weaning to 12 months of age

Heifers from 12 months of age to breeding at 15 months of age

Pregnant heifers from 15 to 24 months of age

First-calf lactating heifers

Cows in early lactation

Cows in mid-lactation

Cows in late lactation

Dry cows

The knowledge required by the veterinarian to provide a nutritional monitoring and advisory service for each of these classes of cattle includes the following:

1. The production objectives to be achieved within each class of animal

2. The nutritional requirements of each class of animal

3. The ingredient analysis and costs of the feeds used

4. The formulation of the diets and the feeding systems used to deliver the diets

5. The diagnosis and prevention of the nutritionally related diseases or problems

A dairy cattle veterinary specialist can acquire the knowledge and the skills to provide a nutritional advisory service that will meet the needs of the typical dairy herd. However, the veterinarian should consult with an experienced dairy cattle nutritionist on a regular basis to ensure that the best advice is being given. This necessitates regular feed analysis and formulation of diets, which should be done in consultation with a competent nutritionist. Programable calculators and computer programers can assist in the formulation of economical complete diets. The nutrient requirements of dairy cattle for growth, maintenance, pregnancy, and lactation are readily available and should be used as guidelines in formulating diets.

NUTRITION OF THE CALF FROM BIRTH TO WEANING AT TWO MONTHS OF AGE

The major objectives during this period are to control the incidence of dietary and infectious diarrheas, to obtain satisfactory growth rates, and to successfully wean the calf at about two months of age. Heifer replacements are expensive; therefore, all available and economical resources should be used and applied to raise the heifer calves in a dairy herd, and they should be given high priority.

The Digestive System of the Newborn Calf

Certain parts of the intestinal tract and their respective digestive enzyme activities have particular nutritional significance; these are reviewed briefly as background for an understanding of digestive disturbances of young calves that are nutritional in origin (Huber 1969).

The Abomasum

In the newborn calf, the abomasum makes up about 70% of the total stomach volume, in contrast to the adult ruminant, in which it makes up only about 8% (Radostits and Bell 1970). In the preruminant calf, liquid food flows through the closed esophageal groove directly into the abomasum, thus bypassing the forestomachs. The abomasum of the newborn calf is capable physically and biochemically of initiating the digestion of milk. It can undergo considerable expansion and hold large quantities of liquid. It secretes rennin, the milk-coagulating enzyme that clots the milk, yielding a casein clot and whey. The whey enters the duodenum within five minutes of feeding, and the casein clot remains in the abomasum. Rennin is also a proteolytic enzyme and is probably responsible for the breakdown of the milk clot in the early life of the calf before it develops any appreciable pepsin HCl proteolytic enzyme activity. The casein clot is degraded gradually by the enzyme action of rennin and/or pepsin and hydrochloric acid, and the partially digested proteins and fat are released at a fairly continuous rate over 24 hours. The main passage into the small intestines and further enzyme action by trypsin, chymotrypsin, and carboxypeptidases present in the pancreatic juice and by other peptidases secreted in the small intestine is followed by absorption from the small intestine as amino acids.

A gradual changeover from rennin to pepsin secretion in the abomasum occurs as the calf grows older. Rennin activity reaches a peak at a pH of 4, whereas the optimum pH for pepsin activity is about 2. Pepsin activity is very slight until the calf is about three weeks of age, at which time it begins to efficiently digest non-milk proteins. Before the calf can digest non-milk proteins (plant proteins, meat meal, and fish by-products), the abomasal juice must attain a pH of 2, and pepsin activity must be adequate.

Intestinal and Pancreatic Enzyme Activity (Fig. 7-1)

Lactase. Lactase is present in adequate amounts in the intestines of the newborn calf, which is well equipped to hydrolyze lactose. The levels of intestinal lactase decrease with age but increase significantly when calves are fed increasing levels of lactose added to whole milk.

Maltase. Intestinal maltase hydrolyzes maltose derived from amylose. The newborn calf has almost no maltase activity, and even at seven weeks of age only slight activity has developed. Based on blood sugar responses after feeding, the digestion of starch in the alimentary tract posterior to the rumen of the calf is very low when compared with the digestion of lactose. Because of the very low levels of amylase and maltase activities in the preruminant calf, it cannot utilize significant levels of dietary starch.

Sucrase. Calves have almost no intestinal sucrase activity at birth and develop little if any in later life. This is in sharp contrast with the pig, which develops enough sucrase activity at about two to three weeks of age for the efficient digestion of some dietary sucrose. In the preruminant calf, there is some intestinal microbial digestion of sucrose, but the extent of utilization of the end products of this bacterial action by the calf is not known.

Pancreatic and Salivary Gland Digestive Enzymes

The pancreas secretes trypsin, chymotrypsin, amylase, and lipase into the intestines. The activities of trypsin and chymotrypsin—the pancreatic protein-splitting enzymes—are low at one day of age but increase to high levels by eight days of age and remain high thereafter. Pancreatic amylase, the starch-splitting enzyme, is secreted in very small quantities in newborn calves, and its activity is still low at nine months of age.

The amount of pancreatic lipase present is low in the calf at birth but increases rapidly to nutritionally adequate levels by eight days of age. This correlates well with the ability of the newborn calf to digest with high efficiency the fat in cows' whole milk and the wide variety of animal and vegetable fats added to milk replacers. However, for maximum digestion, the physical properties of added fats are critical. Their chemical structure influences digestibility; for example, triglycerides containing long-chain saturated fatty acids are not well digested.

Salivary lipase is secreted by the palatine glands of the calf. It hydrolyzes the butyric acid esters of glycerol most effectively and is therefore beneficial in the digestion of tributyrin in butterfat. The content of the enzyme decreases as the calf increases its consumption of roughage but remains high if the calf con-

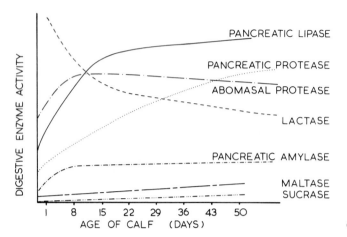

Figure 7-1. The relationship of age and digestive enzyme activity in the young calf.

tinues to consume milk containing triglycerides consisting of butyrate groups. The combination of pancreatic and salivary lipases makes an effective enzyme system for the digestion of fat. There is no significant secretion of lipolytic enzymes by the fundal mucosa of the abomasum, and lipolysis of triglycerides in the abomasum of the preruminant calf is due predominantly to a lipolytic enzyme in saliva (Toothill et al. 1976).

NUTRIENT REQUIREMENTS OF THE CALF BETWEEN BIRTH AND WEANING

The details of the nutrient requirements of the preruminant calf in the first few weeks of life are available (Radostits and Bell 1970; Jacobson 1969; National Research Council 1978). The ingredients of major importance for satisfactory growth are energy, protein, and fat. Cows' whole milk will provide all of the nutrient requirements of the calf from birth to weaning and provides acceptable growth rates. Deficiencies of energy and/or protein are usually associated with the use of inferior-quality milk replacers, which may contain heat-denatured proteins or poorly digestible added nonmilk carbohydrates or proteins. The problems associated with milk replacers will be presented later.

There are marked variations in the estimated protein and energy requirements of calves, particularly in the ruminant stage (Jacobson 1969). These requirements are influenced by rate of gain, body size, age, diet, and other factors. A number of studies have shown that milk replacers, on an air-dry basis, should contain at least 20% crude protein growth and

that protein deposition is increased by even higher levels. The optimum crude protein level for calf starters usually is considered to be about 16%, but lower levels (to about 12%) have often resulted in maximum growth response. Other components of the diet and the rate of gain desired have a major effect on the amount of protein needed in feeds of the young calf. As the rate of growth increases, the optimum ratio of protein to energy increases markedly.

On the basis of data derived from four studies (Jacobson 1969), the average requirements (and range) of the 50-kg. nonruminating calf for digestible energy are 47 kcal. (range, 41 to 52) per kg. body weight for maintenance and 3.3 kcal. (range, 2.7 to 3.8) per g. body weight for gain. The requirements for the ruminating calf weighing 50 to 100 kg. are slightly higher for both digestible energy and protein.

Colostrum

The ingestion of liberal quantities of colostrum by the newborn calf within the first six hours after birth is the most important requirement. Approximately 25% of dairy calves may not voluntarily ingest sufficient colostrum even when they have been left with their dams for the first 24 to 48 hours after birth. This may necessitate the forced feeding of colostrum to all calves as a routine procedure to ensure that a minimum amount has been ingested early enough. Colostrum should be fed for at least three days. Absorption of colostral immunoglobulins ceases by 24 hours after birth, but the continued ingestion of colostrum will provide local intestinal immunity against acute undifferentiated diarrhea.

Storage of Colostrum

Colostrum that is preserved for several days or for up to two to three weeks is practical, economical, and reliable and may assist in the reduction of the incidence of infectious diarrheas because of the presence of colostral immunoglobulins, which provide local immunity (Foley and Otterby 1978). The availability, storage, treatment, composition, and feeding value of surplus colostrum have been reviewed. Surplus colostrum may be considered a cost-free liquid feed for calves, because it is unmarketable for human consumption. Sufficient excess colostrum should be available to feed heifer calves through 28 to 35 days of age. First-calf Holstein heifers and mature cows will yield from 30 to 50 kg. of colostrum from the first five postpartum milkings. With an average of about 44 kg. of colostrum per cow and an average consumption of 11 kg. per calf during the first three days of life, 33 kg. of colostrum would be available per cow for feeding calves over three days of age. Calves commonly have been fed 1.8 to 3.2 kg. of undiluted colostrum daily from day four of life to weaning. With an average daily consumption of 2.5 kg., colostrum from one cow will feed one calf through 16 days of age. If bull calves are sold within several days of birth, sufficient colostrum should be available to feed heifer calves to four weeks of age. Colostrum can be stored economically at ambient temperatures in plastic-lined containers with minimum handling requirements. However, losses to spoilage and undesirable fermentation can limit the shelf-life of stored colostrum. Warm temperatures may enhance putrefactive fermentation, which may be decreased by the use of chemical preservatives such as formic, acetic, and propionic acids and formaldehyde. Although chemical additives have not decreased the total number of microbes, some preservatives have decreased the numbers of coliform bacilli, molds, and yeasts while preserving a greater portion of the nutrient content of colostrum than is possible with natural fermentation. However, some unavoidable nutrient losses occur during storage at ambient temperatures, with and without chemical additives. A given amount of colostrum can replace more than an equal weight of whole milk in calf feeding programs owing to its high content of total solids. Dilution of colostrum diets with water is not necessary, but dilution may provide a more filling diet for calves fed once daily. Dilution with warm water may provide a more acceptable diet to the calf but will not increase calf performance. The amounts of colostrum fed and the rates of dilution should be designed to supply a desirable intake of solids to the calf. Colostrum with a total solid content of 18% can be diluted 2:1 with water to approximate the total solid content of whole milk at 12%. The diluted colostrum is then fed at a rate of 8% of body weight per day.

Whole Milk

Following the three-day colostral feeding period, dairy calves may be fed whole milk, a milk replacer, or a combination of these, depending on preference, availability, and economics.

Whole milk is excellent for use in feeding calves, especially those that are being raised as heifer replacements. Whole milk is usually fed twice daily at a rate of 8 to 10% of body weight, depending on the size of the calf. Small breed calves are usually given the small amount. Calves may be fed solely on whole milk until weaning at 35 to 56 days of age. A calf starter diet containing 16 to 20% protein should be made available in small quantities (100 g./day) beginning the second week of life. This should be increased every several days so that the calf is consuming about 450 g. per day before weaning in addition to small quantities of good-quality hay. Calves should not be weaned until they are consuming about 400 to 600 g. of dry feed per day. When the amount of milk or milk replacer is fed over a shorter period of time (three to four weeks), the calf must be encouraged to eat dry feed at an early age. Early weaning at three to four weeks is a low-cost feeding method that accelerates the transition of the calf from a preruminant to a ruminant. However, some calves do not adjust effectively and are unthrifty for up to several weeks. They may also develop a chronic dietary diarrhea.

Milk Replacers

Milk replacers (substitutes) are used extensively to raise calves for replacements in dairy herds and to fatten calves in vealing operations. These milk replacers are cheaper than cow's whole milk because they consist of skim milk powder and other milk by-products and added fats of animal or vegetable origin, added carbohydrates of vegetable origin, and more recently, added nonmilk proteins (Stobo and Roy 1978). The composition and quality of these milk replacers vary considerably;

whereas many are of good quality, some are nutritionally inadequate and predispose to digestive disturbances, resulting in chronic diarrhea, poor growth rates, secondary starvation, and high morbidity and mortality rates, usually owing to enteric disease (Roy 1969).

This section reviews some of the nutritional aspects of the newborn calf and their relationship to nutritional diarrhea in calves fed milk replacers. Review articles with details on the subject are available (Radostits and Bell 1970; Roy and Ternouth 1972; Roy 1977).

The Digestibility of Nutrients in Calves Fed Milk or Milk Replacers

The apparent digestibilities of the dry matter, nitrogen, and fat of cows' whole milk fed to young calves under 10 days of age are high— 95, 94, and 95% respectively. Based on the nutrient requirements of the newborn calf and the ability of the calf to digest the carbohydrates, protein, and fat in cows' whole milk, the ideal milk replacer for calves up to three weeks of age, which would approximate the quality of cows' whole milk, would contain the following ingredients:

1. Spray-dried skim milk powder derived from liquid skim milk that is preheated prior to drying at a temperature not exceeding 77°C for 15 seconds. This skim milk powder would make up about 75 to 80% of milk replacer.
2. A source of digestible fat, which is mixed and homogenized with liquid skim milk before spray-drying at a level of 15 to 20%.
3. Vitamins A, D, and E; B-complex vitamins; and vitamin B_{12}.
4. Cobalt-iodized salt, copper, iron, and zinc and other trace minerals.

Milk replacers that will support optimum growth of young calves are based on skim milk, which the newborn calf can readily digest. Skim milk is low in butterfat, which is a source of energy and essential fatty acids, and consequently, much of the research with milk replacers for calves is aimed at methods of increasing the energy content by adding nonmilk carbohydrates such as cereal starches and animal or vegetable fats. Whole milk powder contains from 35 to 40% fat, and it has been a challenge to find nonmilk fat that will replace butterfat. Attempts are also being made to replace the high-quality milk protein with less expensive vegetable and animal proteins. Milk replacers that are presently available for young calves usually consist of dried skim milk powder as a base plus varying amounts of dried buttermilk powder, dried whey powder, and a variety of added nonmilk carbohydrates, fats, and proteins.

The quality of milk replacer for calves under three weeks of age depends upon the digestibility of each ingredient and the relative amount of each in the total mixture (Radostits and Bell 1968).

Quality of Skim Milk Powder

Calves under three weeks of age require a diet based on skim milk that has not been severely heated. Only low-temperature preheating of liquid skim milk at 77°C for 15 seconds prior to spray-drying yields a product similar to fresh cow's whole milk. Severe heat treatment (74°C for 30 minutes) of liquid skim milk results in denaturation of the whey proteins (noncasein nitrogen) and failure of the development of a firm milk clot in the abomasum. Many commercially produced skim milk powders designated as high-heat, medium-heat, and roller-dried products yield only soft curds, whereas low-heat powders yield strong curds (Emmons and Lister 1976a, 1976b). The clotting properties of severely heated skim milk are reduced, and flocculent precipitate instead of a firm curd is formed in the abomasum. Abomasal digestion is impaired as a result of reduced acid and enzyme secretion, and undigested casein escapes into the duodenum (Williams et al. 1976; Lister and Emmons 1976). The output of proteolytic enzymes is also reduced, and the overall effect is a reduction in digestibility. Clinically, there is persistent diarrhea, failure to grow, and in some cases emaciation, starvation, and death over a period of two to four weeks. Only the addition of undenatured whey proteins will improve the nutritive quality of heat-denatured skim milk powder (Roy and Ternouth 1972).

Fat Content and Quality. Within a few days of birth, the calf is able to digest a wide variety of animal and vegetable fats added to skim milk–based milk replacers. However, added fats must be homogenized and emulsified for optimum digestion. Low-pressure dispersion of fat in high-fat milk replacers results in the formation of a firm protein-lipid curd in the abomasum that slows the release of nutrients into the intestine and improves overall calf performance (Jenkins and Emmons 1979). When fats are used, anti-oxidants are also necessary to prevent the formation of peroxides, which may contribute to muscular dystrophy due to vitamin E deficiency (Roy 1977).

Nonmilk Carbohydrates and Proteins in Milk Replacers. Because the activities of pancreatic amylase and intestinal maltase and sucrase are very low during the first four weeks of a calf's life, starch (oatmeal, wheat meddlings, and corn flour) and its degradation products should not be included in milk replacers for calves under 28 days of age. The levels of the above enzymes do not increase to significant levels even in older calves, but digestion of added carbohydrates is improved with initiation of rumen function.

Many nonmilk proteins have been examined as possible replacements for skim milk in milk replacers for calves. The most widely available products have been prepared from soybeans (Ramsey and Willard 1975), fish (Huber 1975), single-cell proteins, field beans, peas, rapeseeds, and potato proteins (Stobo and Roy 1978). Replacement proteins must contain the essential amino acids. In general, the apparent digestibility of total dietary nitrogen decreases as the inclusion of nonmilk proteins is increased. The reduction is less in calves over one month of age. The use of soybean in milk replacers results in diarrhea, loss of appetite, muscular weakness, and poor growth rate. The use of highly refined soy protein concentrate in which the trypsin inhibitor and hemagglutinins have been inactivated results in some improvement but is still unsatisfactory. Gastrointestinal allergies characterized by diarrhea, weight loss, and poor growth may occur in preruminant calves receiving diets in which a high proportion of the protein is in the form of soybean flour (Kilshaw and Sissons 1979a, 1979b). Antibodies specific for soybean proteins appear in the serum within two weeks after being on the diet. It would appear that high levels of soybean protein cannot be well utilized by the calf until three to four weeks of age when the abomasum secretes sufficient pepsin-HCl to digest nonmilk proteins. At this time it may be possible to supply up to 40 to 50% of the total protein in milk replacers with highly refined soybean. A similar situation exists with fish protein concentrate, and digestibility also improves with age. Proteolytic enzymes have been added to milk replacers containing nonmilk proteins in an attempt to improve digestibility. However, the proteinases that occur in the calf's gastrointestinal tract, such as pepsin, chymosin, trypsin, and chymotrypsin, hydrolyze milk proteins much better than proteins derived from soybean, rapeseed, or fish sources (Jenkins et al. 1980). The use of certain proteolytic enzymes shows promise as dietary supplementary enzymes for the improvement of the digestibility of nonmilk proteins in calf milk replacers.

Assessment of Milk Replacer Quality. The quality of milk replacers may be evaluated indirectly by animal performance (Fisher 1976), by laboratory analysis of the amount of noncasein nitrogen present in the skim milk powder (Lister 1971), or by the in vitro rennet coagulation of skim milk powder or the milk replacer. The growth rate of calves fed milk replacer may be compared with established growth rates when fed cows' whole milk (Fisher 1976). Calves fed inferior-quality milk replacers will commonly have a persistent diarrhea that responds only to feeding with cows' whole milk. Loss of weight and starvation over a period of three to four weeks occur (Thomson 1965). In large herds where large numbers of calves are being raised, the incidence of diarrhea of infectious origin will be higher than normal.

The concentration of undenatured whey protein (noncasein nitrogen) should not be less than 4 mg./g. of skim milk powder for optimum abomasal curd formation. The rennet coagulability of the skim milk powder or the reconstituted milk replacer may also be used. A few drops of rennet are added to 15 ml. of reconstituted milk replacer, and the degree of clotting that occurs from 20 seconds to two minutes later is evaluated using whole milk as a control (Johnson and Leibholz 1976). Whole milk clots in 22 to 37 seconds; low-heat spray-dried skim milk clots in 30 to 47 seconds; and high-heat spray-dried skim milk does not clot, even after 15 minutes.

There is no reliable relationship between the concentration of whey protein nitrogen and the rennet coagulability of the reconstituted milk replacer (Lister and Emmons 1976). Milk replacers may contain adequate levels of whey protein nitrogen but fail to clot when mixed with rennet.

The in vitro rennet coagulation of reconstituted skim milk powder is affected by several factors (Emmons and Lister 1976a). Curd firmness is increased by lower pH of the skim milk powder over a range of 5.6 to 6.6, higher concentration of skim milk solids over a range of 5 to 20%, high concentrations of rennin, lower temperatures of heat treatment of liquid skim milk prior to spray-drying, and higher temperature of coagulation—37 vs. 30°C. Reconstitution of the powder in water above 56°C for two minutes remarkably reduces the firmness of the curd. Thus, when protein nitrogen is neither an acceptable index of rennet coagulability of milk replacers nor a reliable index for selecting commercially produced skim milk powders with good rennet coagulability. Coagulation testing conditions are now recommended for the laboratory evaluation and comparison of powders and milk replacers.

In summary, chronic diarrhea and unthriftiness may occur in calves under three weeks of age being fed a milk replacer. The digestibility of the ingredients of the milk replacer is dependent on the quality of the ingredients and age of the calf. The ingredient composition of the milk replacer must be obtained from the manufacturer, and simple laboratory tests are available to evaluate the suitability of the product for calves. The other common causes of diarrhea and unthriftiness must be excluded by clinical and laboratory examination. Calves can be reared successfully on good-quality milk replacers offered immediately following the colostral feeding period, and producers should be encouraged to use high-quality milk replacers.

WEANING CALVES

Calves should be weaned only when they are ready to be weaned. They should be eating at least 450 g. of dry feed daily—primarily a high-protein calf starter and some good-quality hay (Kertz et al. 1979). They should be ruminants before they are weaned. Limited whole milk or milk replacer feeding systems with early weaning at three to four weeks of age may be successful under excellent management conditions. However, under most practical conditions it is uneconomic to wean heifer replacement calves too early. They may not adjust to the dry feed quickly and effectively and may become unthrifty for several weeks.

The trend toward early weaning, rapid growth, and early breeding stresses the importance of good calf starter ration. The starter should be fresh daily and palatable, with the grains cracked or rolled and nutrient composition of 20% protein, 70% total digestible nutrients (TDN), and added vitamins and minerals. At weaning time the calf should be consuming approximately 0.5 to 0.7 kg. of calf starter per day, which will increase rapidly after weaning when offered free choice. The amount can be limited to 2 kg. per calf per day and can be fed along with good-quality hay and free-choice water until the calf is six months of age.

HOUSING FOR CALVES

A major determinant of successful calf rearing is adequate comfortable housing, the details of which are presented in the section under housing of dairy cattle. In the context of the nutrition of the young calf, it should be emphasized that cold housing will increase the nutrient requirements, especially energy, by as much as 25% during the winter months. The intake of liquid diets must be increased for calves raised outdoors in calf hutches or in cold unheated calf barns.

MONITORING CALF PERFORMANCE FROM BIRTH TO WEANING

Insufficient attention has been given to monitoring the performance of calves. Ideally, calves should be weighed at birth and weekly thereafter until weaning. Body weight gain is usually minimal during the first week of life, but gains of 300 to 500 g./day, depending on the breed of the calf, should occur after the second week of life and until weaning. Decreased growth rates are associated with a decreased whole milk intake, inferior milk replacers, and subclinical diseases such as chronic diarrhea and enzootic calf pneumonia.

REARING CALVES ON PASTURE

In many countries where grass is plentiful for several or more months of the year, young calves can be reared successfully on grass beginning shortly before or after being weaned from milk or milk replacer.

In New Zealand and to a lesser extent in Britain, most calves born in the spring are routinely placed on pasture soon after birth. Successful rearing of dairy calves on pasture can also be achieved in North America. Calf performance on pasture, with few exceptions, has equaled or surpassed indoor rearing and has produced healthier, thriftier calves (Gorrill 1964).

Several factors are important for the successful rearing of young calves on pasture. The quantity and quality of grass available are of utmost importance owing to the highly selective nature of grazing calves. Young calves will tend to starve themselves on unsuitable pastures unless they receive a supplemental concentrate. Digestibility trials reveal that calves from three to five weeks of age can utilize approximately 75% of herbage dry matter. Compared with indoor feeding of hay and concentrates, pasture rearing has resulted in calves ruminating at an earlier age and developing greater rumen size and capacity. Pasture quality can also alter the response of calves to concentrate feeding. Calves on excellent pasture alone can make greater live-weight gains than calves on poorer pasture with supplementary grain feeding. Under conditions of poor pasture, low level of nutrition, and adverse weather conditions, young calves are highly susceptible to parasitic gastroenteritis, which will cause severe unthriftiness.

Dairy calves can be turned out to grass at either three or four months of age under a leader-follower rotational grazing system during the summer months and can gain 0.55 to 0.74 kg./day while receiving a daily grazing supplement of about 1.8 kg. of concentrate (Poole 1981). The followers can be yearling cattle and sheep.

The major problems in rearing young calves on pasture include insufficient good-quality grass to support optimum growth, mineral deficiencies—particularly the trace minerals, parasitic gastroenteritis, and lungworm pneumonia.

Assessment of the nutritive value of pasture for young calves is a practical problem. Spring-born calves that have received cows' whole milk or a good-quality milk replacer until weaning at six to eight weeks of age will perform well on lush spring pasture. The performance of the calves must be monitored regularly by visual observation or preferably by monthly weighings. When grass is not plentiful or is of less than good quality, calves should be maintained on milk replacer for longer periods and supplemented with concentrate while on pasture.

A salt-mineral mixture must be provided for young calves on pasture. The composition of the mineral mixture depends on the mineral content of the forages and soil in the area. There are seven major or macro-minerals—calcium, phosphorus, potassium, sodium, chlorine, magnesium, and sulfur—and eight trace or microminerals—iron, iodine, zinc, copper, manganese, cobalt, molybdenum, and selenium. The minerals that are commonly deficient in cattle grazing native unsupplemented pastures are phosphorus, copper, and cobalt. The subject of microminerals for ruminant animals has been reviewed (Hansard 1983). Mineral deficiencies are particularly common in cattle of all ages grazing in the tropics (McDowell et al. 1983). Lack of good-quality pasture and multiple mineral deficiencies are major factors in the poor growth rates and prolonged delayed onset of puberty in calves grazing in tropical countries. It is not uncommon for dairy heifers to have their first calf at three to four years of age.

The control of parasitic gastroenteritis in calves that are pastured during the grazing seasons in countries with a temperate climate is now possible. Strategic chemotherapy involving the use of anthelmintics at selected times combined with various systems of grazing management have been successful (Armour and Ogbourne 1982). In the Northern Hemisphere, in the so-called Weybridge "dose and move" system, young cattle are dosed with an anthelmintic in late spring before the infection pressure is high and then moved to a pasture ungrazed by cattle since the previous autumn. Grazing management systems used to control bovine ostertagiasis have included rotational grazing of cattle, alternate grazing of cattle with different host species, or integrated rotational grazing of different age groups of cattle. Improved live-weight gains have also been reported when susceptible dairy calves were rotationally grazed on permanent pastures and followed by replacement heifers. The success of this system, known as the leader-follower system, depends on the careful management of the paddocks grazed by the calves and on the assumption that two- to three-year-old dairy heifers are immune to infection with *O. ostertagi*. Thus, the calves are only permitted to graze the upper leafy part of the herbage before being moved onto the next paddock, thus avoiding the mass of third-stage larvae thought to be concentrated in the lower quartile of the herbage and subsequently ingested by the incoming immune heifers. In the Southern Hemisphere, the same principles have been used for the control of ostertagiasis, and the reservation of safe pasture at times of the year when levels of infestation are known to be increasing has been the method widely advocated in areas such as Australasia.

Review Literature

Foley, J.A. and Otterby, D.E. Availability, storage, treatment, composition and feeding value of surplus colostrum: A review. J. Dairy Sci., 61:1033–1060, 1978.

Huber, J.T. Development of the digestive and metabolic apparatus of the calf. J. Dairy Sci., 52:1303–1315, 1969.

Jacobson, N.L. Energy and protein requirements of the calf. J. Dairy Sci., 52:1316–1321, 1969.

Kertz, A.F., Prewitt, L.R. and Everett, J.P. An early weaning calf program: Summarization and review. J. Dairy Sci., 62:1835–1843, 1979.

Nutrient Requirements of Dairy Cattle. Fifth Revised Edition 1978. National Research Council. National Academy of Sciences, Wash., D.C.

Radostits, O.M. and Bell, J.M. Nutrition of the preruminant dairy calf with special reference to the digestion and absorption of nutrients. A review. Can. J. Anim. Sci., 50:405–452, 1970.

Ramsey, H.A. and Willard, T.R. Symposium: Recent advances in calf rearing. Soy protein for milk replacers. J. Dairy Sci., 58:436–441 1975.

Roy, J.H.B. The composition of milk substitute diets and the nutrient requirements of the pre-ruminant calf. Basel, F. Hoffmann-La Roche and Co. A.G., 1977.

Roy, J.H.B. and Ternough, J.H. Nutrition and enteric diseases in calves. Proc. Nutr. Soc., 31:53–60, 1972.

References

Armour, J. and Ogbourne, C.P. Bovine ostertagiasis: A review and annotated bibliography. Miscellaneous publication No. 7 of the Commonwealth Institute of Parasitology. Commonwealth Agricultural Bureau, 1982, pp. 1–93.

Emmons, D.B. and Lister, E.E. Quality of protein in milk replacers for young calves. I. Factors affecting in vitro curd formation by rennet (chymosin, rennin) from reconstituted skim milk powder. Can. J. Anim. Sci., 56:317–325, 1976a.

Emmons, D.B., Lister, E.E. and Campbell, D.L. Quality of protein in milk replacers for young calves. III. Rennet coagulation and undenatured whey protein nitrogen content of skim milk powders and commercial milk replacers. Can. J. Anim., Sci., 56:335–338, 1976b.

Fisher, L.J. An evaluation of milk replacers based on the growth rate, health and blood chemistry of Holstein calves. Can. J. Anim. Sci., 56:587–594, 1976.

Foley, J.A. and Otterby, D.E. Availability, storage, treatment, composition and feeding value of surplus colostrum: A review. J. Dairy Sci., 61:1033–1060, 1978.

Gorrill, A.D.L. Pasture rearing and milk-replacer feeding of dairy calves. Can. J. Anim. Sci., 44:235–247, 1964.

Hansard, S.L. Microminerals for ruminant animals. Nutrition Abstracts and Reviews. Series B. Livestock feeds and feeding. 53:1–24, 1983.

Huber, J.T. Development of the digestive and metabolic apparatus of the calf. J. Dairy Sci., 52:1303–1315, 1969.

Huber, J.T. Fish protein concentrate and meal in calf milk replacers. J. Dairy Sci., 58:441, 1975.

Jacobson, N.L. Energy and protein requirements of the calf. J. Dairy Sci., 52:1316–1321, 1969.

Jenkins, K.L. and Emmons, D.B. Effect of fat dispersion method on performance of calves fed high-fat milk replacers. Can. J. Anim. Sci., 59:713–720, 1979.

Jenkins, K.J., Mahadevan, S. and Emmons, D.B. Susceptibility of proteins used in calf milk replacers to hydrolysis by various proteolytic enzymes. Can. J. Anim. Sci., 60:907–914, 1980.

Johnson, R.J. and Leibholz, J. The flow of nutrients from the abomasum in calves fed on heat-treated milks. Aust. J. Agric. Res., 27:903–915, 1976.

Kertz, A.F., Prewitt, L.R. and Everett, J.P. An early weaning calf program: Summarization and review. J. Dairy Sci., 62:1835–1843, 1979.

Kilshaw, P.J. and Sissons, J.W. Gastrointestinal allergy to soybean protein in preruminant calves. Antibody production and digestive disturbances in calves fed heated soybean flour. Res. Vet. Sci., 27:361–365, 1979a.

Kilshaw, P.J. and Sissons, J.W. Gastrointestinal allergy to soybean protein in preruminant calves. Allergic constituents of soybean products. Res. Vet. Sci., 27:366–371, 1979b.

Lister, E.E. Effects of heat treatment of skim milk powder and levels of fat protein in milk replacer diets on the growth of calves. Can. J. Anim. Sci., 51:735–742, 1971.

Lister, E.E. and Emmons, D.B. Quality of protein in milk replacers for young calves. 2. Effect of heat treatment of skim milk powder and fat levels on calf growth, feed intake and nitrogen balance. Can. J. Anim. Sci., 56:327–333, 1976.

McDowell, L.R., Conrad, J.H. and Ellis, G.L. Mineral deficiencies, imbalances and diagnosis: Part 1. Feedstuffs. September 12, 1983, pp. 31, 34, 35, 38, 40.

National Research Council. National Academy of Sciences. Nutrient Requirements of Domestic Animals No. 3. Nutrient Requirements of Dairy Cattle, 5th Ed., 1978.

Poole, D.A. The effect of age at which spring-born calves are introduced to pasture. J. Agric. Sci. U.K., 97: 433–435, 1981.

Radostits, O.M. and Bell, J.M. The digestibility of nutrients by newborn calves fed milk replacer. Can. J. Anim. Sci., 48:293–302, 1968.

Radostits, O.M. and Bell, J.M. Nutrition of the preruminant dairy calf with special reference to the digestion and absorption of nutrients. A review. Can. J. Anim. Sci., 50:405–452, 1970.

Ramsey, H.A. and Willard, T.R. Symposium: Recent advances in calf rearing. Soy protein for milk replacers. J. Dairy Sci., 58:436–441, 1975.

Roy, J.H.B. Diarrhea of nutritional origin. Proc. Nutr. Soc., 28:160–170, 1969.

Roy, J.H.B. The composition of milk substitute diets and the nutrient requirements of the pre-ruminant calf. Basel, F. Hoffmann-La Roche and Co. A.G., 1977.

Roy, J.H.B. and Ternouth, J.G. Nutrition and enteric diseases in calves. Proc. Nutr. Soc., 31:53–60, 1972.

Stobo, I.J.F. and Roy, J.H.B. The use of non-milk proteins in milk substitutes for calves. World Animal Rev., 25:18–24, 1978.

Thomson, R.G. Emaciation in calves fed artificial diets. Can. Vet. J., 8:242, 1965.

Toothill, J., Thompson, S.Y. and Edwards-Webb, J.D. Studies on lipid digestion in the preruminant calf. The source of lipolytic activity in the abomasum. Br. J. Nutr., 36:439–447, 1976.

Williams, V.J., Roy, J.H.B. and Gillies, C.M. Milk-substitute diet composition and abnormal secretion in the calf. Br. J. Nutr., 36:317–335, 1976.

THE HEIFER CALF FROM WEANING TO NEAR CALVING

The major objectives during this period are to ensure that the heifer calf develops quickly as a ruminant and grows rapidly enough to be bred at 15 months of age in order to calve at 24 months of age. Good-quality forages are required throughout this period. A grain supplement with added vitamins and minerals is required during the period of rapid growth (two months to 18 months of age). The common problems during this period include inferior growth rates due to undernutrition, especially a lack of energy, and nutritional osteodystrophy due to a dietary deficiency or relative imbalance of calcium, phosphorus, and vitamin D, especially in calves raised indoors. Poor growth rates will usually result in delayed onset of estrus, delayed breeding, and calving at 28 to 30 months of age instead of 24. Experimentally, heifers calving for the first time at 20 months produce more over three lactations than heifers calving at 27 months (Gardner et al. 1977). This means that in well-managed herds, well-fed, well-grown-out heifers may be bred at an early age. Early-bred heifers may have more calving difficulties and produce less in the first lactation than heifers bred later. However, the total production over the succeeding three lactations is greater if the animals are well fed after calving (Schultz 1969).

The desirable weights for heifers at calving are: for Holsteins and Brown Swiss, 520 to 575 kg.; for Ayrshires and Guernseys, 450 to 500 kg.; and for Jerseys, 375 to 400 kg. These weights can be reached at 24 months with an average daily gain of 0.73, 0.68, and 0.50 kg. respectively for the three groupings (Table 7-1; Figs. 7-2 to 7-5).

Purebred and commercial dairymen describe a "big cow" as one that has both weight and height, terms that are used to describe a heifer that is "well-grown for age." The height of a cow is determined by the length of body—a major dimension for body capacity—and the length of leg. A longer leg allows the udder to be held higher off the ground for cleanliness, ease of milking, and prevention of injury. The desirable height at the withers of two-year-old heifers in the three groups mentioned previously is 137 to 142 cm., 132 to 137 cm., and 125 to 130 cm. respectively. The genetic trait for size is highly inherited, and visible improvement can be expected in one generation. However, increased size is not realized from breeding unless the management, feeding, and health programs are given high priority.

The usual growth pattern for a dairy heifer of a large breed is to peak at close to 1 kg. of weight gain per day at five to six months of age, followed by progressive reduction to 0.45 kg. at 14 to 16 months of age.

There is a direct relationship between average daily gain and total dry matter intake. The amount of dry matter a heifer will consume depends on the availability and quality of the feed. Feeding trials indicate that the dry matter intake of excellent forage by heifers weighing up to 450 kg. may not average over 1.7% of body weight (Table 7-2).

From eight weeks to 10 months of age, because of limited capacity to consume forage, the heifer will require an average of 2 kg. of grain ration per day. Occasionally, when the forage is limited or the quality is slightly better than straw, 3 kg. of grain ration will be necessary. Heifers at this age may receive limited silage, but most good dairymen prefer the bulk of the forage to come from hay, because the moisture of silage can reduce the amount of dry matter a young heifer can consume. Pasture should be limited to not more than 50% of the total forage intake, and the grain ration should be continued. At this stage of the growth curve, the grain ration should be highly concentrated, the energy level at 72% TDN (or higher), and the protein at 14 to 18%. The grain ration should complement the forage ration and also should contain the essential salt, minerals, and vitamins (Table 7-3). Usually, the dairy ration being fed to the milking herd proves to be adequate for these heifers.

Heifers at 10 to 16 months of age can become more dependent on pasture and silages for their forage requirement. However, they must receive an adequate supply of energy, protein, minerals, and salt to keep growing, to show heats, and to conceive. Feeding 1 to 2 kg. of a grain ration per head per day will meet these objectives.

The period from 16 months to calving is a "tricky" feeding period because the objective is to keep the heifer in a good growing condition without allowing her to become overly fat. A common cause of dystocia is excessive fat in the pelvic area—and not the fault of the sire. Bulls that sire abnormally large calves may create problems, but properly conditioned heifers can be bred to bulls that have a rating of at least +6 for size. Excess fat on a heifer is often linked with postcalving health problems and a reduction in milk production in the first lactation.

Maturing heifers can adapt to any forage when fed on a free-choice basis. With good-quality hay or grass forage (protein 14% DM or better), heifers may not require a grain ration. However, if the forage protein falls below 10%, a supplement is warranted. Heifers on heavy corn silage feeding will make good use of the extra energy if fed 0.5 to 1 kg. per day of a high-protein supplement (32 to 44%). In all feeding programs, older heifers may have to be restricted on high-quality roughage, particularly corn silage programs, to keep their "dairy-like" figures or dairy character.

Lush green pastures are excellent for providing adequate daily gains from late May until mid-August. With no apparent change in the quality of pasture, the average daily gain will drop dramatically in August and continue to decline until October 1, when it reaches zero. Supplementary feeding of forage and grain should start in August and continue until stabling, especially for the 10- to 16-month-old heifers.

Table 7-1. GROWTH GUIDES FOR REPLACEMENT HEIFERS

| Age in Months | Ayrshire and Guernsey | | Brown Swiss and Holstein | | Jersey | |
	Ht. at Withers (cm.)	Wt. (kg.)	Ht. at Withers (cm.)	Wt. (kg.)	Ht. at Withers (cm.)	Wt. (kg.)
Birth	70	30	75	42	66	25
1	76	40	78	54	72	32
2	84	55	86	73	78	50
4	94	97	100	127	88	85
6	106	142	112	182	100	132
8	111	187	118	235	105	170
10	115	230	123	280	110	207
12	119	270	127	323	112	240
14°	122	310	130	366	115	268
16°	127	350	133	388	118	295
18	129	390	136	450	120	316
20	132	430	138	488	124	340
22	135	465	141	525	127	365
24	137	500	142	575	130	390

°Size and age for breeding.

Bred heifers in the last two months of pregnancy will require roughage, grain, and minerals similar to dry cows. Being housed with the milking herd or in close proximity will enable the heifer to develop immunity to pathogens in the environment. This can also serve as a training period for milking parlors, milking routine, teat dipping, and grain ration (lead feeding).

Additional requirements for successful rearing of heifer replacements include:

1. Adequate space. Housed heifers should

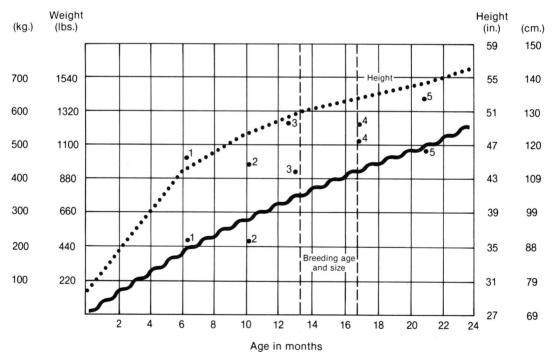

This growth chart shows how to use the graph. Heifer No. 1 is 6½ months old. She is 45 inches tall and weighs 440 pounds. On the graph, she is at the desired height and weight, so we would say she is well-grown and in the right condition.
Heifer No. 2 is 10 months old. She is 45 inches tall and slightly above 440 pounds. Both readings are below the line for her age but spaced to indicate good condition. This heifer is just too small. If the heifers were penned together, a visitor would be impressed by both. However, on the graph, Heifer No. 2 cannot hide. Her lack of size stands out.
Heifer No. 3 is alright for stature, but is too fat. No. 4 is short and fat. Heifer No. 5 lacks height but has desirable weight. Generally, this graph demonstrates typical lack of height but adequate weight.

Figure 7-2. Explanation of heifer growth chart for Holstein and Brown Swiss heifers, height and weight according to age. (From Clapp, J.H. Hoards' Dairyman, Sept. 25, 1981, pp. 1250–1251.)

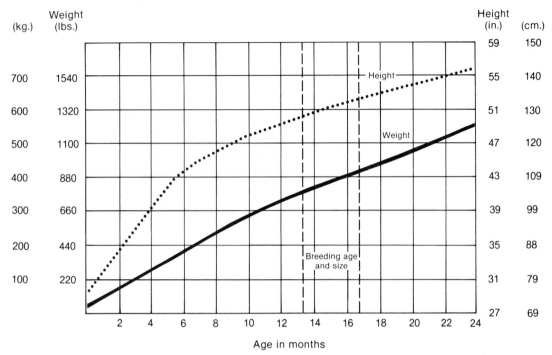

Figure 7-3. Heifer growth chart for Holstein and Brown Swiss heifers, height and weight according to age. (From Clapp, J.H. Hoards' Dairyman, Sept. 25, 1981, pp. 1250–1251.)

have sufficient space and bedding to be comfortable and to be easily seen daily by the attendant.

2. Regular control of lice, warbles, and internal parasites. In large herds, heifers are usually not monitored as carefully as lactating cows, and a regular examination and treatment for lice and parasites should be part of the routine activities.

3. Vaccination schedule. Heifers should be

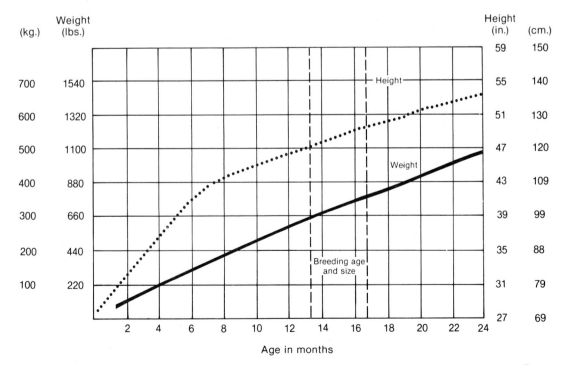

Figure 7-4. Heifer growth chart for Ayrshire and Guernsey heifers, height and weight according to age. (From Clapp, J.H. Hoards' Dairyman, Sept. 25, 1981, pp. 1250–1251.)

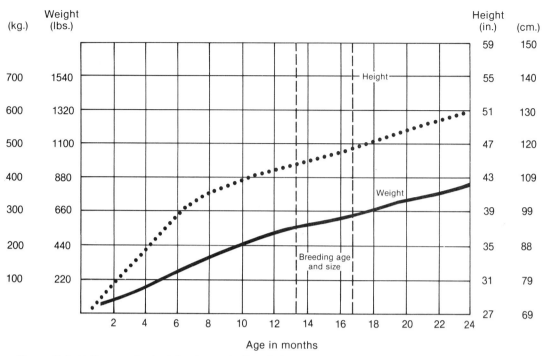

Figure 7-5. Heifer growth chart for Jersey heifers, height and weight according to age. (From Clapp, J.H. Hoards' Dairyman, Sept. 25, 1981, pp. 1250–1251.)

vaccinated for the economically important diseases that may occur in the area. These include infectious bovine rhinotracheitis, the clostridial diseases, leptospirosis, and the infectious causes of diarrhea in newborn calves.

4. Reticular magnet at 15 months of age for control of traumatic reticuloperitonitis.

5. Dehorning by at least four months of age.

6. Removal of supernumerary teats by eight months of age.

7. Selection of heifer replacements. If the heifers entering the herd are expected to contribute to substantial genetic improvement of the herd, rigid selection and culling must be practiced. Heifers with low potential based on visual appraisal or on their pedigree can be removed at a young age. However, the most accurate selection can be accomplished from

Table 7–2. ESTIMATED FORAGE INTAKE FOR DAIRY HEIFERS FED AVERAGE-QUALITY FORAGE

Heifer Weight (kg.)	Forage DM Intake (% of body weight)
90	0.53
160	1.00
250	1.50
325	1.60
400	1.60
450	1.50

midway through the first lactation. At that time, production, test, and type information is available. Heifers should classify as "Good" or better and be projected higher than the herd average to stay in the herd. However, to be herd improvers, they must eventually exceed the herd average in milk and fat production and develop "Good Plus" or better for type. Where heifers are sired by Plus Proven bulls and are born to dams in the top one half of the herd, the average culling rate of heifers will be 50%, or the herd will have no overall improvement. With less qualified parentage, the culling rate will be higher. Very discriminating breeders will select only 15 to 20% of their heifers to stay in the herd.

8. Selection of service sire for heifers. A heifer in-calf to a Plus Proven bull has more merit for selection as a herd replacement and has more appeal to a prospective buyer compared with a similar heifer in-calf to "just a bull." Service sires should be chosen that will improve production and type and have an acceptable rating for ease of calving and conception rate. Select sires in the following order:

(1) A bull proven in many herds as a plus in milk production, type, and fat percentage

(2) A bull proven in many herds as at least plus in the categories where there are

Table 7-3. DAILY NUTRIENT REQUIREMENTS FOR EARLY
CALVING DAIRY HEIFERS (LARGE BREEDS)

Wt (kg.)	Feed (DM) (kg.)	C. Prot. (kg.)	TDN (kg.)	Minerals		Vitamins	
				CA (G.)	P (G.)	A (1000 IU)	D (IU)
75	2.10	0.341	1.80	19	10	3.2	495
100	2.80	0.402	2.10	23	12	4.2	660
150	4.00	0.528	2.88	24	14	6.4	990
200	5.20	0.640	3.56	26	18	8.5	1320
250	6.30	0.719	4.19	28	20	10.6	1650
300	7.20	0.782	4.73	30	22	12.7	1980
350	8.00	0.841	5.20	32	23	14.8	2310
400	8.60	0.876	5.61	33	24	17.0	2640
450	9.10	0.892	5.82	34	25	19.1	2970
500	9.50	0.916	6.35	37	26	21.2	3300
550	9.80	0.928	6.62	42	30	42.0	3630
600	10.00	0.950	6.50	45	32	46.0	3960

(From National Research Council. National Academy of Sciences. Nutrient Requirements of Domestic Animals No. 3. Nutrient Requirements of Dairy Cattle. 5th Revised Edition, 1978.)

weaknesses in the heifer and/or her pedigree

(3) A selected young sire in a bull proving program

THE DAIRY COW DURING THE LACTATION-PREGNANCY CYCLE

The production objectives during lactation are for the cow to reach peak yield and persistency according to her genetic potential and the nutritional allowance. The optimum targets of live-weight changes and body condition during the lactation cycle include: minimum losses in early lactation commensurate with maximum yield; adequate body condition and live-weight change at first service; adequate body condition score at calving; and increases in total body weight of young cows to ensure achievement of full mature size. Another major objective is to minimize the occurrence of metabolic and digestive diseases that are commonly associated with high-level grain feeding during the dry period and during early lactation. This necessitates that changes in feed be made gradually, since marked changes in feed composition commonly lead to simple indigestion that in turn may result in metabolic diseases such as parturient hypocalcemia and primary acetonemia. Thus, the feeding of dairy cows must be consistent and according to needs, which requires dedicated personnel.

Intensive Grassland Feeding

In grassland countries, the major source of feed is grass. The growing season extends over several months, and as long as grass is available the cows graze on pasture. Only limited amounts of hay and concentrates are fed. The feed costs of grass are relatively cheap. The major developments in grassland dairy farming include new grass varieties, increased use of fertilizers, and intensification such as "zero" grazing and strip grazing.

Levels of milk production in tropical countries where dairy cows are fed almost totally on pasture will average from 1000 to 2000 kg. of milk per cow per lactation. It is possible for dairy cattle in tropical countries to yield 3000 kg. of milk per lactation if they are fed high-quality forage and some crop residues (Payne 1981). Some specialized dairy cattle can produce levels up to 6000 kg., but these are unusual.

The animal health problems that have developed with intensified grassland farming include the following:

1. Over-reliance on grass and more particularly its conserved products may, especially in the dairy cow, result in a restriction of dry matter intake and a degree of underfeeding that, apart from having adverse effects on production, can contribute to the occurrence of ketosis in clinical or subclinical form.

2. Because a high proportion of the diet is derived from a single plant source, the composition of the diet tends to be unbalanced, and the imbalance may be exaggerated by heavy fertilizer use. Disorders that may be attributable to this feature include hypomagnesemia, problems of infertility due to undernutrition, and nitrate toxicity.

3. Reliance on farm feeds produced intensively with the heavy use of inorganic fertilizer can exacerbate trace and other mineral deficiencies characteristic of the soil area. Elements that may be involved are copper, cobalt, manganese, selenium, and magnesium.

4. Intensified grazing systems increase the risk of parasite infection.

5. The need to dispose of slurry on grasslands increases the risk of spread of diseases such as salmonellosis, leptospirosis, and cysticercosis.

In summary, dairy cows are more likely to be subjected to a nutritional deficiency or imbalance when they are at pasture than when they are confined and fed a complete prepared diet. Most of these problems are nutritional deficiencies of energy, protein, water, minerals, or trace elements, although occasionally excessive intake may result in poisoning or disease. In every case, however, the disease may be considered as an imbalance between input, throughput, and output requirements, and it may be corrected by means of an alteration in one of these three variables.

Milk Production in the Tropics

There is considerable interest in milk production in the tropics and subtropics (30°S to 30°N), particularly in developing countries. Some veterinarians have participated in educational and extension programs in an attempt to increase milk production in tropical countries that are densely populated and where there are large areas of marginal land that could be developed with sown pastures.

There is a notion that the tropical countries have an abundance of green grass year round that should support high levels of milk production. This is not necessarily so.

Livestock production is seriously retarded in the tropics as compared with temperate climates (Abou-Akkada 1982). The key factor limiting animal production is inadequate nutrition of livestock maintained under tropical conditions. Some of the causes of lowered production include heat stress, which decreases feed intake; high environmental temperature, which may decrease dry matter digestibility by ruminants; natural grazing lands of low productivity; and the slow development of improved pasture and irrigated forage because of limitations imposed by technical, economic, and human factors. Mineral deficiencies are also common (Conrad et al. 1982), and the pastures are low in energy and protein.

One of the striking differences between tropical and cultivated temperate grasses is that tropical grasses are less digestible at all stages of growth (Milford and Minson 1966). The animal intakes of some tropical grasses

and legumes are similar to those of temperate herbages, particularly when both are young. However, when mature, the animal intakes of many tropical grasses are low. This is a major reason for the observed low level of animal production during the nongrowing season. To raise production at this time, it is necessary to increase the amount of feed eaten. Also, since plant growth is then usually limited by temperature and soil moisture, other management practices are necessary. Irrigation, pasture conservation, supplementary feeding, or the growing of special arable crops to increase the amount of good-quality feed available during the nongrowing season will help to even out the marked seasonal patterns in animal production.

The low protein percentage of mature pastures is a second major reason for low levels of animal production. In many cases, this is the primary limiting factor. The protein shortage can be alleviated by supplementation with a protein concentrate or urea plus molasses.

A striking difference between temperate and tropical pastures is that at similar stages of growth, tropical grasses have considerably lower crude protein percentages than temperate species. With well-managed temperate pastures, animal production is rarely limited by lack of dietary protein, whereas in the tropics, deficiencies of protein may limit animal production for much of the year (Whiteman 1980).

Because of the high nutritional requirements of the lactating dairy cow, tropical pastures alone cannot support high levels of milk production (Stobbs 1971). On tropical pastures in Australia, average production per cow seldom exceeds 8 to 9 kg. per day. By comparison, milk yields per cow in temperate areas are considerably higher, although it is difficult to find data for annual yields from pasture alone without supplementary or winter stall feeding (Whiteman 1980). Temperate pastures alone can support milk yields between 15 to 20 kg. per cow per day.

While legume-based tropical pastures are adequate for beef production, they are severely limiting for high milk yields per cow. Since energy intake is the major limitation, milk yields can be readily increased by feeding grain supplements in direct competition with human or nonruminant feeding requirements. Thus if we want dairy production in the tropics, we must accept lower production per animal. However, by taking advantage of the dry matter yield potential of tropical pastures, we can achieve respectable milk yields per hectare by correct pasture management to maintain high stocking rates compatible with maintaining an adequate legume content.

Another factor of importance in milk production in the tropics is the breed of animal used. In view of the limitation of tropical pastures, one must question the expense and effort put into the importation of high-yielding temperate dairy breeds and cross-breeding programs, whose potential can only be achieved by the substitution of valuable grain and by-products. Far more advantage is likely to be achieved by sound development of tropical pastures, whose potential may more closely match the genetic potential for milk yield of locally adapted breeds. Pasture improvement must be the first priority. Once adequate forage resources are provided, then further gain may be achieved through breeding and other management practices (Whiteman 1980).

Combination of Pasture, Preserved Forages, and Concentrates

In countries where utilizable pasture is available for only a few months each year, dairy cows have traditionally been fed conserved forages (hay, silage) and concentrates (grain and protein supplements) during the winter months. Well-managed, high-quality pasture has the potential to supply a major portion of the nutrient needs of cows of moderate production. Dairy cows grazing high-quality pastures without concentrate supplementation can produce 20 kg. of milk daily at the peak of their lactation. High-quality pasture combined with modest amounts of concentrate can support high milk yields reasonably well (Salinas et al. 1983). A wide variety of housing, feedstuffs, and feeding systems has developed, depending on the geographic location and the crops that can be grown in a particular locality. Where the winters are cold, the cows may be fed and housed indoors for several months of the year. The housing will vary from individual stanchion-tied stalls to free-stall and loose housing with natural ventilation to complete climate-controlled dairy barns. In semi-tropical areas like Florida and California, the cows may be kept outdoors year round in loose-housing conditions but in total confinement in large paddocks or corrals often covered with a roof for protection from excessive solar heat.

Concurrent with the development of elaborate and completely automated housing and feeding systems, largely because of the pressure of economics, there has been tremendous progress in the breeding and selection of high-producing cows. Furthermore, until the energy crisis of the mid-1970s, there was a potential oversupply of the cereal grains, corn crops, and high-protein feeds like soybeans that provided high nutrient–density feeds required for high milk production. A major thrust in the dairy industry has been to select for "super-cows" that produce large quantities of milk efficiently. This in turn has created a vicious circle. New feeding systems and even different feedstuffs had to be developed in order to satisfy the nutrient requirement of this high-producing cow and to minimize feed-related animal health problems. The challenge has been to develop a combined feeding, breeding, and housing system that will produce milk at the lowest cost per unit of milk. Major problems have included the availability and the high cost of feeds and the search for a reliable automated feeding system that will deliver the optimal amount of feed to each cow according to her production ability. The feed-related animal health problems in dairy cattle include underfeeding cows that have a genetic potential to produce more milk, overfeeding cows that lack the genetic potential to produce milk efficiently, and inadequately balanced diets.

Nutrient Requirements of Lactating Cows

The nutrient requirements of lactating cows are available in the publication, "Nutrient Requirements of Dairy Cattle," Fifth Revised Edition, 1978, the National Research Council. This publication provides the nutrient requirements for all classes of dairy cattle such as growing heifers, lactating cows, dry cows, and dairy bulls. The nutrient requirements for lactating cows are given as maintenance requirements based on body weight plus the recommended nutrient allowances for different levels of milk production. The publication also provides the recommended nutrient content of rations for dairy cattle and instructions for formulating dairy rations (Tables 7–4 and 7–5).

The first step in formulating a ration is to calculate the nutrient requirements for the cow, or group of cows, to be fed. This will vary with the size and age of the cow, the amount of activity, and the amount and fat content of milk produced. The next step is to calculate the total nutrient composition of the feeds available and determine which other feedstuffs and

Table 7-4. DAILY NUTRIENT REQUIREMENTS OF LACTATING AND PREGNANT COWS

Body Weight (kg.)	Feed Energy				Total Crude Protein (g.)	Calcium (g.)	Phosphorus (g.)	Vitamin A (1000 IU)
	NE$_l$ (MCAL.)	ME (MCAL.)	DE (MCAL.)	TDN (KG.)				
Maintenance of Mature Lactating Cows[a]								
350	6.47	10.76	12.54	2.85	341	14	11	27
400	7.16	11.90	13.86	3.15	373	15	13	30
450	7.82	12.99	15.14	3.44	403	17	14	34
500	8.46	14.06	16.39	3.72	432	18	15	38
550	9.09	15.11	17.60	4.00	461	20	16	42
600	9.70	16.12	18.79	4.27	489	21	17	46
650	10.30	17.12	19.95	4.53	515	22	18	50
700	10.89	18.10	21.09	4.79	542	24	19	53
750	11.47	19.06	22.21	5.04	567	25	20	57
800	12.03	20.01	23.32	5.29	592	27	21	61
Maintenance Plus Last 2 Months of Gestation of Mature Dry Cows								
350	8.42	14.00	16.26	3.71	642	23	16	27
400	9.30	15.47	17.98	4.10	702	26	18	30
450	10.16	16.90	19.64	4.47	763	29	20	34
500	11.00	18.29	21.25	4.84	821	31	22	38
550	11.81	19.65	22.83	5.20	877	34	24	42
600	12.61	20.97	24.37	5.55	931	37	26	46
650	13.39	22.27	25.87	5.90	984	39	28	50
700	14.15	23.54	27.35	6.23	1035	42	30	53
750	14.90	24.79	28.81	6.56	1086	45	32	57
800	15.64	26.02	30.24	6.89	1136	47	34	61
Milk Production—Nutrients Per Kg. Milk of Different Fat Percentages								
(% Fat)								
2.5	0.59	0.99	1.15	0.260	72	2.40	1.65	
3.0	0.64	1.07	1.24	0.282	77	2.50	1.70	
3.5	0.69	1.16	1.34	0.304	82	2.60	1.75	
4.0	0.74	1.24	1.44	0.326	87	2.70	1.80	
4.5	0.78	1.31	1.52	0.344	92	2.80	1.85	
5.0	0.83	1.39	1.61	0.365	98	2.90	1.90	
5.5	0.88	1.48	1.71	0.387	103	3.00	2.00	
6.0	0.93	1.56	1.81	0.410	108	3.10	2.05	
Body Weight Change During Lactation—Nutrients Per Kg. Weight Change								
Weight loss	−4.92	−8.25	−9.55	−2.17	−320			
Weight gain	5.12	8.55	9.96	2.26	500			

[a]To allow for growth of young lactating cows, increase the maintenance allowances for all nutrients except vitamin A by 20% during the first lactation and 10% during the second lactation.

(From National Research Council. National Academy of Sciences. Nutrient Requirements of Domestic Animals No. 3. Nutrient Requirements of Dairy Cattle. 5th Revised Edition, 1978.)

mineral mixtures must be used to meet the requirements of the cows. It is customary to begin with a consideration of the available roughages (hay, silage), because they are the least expensive source of nutrients for lactating dairy cows. This is followed by selection and formulation of the concentrate mixture, which usually contains grains, protein supplements, minerals, vitamins, and perhaps additives such as buffers.

The major determinants of total milk yield for a lactation are peak milk yield and persistency of production. Peak milk yield is more critical in determining total milk yield for the lactation than is persistency of milk production if persistency is near normal. For example, for each 1-kg. increase in peak milk production

there is a 200-kg. increase in total milk yield for the lactation. Thus, any nutrient deficiency that decreases peak milk production greatly reduces total production during the lactation. The two nutritional factors that are most likely to limit milk production are energy and protein.

The major nutritional considerations for the dairy cow throughout the lactation-pregnancy cycle and the reasons for their importance are as follows:

Dry Matter Intake

Total dry matter intake is a major factor that limits milk production in cows with the genetic potential to be high producers. Dry matter intakes may not exceed 1.5% of body weight immediately after calving but can reach 3.5 to 4.0% of body weight by 12 to 15 weeks of lactation in cows fed high-quality forage. Dry matter intake usually lags behind peak milk production by a few weeks (Fig. 7-6).

Dairy cows early in lactation are unable to consume sufficient dry matter to support maximal milk production (Clark and Davis 1980). Body fat is mobilized to supply energy during this period. However, mobilization of total body protein is minimal, and rapid depletion of mobilizable protein occurs during periods of negative nitrogen balance (Botts et al. 1979).

During the early stages of lactation, the demand for nutrients by the mammary gland is extremely great in the high-producing cow. As the cow goes from a nonlactating state to peak milk production of 35 to 50 kg. daily, the nutrient requirement of the cow increases 300 to 700% as a direct result of requirements by the mammary gland for milk production. The most critical period for nutrient supply to the high-producing cow is from parturition until peak milk production, which usually occurs four to 10 weeks post partum. For cows to survive this critical period without severe metabolic problems and to attain their peak milk production, it is essential that a diet properly balanced in all nutrients be fed ad libitum.

Even when such feeding recommendations are followed, lactating cows suffer from a shortage of energy and protein because maximum intake of dry matter does not occur until after the cow has peaked in milk production. During the time that feed intake lags behind milk production, nutrient intake may not be adequate to meet the needs of the mammary gland for milk production, even though the cow is being fed according to recommended guidelines. Therefore, feeding the high-producing cow in early lactation presents a special problem, because often she is either not offered adequate amounts of feed or cannot consume enough feed to supply the energy and protein needed for maximum milk production. When the cow's requirement for energy and protein is greater than the intake from feed, she draws from body stores of fat and protein to supply energy and amino acids for milk production. Although it is normal for high-producing cows to lose body weight in early lactation, the energy and especially protein available from body stores can supply only a limited amount of her needs. If the cow has to rely too heavily on body stores of energy and protein, either milk production will be held to the level of nutrient availability or metabolic disease such as ketosis will develop.

The level of body fat at calving may have a negative effect on feed intake after calving (Garnsworthy and Topps 1982a). Dairy cows that are thinner at calving are able to increase their intake of dry matter after calving at a faster rate than fatter cows, and the delay between peak milk yield and maximum dry matter intake is shorter. Thus the level of body fat at calving has an inhibitory effect on feed intake during early lactation if cows are fed a high-energy diet ad libitum. The inhibitory effect may be due to the release of excess quantities of free fatty acids (Garnsworthy and Topps 1982b). Under these conditions, it is not necessary to fatten cows before calving, provided body condition score at calving is not likely to be lower than 1.5 to 2.0 out of 4.

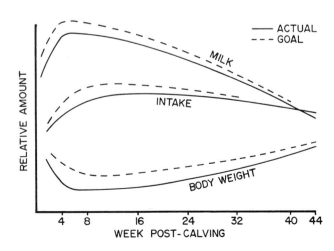

Figure 7-6. Typical changes (———) in milk production, dry matter intake, and live body weight within weeks after calving; suggested goals represented by (----).

Table 7-5. RECOMMENDED NUTRIENT CONTENT OF RATIONS FOR DAIRY CATTLE

Nutrients (Concentration in the feed dry matter)	Lactating Cow Rations Daily Milk Yields (KG.)				Nonlactating Cattle Rations					Maximum Concentrations (All Classes)
Cow WT. (KG.) ≤400 / 500 / 600 / ≥700	< 8 / <11 / <14 / <18	8-13 / 11-17 / 14-21 / 18-26	13-18 / 17-23 / 21-29 / 26-35	>18 / >23 / >29 / >35	Dry Pregnant Cows	Mature Bulls	Growing Heifers and Bulls	Calf Starter Concentrate Mix	Calf Milk Replacer	
Ration No.	I	II	III	IV	V	VI	VII	VIII	IX	Max.
Crude protein, %	13.0	14.0	15.0	16.0	11.0	8.5	12.0	16.0	22.0	—
Energy										
NE_l, Mcal./kg.	1.42	1.52	1.62	1.72	1.35	—	—	—	—	—
NE_m, Mcal./kg.	—	—	—	—	—	1.20	1.26	1.90	2.40	—
NE_g, Mcal./kg.	—	—	—	—	—	—	0.60	1.20	1.55	—
ME, Mcal./kg.	2.36	2.53	2.71	2.89	2.23	2.04	2.23	3.12	3.78	—
DE, Mcal./kg.	2.78	2.95	3.13	3.31	2.65	2.47	2.65	3.53	4.19	—
TDN, %	63	67	71	75	60	56	60	80	95	—
Crude fiber, %	17	17	17	17a	17	15	15	—	—	—
Acid detergent fiber, %	21	21	21	21	21	19	19	—	—	—
Ether extract, %	2	2	2	2	2	2	2	2	10	—
Minerals b										
Calcium, %	0.43	0.48	0.54	0.60	0.37	0.24	0.40	0.60	0.70	—
Phosphorus, %	0.31	0.34	0.38	0.40	0.26	0.18	0.26	0.42	0.50	—
Magnesium, %c	0.20	0.20	0.20	0.20	0.16	0.16	0.16	0.07	0.07	—
Potassium, %	0.80	0.80	0.80	0.80	0.80	0.80	0.80	0.80	0.80	—
Sodium, %	0.18	0.18	0.18	0.18	0.10	0.10	0.10	0.10	0.10	—
Sodium chloride, %d	0.46	0.46	0.46	0.46	0.25	0.25	0.25	0.25	0.25	5
Sulfur, %d	0.20	0.20	0.20	0.20	0.17	0.11	0.16	0.21	0.29	0.35
Iron, ppm d,e	50	50	50	50	50	50	50	100	100	1000
Cobalt, ppm	0.10	0.10	0.10	0.10	0.10	0.10	0.10	0.10	0.10	10

							Maximum safe level
Copper, ppm[d,f]	10	10	10	10	10	10	80
Manganese, ppm[d]	40	40	40	40	40	40	1000
Zinc, ppm[d,g]	40	40	40	40	40	40	500
Iodine, ppm[h]	0.50	0.05	0.50	0.50	0.25	0.25	50
Molybdenum, ppm[i,j]	—	—	—	—	—	—	6
Selenium, ppm	0.10	0.10	0.10	0.10	0.10	0.10	5
Fluorine, ppm[j]	—	—	—	—	—	—	30
Vitamins[k]							
Vit A, IU/kg.	3200	3200	3200	3200	2200		3800
Vit D, IU/kg.	300	300	300	300	300		600
Vit E, ppm	—	—	—	—	—	—	—

[a] It is difficult to formulate high-energy rations with a minimum of 17% crude fiber. However, fat percentage depression may occur when rations with less than 17% crude fiber or 21% ADF are fed to lactating cows.

[b] The mineral values presented in this table are intended as guidelines for use of professionals in ration formulation. Because of many factors affecting such values, they are not intended and should not be used as a legal or regulatory base.

[c] Under conditions conducive to grass tetany (see text), should be increased to 0.25 or higher.

[d] The maximum safe levels for many of the mineral elements are not well defined; estimates given here, especially for sulfur, sodium chloride, iron, copper, zinc, and manganese, are based on very limited data; safe levels may be substantially affected by specific feeding conditions.

[e] The maximum safe level of supplemental iron in some forms is materially lower than 1000 ppm. As little as 400 ppm added iron as ferrous sulfate has reduced weight gains (Standish et al., 1969).

[f] High copper may increase the susceptibility of milk to oxidized flavor (see text).

[g] Maximum safe level of zinc for mature dairy cattle is 1000 ppm.

[h] If diet contains as much as 25% strongly goitrogenic feed on dry basis, iodine provided should be increased two times or more.

[i] If diet contains sufficient copper, dairy cattle tolerate substantially more than 6 ppm molybdenum (see text).

[j] Maximum safe level of fluorine for growing heifers and bulls is lower than for other dairy cattle. Somewhat higher levels are tolerated when the fluorine is from less-available sources such as phosphates (see text). Minimum requirement for molybdenum and fluorine not yet established.

[k] The following minimum quantities of B-complex vitamins are suggested per unit of milk replacer: niacin, 2.6 ppm; pantothenic acid, 13 ppm; riboflavin, 6.5 ppm; pyridoxine, 6.5 ppm; thiamine, 6.5 ppm; folic acid, 0.5 ppm; biotin, 0.1 ppm; vitamin B_{12}, 0.07 ppm; choline, 0.26%. It appears that adequate amounts of these vitamins are furnished when calves have functional rumens (usually at 6 weeks of age) by a combination of rumen synthesis and natural feedstuffs.

(From National Research Council. National Academy of Sciences. Nutrient Requirements of Domestic Animals No. 3. Nutrient Requirements of Dairy Cattle. 5th Revised Edition, 1978.)

Energy Concentration of Feed and Intake

A corollary to the problem of dry matter intake is the inability of the dairy cow to consume sufficient energy during the first six to eight weeks of lactation. During this period, the cow mobilizes body fat stored during the previous late lactation and the dry period to supplement the energy component of the feed. Considerable effort goes into finding economic methods of maximizing energy intake and at the same time minimizing diseases associated with high-energy feeds.

To ensure maximum intake of feed after calving and to attain the highest peak milk production, the diet should be high in energy but should contain sufficient fiber to maintain normal rumen function and normal milk fat percentage. A minimum of 17% crude fiber in the diet has been suggested for lactating and dry cows. Grinding, pelleting, or fine chopping of the roughage will lower the effectiveness of the fiber, and thus the physical form of the roughage should be coarse enough to prevent any adverse effects that processing might have on fiber.

The effects of varying the proportions of forage to concentrate in the diets of dairy cows have been reviewed (Broster et al. 1977). In general, they concluded that raising the proportion of concentrate in the diet until it reaches approximately 60% of total ration dry matter increases milk yield and feed intake of cows in early lactation. Milk fat test is reduced as grain feeding increases.

In general, cows will consume the most energy when the dry matter of the diet consists of 40 to 55% good-quality forage and 55 to 60% concentrate (Spahr 1977). The risks of the cow going off feed or of having a reduced milk fat percentage are increased as the proportion of concentrate in the ration is increased above 60% (Miller and O'Dell 1969). However, high intake of feed and above-average milk production can be obtained when the ration contains 50 to 60% concentrate and 40 to 50% roughage (Fig. 7-7). Some workers suggest that there is no need to go above 50 to 55% concentrate in the diet because of depressed milk fat test, more off-feed problems, other metabolic and digestive diseases, and impaired ability to mobilize body tissue reserves to supplement dietary energy (Wangsness and Muller 1981). The feed intake, milk yield, and composition responses of cows in first lactation—when offered complete feeds of contrasting forage and concentrate proportions—

are basically similar to those of multiparous cows (Macleod et al. 1983).

Protein Concentration of Feed and Total Intake

The requirement for crude protein is defined as the minimum amount of protein that will support maximum milk production. The protein requirements during the first 12 to 15 weeks of lactation are higher than those in later lactation. Because of the high cost of protein supplements, they must be used judiciously in order to maximize income over feed costs.

The large nutritional stress placed on the high-producing cow, in combination with greatly increased costs of protein supplement, has stimulated reevaluation of protein requirements of cows in early lactation. The producer should determine if it is economic to feed a diet containing more than 14% crude protein in early lactation. In some situations, the best choice may be to feed a diet containing 13% from week 14 of lactation onward; it is uneconomic to feed a level of 17% (Barney et al. 1981a, 1981b). The concentration of crude protein in the diet of multiparous cows can be reduced from 17 to 13.5% after eight weeks postpartum without significantly reducing their milk production during weeks nine to 12 of lactation; the crude protein can be reduced for primiparous cows beginning at one month after calving (Roffler and Thacker 1983). Recent development of new systems to express protein requirements has placed emphasis not only on the protein content of the diet but also on the rumen degradability of the protein. There is a separate requirement of nitrogen for rumen bacteria (ruminal degradable protein) and for amino acids reaching the cow's small intestine above the amount supplied by ruminal microflora. Utilization of protein is inefficient when rumen ammonia rises above that required by rumen microbes (Satter and Roffler 1975). Therefore, interest in ruminal bypass of protein has been stimulated to meet the animal's protein requirement with a minimum waste of protein. Decreasing dietary protein degradability at 14% crude protein increases milk production in dairy cows in early lactation (Forster et al. 1983).

There are also good indications that providing combinations of nonprotein nitrogen and rumen-undegradable protein might best support protein needs for high milk production as well as yield greatest profits (Kung and Huber 1983). The major reasons for feeding nonprotein nitrogen (NPN)—e.g., urea—are to

Figure 7-7. Theoretical visualization of some of the possibilities in milk production resulting from different proportions of forages and concentrates. With high proportions of forage, digestible energy intake normally limits production; whereas with proportions of grain, metabolic problems limit production. Both types of limitations vary widely with specific conditions; thus each is a family of curves. Theoretically, if conditions are proper, it should be possible to obtain maximum cow performance with diets varying from almost complete forage to nearly all grain. (From Wangsness, P.J. and Muller, L.D. Maximum forage for dairy cows: Review. J. Dairy Sci., 64:1–13, 1981.)

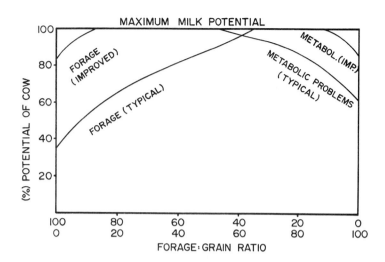

reduce the need for preformed protein supplements when the supply is not adequate or because of an economic advantage in the use of NPN. Supplements of NPN add only nitrogen to the diet unless they are complexed with starch or fortified with minerals. If rumen bacteria do not use NPN for protein synthesis, it is of no benefit to the animal and represents a waste of nitrogen. In contrast, preformed protein supplies protein, energy, and minerals. Nonprotein nitrogen is used most efficiently when small quantities are added to low-protein, high-energy rations.

High-producing cows should not be fed NPN in early lactation if maximum production is to be obtained. However, after the peak in milk yield, when production decreases to about 20 kg. daily, NPN can supply a portion of the nitrogen requirement without decreasing production. When NPN is added to the ration, recommended guidelines should be followed. Supplemental urea should not exceed 1.5% of the concentrate mixture.

Crude Fiber Concentration of Feed

The level of crude fiber should be maintained at 17% or more in order to maintain a satisfactory butterfat test. This means that every economical effort must be made to ensure a high level of intake of roughages.

A low score on the butterfat test indicates poor efficiency of energy utilization for milk production, resulting in greater deposition of energy into adipose tissue instead of into milk. Cows fed relatively high–roughage diets maintain a normal fat test but do not produce maximum quantities of milk (Zanartu et al.

1983). Cows fed large quantities of concentrates can express maximum milk production, but depression of milk fat production is common. Also, large quantities of concentrates fed too quickly may cause one of several digestive disorders.

Thus, a major challenge for the dairyman is to feed the cow sufficient roughage to maintain a normal fat test and sufficient concentrate to obtain the yield of milk genetically capable by the cow.

Mineral Composition of Feed and Total Intake of Minerals

The mineral requirements for dairy cattle during lactation and the dry period are well established. All minerals should be added to the concentrate portion of the diet because dairy cattle will not voluntarily consume their nutritional requirements when the minerals are provided on a free-choice basis (Coppock et al. 1981). Dry cows should receive a diet low in calcium to minimize the incidence of milk fever. All feedstuffs should be analyzed regularly for mineral composition to ensure that a mineral deficiency does not occur. This is particularly important for the trace minerals.

Selenium and vitamin treatments do not reduce the high incidence of retained fetal membranes and have no beneficial effects on health and reproductive performance in dairy cows not deficient in selenium or vitamin A (Ishak et al. 1983).

Vitamin Concentration of Feed

The vitamin requirements are important and are usually easily and economically provided through the concentrate mixture.

Water

Milk contains 85 to 87% water, and the provision of an unlimited supply of clean drinking water—with continuous access—is recommended. Water intake can be affected by the physiological condition and stage of growth of the animal, ambient temperature, relative humidity, wind velocity and rainfall, quantity of dry matter consumed, composition of the diet, frequency and periodicity of watering, and mineral composition of the water (Commonwealth Agricultural Bureau 1980; Murphy et al. 1983).

Total Cost of Feed and Milk Production

Feed is the largest component cost of milk production; therefore, the cost of feed and the total cost of milk production per 100 kg. of milk should be calculated and assessed regularly. Marked increases in the price of feedstuffs without a concurrent increase in the income from milk may require major changes in feed formulation or the size of the herd. It may be more profitable to feed fewer cows.

THE NUTRITIONALLY RELATED DISEASES OF THE DAIRY COW THROUGHOUT THE LACTATION CYCLE

Lactation Periods

The lactation cycle of the dairy cow can be divided into four periods; early, middle, and late lactation and the dry period. The production objectives and the nutrient requirements are different for each period. Also, during each period, major metabolic changes occur that account for changes in milk production, shifts in body weight and feed intake, and the occurrence of certain metabolic or digestive diseases. The relationships between the periods of the lactation cycle, the energy status, and the occurrence of the common metabolic diseases are shown at the bottom of the page.

The salient features of the etiology, occurrence, and prevention of the nutritionally related diseases or suboptimal performance in dairy cows are summarized in Table 7-6.

The limiting nutrient is usually energy—especially for high-producing cows in which considerable amounts of forage comprise the diet. Even with a high-quality forage, the major limitation in nutrients to support milk production is often daily intake of energy (Wangsness and Muller 1981). Milk production peaks early in lactation, and cows will usually attempt to satisfy their energy needs by eating more until a minimum is reached. However, because of a delay in the intake response, cows must mobilize body reserves to support high milk production (Fig. 7-8).

The amount of energy required by lactating cows varies widely, depending on body size and level of milk production. Milk production usually peaks about six to eight weeks following parturition and then gradually declines during the remainder of the lactation period. It is difficult to fulfill the energy requirements of the high-producing cow in early lactation because of the large energy demands of high production, and maximum dry matter intake does not occur until about 12 to 14 weeks of lactation. Therefore, high-producing cows frequently lose weight in early lactation because they utilize body fat as a source of energy. A drop in the lactation curve in early lactation—

	Lactation Periods			
	EARLY	MIDDLE	LATE	DRY
No. weeks of lactation	0–10 (period of peak milk production)	10–20	20–24	44–52
Energy status	Negative balance and weight loss	Balance	Positive balance and restore weight loss	Maintain balance
Common diseases	Fat cow syndrome, milk fever, hypomagnesemia, simple indigestion, downer cow, left side displacement of abomasum, right side displacement of abomasum, cecal dilatation, primary acetonemia, postparturient hemoglobinuria, delayed onset of estrus, early lactation drop in milk production			Fat cow syndrome

Table 7–6. SALIENT FEATURES OF THE ETIOLOGY, OCCURRENCE, AND PREVENTION OF NUTRITIONALLY RELATED DISEASES OR SUBOPTIMAL PERFORMANCE IN DAIRY COWS

Disease or Suboptimal Performance	Etiology	Occurrence	Prevention
Simple indigestion	Change of feed a few days before or at parturition	Within a few days after calving	Avoid marked changes in nature of feed in peri-parturient cows
Fat cow syndrome	Excessive intake of energy during dry period	Within a few days before, but most commonly a few days after, calving	Feed for maintenance and pregnancy during dry period. *Feed dry cows separately.* Monitoring body condition score
Parturient hypo-calcemia (milk fever)	High calcium intake dur-ing dry period	Within 48 hours before or after calving. Mid-lactation cases occur too	Low-calcium diets during dry period. Injection of vitamin D metabo-lites before calving
Hypomagnesemia (lactation tetany)	Relative deficiency of dietary magnesium in lush pasture; stress of cold weather	Within first few weeks after calving	Supplement diet with magnesium at strategic times
Downer cow	Complication of milk fever (traumatic injuries, prolonged recumbency)	Recumbent cases of milk fever fail to rise fol-lowing treatment with calcium	Recognize and treat cases of milk fever in first stage
Left side displacement of abomasum	Uncertain. Epidemiologi-cally related to feed-ing grain before calving	Within a few days to a few weeks after calving	Unreliable. Feed liberal quantities of low-energy forage during dry period; begin feeding grain only 10 days to 2 weeks pre-partum and provide exercise
Right side displacement and torsion of abomasum	Uncertain. Epidemiologi-cally related to high grain feeding in early lactation	Usually 2 to 3 weeks after calving	Ensure high intake of high-quality forage in early lactation
Cecal dilation and torsion	Uncertain. May be re-lated to high grain feeding in early lacta-tion	Usually within 2 to 4 weeks after calving	Ensure high intake of high-quality forage in early lactation
Primary acetonemia	Insufficient energy intake due to physical inability to consume, lack of energy in diet, or secondary disease affecting appetite	Usually 2 to 6 weeks after calving just prior to peak milk produc-tion	Ensure an increasing plane of energy intake in early lactation.
Postparturient hemo-globinuria	Deficiency of phosphorus intake	2 to 6 weeks after calving	Ensure adequate level of phosphorus in diet
Early lactation drop in milk production	Insufficient intake of energy and low body condition score at calv-ing, thus providing no body fat for mobiliza-tion	6 to 8 weeks after calving	Ensure adequate intake of energy and protein during first 6 to 8 weeks after calving
Suboptimal milk pro-duction of herd	Insufficient intake of energy or protein or mineral deficiency because of lack of surveillance of feed quality	Usually noticed in early to mid-lactation	Constant awareness of quality and intake of feed
Delayed onset of estrus	Inadequate heat detec-tion. May be related to inadequate energy intake and excessive loss of body weight in early lactation	8 to 10 weeks after calving	Provide good heat detec-tion of cows beginning 40 days after calving. Monitor body condi-tion, adequate energy intake too

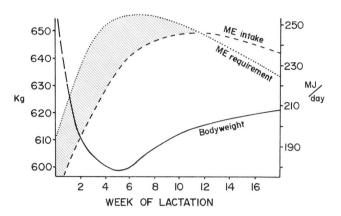

Figure 7-8. Metabolizable energy intakes and calculated requirements in a group of 18 cows in the first 18 weeks of lactation. (From Roberts, C.J. Fat mobilization of high-yielding dairy cows in early lactation. Proc. XII World Congress on Diseases of Cattle. The Netherlands. pp. 501–507, 1982.)

early lactation drop—is usually associated with insufficient intake of concentrates. This early lactation drop cannot be entirely prevented in high-producing cows that milk beyond their feed capacity, but it can be delayed or reduced by feeding more concentrates. Several different feeding systems have been developed for lactating cows, depending on the production level of the cows, the size of the herd, and the housing systems used. The major objective is to feed the optimum amounts of grain and hay that will produce the desired amount of milk according to the cow's potential. Thus, "challenge feeding" was widely adopted. The basic concept is to feed more grain and thus more energy to lead the cow to highest production rather than limiting grain to the amount of milk produced. Free-choice, or unlimited, grain feeding became a common practice on dairy farms. However, high-level grain feeding is associated with several problems. The use of unrestricted levels of grain reduces the intake of forage, which reduces the intake of crude fiber and physical bulk or roughage. A reduction in crude fiber causes a drop in butterfat. As the level of grain feeding increases, the digestibility decreases. Digestive disturbances such as simple indigestion, right side displacement of the abomasum, and cecal dilatation are epidemiologically associated with feeding large quantities of grain and insufficient forage to dairy cows in the late part of the dry period and in early lactation.

Voluntary food intake is critical (Broster and Alderman 1977). In early lactation, daily dry matter intake may amount to only 1.5% of live weight per day. It reaches a peak about 12 to 15 weeks after calving, attaining a level of about 3.6% and an average over weeks one to 18 of 3.0%. The intake is affected by the size and milk yield of the cow. The larger and higher-yielding cow may be expected to eat more than the average cow. Intake is also affected by diet composition. For diets of low digestibility (high proportions of forages), intake is controlled by rumen capacity and the rate of passage of feed through the stomachs and digestibility. For diets of high digestibility and for high milk production (concentrates), metabolic factors play an increasing role in the control of voluntary intake. Excessive intake of grain will result in greater risks of acidosis and simple indigestion without any improvement in energy intake or milk yield. Such risks may be reduced by frequent feeding of concentrates, with continuous availability of roughage. Conserved forages such as field-dried hay, artificially dried forage, and grass, or legume silage, corn silage, rape, and kale silage should be used to their maximum in the diet of dairy cows (Ekern and Macleod 1978). In high-yielding dairy cows, conserved forages support high-concentrate feeding during early lactation, maintain optimum rumen metabolism, and sustain high levels of milk production throughout the lactation cycle.

The major factors that regulate feed intake in the cow are the size and physiological state of the animal, the composition and physical form of the diet, and the amount of access to the feed (Bines 1976). The size of the animal is critical in determining the volume of the abdominal cavity, which in turn limits the volumetric expansion of the rumen during eating. For diets of low digestibility, intake is regulated by rumen capacity, rate of passage, and dry matter digestibility, whereas metabolic size, production, and digestibility are the controlling influences on intake of rations of higher digestibility.

The level of feed intake and the efficiency of energy utilization also vary, depending on the stage of the pregnancy-lactation cycle (Bines 1976). In early lactation, feed intake gradually increases but at a rate that is slower in terms of energy input than the increasing rate of energy output in milk. This leads to a considerable loss in body weight, which is only replaced in later lactation when milk yield starts to fall while appetite remains high. The mobilization of body tissue to meet requirements of lactation is a biologically insufficient process. The lag between peak milk yield and peak feed intake is greater in the first than in subsequent lactations. The causes of this lag in feed intake in early lactation are not clear but could include the presence of abdominal fat associated with pregnancy. Also, the rate of metabolism in the rumen and tissues takes time to adapt after calving. The practice of "steaming-up" a cow to get her fat at the time of calving actually depresses intake during the critical early part of lactation when intake should be maximized. Pregnancy produces a measurable increase in appetite, and during the dry period the energy intake must be reduced to avoid the fat cow syndrome.

The composition of the diet and the frequency of feeding will influence rumen metabolism and feed intake (Kaufmann 1976). A certain ratio between roughage and concentrates is necessary rather than depending exclusively on an increase in the amount of concentrates for meeting the energy requirements at high levels of production. High amounts of roughage lead to a relatively high pH in the rumen, which promotes cellulolytic activity, whereas a high amount of concentrates and a low pH promote amylolytic activity. In high-producing cows there is a need for at least 20% crude fiber in the dry matter of the diet to maintain a ratio of acetic to propionic acid of 3:1 in the rumen. This is necessary to maintain a normal butterfat content of the milk and to avoid acidosis. Increasing the frequency of feeding from twice daily up to six to 14 times daily will also maintain the optimum ratio of volatile fatty acids and result in an increase in milk production without a decrease in butterfat concentration. The addition of fat at a level of 3 to 5% to the diet of high-producing dairy cows will maintain and sometimes even increase the level of milk fat (Palmquist and Jenkins 1980). The added fat increases the energy intake of high-producing cows, which allows a reduction in the amount of grain feeding and an increase in the amount of forage intake—both of which prevent depression of milk fat.

The efficiency of utilization of feed energy for milk production could be improved by minimizing the cyclic variation in live weight, which has traditionally been accepted as an essential part of the pregnancy-lactation cycle in the high-producing dairy cow. Methods are being examined for the manipulation of the composition of the diet to enable the cow to consume enough feed in early lactation to meet the requirements for milk production. By feeding to appetite and altering the composition of the diet to enable live weight to be maintained at a constant value, reliance on body tissue withdrawals for maintenance of milk yield will be reduced to a minimum, thus improving the overall efficiency of production. The level of live weight maintained should be such that the cows are not fat, because this would depress intake in the critical early phase of lactation. Some allowance will have to be made during later pregnancy for the developing fetus and also for the younger animal that is still growing. Beyond this, any change in live weight during lactation is biologically wasteful.

In dairy cows at the beginning of lactation, an increased energy demand is accompanied by an increased feed intake, but a failure to regulate energy balance is usually observed at the beginning and end of lactation (Journet and Remond 1976). The deficit of energy during these two periods depends not only on the milk production of the cow but also on the energy concentration and on the "ingestibility" of the diet. With good-quality roughage like leafy grass and mature and finely chopped corn silage, or with pelleted, dehydrated grass and legumes, cows can better adjust their intake to their needs when a limited quantity of concentrate is given during the first part of lactation. They are also able to reconstitute body reserves during the second part of lactation from an excess of energy intake from this roughage. Consideration of these facts is very important if in the future sufficiently highly productive cows are to better utilize roughages and produce milk without an excess of concentrate, and if simpler methods of group feeding are to be promoted.

The type of carbohydrate and nitrogen included in the diet as well as the ratio of nitrogen to energy will influence the amount of milk produced and the efficiency of feed utilized by the high-producing cow. High-producing dairy cows should not be fed nonprotein nitrogen in early lactation. However, when milk yield decreases to less than 20 kg. daily, nonprotein nitrogen can be included in the diet as guidelines recommend (Wangsness and Muller

1981). Proteins that are both degradable and nondegradable in the rumen should be included in the diet, but an excess of either will reduce milk production and efficiency of feed utilization.

The incorporation of buffering agents into dairy cattle rations will help to prevent or alleviate problems that result from a lowering of rumen pH in cows fed on high-level grain rations. The most commonly used buffering agents are sodium bicarbonate and magnesium oxide, and both will maintain milk fat content for cows receiving high-grain diets (Clark and Davis 1980). Sodium bicarbonate increases the acetate to propionate molar ratios in the rumen, which maintains or increases butterfat test of milk. Levels of 1.5 to 2.0% sodium bicarbonate and 0.75 to 1.0% magnesium oxide of the grain mixture, or 0.75 to 1% and 0.30 to 0.5% of the total diet respectively are recommended (Chalupa and Kronfeld 1983).

The role of the computer has become widespread in the application of the principles of dairy cattle nutrition to practical feeding programs (Jones et al. 1978). Linear programming has been used to develop least-cost or maximum-profit rations. In other situations, computers have been useful in selecting the most appropriate concentrate supplements for dairy herds to complement the forage program. It is possible to develop concentrate supplements that are specific to the needs of individual dairymen. Also, the results demonstrate that the National Research Council recommendations used in formulating dairy diets will maintain milk production over various yields and allow cows an opportunity to attain their potential production.

One of the most difficult concepts in the study of nutrition is to be able to visualize how all the factors that influence the flow of nutrients into the milk exert their particular pressure and at what point in the process. This can be done by construction of a computer simulation model that must be based on a well-defined flow chart (Fig. 7–9) and one of these relating to dairy cow nutrition is set out below (Bywater and Dent 1976). It brings together the major factors affecting milk production and enters them one by one into a system with feed available at one end and milk produced at the other. If each of the controlling factors can be quantitated, the output of the system can be measured. Without any knowledge of any of these factors, the estimate of output must be largely conjectural.

Dry Period

To attain greatest milk yield, a cow should be given a 50- to 60-day dry period (Clark and Davis 1980). This allows the mammary gland to involute and prepare for subsequent lactation.

When cows are to be dried off, the feeding of grain and high-quality hay should be stopped, milking is ceased, and the mammary gland should be treated with dry cow antibiotic therapy according to the presence or absence of subclinical mastitis in each quarter as determined by the California Mastitis Test.

Proper feeding of the dairy cow during the dry period is essential for best performance. Maximum dry matter intake and milk production can be obtained if cows are fed during the dry period so that they are in good body condition without becoming excessively fat. Conditioning of the cow should start near the end of lactation, because the overall efficiency of converting metabolizable energy of feed to body tissue is higher for lactating cows (61.6%) than for nonlactating cows (48.3%) (Moe et al. 1971). Overfeeding during the dry period is more common than underfeeding, because in many situations dry cows are group-fed with lactating cows. Fat cows resulting from overfeeding are more susceptible to calving difficulties, metabolic disorders, and infectious diseases (Morrow 1976). Excess fat on the cow can reduce feed intake after calving, possibly by restricting gastrointestinal capacity and by the release of larger than normal amounts of free fatty acids into the blood (Fig. 7–10), thereby depressing appetite (Bines 1976). Depressed feed intake after parturition may result in a marked shortage of nutrients, thus reducing milk production or leading to metabolic disease such as the fatty liver syndrome or severe ketosis.

The nutritional objectives during the dry period depend in part on the body condition of the cow at the end of lactation. Under optimum conditions, cows should be dried off in good bodily condition (body condition score of 2.5 out of 5) and reach a score of 3.5 to 4 out of 5 at calving.

The diets fed to dry cows should be formulated to minimize the incidence of milk fever, fat cow syndrome, displaced abomasa, and simple indigestion following parturition. Cows that have had a long calving to conception interval (150 to 180 days or longer) may have a dry period lasting three to four

X = controlled by

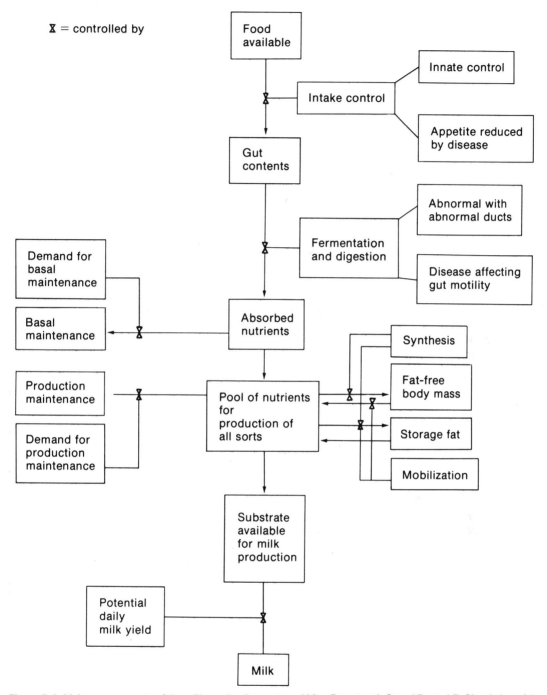

Figure 7-9. Major components of the milk production system. (After Bywater, A.C. and Dent, J.B. Simulation of the intake and partition of nutrients by the dairy cow. 1. Management control in the dairy enterprise; philosophy and general model construction. Agricultural Systems, 1:245-260, 1976.)

months and are likely to become excessively fat, which may result in the fat cow syndrome. These cows need extra surveillance of their body condition score throughout the dry period and appropriate changes in the diet to avoid excessive weight gain. The nature and amount of the diet fed to dry cows is of particular importance because several economically important metabolic and digestive diseases that occur at the time of parturition or

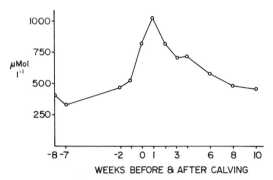

Figure 7-10. Mean plasma free fatty acid concentrations in cows before and after calving. (From Roberts, C.J. Fat mobilization of high-yielding dairy cows in early lactation. Proc. XII World Congress on Diseases of Cattle. The Netherlands. pp. 501–507, 1982.)

shortly thereafter have their origins during the dry period. The nutrient allowances of the pregnant dry cow must meet the needs for maintenance, pregnancy, and excessive loss of body weight during the previous lactation. The length of the first dry period of dairy cows is most critical. Mature dairy cows do not need dry periods as long as first-calf heifers, which require a longer dry period because their peak yield usually persists longer than mature cows and because of their requirements for continued growth.

During early and mid-lactation, high-producing dairy cows lose considerable body weight, most of which should be restored during late lactation. Dairy cows use feed more efficiently during lactation than when dry and thus it takes less energy to restore body weight during the last two or three months of lactation than it does during the dry period (Moe et al. 1971, 1972). Overfeeding grain during the end of lactation and then feeding to maintain this condition during the dry period appears to be nutritionally sound and practical. Feeding extra grain according to the body condition score of the cow while still in milk or feeding a high-energy ration to all milking cows would be methods to have them in good condition at the end of lactation.

The fat cow syndrome is caused by an excessive intake of energy during late lactation and the dry period (Morrow 1976). Feeding excessive quantities of corn silage and high-quality hay crop forages is a major cause. In some instances, grain feeding is begun too far ahead of calving in an attempt to condition the cow for a heavy lactation such as is practiced in the "lead-feeding" system for high-producing cows. Clinically, fat cows are obviously overconditioned at the time of calving (Mor-

row et al. 1979). Within a few days after calving, they are inappetent or totally anorexic. Those that are only inappetent will require about one week to begin eating and milking normally. The prognosis is poor for those that are totally anorexic, and the case fatality rate is high. Prevention depends on the avoidance of excessive energy intake during the dry period. There is no need to provide excess energy before parturition (Gardner 1969a, 1969b; Gardner and Park 1973). Experimentally, high-energy feeding for eight weeks during the dry period results in overconditioning. However, the overconditioning does not greatly alter the pre- and postpartum body weight change, feed intake, or blood metabolites (Fronk et al. 1980). The hepatic lipid content increases from 9.8% in normal cows to 12.5% in overconditioned cows. The incidence of periparturient diseases was greater in the overconditioned cows.

The control of parturient paresis has been attempted by feeding diets low in calcium during the last four to five weeks of the dry period (Jonsson 1978). With a high-calcium prepartum diet, calcium homeostasis is governed mainly by absorption from the intestinal tract. Calcium mobilization from bone is of minor importance as the high dietary intake of calcium stimulates secretion of thyrocalcitonin. The sudden increase of calcium outflow to milk at calving and impaired gastrointestinal function result in a fall in the level of calcium. If the prepartum diet is of low calcium content, mobilization of calcium from bone—mediated by stimulation of the parathyroid glands—plays a more important part in calcium homeostasis (Yarrington et al. 1977). When the sudden increase of calcium outflow to the udder occurs, any impairment of gastrointestinal function at parturition does not influence the plasma pool significantly. However, the published results are conflicting. Experimentally, a prepartum diet very low in calcium (below 15 to 25 g./day) is associated with a low incidence of milk fever (Wiggers et al. 1975), but such low levels are difficult to achieve under the practical situation on most dairy farms, which produce leguminous hays that contain a high level of calcium. The feeding of prepartum diets that provide no more than 100 to 125 g. of calcium/day has been advocated (Jorgensen 1974), but in other field trials that compared 37, 75, and 150 g. of calcium/day there was no evidence that the low levels provided reliable protection (Jonsson 1978). The risk of skeletal demineralization from low levels of calcium over prolonged periods must also be considered.

The acidification of prepartum diets with salt supplements such as mixtures of calcium chloride and aluminum and magnesium sulfate or calcium carbonate has reduced the incidence of milk fever (Dishington 1975). The most promising results have been obtained by dispersing on hay a solution of calcium chloride (33 g. $CaCl_2.2H_2O/L.$ of water) followed by a solution of aluminum and magnesium sulfates (<130 g. $Al_2(SO_4)_3. 16H_2O$ and 80 g. $MgSO_4/1.5$ L. of water). This acid diet is given during the last four weeks before parturition. As an alternative, 100 g. of $CaCO_3$ added to the diet provides the best effect (Jonsson 1978). The administration of 100 g. of NH_4Cl daily for three weeks prior to parturition will significantly reduce the incidence of milk fever. Additional methods for the prevention of milk fever include: supplementation of the diet with high levels of vitamin D for several days before calving, the administration of calcium salts a few days before calving, or the parenteral administration of vitamin D_3 and its analogues.

The possible uses of vitamin D_3 or its analogues for the prevention of milk fever in dairy cows are as follows:

1. Vitamin D_3 (cholecalciferol)—1 million units/45 kg. B.W., I.M. two to eight days before expected date of parturition

2. 25-hydroxycholecalciferol (25-OHD$_3$)—8 mg. I.M. three to 10 days before expected date of parturition (may be repeated at weekly intervals at 4- to 8-mg. doses)

3. 1-alpha-hydroxycholecalciferol—250 μg. I.M. within two hours after calving

There is some limited evidence that the feeding of excessive quantities of grain during the dry period predisposes to *left side displacement of the abomasum* (Coppock et al. 1972). Forage should constitute at least 60% of the total dry matter intake, and the daily intake of concentrate should not exceed 1.0% of body weight during the last two to three weeks of the dry period.

When an increased incidence of displaced abomasa is encountered, the following feeding procedures should be ensured:

1. Separate dry cows from the milking herd so that their feed intake can be controlled

2. Feed only hay, haylage, or pasture (when available)

3. If corn silage is fed as the only forage, limit the intake to 1.5 lb./100 lb. B.W. daily. This diet must be supplemented with protein, minerals, and vitamins to meet the requirements according to the size of the cow.

Prepartum Management

In preparation for parturition, about 10 days before calving, the diet of pregnant cows should be gradually shifted to free-choice good-quality hay, and concentrate feeding should begin so that an amount equivalent to 1% B.W. per day is being consumed at parturition. This is gradually increased to peak levels about three to four weeks after calving. Each cow should be placed in a well-bedded maternity box–stall for at least six days before calving. Maternity pens should measure at least 12 feet square; one pen per 16 cows in the herd should be available so that all cows calve in a box-stall. Such accommodation will allow effective surveillance of the cow throughout the periparturient period. Obstetrical assistance is more easily provided if necessary, the early signs of milk fever are more easily recognized, and there are fewer complications and traumatic injuries associated with slipping, which may occur during the increased activity of parturition and the recumbency of milk fever. A maternity pen containing a cow expected to calve is a constant focal point for the dairyman that will pay dividends by minimizing the incidence and severity of diseases associated with parturition.

In summary, the major nutritional problems during the dry period include excessive energy resulting in the fat cow syndrome and diets high in calcium that predispose to parturient paresis. This is in contrast to the relative lack of energy intake that occurs in early and mid-lactation.

Body Condition Scoring

In early lactation, the dairy cow loses body weight because of a negative energy balance. In mid-lactation, the cow will stabilize body weight, and in late lactation, she will usually begin to gain weight. During the dry period, she may gain an excess of weight, which is uneconomical and may result in metabolic disease, such as the fat cow syndrome immediately after parturition, and subsequent reduced reproductive performance.

The ideal body condition for pregnant, nonlactating dairy cows that allows them to attain maximal milk production and minimal metabolic disorders during the subsequent lactation has not been defined. Recommendations for satisfying the nutritional requirements of dairy cows are based on maintenance needs of a cow at a given body weight and with additional needs for milk production or gestation or both. The use of scales to weigh cows at such critical times as parturition, mid- and late lactation, and drying off could be an effective method of monitoring body weight and assessing the need for more or less feed to avoid undernutrition or overnutrition. However, very few producers weigh cows regularly.

Body condition scoring is a simple, practical, and accurate method of assessing the general nutritional status of the dairy cow during any given stage of the production cycle, especially the last third of lactation and the dry period, in preparation for parturition and subsequent lactation. The scoring system is an accurate and practical means of determining the degree of fitness in dairy cows, independent of cow frame size.

The body condition of cows is scored by visual inspection and palpation of the loin area and tailhead of the animal. The degree of fatness over these areas is assessed, and a score from 0 to 5 is given. An alternative system, based on similar criteria but scoring 1 to 8, is shown in Figure 7–11. The following scoring method is recommended (Ministry of Agriculture, Fisheries, and Food):

◻ Stand directly behind the cow to score both areas
◻ Score the tailhead area by feeling the amount of fatness. This gives a better estimate than visual inspection alone because of the set of tailhead and thickness of coat. Always use the same hand
◻ Score the loin area in a similar way, using the same hand, when the cow is relaxed
◻ Assess the scores to the nearest half point. Cows must be handled for accurate assessment of half score points
◻ Adjust tailhead score by half a point if it differs from the loin score by one point or more
◻ The adjusted tailhead score is used as the condition score

The characteristics of cows with body condition scores from 0 to 5 are recorded as shown in Table 7–7 (Wildman et al. 1982; Lowman et al. 1976).

The suggested target condition scores for the critical times are as follows:

Calving—Body condition score should be 3.5

First service—Body condition score should be 2 to 2.5

Drying-off—Body condition of 3 is optimum

There are relationships between certain production characteristics of dairy cows and body condition scores (Wildman et al. 1982). Cows with a significant increase in body condition during lactation are less efficient producers and have a longer calving to conception interval and a high body condition score at the end of lactation.

The body condition score at calving is the most important score. Cows in good but not fat condition at calving will supplement their nutrient intake in early lactation through fat mobilization. The cow should then be allowed to replenish body condition in late lactation after tissue mobilization in early lactation. It is more efficient to gain body condition during lactation than in the dry period. The cow's appetite is also greater during lactation, making it easier to replenish condition through feeding forage, whereas feeding for tissue gain during the dry period will usually require higher concentrate feeding.

FEEDING SYSTEMS

Even when the guidelines of the nutrient requirements of the dairy cow throughout the lactation-pregnancy cycle are followed, a major practical problem is the actual feeding of the animal. The history and current state of the art of feeding systems in dairy cows has been reviewed (Coppock et al. 1981).

Twenty-five years ago, pasture was the dominant forage used for dairy cows. This was followed by widespread use of hay and silage; cows were fed liberal quantities of forage, and grain mixtures were fed primarily while the cow was being milked. In the 1950s and 1960s it was found that milk yield could be increased if additional concentrates were fed. This led to the concept of "challenge feeding" in which cows could be fed sharply increasing amounts of concentrates during early lactation until peak yield and the limit of appetite was reached. Then adjustments were made to follow the decline in the lactation curve. The response in milk yield led to the recognition that the genetic ability to produce large quantities of milk was widespread in the dairy cow population. This was exploited by breed associations and breeding centers and led to the development of the high-yielding dairy cow.

Concurrent with the development of challenge feeding and genetic selection of super cows, technological developments improved the efficiency of the milking process, and it

Table 7–7. CLINICAL FINDINGS OF BODY CONDITION SCORES IN CATTLE

Score	5	4	3
Condition	Grossly fat	Fat	Good
Tailhead Area	Tailhead buried in fatty tissue. Skin distended. No part of pelvis felt even with firm pressure	Folds of soft fatty tissue present. Patches of fat apparent under skin. Pelvis felt only with firm pressure	Fatty tissue easily felt over the whole area. Skin appears smooth but pelvis can be felt
Loin Area	Folds of fatty tissue over transverse processes. Bone structure cannot be felt	Transverse processes cannot be felt even with firm pressure. No depression visible in loin between backbone and hip bones	End of transverse processes can be felt with pressure, but thick layer of tissue on top. Slight depression visible in loin

Score	2	1	0
Condition	Moderate	Poor	Very poor
Tailhead Area	Shallow cavity lined with fatty tissue apparent at tailhead. Some fatty tissue felt under the skin. Pelvis felt easily	Cavity present around tailhead. No fatty tissue felt between skin and pelvis, but skin is supple	Deep cavity under tail and around tailhead. Skin drawn tight over pelvis with no tissue detectable in between
Loin Area	Ends of transverse processes feel rounded, but upper surfaces felt only with pressure. Depression visible in loin	Ends of transverse processes sharp to touch and upper surfaces can be felt easily. Deep depression in loin	No fatty tissue felt. Shapes of transverse processes clearly visible. Animal appears emaciated

(From the Ministry of Agriculture, Fisheries, and Food, 1976. (MAFF Crown Copyright©)

soon became clear that high-producing cows could not consume an adequate amount of concentrate in the milking parlor to reach peak milk yield. The economic pressures to improve the efficiency of labor and to increase the size of the herd also created feeding problems. If feeding operations could be mechanized and automated more completely, labor productivity would be improved and more time would be available for other work. Feeding the concentrate mixture individually to each cow according to expected milk production was reasonably successful but a time-consuming practice.

The success of challenge feeding led to "lead feeding," which is the practice of increasing grain feeding beginning about three weeks prepartum to 1 to 1.5% of body weight by the expected date of parturition. This seemed like a reasonable method to adjust cows to high levels of grain feeding before parturition so that they would be able to consume large amounts after calving. However, there was no experimental evidence that lead feeding was beneficial. In fact, it had deleterious effects. Forage consumption was severely depressed near parturition, which appeared to induce digestive disorders such as simple indigestion and displacement of the abomasum. A more economically important disease complex, however, was the development of the fat cow syndrome due to the consumption of energy above the requirements of the dry-pregnant cow. Thus, lead feeding was not successful.

The trend toward larger herd size and handling cows in groups has reduced attention to feeding individual cows. Providing sufficient grain for high-producing cows and allocating grain according to requirements is a major problem on many dairy farms.

With the continued development and emphasis on improved efficiency and throughputs of milking parlors, high-producing cows cannot consume adequate grain in the parlor to reach and maintain high milk production. The amount of grain consumed per minute is

WHAT'S THE SCORE ON YOUR

Over the past few years, much of the research work at the Ellinbank Dairy Research Station, near Warragul, has revolved around pre-calving and post-calving problems in dairy cattle.

One of the most significant developments to evolve from this research is a system of "scoring" that will be a valuable aid to farmers in assessing the condition of their dairy cows.

Scoring is in numbers, from "1" to "8", and the range is from emaciated cattle (Score No.1) through to very fat (Score No. 8). The condition scoring system is mainly based on different amounts of fat around the base of the tail and

over the hips and back.

David Earle, a young research officer at the Station, told Unigate Farmer why the system was developed.

He said that the problem encountered was that people had different ideas of cow condition and used different terms to describe it. The scoring system overcame this language problem and helped farmers to make a confident assessment of cow condition. If a farmer could assess the body condition of his cows he could control their condition to ensure that feed was used efficiently and a high production per cow was achieved. David explained the research work

into feeding cows that has been carried out at Ellinbank. Experiments conducted over the past five years on feeding dry cows included feeding hay, grass and grain. From these experiments it was found that the type of ration was not important, so researchers at Ellinbank then looked at overseas experiments which had shown benefits from generously feeding dry cows.

David said that the overseas research did not show whether it was the live weight gains before calving or the body condition of cows at calving which was important.

"We conducted our own

experiments and firstly found that cows which had large live weight gains before calving produced no more milk or fat in lactation than cows which had smaller live weight gains and calved in the same condition," said David.

"We then did an experiment to see if a live weight gain before calving was necessary.

"Some cows were maintained at a constant live weight before calving and even though they lost body condition because of calf growth they still produced as well as cows which calved in the same condition but had large live weight gains before calving.

"In a further experiment looking at

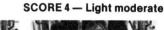

SCORE 1 — Emaciated

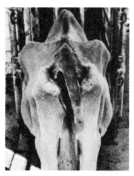

Very little flesh over the skeleton. Cow has a tucked-up appearance.

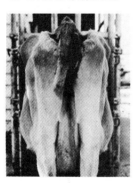

SCORE 2 — Very poor

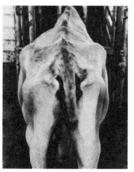

Area around base of tail is deeply sunken. Backbone, hips, pins and ribs are very prominent.

SCORE 3 — Poor

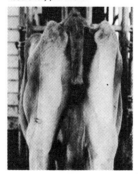

Area around base of tail is sunken. Backbone, hips and pins are prominent.

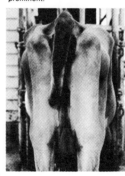

SCORE 4 — Light moderate

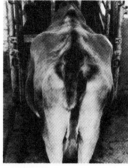

Area around base of tail is only slightly sunken. Slight fat covering over pins, hips, ribs and backbone.

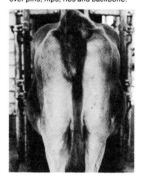

Feeding dry cows

Cows calving in Score 5 condition will produce to their full potential on pasture. Cows calving in Score 3 condition will produce 10% less milkfat over their lactation.

It is not necessary to calve cows in Score 6, 7 or 8 condition; milk production would not be improved.

If cows calve in Score 5 condition, increases in weight approaching calving are not necessary. However, restricting cows in the early stage of the dry period followed by more generous feeding in the last four to six weeks before calving achieves:

• better control over condition of the cows.

• a saving in the amount of feed required.

In any system of feeding dry cows, first and second-calvers need preferential treatment. Regardless of condition at calving, cows must be fully fed after calving to ensure optimum milk production.

Figure 7-11. What's the score on your dairy herd? (Reprinted from Unigate Farmer, Vol. 9, No. 10, December 1976.)

DAIRY HERD

the effect of calving cows in different body conditions, researchers found that if cows calved in poor condition they would produce 10 percent less milk fat than cows in moderate condition,'' David said.

Research work at Ellinbank has therefore shown that the condition of cows at calving is important.

But how the cow reaches that condition is not important. Experiments are now looking for the condition score which will be most profitable for farmers to calve their cows in.

Researchers also want to find out if milk production losses due to feed shortages after calving can be

reduced by calving cows at higher condition scores.

This is why the scoring system has been so useful.

David said the system is accurate enough for research purposes and practical for farmers.

The scoring system has been introduced to discussion groups by Dairy Husbandry Officers, and now many farmers in South and West Gippsland are using the method.

The Department of Agriculture has produced 3000 booklets on the system and is using Field Days to discuss cow condition with farmers.

● Photographs below are reproduced from the Department's booklet

THE INDICATORS

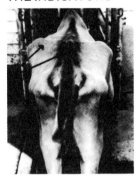

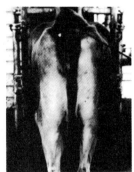

Amount of fat on backbone, hips and ribs.

Amount of fat around base of tail and prominence of pin bones.

SCORE 5 — Moderate

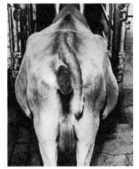

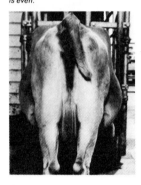

Area around base of tail is filled out. Fat covering over pins, hips and ribs is even.

SCORE 6 — Heavy moderate

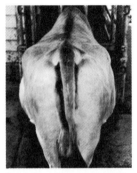

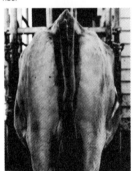

Description as for moderate condition but more fat cover on back and over ribs.

SCORE 7 — Fat

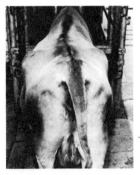

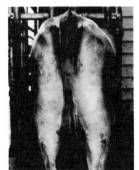

Considerable fat layer on pins, hips, ribs and on back.

SCORE 8 — Very fat

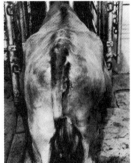

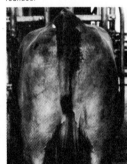

Heavy covering of fat over whole body. Animal looks smooth and rounded.

Some rules of thumb

- Cows more than four weeks from calving can be maintained on about 7 kg of reasonably good hay per day or about three hours of grazing of good quality pasture.
- Cows within four weeks of calving can be

maintained in Score 5 condition by being fed about 11 kg of reasonably good hay or by grazing of good quality pasture for four or five hours.

- About five weeks of unrestricted grazing is required to improve the condition score by 1 near calving time. Thus a cow in

Score 3 condition will need about 10 weeks of unrestricted grazing to reach Score 5.

This a rough guide. Choose the ration according to your own assessment of the condition of your cows at any time.

Figure 7-11. Continued

influenced by several factors, including production and body size, pelleting, fineness of grind and water content, breed, housing systems, and the amount fed.

The feeding systems that are currently in use include the conventional stanchion, individual cow feeding using electronic delivery systems, combined free-stall bunk feeding and milking parlor, and group feeding of complete rations.

The usual procedure in the conventional stanchion or tie-stall barn is to offer cows free-choice forages plus a grain mixture fed individually according to feeding guides that reflect the quality and quantity of forage eaten by the herd and individual requirements for energy based on lactation number, body size, milk quantity, milk fat content, and gestation (Coppock 1977). However, even when a concentrate mixture is allocated carefully, a serious limitation of this system is the inaccuracy of predicting forage intake of individual cows and individual cow variation in forage preference even if the herd intake is known. Thus, the accuracy with which energy and other nutrients can be provided through the concentrate mixture has never been precise even in a system where it seemed possible.

With the advent of the combination of free-stall housing with a milking parlor, rapid developments in parlor automation reduced the time spent by cows in the parlor so that high producers do not have enough time to eat their required grain, even if they have the appetite to do so. To resolve this problem, dairymen add a base amount of grain to the forage, which is fed outside in a bunk. However, this may aggravate the problem as low producers receive too much energy and high producers receive an insufficient amount. The fat cow syndrome has also been associated with bunk and parlor feeding.

Another approach is to provide the concentrates on an individual basis through a protected stall with an enclosed box. Individual cows are equipped with a magnet on a neck collar that activates a small auger that delivers feed at a predetermined rate. As long as the cow has her head in the feeder, grain is delivered slowly (Owens et al. 1978). The magnet is placed on the cow at calving and removed at 13 to 15 weeks of lactation or when production is dropping. Problems include overeating, a decrease in forage intake, aggressive behavior by dominant cows, and a lower fat content of milk. In another system, cows are equipped with an electronic device on a neck collar that allows them to open a door

for access to a manger of feed. The system is designed so that a particular cow is allotted a predetermined amount of concentrate per day based on production, but the cow must return to the feeder at least once every six hours to obtain her full programed ration (Frolisch et al. 1978). With the electronic system, cows receive concentrate several times daily, which increases daily milk production and maintains butterfat concentration. However, any system designed to allocate concentrate individually and forages ad libitum suffers the same imprecision as described earlier for stanchion barn feeding systems. These three systems of supplementing concentrate will have greatest merit in loose housing systems where grouping is not feasible.

Complete Ration—Group Feeding System

In this system, cows are housed and fed in groups according to the amount of daily milk production. The herd must be large enough to justify grouping. The cows are moved from one group to another as their daily milk production declines throughout lactation. There are usually at least three groups: *early lactation, mid- and late lactation,* and the *dry group.* The objective is to provide a complete ration that will provide the nutrient requirements necessary for the "average" cow in that particular group. The term "complete ration" is used to define a quantitative blend of all diet ingredients mixed thoroughly enough to prevent separation and sorting, formulated to specific nutrient levels, and offered ad libitum. The roughages and concentrates are mixed together. To achieve maximum income above feed cost, the rations should be consumed in large quantities, contain a high concentration of utilizable nutrients, contain sufficient fiber to avoid depressed milk fat percentage, and contain feed ingredients formulated on least cost (Spahr 1977).

The *advantages* of complete rations include the following:

1. No expression of choice among feeds is permitted. The feed is a uniform blend

2. High production levels can be obtained in both experimental and commercial herds

3. Free-choice mineral supplements are unnecessary

4. Complete rations coupled with lactation groups allow for special formulation for high-producing cows who cannot consume enough feed energy to sustain their production

5. Complete rations fed ad libitum result in

few digestive upsets early in lactation because the concentrates are mixed thoroughly with the roughages

6. Nonprotein nitrogen compounds, especially urea, are metabolized more efficiently when consumed several times a day in small quantities along with an energy source that contains starch

7. A complete ration with forage base of silage serves to dilute and mask the flavor of unpalatable ingredients such as urea

8. They are labor-efficient

9. By the provision of a specific and obligatory ratio of forage to concentrate, the depression of milk fat can be minimized by ensuring a constant level of crude fiber

10. Feeding concentrate in the parlor is unnecessary. Advantages of this include: No parlor grain feeding equipment is necessary; cows are quieter during milking and defecate less; there is less feed dust in the parlor; movement out of the parlor is quicker because cows do not delay to finish eating; and more cows per man are possible because parlor operators do not spend time dispensing grain

11. It is possible to mechanize a conventional tie-stall barn for complete rations

12. The total diet can be formulated quantitatively

The *disadvantages* of complete rations include:

1. Roughage stored in bales or long form must be chopped before it can be blended with silage or grain

2. Mixing equipment is expensive

3. Many barns are not easily redesigned for group feeding

4. They are not yet economically feasible in small herds

The *advantages* for grouping herds fed complete rations include:

1. Production groups allow cows to move to higher-forage–lower-energy diets as lactating progresses and production declines. This should minimize the occurrence of the fat cow syndrome

2. Production groups allow lower-producing cows to be fed a less expensive diet

3. When cows are grouped and fed by production, the highest-producing group can be fed a diet with a higher concentration of those nutrients for which the cow has limited capacity for storage. A high-energy diet fed in early lactation should minimize the period of negative energy balance and perhaps result in improved reproductive performance

4. Heat detection and other features of herd management are simplified if cows are grouped by production and/or stage of lactation

5. More uniform milk-out in the parlor will occur if cows are grouped by production

6. It is impossible to switch cows from a high-forage complete ration to a high-energy complete ration within a few days post partum without experiencing digestive disturbances

The *disadvantages* of grouping herds fed complete rations include:

1. Labor and time are required periodically to regroup cows

2. Housing and facilities required for grouping may be uneconomic for a particular herd

3. A significant drop in milk production may occur when cows change groups from high-energy to lower-energy diets. This may be due to the combined effects of a change in diet and a social change

4. More feed analyses and ration formulations may be necessary than when one lactating-cow ration is used

FORMULATION OF DAIRY CATTLE RATIONS

Proper feeding is the cornerstone of a successful dairy operation, because feed costs account for over one half of the total costs of milk production. Milk yield per cow and cost of feed have by far the greatest influence on profitability of milk production. Therefore, for a profitable dairy enterprise it is necessary to have cows with a high genetic potential for milk production that are fed to achieve the greatest output of milk at the most economical cost. A balanced ration is essential for optimum performance. A shortage or an imbalance in the supply of energy, protein, vitamins, or minerals may subject the cow to nutritional stress, resulting in metabolic disorders or decreased milk production. Requirements for these nutrients depend largely on milk yield, milk composition, and body weight, with milk yield having by far the greatest influence in the high-producing dairy cow.

Superior feeding and management leading to a high nutrient intake is generally a major reason for high herd yield (Fredeen et al. 1982; Bowman et al. 1980; Martin et al. 1978). The variability in feeds and feeding management account for the observed major differences in milk production between herds. Surveys of feeding management practices of dairy herds in Canada reveal that nutrition is a major determinant of milk production. High average herd milk yield was associated with high average nutrient intake, specifically energy and protein (Fredeen et al. 1982). Owners of high-producing herds demonstrated superior feeding and management. High nutrient intake in early lactation was associated with special efforts to increase intake and maintain cow health during the periparturient period. Higher proportions of concentrate were fed after calving. Dry cows were more often separated from lactating cows, and rations were more frequently balanced in response to changes in type and quality of forage fed in high-yielding herds.

The nutrition of the dairy cow is of primary importance in explaining variation in herd average 4% FCM production and income over feed costs (Bowman et al. 1980). The management factor associated with the largest amount of variation in production and income per cow was the amount of meal fed per cow.

To optimize the level of production in many dairy herds, the level of nutrition must be improved. In a survey of the feeding and management practices of Saskatchewan dairy herds classified according to milk production levels, the following feeding and management practices are considered to limit production in low-producing herds (Martin et al. 1978):

1. The total daily feed per cow was lower in low-production herds than in high-production herds
2. The intake of crude protein was lower in low-production herds than in high-production herds
3. Replacement heifers in low-production herds were fed significantly less crude protein, energy, calcium, and phosphorus than those in high-production herds
4. The intake of copper and zinc was marginal or deficient in all herds
5. Mature body weight, calving interval, and age at first breeding were similar in both groups
6. The incidence of mastitis was higher in low-production herds
7. Use of herd health and other advisory services was associated with high-production herds

The nutritional part of a dairy herd health program provided by a veterinarian would include the following:

1. Be knowledgeable about the nutritionally related diseases of dairy cattle

2. Monitor and assess the incidence of these diseases in the herd
3. Be knowledgeable about the nutrient requirements of dairy cattle during growth, for maintenance, for pregnancy, and for lactation
4. Understand the feeds and feeding systems used on the particular farm and identify problem areas. This should be assessed monthly. Feed analyses should be done on each new batch of farm-grown grains

Formulation of rations for dairy cattle by computer has had a marked effect on feeding practices in recent years (Erdman et al. 1980). Many commercial feed companies use linear programing methods to determine ingredient formulas for their concentrate mixes (Black and Hlubik 1980). Computer-formulated concentrate mixes for dairy cattle are efficacious, and cost savings are realized from feeding them to lactating cows. Similarly, least-cost complete dairy rations are economical.

The basic nutrient requirements built into computer-formulated programs are taken from the latest National Research Council bulletin, *Nutrient Requirements of Dairy Cattle*. Additionally, requirements for crude protein and net energy for lactation; for maintenance; and for milk production, based on body size and amount of fat content of milk produced, are included in the matrix. The program must satisfy both sets of constraints. This allows the program to operate efficiently whether the ration ingredients are fed separately to individual cows or groups of cows or are fed as a complete ration ad libitum to groups of cows with similar nutrient requirements. The only mineral requirements built into the program are for calcium and phosphorus. However, the program does list the calculated concentrations of minerals provided by the ration along with the National Research Council recommendations for comparison. The computer program selects the milk production at which the value of milk equals the cost of energy needed to produce it and formulates a ration for that milk production. Thus, rather than formulating a least-cost ration, a ration is formulated that maximizes income above feed costs. Since feed is the largest single expense in milk production, it has the greatest potential effect on profit.

Computerized ration formulation programs once relied on the mail, but they can now be accessed with remote computer terminals. *A dairyman is more likely to implement recom-*

mendations from the computer if answers to his questions are immediate rather than days or weeks later. Computer terminals now make it possible to obtain ration formulations directly by connecting with the central computer over telephone lines. Prices of available feed ingredients, size of cow, milk fat test, milk price, and milk production response curve are typed on the keyboard of the terminal and sent to the computer, which has ration requirements, feedstuff composition, and other programs on file. The central computer calculates the optimum ration formula data and prints it out on paper at the remote terminal or on a TV-type screen.

If a ration needs modification to make it compatible with equipment or management practices on individual farms, changes in ingredient constraints or other input data can be sent to the central computer, and another ration will be returned within a minute. When several rations are needed for individual cows or groups of cows with varying body weights, fat tests, and production, or at varying stages of lactation within a herd, they are easily obtained with simple changes in the input data for each successive ration (Bath and Bennet 1980). Also, once the basic input data are sent to the central computer, they can be stored for future use. These data can be retrieved, corrected to fit current conditions, and used for ration formulation without re-entering all the original input data. The program is simple to run. An hour or two of training is adequate for extension agents, veterinarians, and dairymen to become competent in the use of the program or computer terminals. Ultimately, computer-formulated ration service will be offered at dairy records centers, which will provide monthly print-outs containing reproductive performance, milk production, feed costs, somatic cell counts, and action lists (cows to calve, cows to dry, cows to breed, cows to check for pregnancy, and potential culls).

The programable calculator should be considered as a supplement to, and not a substitute for, larger computers. The calculator can be taken directly to the farm and used to help solve simple management problems at low cost. Rations can be formulated and management decisions made for individual situations quickly and accurately. In consulting with dairymen, ration deficiencies can be determined and new rations formulated in a short time. Because of limited data storage, programable calculators cannot do the genetic evaluations and formulations of least-cost rations currently done in large computers. Also, Dairy Herd Improvement records cannot be kept on programable calculators (Linn and Spike 1980).

Review Literature

Baile, C.A. and Della-Fera, M.A. Nature of hunger and satiety control systems in ruminants. J. Dairy Sci., 64:1140–1152, 1981.

Broster, W.H. Effect on milk yield of the cow of the level of feeding before calving. Dairy Sci. Abstr., 33: 253–270, 1971.

Broster, W.H. Effect on milk yield of the cow of the level of feeding during lactation. Dairy Sci. Abstr., 34:265–288, 1972.

Broster, W.H. and Swan, H. Feeding strategy for the high yielding dairy cow. EAAP Publication No. 25, Granada Publishing, London, 1979.

Chalupa, W. Rumen bypass and prolactin of protein and amino acids. J. Dairy Sci., 58:1198–1218, 1975.

Clark, J.H. Lactational responses to postruminal administration of proteins and amino acids. J. Dairy Sci., 58: 1178–1197, 1975.

Clark, J.H. and Davis, C.L. Some aspects of feeding high producing dairy cows. J. Dairy Sci., 163:873–885, 1980.

Commonwealth Agriculture Bureau. The Nutrient Requirements of Ruminant Livestock, 1980.

Coppock, C.E., Bath, D.L. and Harris, B., Jr. From feeding to feeding systems. J. Dairy Sci., 64:1230–1249, 1981.

Hogan, J.P. Quantitative aspects of nitrogen utilization in ruminants. J. Dairy Sci., 58:1164–1177, 1975.

Huber, J.T. and Kung, L., Jr. Protein and nonprotein nitrogen utilization in dairy cattle. J. Dairy Sci., 64: 1170–1195, 1981.

Miller, W.J. Mineral and vitamin nutrition in dairy cattle. J. Dairy Sci., 64:1196–1206, 1981.

Miller, W.J. and O'Dell, G.D. Nutritional problems of using maximum forage or maximum concentrates in dairy rations. J. Dairy Sci., 52:1144–1154, 1969.

Moe, P.W. Energy metabolism of dairy cattle. J. Dairy Sci., 64:1120–1139, 1981.

National Research Council. National Academy of Sciences. Nutrient Requirements of Domestic Animals No. 3. Nutrient Requirements of Dairy Cattle. 5th Revised Edition, 1978.

Satter, L.D. and Roffler, R.E. Nitrogen requirement and utilization in dairy cattle. J. Dairy Sci., 58:1219–1237, 1975.

Tyrrell, H.F. and Moe, P.W. Effect of intake on digestive efficiency. J. Dairy Sci., 58:1151–1163, 1975.

Waldo, D.R. and Jorgensen, N.A. Forages for high animal prolactin: Nutritional factors and effects of conservation. J. Dairy Sci., 64:1207–1229, 1981.

Wangsness, P.J. and Muller, L.D. Maximum forage for dairy cows: Review. J. Dairy Sci., 64:1–13, 1981.

References

Abou-Akkada, A.R. Some aspects of ruminant feeding in the tropics. In: Animal Production in the Tropics. M.K. Yousef (Ed.). Praeger Scientific, New York, 1982, pp. 29–42.

Barney, D.J., Grieve, D.G., Macleod, G.K. et al. Response of cows to a reduction in dietary crude protein from 17 percent to 13 percent during early lactation. J. Dairy Sci., 64:25–33, 1981a.

Barney, D.J., Grieve, D. G., Macleod, G.K. et al. Response of cows to dietary crude protein during midlactation. J. Dairy Sci., 64:655–661, 1981b.

Bath, D.L. and Bennett, L.F. Development of a dairy feeding model for maximizing income above feed cost with access by remote computer terminals. J. Dairy Sci., 63:1379–1389, 1980.

Bines, J.A. Regulation of food intake in dairy cows in relation to milk production. Livestock Prod. Sci., 3: 115–118, 1976.

Black, J.R. and Hlubik, J. Basics of computerized linear programs for ration formulation. J. Dairy Sci., 63: 1366–1378, 1980.

Botts, R.L., Hemken, R.W. and Bull, L.S. Protein reserves in the lactating dairy cows. J. Dairy Sci., 62:433–440, 1979.

Bowman, J.S.T., Morley, J.C., Kennedy, B.W. et al. The dairy herd management system and farm productivity. Can. J. Anim. Sci., 60:495–502, 1980.

Broster, W.H. and Alderman, G. Nutrient requirements of the high yielding cow. Livestock Prod. Sci., 4:263–275, 1977.

Bywater, A.C. and Dent, J.B. Simulation of the intake and partition of nutrients by the dairy cow. 1. Management control in the dairy enterprise; philosophy and general model construction. Agricultural Systems, 1:245–260, 1976.

Chalupa, W. and Kronfeld, D. Buffers for dairy cattle. Animal Nutrition and Health, May-June, 1983.

Clark, J.H. and Davis, C.L. Some aspects of feeding high producing dairy cows. J. Dairy Sci., 63:873–885, 1980.

Commonwealth Agricultural Bureau. The Nutrient Requirements of Ruminant Livestock. 1980.

Conrad, J.H., McDowell, L.R. and Loosli, J.K. Mineral deficiencies and toxicities for grazing ruminants in the tropics. In: Animal Production in the Tropics. M.K. Yousef (Ed.). Praeger Scientific, New York, 1982, pp. 73–106.

Coppock, C.E. Feeding methods and grouping systems. J. Dairy Sci., 60:1327–1336, 1977.

Coppock, C.E., Bath, D.L. and Harris, B.J. From feeding to feeding systems. J. Dairy Sci., 64:1230–1249, 1981.

Coppock, C.E., Noller, C.H., Wolfe, S.A. et al. Effect of forage concentrate ratio in complete feeds fed ad libitum on feed intake prepartum and occurrence of abomasal displacement in dairy cows. J. Dairy Sci., 55:783–789, 1972.

Dishington, I.W. Prevention of milk fever (hypocalcemic paresis puerperalis) by dietary salt supplements. Acta Vet. Scand., 16:503–512, 1975.

Ekern, A. and Macleod, G. The role of conserved forages in the nutrition of the dairy cow. Livestock Prod. Sci., 5:45–56, 1978.

Erdman, R.A., Botts, R.L., Hemken, R.W. et al. Effect of dietary sodium bicarbonate and magnesium oxide on production and physiology in early lactation. J. Dairy Sci., 63:923–930, 1980.

Forster, R.J., Grieve, D.G., Buchanan-Smith, J.G. et al. Effect of dietary protein degradability on cows in early lactation. J. Dairy Sci., 66:1653–1662, 1983.

Fredeen, A.H., Macleod, G.K., Grieve, D.G. et al. Differences in feeding and management associated with milk yields in Ontario dairy herds. Can. J. Anim. Sci., 62:449–458, 1982.

Frolisch, R.A., Harshberger, K.E. and Olver, E.F. Automatic individual feeding of concentrates to dairy cattle. J. Dairy Sci., 61:1789–1792, 1978.

Fronk, T.J., Schultz, L.H. and Hardie, A.R. Effect of dry period overconditioning on subsequent metabolic disorders and performance of dairy cows. J. Dairy Sci., 63:1080–1090, 1980.

Gardner, R.W. Interactions of energy levels offered to Holstein cows prepartum and postpartum. I. Production responses and blood composition changes. J. Dairy Sci., 52:1973–1984, 1969a.

Gardner, R.W. Interactions of energy levels offered to Holstein cows prepartum and postpartum. II. Reproductive performance. J. Dairy Sci., 52:1985–1987, 1969b.

Gardner, R.W. and Park, R.L. Effects of prepartum energy intake and calcium to phosphorus ratios on lactation response and parturient paresis. J. Dairy Sci., 56:385–389, 1973.

Gardner, R.W., Schuh, J.D. and Vargus, L.G. Accelerated growth and early breeding of Holstein heifers. J. Dairy Sci., 60:1941–1948, 1977.

Garnsworthy, P.C. and Topps, J.H. The effect of body condition of dairy cows at calving on their food intake and performance when given complete diets. Anim. Prod., 35:113–119, 1982a.

Garnsworthy, P.C. and Topps, J.H. The effects of body condition at calving, food intake and performance in early lactation on blood composition of dairy cows given complete diets. Anim. Prod., 35:121–125, 1982b.

Ishak, N.A., Larson, L.L., Owen, F.G. et al. Effect of selenium vitamins and ration fiber on placental retention and performance of dairy cattle. J. Dairy Sci., 66:99–106, 1983.

Jones, G.M., Wildman, E.E., Wagner, P. et al. Effectiveness of the dairy cattle feed formulation system in developing lactating rations. J. Dairy Sci., 61:1645–1651, 1978.

Jonsson, G. Milk fever prevention. Vet Rec., 102:165–169, 1978.

Jorgensen, N.A. Combating milk fever. J. Dairy Sci., 57: 933–944, 1974.

Journet, M. and Remond, B. Physiological factors affecting the voluntary intake of feed by cows: A review. Livestock Prod. Sci., 3:129–146, 1976.

Kaufmann, W. Influence of the composition of the ration and the feeding frequency on pH regulation in the rumen and on feed intake in ruminants. Livestock Prod. Sci., 3:103–114, 1976.

Kung, L., Jr. and Huber, J.T. Performance of high-producing cows in early lactation fed protein of varying amounts, sources, and digestibility. J. Dairy Sci., 66:227–234, 1983.

Linn, J.G. and Spike, P.L. Programmable calculators and their application to feeding and management of dairy cattle. J. Dairy Sci., 63:1390–1394, 1980.

Lowman, B.G., Scott, N.A. and Somerville, S.H. Condition scoring of cattle. East Scotland Coll. Agric. Bull. No. 6, 1976.

Macleod, G.K., Grieve, D.G. and McMillan, I. Performance of first lactation dairy cows fed complete ration of several rations of forage to concentrate. J. Dairy Sci., 66:1668–1674, 1983.

Martin, L.J.F., Christensen, D.A. and Armstrong, K.R. Feeding and management in Saskatchewan dairy herds classified according to milk production level. Can. Vet. J., 19:331–334, 1978.

Milford, R. and Minson, D.J. The feeding value of tropical pastures. In: Tropical Pastures. W. Davies and C.L. Skidmore (Eds.). Faber and Faber Ltd., London, 1966. pp. 106–114.

Miller, W.J. and O'Dell, G.D. Nutritional problems of using maximum forage or maximum concentrates in dairy rations. J. Dairy Sci., 52:1144–1154, 1969.

Ministry of Agriculture, Fisheries, and Food. Condition scoring of dairy cows. Leaflet 612, 1978.

Moe, P.W., Flatt, W.P. and Tyrrell, H.F. Net energy value of feeds for lactation. J. Dairy Sci., 55:945–958, 1972.

Moe, P.W., Tyrrell, H.F. and Flatt, W.P. Energetics of body tissue mobilization. J. Dairy Sci., 54:548–553, 1971.

Morrow, D.A. Fat cow syndrome. J. Dairy Sci., 59:1625–1629, 1976.

Morrow, D.A., Hillman, D., Dade, A.W. et al. Clinical investigation of a dairy herd with the fat cow syndrome. J. Am. Vet. Med. Assoc., 174:161–167, 1979.

Murphy, M.R., Davis, C.L. and McCoy, G.C. Factors affecting water consumption by Holstein cows in early lactation. J. Dairy Sci., 66:35–38, 1983.

National Research Council. National Academy of Sciences. Nutrient Requirements of Domestic Animals No. 3. Nutrient Requirements of Dairy Cattle. Fifth Revised Edition. 1978.

Owens, M.J., Muller, L.D., Rook, J.A. et al. Evaluation of magnetic grain feeder for lactating dairy cows. J. Dairy Sci., 61:1590–1597, 1978.

Palmquist, D.L. and Jenkins, T.C. Fat in lactation rations. Review. J. Dairy Sci., 63:1–14, 1980.

Payne, W.J.A. The desirability and implications of encouraging intensive animal production enterprises in developing countries. In: Intensive Animal Production in Developing Countries. British Society of Animal Production Occasional Publication No. 4. A.J. Smith and R.G. Gunn (Eds.), pp. 1–9.

Rickaby, C.D. A review of the nutritional aspects of complete diets for dairy cows. A.D.A.S. Quarterly Review, 29:51–70, 1978.

Rickaby, C.D. Developments in complete diet feeding of dairy cows. A.D.L.S. Quarterly Review, 34:195–211, 1979.

Roberts, C.J. Fat mobilization of high-yielding dairy cows in early lactation. Proc. XII World Congress on Diseases of Cattle, The Netherlands, pp. 501–507, 1982.

Roffler, R.E. and Thacker, D.L. Influence of reducing dietary crude protein from 17 to 13.5 percent on early lactation. J. Dairy Sci., 66:51–58, 1983.

Salinas, H.G., Stringer, W.C., Kesler, E.M. et al. Performance of dairy cows in midlactation fed high quality grass pasture and concentrate at three percent of energy requirements. J. Dairy Sci., 66:514–519, 1983.

Satter, L.D. and Roffler, R.E. Nitrogen requirement and utilization in dairy cattle. J. Dairy Sci., 58:1219–1237, 1975.

Schultz, L.H. Relationship of rearing of dairy heifers to mature performance. J. Dairy Sci., 52:1321–1329, 1969.

Spahr, S.L. Optimum rations for group feeding. J. Dairy Sci., 60:1337–1344, 1977.

Stobbs, T.H. Limitation to dairy production in the tropics. Tropical Grasslands 5:139–303, 1971.

Wangsness, P.J. and Muller, L.D. Maximum forage for dairy cows: Review. J. Dairy Sci., 64:1–13, 1981.

Whiteman, P.C. Tropical Pasture Science. Oxford University Press, Oxford, 1980.

Wiggers, K.D., Nelson, D.K. and Jacobson, N.L. Prevention of parturient paresis by a low-calcium diet preparation: A field study. J. Dairy Sci., 58:430–431, 1975.

Wildman, E.E., Jones, G.M., Wagner, P.E. et al. A dairy cow body condition scoring system and its relationship to selected production characteristics. J. Dairy Sci., 65:495–501, 1982.

Yarrington, J.T., Capen, C.C., Black, H.E. et al. Effects of a low calcium prepartal diet on calcium homeostatic mechanisms in the cow: Morphologic and biochemical studies. J. Nutr., 107:2244–2256, 1977.

Zanartu, D., Polan, C.E., Ferreri, L.E. et al. Effect of stage of lactation and varying available energy intake on milk production, milk composition, and subsequent tissue enzymic activity. J. Dairy Sci., 668:1644–1652, 1983.

Housing

INTRODUCTION

In countries with several months of freezing winter weather each year and where access to grazing pastures is limited to a few months of the year, or in heavily populated areas where dairy cows are hand-fed because of the high costs of land, cows are housed in a variety of barn types ranging from outdoor corrals to free-stall barns to traditional stall (or stanchion) barns (Hoglund and Albright 1970; Bakken 1981). In temperate zones, stanchion barns with pail or pipeline milkers and free-stall barns with milking parlors predominate. In tropical countries, the cows are on pasture most of the time and are milked in parlors.

Previous to 1950, dairy farming was labor-intensive. Cows were fed individually in stanchion-type stalls, they were milked in their individual stalls, and the barn was cleaned by hand at least once daily.

Major changes in the housing of dairy cattle

have occurred in the last 30 years in those countries where cattle are housed throughout the winter months. Dairy herds have become progressively larger, and producers have introduced labor-saving systems of feeding, milking, manure disposal, and handling and caring for cows and young stock (Martin 1982; Nolt et al. 1981).

The basic objective of dairy buildings and equipment is to provide a system that will give cattle the opportunity to be housed, fed, and milked and to reproduce efficiently. The system is interrelated with almost every other aspect of dairy management. It involves a major capital investment, and building costs are normally the third largest production cost in dairy operations. The system also determines labor efficiency. Decisions regarding dairy housing and facilities have long-term effects on the dairy operation, because the expected life of most buildings is 20 or more years and that of equipment, five to 15 years. Major changes within these periods are expensive. These factors stress the importance of thorough planning before old systems are remodeled. Many existing systems are examples of poor planning and design. They are characterized by low labor efficiency, inadequate drainage because of poor site selection, high maintenance costs, and lack of flexibility for expansion or changes. These problems have been accentuated because of the changes that have occurred in recent years, that is, increasing herd size and new technical developments in feeding, milking, and waste handling systems. Recent advances make it possible to confine and house large numbers of dairy cows and to feed and milk them efficiently to achieve high levels of milk production.

There has been a notable lack of research in the design and economics of dairy cattle housing and equipment industries have often designed and built facilities on a trial and error basis, based on previous experience and intuition.

The veterinarian should be aware of the housing and environmental factors that affect health and production in the dairy herd. The effects of housing and environment are complex, and there is usually no simple solution to a particular problem. For this reason, the interdisciplinary team approach should be used to identify and solve problems. Agricultural engineers with experience in animal housing and ventilation systems should be consulted, and the veterinarian and the engineer should visit the farm together. Detailed observations should be recorded, ventilation tests conducted, and a clear report of the recommendations given to the farmer (Anderson and Bates 1982a, 1982b).

A check list of the criteria needed to design any agricultural animal housing for comfort and productivity, which are applicable to dairy housing, includes the following (Hazen 1971):

□ *Site planning*: Placement, legal, public relations

□ *Services to and from the facility*: Electric power, water, transportation and access, communication, emergency services, feed storage and handling, required fuels, waste handling, drainage, animal disposal

□ *The facility*: Climate control, space allocation, basic design, sanitation and contamination control, special equipment, instrumentation, animal behavior

□ *Economics*: The construction costs are of paramount importance

Dairy housing systems should be designed so that cows are fed, handled, observed, and protected properly. The need to feed cows properly is top priority. The role of housing is to make it possible for cows to receive the proper amounts of roughages, concentrates, vitamins, minerals, and water. An inadequate feeding system can be a major cause of low production or of overfeeding. Next in importance is being able to handle cows as effortlessly as possible. With varying degrees of frequency, cows must be detected in heat, identified, sorted out and bred, treated for disease, confined for a variety of reasons, moved to calving stalls, examined by the veterinarian, and have their feet trimmed if necessary. Housing systems must enable the herdsman to observe cows in heat and to observe appetite, general health, and accurate identification of the animals. Housing systems must also protect cattle from inclement weather such as heat, cold, wind, rain, snow, and excessive humidity, and from excessive build-up of manure.

The environmental factors that affect health and the efficiency of production in housed dairy cattle include air quality, floor and bedding, space allowance, feeding and milking systems, manure storage and disposal, animal traffic flow and ease of handling, and degree of comfort for people working in the facility. Dairymen are seeking control of all aspects of the environment in their production facilities (Martin 1982).

The complete confinement of a dairy herd for several months each year is associated with many health and production problems, some of which include the following:

1. Endemic respiratory disease in calves raised indoors in close proximity to adult cows housed in poorly ventilated barns. Adult cattle are able to tolerate inadequately ventilated barns much more effectively than young calves, which are highly susceptible to enzootic calf pneumonia. Outbreaks of acute respiratory disease occur sporadically in adult cows kept indoors throughout the winter months in countries like Canada, the U.S., and the U.K.

2. Lameness due to diseases of the feet such as sole ulcer and foot rot associated with the quality of floors (Blom 1982). Acute traumatic injuries of the musculoskeletal system are associated with slippery floors (the downer cow syndrome). The level of the floor of the feeding manger relative to the floor of the stall may be associated with traumatic injuries of the legs, feet, and udder (Gjestang 1978, 1982). A feeding level 16 cm. above the stall floor results in the least injuries. A low feeding level forces cattle to spread their legs during eating, which may predispose to development of lesions of the feet.

3. An increased incidence of peracute coliform mastitis associated with unsanitary conditions because of excess accumulation of manure on cows with inadequate bedding or the use of contaminated bedding such as sawdust or shavings.

4. Inefficient circulation of cows between feeding, lounging, and milking because of inadequate design of the floor plan.

5. Insufficient space for each age group of animals in the herd, which results in overcrowding and allows for the spread of infectious diseases.

6. Feeding system problems. Failure to provide separate feeds and feeding systems so that groups of cows can be fed according to their needs may lead to over- or undernutrition.

7. Inadequate system and visibility for the detection, identification, and handling of cows in heat. This results in suboptimal reproductive performance.

8. Inadequate number of maternity box stalls for cows that are due to calve. Cows calving in well-bedded box stalls are less prone to traumatic injuries associated with slipping, falling, and recumbency due to parturient paresis. Calves born in clean, well-bedded box stalls have every opportunity to obtain liberal quantities of colostrum early in life.

9. Inadequate housing for newborn calves, which results in an increase in the incidence of infectious diseases such as pneumonia and enteritis.

10. Inefficient animal movement systems in the milking parlor, which result in overmilking and an increase in the incidence of mastitis.

11. Inadequate, inefficient and dangerous waste disposal systems. Manure gas poisoning may occur during emptying of manure pits, which may release large quantities of H_2S.

12. Lack of suitable animal holding and handling facilities for routine procedures and regular clinical examination by the veterinarian, i.e., pregnancy diagnosis, foot trimming, vaccination, artificial insemination.

13. Bedding. The availability and choice of suitable bedding material such as straw, wood shavings or sawdust, soil, or sand can be a problem. The bedding must be kept clean and dry. Modern manure disposal systems are based on handling only feces and urine (liquid slurry).

TYPES OF DAIRY HOUSING

The advancements in housing systems during the past 25 years have been described (Bickert and Light 1982). New concepts in barns, feeding systems, milking facilities, and manure handling have dramatically increased the productivity of dairy farm labor.

The dairy housing systems in use include the conventional individual stanchion or tie-stall barn, the free-stall, and the corral or the drylot system. For northern climates with long, cold winters, the stanchion or free-stall barns offer much in the way of ease of cow handling, mechanized manure removal, low-labor feeding if mechanized carts are used, and reasonably efficient milking, except that the milker must stoop to do the work. Stanchion barns are used extensively as housing and protection from inclement weather. During the winter months, the cows are confined inside throughout the day and night except for a brief period each day when the barn is cleaned and the cows are allowed outside for exercise and observation for heat. In the summer months, the cows are usually outside on pasture throughout the day and night and are brought in only for milking and feeding. In some situations, the cows are kept inside throughout the day during the summer and allowed outside during the night. This variation has increased milk production, improved heat detection, kept flies away from the cows, and improved the nutritional status. This suggests that improved control of the cows will result in improved performance.

Problems in stall barns include tying and untying cows; distribution of feed and bedding; difficulty in installing modern pipeline milking systems, which result in stable milking vacuum; stooping to milk; and the difficulty of detecting heat.

The loose-housing systems include the open-lot loafing shed and the free-stall variety. In the open-lot loafing shed system, the cows lounge and rest on a manure-straw pack and are fed in a feed bunk with or without feeding in the milking parlor. It is an inexpensive, labor-efficient system, but cows are usually dirty because they rest on manure packs.

The free-stall system is now a widely accepted development that offers fewer injuries to cows, lower bedding requirements, cleaner cows, and more concentrated housing in terms of square area of building or lot space per animal. The alleys between the rows of free stalls must be scraped of manure daily to prevent slippery floors and dirty cows. Fully slatted floors can be a major problem if the surfaces of the slats are abrasive or have sharp edges that traumatize the sole of the claw.

Other problems of free-stall housing include dimensions and design of the stall, which are critical in order to keep them clean and to minimize injury; difficulty of obtaining and handling comfortable bedding; and poor overall barn design, which does not permit easy flow of cow traffic and ease of cleaning alleyways (Harper 1983).

Observations of dairy cows housed in tie-stalls versus those in loose housing indicate that the incidence of disease and injury is lowest when the animals have soft bedding in the lying area and free access to open air. Closed cow barns with slatted floors or concrete floors with no bedding in the lying area result in a high incidence of disease and injury regardless of whether the animals are loose or tied (Ekesbo 1966).

There are marked differences in the behavior of cows housed in free stalls compared with conventional tie stalls. There is a marked increase in standing during estrus in free-stall cows. Older cows in free stalls rest several hours more per day than cows of a comparable age group in tie stalls (Pollock and Hurnik 1979). There is no difference between the two housing systems in their effect on ovarian function.

Changing from one housing system to another or increasing the size of the herd can affect milk production per cow (Norell and Appelman 1981). The loss of production is a function of the change in housing system and herd management during and immediately after expansion. Changing from stanchion to free-stall housing may result in a decrease of 200 kg. of milk per cow. Production may also decline following the introduction of a herd into a new barn.

The corral or drylot system is commonly used in hot southern climates where cows are not placed on pasture daily. The cows are totally confined throughout the year. Protection from heat is usually provided by some type of shade. The cows are fed in feed bunks and milked in milking parlors. The drylot area may be a well-drained ground surface or may be completely paved. Regular scraping of the earthen lots is necessary to remove manure build-up, and the paved lots may be flushed regularly. These drylots offer excellent confinement and handling facilities for large dairy herds in southern climates. Other characteristics of these large drylot operations might include centralized feed storage and processing, a controlled method of feeding, large amounts of lot space per cow, lock-up feeding mangers in which many cows can be locked by head gates for feeding or veterinary examination, treatment and hospital pens, good cow identification and location systems, smooth cow movement patterns, and efficient milking systems.

There are many different types of dairy housing systems. They are chosen for a variety of reasons, including climate, economics, management style, tradition, or other factors. It seems evident that there is no single best system. Just about anything will work if the farmer or manager wants it to work, and even the most well-planned system will be of little value if it is not operated properly. The system must be designed to provide as much control as is possible over what the cow does and what is done for her. The system must enable the farmer to feed, handle, observe, and protect the cows as efficiently as possible (Saloniemi 1980).

REQUIREMENTS AND CONSIDERATIONS FOR A DAIRY BARN THAT MAINTAINS A HIGH LEVEL OF HEALTH AND PRODUCTION

The basic requirements include the following:

1. *Thermal comfort.* It must not be too cold or too hot to interfere with production. Me-

chanical or natural ventilation should minimize condensation and chilling or heat stress.

2. *Physical comfort.* The lounging and feeding facilities should be comfortable and not cause traumatic injuries to the animals.

3. *Disease control.* The stocking density, feed and water system, and manure disposal system should be conducive to effective infectious disease control.

4. *Behavioral satisfaction.* Animals should be able to walk around, lie down, and perform their biological functions without significant restriction.

The following section will outline the housing and environmental factors that may affect the health and production of dairy cattle and the control measures that are available. Unfortunately, both basic and applied research into the diseases associated with housing and environment have lagged behind the rapid developments in dairy cattle housing that have occurred in the last 25 years. Consequently, many of the observations are not well documented, and the recommendations have not been field tested.

Behavior of Lactating Dairy Cows During Total Confinement

The behavior of dairy cattle has been reviewed (Arave and Albright 1981). The daily pattern of behavior and duration of various activities of confined cows appear similar to the pattern and duration of activities in field-grazed and partially confined cattle (Hedlund and Rolls 1977). The behavior of dairy cows during a 24-hour period may indicate the housing requirements. The total amount of time lying per 24 hours for cattle averages 11 hours (range 9 to 13 hours) on pasture, 11 to 11.5 hours for loose or free-stall housing, and 12 hours for stanchion stalls. Observations of dairy cows in total confinement reveal that during 15 hours of daytime, they spent an average of 45% of the time lying, 26% eating, and 22% ruminating, 1% drinking, and 2% socializing (Hedlund and Rolls 1977). Periods of eating, drinking, and social activity are most intense during and shortly after the morning and afternoon milking and feeding times. Conversely, periods of greatest recumbency, rumination, and rest occurred between feeding time from mid-day to late afternoon.

These observations indicate that cows spend about 50% of a 24-hour day lying down, which emphasizes the importance of comfortable stalls regardless of the system used. Cattle ruminate a total of four to nine hours per day in 15 to 20 periods, and 65 to 80% of this time is spent in the recumbent position. Active sleep occurs in the cow only when she is lying down.

Lactating dairy cattle are susceptible to a total change in environment (Hodges et al. 1978). Movement of a lactating herd from one environment to a totally different one, with changed methods of feeding, milking, and housing, can adversely affect milk yield and milk composition for several days following the change (Saloniemi and Nasi 1981).

Sufficient Space

A major problem in dairy herds during the housed period is the lack of sufficient space for each group of animals according to age and production. A dairy herd that raises all of its herd replacements requires space for the following groups (Martin 1973):

1. *Dry cows:* Should be housed and fed separate from the lactating cows.

2. *Calving cows:* Maternity box stalls for cows due to calve. The number depends on the size of the herd and the calving schedule. One box stall per 25 cows is desirable. Box stalls should have a sand or earthen floor and be well bedded with a deep straw pack. Cows that develop milk fever and the downer cow syndrome are more easily managed in well-bedded box stalls than in individual tie stalls, where secondary complications are common because the downer cow usually slips back into the gutter.

3. *Calves:* Individual stalls for newborn calves under one month of age. Group pens for calves over one month of age.

4. *Heifers:* Two months old through 12 months and 12 months old through 18 months.

5. *Mature heifers:* 18 months old to calving.

6. *Lactating cows:* May be grouped according to amount of production or stage of lactation.

Grouping Dairy Cows

During the past 25 years, the average size of dairy herds in North America and the United Kingdom has increased fourfold. Coincidental with increases in average herd size has been a trend toward housing cows in groups. Growth in herd sizes has created a need to alter conventional practices of reproductive management to increase efficiency of estrus detection, artificial insemination, cow handling, and record keeping. It has been necessary to develop management procedures to capitalize on increased income generated during a cow's lifetime when calving intervals are maintained at 12 months or less. Increased herd sizes also have resulted in increases in problems of herd health, at least partially potentiated by management practices adopted to cope with more cows per herd (Britt 1977).

Several practices in the management of dairy herds lend themselves to group management; the most obvious are feeding and reproductive management. Cows can be categorized into five reproductive classes as follows:

1. Early postpartum cows, prebreeding
2. Breeding group
3. Pregnant cows, lactating
4. Pregnant cows, nonlactating
5. Problem cows, open more than 100 days

Group management of reproduction can be compatible with group feeding, herd health, and milking management. Energy density of complete rations can be varied for high production (Group I), low production (Group II), or dry cows (Group III). Herd health programs can be concentrated on cows around calving and those in early lactation. Cows in early lactation are more likely to develop metabolic diseases, and preventive measures can be centered on cows in Groups I and III. Mastitis prevention and control is also compatible with grouping for reproduction, since cow-side detection tests can be more frequent in postpartum cows, and dry cow therapy can be administered as cows move into the dry group. Vaccinations may be recommended only for nonpregnant cows; thus, only certain cows in Group I may be subjected to these procedures. Reproductive group management also provides an opportunity to conduct other practices that may enhance cow performance. The provision of shade for cows housed outdoors in hot climates increases milk yield and conception rates.

A major practical problem in managing dairy cows in large groups is the accurate identification of each cow. Several methods are available, including neck chain tags, rubber ear tags, ankle tags, and freeze branding of the hair coat. The advantages and disadvantages of each have been reviewed (Hoover 1978). The use of an electronic system in which a central detector can identify electronic devices implanted in animals seems to be the next development.

Floor Surface

The floor surfaces in dairy barns include the old style wooden platforms in stanchion stalls, concrete floors in stanchion stalls, and solid concrete or slatted floors in alleyways. The ideal floor surface for dairy cows that are housed in total confinement for several months each year is unknown. Veterinarians and dairy producers feel that foot lesions in dairy cows are initiated by the constant daily contact of the feet with floor surfaces that are excessively rough, abrasive, and uneven. The edges of the slats of slatted floors may be sharp or rough and may be a source of traumatic injury.

Alleyways or lanes leading from the barn to the pasture may be poorly drained, may be continuously covered with wet manure, and may contain small stones, which may cause traumatic injury.

Severe traumatic injuries of the limbs can occur as a result of alleyway floors that are slippery because of an excessively smooth finish or because of the presence of a cover of urine, water, and manure.

Lameness in Dairy Cattle

Lameness in dairy cattle is a major cause of financial loss and inconvenience to dairy farmers and of pain and discomfort to cows. Next to mastitis and reproductive failure, lameness is an important cause of involuntary culling in dairy herds. One survey reveals that up to 6.48% of dairy cows may be culled for lameness (Russell et al. 1982).

Surveys of lameness in dairy cows reveal an average incidence ranging from 4.7 to 30%. A survey of the number of treatments for lameness in 21,000 dairy cows from 185 herds showed an average incidence of 25% (Whitaker et al. 1983). An annual incidence of up to 60% has been suggested if all treatments given by the farmer and the veterinarian are included (Eddy and Scott 1980). However, the national average is about 5% per annum.

There has been a notable lack of basic and applied research in lameness in cattle, and consequently there is a lack of reliable literature on the subject. One major problem has been the lack of a consistent nomenclature with which to describe the several different lesions of the feet of cattle. There is now some agreement for an international nomenclature on the diseases of the ruminant digit, which should improve the scientific communications on the subject (Weaver et al. 1981).

Lameness occurs in both pastured and housed dairy cattle but appears to be a greater problem in housed animals. In New Zealand, an incidence of 14% was reported in a study of four herds (Dewes 1978).

The epidemiologic features of lameness in dairy cattle include the following:

1. Approximately 85% of cases of lameness in

dairy cattle are due to lesions of the feet; 15% are due to lesions elsewhere on the limb.

2. Most foot lesions (80 to 85%) occur in the hind feet, and 85% affect the lateral claw. This may be associated with the design of stalls that force cows to stand with their hind feet in the gutter, which contains urine and manure, resulting in constant wetting of the feet.

3. Most cases of foot and leg lameness occur in mature cows from six to eight years of age. Young cows do not appear to be as susceptible.

4. Most cases of lameness occur in cows during the first three months of lactation, which has serious economic consequences. Lame cattle do not eat normally, they may not exhibit estrus normally, they lose weight, and they may develop metabolic disease. The greater occurrence of foot lameness during early lactation suggests that nutrition may predispose to the lesions, but there is no documented information to support the relationship. The feeding of large amounts of concentrate to support high milk production during the first six to eight weeks of lactation may predispose to laminitis and the development of foot lesions, but this is also not supported by critical field or experimental observations.

5. An assessment of the economic effects suggests that the average annual cost of a 100-cow herd is £1175 (approximately $1500 U.S. 1984).

6. The most common foot lesions causing lameness in dairy cows are foul-in-the-foot, white line disease, sole ulcer (Toussaint Raven 1973), punctured sole, and underrun heel (Russell et al. 1982). Interdigital papillomas may occur in epidemics in dairy cattle herds, involving up to 70% of animals (Rebhun 1982). Affected herds are confined in free-stall housing. The lesions are painful and cause severe lameness, weight loss, decreased milk production and difficulty in heat detection. The epidemiology suggests an infectious viral papillomatosis.

7. There may be a relationship between the season of the year and certain foot lesions. Rainfall may predispose cows to certain foot lesions because of constant wetting (Eddy and Scott 1980). The wet conditions of winter and the dry conditions of summer appear to be associated with lameness, although the types of lesions differ (Baggott and Russell 1981). In some surveys, sole ulcers of dairy cattle were more common during the summer months when cattle spent the most hours on pasture (St. Pierre et al. 1982).

8. Trauma is the major cause of leg lesions, of which the common ones are arthritis, tendonitis, peripheral nerve paralyses (peroneal and obturator), ischemic necrosis of muscle, and rupture of the gastrocnemius muscle and tendon.

9. There is a widespread hypothesis that traumatic injuries caused by continuous contact of the feet with certain floor surfaces or outside alleyways are a major factor predisposing to the variety of foot lesions in the dairy cow (Russell et al. 1982). However, there is no definitive information available on the cause and effect relationship between the ground surface and foot lesions in dairy cows. For example, the pathogenesis of sole ulcer in cattle is probably dependent on a wide range of factors, which remain unexplained (Martig 1983). In a study of lameness in four New Zealand herds, excessive wear of the soles was considered to be a common cause of lameness in two-year-old Friesian heifers (Dewes 1978). Lameness in older cattle frequently resulted from lesions in the interdigital spaces of soft tissue structures and usually occurred two to 12 weeks after calving. Excessive wear of the sole resulted when animals walked some distance in wet conditions and after abrasive materials had accumulated on concrete holding yards.

10. Lameness may be more common in certain heavy breeds such as the Holstein-Friesian than in lighter breeds like the Ayrshire, Guernsey, and Jersey. Some of these differences may be due to different growth and wear rates of hoof horn (Prentice 1973; Glicken and Kendrick 1977).

Control of Lameness in Dairy Cattle

The control of lameness in dairy cattle is largely empirical and based on field observations. The following guidelines are recommended:

1. *Floor surface texture:* The floor surfaces of the barn and the outside alleyways where cows either stand or walk for long periods must be nontraumatic.

2. *Sanitation:* Floor surfaces and alleyways must be cleaned as necessary to remove collections of urine, water, and manure, which contribute to constant wetting of the feet.

3. *Clinical examination:* All lame cows should be examined and treated as soon as possible. Isolation in a well-bedded hospital pen for several days may be necessary. A record of each lame cow and the diagnosis should be kept.

4. *Foot bath:* Foot baths containing formaldehyde or copper sulfate solution have often been advocated to control foot disease in cattle

(Davies 1982). However, the recommendations are empirical because no documented information exists on the effectiveness of foot baths for the control of diseases of the feet of cattle. Regular use of a foot bath should be encouraged in herds with a high incidence of interdigital disease, heel erosion, and solar ulceration. With a foot bath containing 1% formalin (1 part formalin:39 parts of water), the cows can be walked through the bath after each of four successive milkings; this is repeated weekly (Davies 1982). However, results have been variable, which may be due to the accumulation of excessive amounts of feces on the feet of the animals, thus rendering the solution ineffective. Another reason may be that the lesions are not caused primarily by infectious agents. It would appear logical that for maximum effect in problem herds, the feet of the animals should be cleaned with a pressurized spray of water before being walked through the foot bath.

Foot baths should be located in a passageway 1.0 to 1.2 m. wide on the return route from the milking parlor. It is useful to have two baths in series, the first containing water to wash the feet and reduce contamination of the astringent in a second bath. The specifications for a foot bath are: at least 300 cm. long; 100 cm. wide at the top; 60 cm. wide at the bottom, in order to reduce the amount of solution used; 30 cm. deep; sloping ends to permit emptying with a brush; nonslip surface; solution depth of 17 cm.; exit area sloping back to the bath to reduce the loss of solution. It should open onto a large clean area, to prevent immediate recontamination of feet with feces. Astringent chemical solutions of either 5% copper sulfate or 5% formalin should not be used more than twice a week, even for herds with very soft feet, and less frequently as the feet harden. The skin of the coronary band and the soft tissues of the claw should be monitored in representative cows for evidence of chemical injury.

5. *Regular foot trimming:* The feet of all cows should be examined and trimmed if necessary at least once annually. The claws of the hind feet of housed cattle should be examined and trimmed if necessary midway through the housing period. Under-running of the bulbar horn (erosio ungulae) and pododermatitis circumscripta (Rusterholz sole ulcer) are more common in housed cattle and can be controlled by preventive hoof trimming (Anderson and Lundstrom 1981). Commercial foot trimmers are now becoming popular. They will visit the farm with a hydraulic table

and foot trimming instruments and trim the feet of all cattle in the herd during one visit. Veterinarians can also supply this kind of service as part of a herd health program. However, some field trials indicate that routine foot trimming does not significantly reduce lameness (Arkins and Hannan 1982).

Stall Design

The length and width of stanchion stalls and free stalls are critical. Stalls that are too short for large cows are uncomfortable and can result in traumatic injuries such as lesions on the skin of the udder and legs (Nasi and Saloniemi 1981). When the stalls are too long, feces and urine are allowed to fall into them, and the cows become dirty. Specification guidelines for the design and measurements of free stalls are available (Light 1973). The incidence of traumatic injuries to the skin of the udder and legs may decrease following renovation and improvement of the design of the cow barn (Nasi and Saloniemi 1981). Teat injuries are more common in barns with short-standing stalls than in longer stalls (Koskiniemi 1982).

The number of free stalls recommended per cow usually is 1.1. However, this can be reduced by over 30% without loss of comfort or production (Friend et al. 1977).

Animal Handling

Ease of handling and moving animals from one part of the barn to another is important. Cows may be moved from one group to another according to production.

Bedding

Bedding materials used for dairy cattle include cereal grain straws, wood shavings and sawdust, fresh topsoil, and sand. Rubber mats without any bedding are also used in stanchion confinement stalls. In stanchion stalls with wooden or concrete floors, straw is most commonly used; occasionally rubber mats are used. In free-stall housing, fresh topsoil, sand, or straw is commonly used. Dairy cows in free stalls prefer compressible materials compared with carpets and rubber mats (Natzke et al. 1982). Fresh sawdust may be contaminated with *Klebsiella* sp., which is a potential cause of peracute mastitis (Newman and Kowalski 1973).

Feed Storage

The storage of feed is a major chore.

Feeding large amounts of high-quality forages supplemented with grain, protein, vitamins, and minerals is the basis of profitable milk production. The total yearly dry matter feed intake of a dairy cow is about nine tons, and feeding systems must be designed to store, process, and deliver this volume of material efficiently. The major objectives in the design of a feed storage and handling system are to maintain feed quality, to allow easy handling of feed materials, and to properly proportion the feed ingredients to meet the nutritional needs of cows and replacement animals.

Forages are the largest volume feed ingredient and are commonly grown on the farm. Forage storage structures should be selected based on the types and volumes of forages, initial cost, operating cost, ease of fitting into the handling system, and labor required for filling and emptying. In temperate climates, dry hay storage and silos are the main structures. Dry hay is usually stored under post or metal frame buildings to provide protection from precipitation. Upright oxygen-limiting and conventional concrete stave silos and horizontal pit silos are used for the storage of silage, haylage, or high-moisture grains. Proper management of these is necessary to minimize spoilage.

The major health concern with the storage of forages is spoilage and the development of molds, which may result in dicumarol poisoning in the case of sweet clover hay or silage. The preparation and storage of large amounts of sweet clover hay or silage with a minimum of spoilage by dicumarol-producing molds is a major unsolved problem. Every effort must be made to avoid spoilage.

Feeding Systems

The various feeding systems used in dairy herds were presented in the section on dairy cattle nutrition.

Linear feedbunk space requirements for dairy cattle have ranged from 0.67 to 0.76 m./cow. However, depending on the type of feed and the total time the animals have access to it, 0.2 m. in feedbunk space may be adequate. A reduction in the allocation of feedbunk space would make it possible to build smaller, cheaper housing or to convert existing buildings to accommodate more cows (Collis et al. 1980). A reduction in feedbunk space from 105 cm. per cow to 15 cm. per cow did not change the mean number of visits by the cow to the feedbunk, the amount of aggressive behavior, the milk yield, or the general activity of the cows (Collis et al. 1980). The development of complete dairy rations makes such renovations possible.

Water Supply

Adequate drinking water supplies should be available at all times. In stanchion stall systems, a water bowl is usually located in each stall. In loose-housing, free-stall and open corral systems, an adequate number of water bowls or tanks must be located near the feed bunks. The area around water tanks must be well drained to provide for water spillage.

The effect of a marked reduction in water intake by lactating dairy cows has been examined (Little et al. 1980). A restriction of 50% of voluntary water intake can reduce milk production by 50% and body weight by 14% after four days. The restricted cows behave aggressively around the water tank and spend less time lying down than cows with an unrestricted supply. When lactating dairy cows are allowed 90% of voluntary water intake, the effects are much smaller and difficult to detect. However, changes in behavior around the water tank are still noticeable.

Effects of Environmental Stress on Dairy Cattle

Environment directly and indirectly influences survival and productivity of dairy animals. The degree of environmental impact is modified by stage of life cycle and adaptation of given breeds and species. Environmental factors include direct effects of air temperature, humidity, wind speed, and solar radiation on animals. Indirect effects of feed quality and quantity also influence the effect of the environment. Dairy calves are relatively cold-sensitive at birth. Lactating dairy cows generally are more heat-sensitive and cold-resistant. The effects of heat stress on dairy cattle include a decreased birth weight of calves, lowered milk production, delayed involution of the uterus, and delayed onset of estrus (Collier et al. 1982).

The effects of age and physiological state on critical temperatures of dairy cattle are shown as follows (Collier et al. 1982):

	Critical Temperatures (°C)	
	Lower	Upper
Calf (4 L. milk/day)	13	26
Calf (50–200 kg., growing)	−5	26
Cow (dry and pregnant)	−14	25
Cow (peak lactation)	−25	25

Critical temperature is defined as the lowest or highest temperature at which an animal can maintain normal body temperature without altering basal metabolic rate.

There are several potential metabolic health problems and related interactions of heat stress and nutrition that might occur from physiological responses of dairy cattle to heat stress. Energy and nutritional deficits, respiratory alkalosis, ketosis, and ruminal acidosis are related to heat stress–induced alterations in nutrient metabolism and balance. Nutritional metabolic changes include alteration in (1) feed consumption and energy metabolism, (2) protein metabolism, (3) water balance, (4) metabolism of electrolytes and associated acid-base balance, and (5) endocrine status. Heat stress in dairy cattle will result in decreased feed intake, increased water intake, increased respiratory rate, and changes in electrolyte and acid-base balance (Collier et al. 1982).

As environmental heat load approximates body temperature, sensible avenues of heat loss (ie., radiation, conduction, and convection) are compromised, leaving only evaporative heat loss as the major route of heat dissipation in the cow. This leads to dramatic decreases in roughage intake and rumination. Decreases in roughage intake contribute to decreased volatile fatty acid production and may contribute to alteration in the ratio of acetate propionate. Rumen pH also declines during heat stress. Rumen water content increases, and osmotic pressure of rumen fluid declines during heat stress owing to increased water intake. Electrolyte concentrations, in particular sodium and potassium, also are reduced in rumen fluid of heat-stressed cattle. The decreases in sodium and potassium are related to increases in urinary sodium loss and skin potassium loss as well as a decline in plasma aldosterone and an increase in plasma prolactin. Increasing the concentration of potassium in the diet of heat-stressed cattle increased milk production and reduced plasma prolactin. The reduction in thyroxine, growth hormone, and glucocorticoid concentrations in chronically heat-stressed cattle appears to be related to decreases in basal metabolism during heat stress.

Heat stress also causes a measurable decrease in uterine blood flow, which is associated with decreased conception, reduced fetal growth in late pregnancy, and altered placental function. Alterations of conceptus function by heat stress during late pregnancy may have carryover effects into the postpartum period on milk yield and reproductive performance.

The effects of environment on the nutrient requirements of dairy cattle have been reviewed (National Research Council 1981). The feasibility both from the standpoint of economics and biological efficiency for supplying additional feed for higher maintenance needs of calves and heifers of dairy breeds under hot or cold conditions is not clear at this time. It seems that except under extreme circumstances for calves or heifers in later stages of pregnancy, added feed is not practical because compensatory gains in other periods will occur. In the lactating cow producing over 6000 kg. of milk per lactation, there may be an indication for adjustments in feeding during cold periods. If the kilogram of milk per megacalories of estimated net energy consumed exceeds 0.8, the offering of more feed will usually be profitable. This means it is practical to increase feeding when environmental temperature is below 0°C.

The effects of the stress of hot or cold conditions can be alleviated by environmental modifications such as ventilated and heated barns in the case of cold conditions and sun shades in the case of hot conditions. An additional alternative to more feed or housing is to change the genotype of the animal (Freeman 1975). The estimates for heritability of feed efficiency in dairy breeds range from 0.12 to 0.48, indicating that genetic progress could be made in selection for increased gross feed efficiency—a trait that is phenotypically and genotypically related to the traits of milk yield and feed intake.

Barn Environment

Structures to alter the environment for lactating cows have ranged from fully insulated, mechanically ventilated and, sometimes, heated buildings in cold areas to simple sun shades and windbreaks in warmer areas. Buildings that covered the resting and feeding areas of loose housing systems usually had at least one side open. Winter moisture control in those facilities was marginal, but problems from excess moisture were minimized by the open side, and cows had access to outside lots.

With the advent of free-stall housing with total confinement and decreased building area per animal, the needs for moisture and temperature control changed. One solution was warm free-stall housing—insulated structures with mechanical ventilation in which warm environments similar to those in properly ventilated and insulated barns were maintained.

Mature dairy cows can thrive, produce, and reproduce well in a remarkably wide range of temperatures. Low temperatures stimulate appetite, resulting in increased feed consumption to offset the increased animal heat losses. Cold weather has a limited impact on the milk production of dairy cows (Hahn 1981). For cows that receive adequate diets, the milk production declines 0.25 kg./cow for each 10°C below 5°C. The estimated increased daily feed requirement (to offset reduced feed digestibility and increased heat loss in cold weather) is equivalent to 1 kg. hay/10°C decline in temperature below 5°C. High humidity with cold can be detrimental to productivity because of its association with fogging and condensation, thereby reducing the insulating value of the cow's hair coat. In the colder areas of North America, mature dairy cows may be kept in totally enclosed barns in which mechanical ventilation is necessary and supplemental heat may or may not be necessary, depending on the degree of ventilation heat deficit. In very cold climates, complete success with a controlled environment system requires substantial supplemental heat to control humidity. In less cold areas, a modified environment (almost-closed barns) system has evolved and is successful (Turnbull 1973). In cold climates, properly designed and managed natural ventilation systems can be used instead of mechanical sytems to provide a very satisfactory thermal environment for dairy cattle. In cold weather, the amount of insulation and proper ventilation management are primary factors in providing desirable barn conditions (Kammel et al. 1982). Natural ventilation systems will save about 25 kwhr. of electricity per cow per month. Control over inlet and outlet areas on insulated buildings with a sufficient animal population allows the farmer to maintain temperature far above outside winter conditions and still allow a large enough air flow to remove excess moisture. During summer conditions, large open inlet and outlet areas allow large air flows across the building, providing greater animal comfort than outside.

Specific diseases of the respiratory tract, like infectious bovine rhinotracheitis, do occur sporadically in housed dairy cows, and outbreaks may be associated with a breakdown in ventilation. However, endemic respiratory disease is not a problem in housed dairy cows as it is in housed dairy calves, which are highly susceptible to enzootic calf pneumonia associated with inadequate ventilation, high humidity, dampness, and inadequate nutrition.

Heat Stress

Heat stress may decrease milk production in dairy cattle by as much as 25% (Barth 1982). The prevention of severe heat stress is one of the most significant modifications of the external environment that can be made to maintain reproductive performance in dairy cattle. The provision of shade, spray cooling, evaporative cooling, and other low-cost alternatives in common use are strongly recommended to protect breeding females from thermal stress. This protection should guard the female against temperatures exceeding approximately 30°C for any sustained period of days, beginning with the estrus cycle prior to breeding and extending through gestation to parturition (Stott et al. 1972). The performance of lactating dairy cattle is significantly improved during the hot summer in the southwestern United States by providing an evaporatively cooled shade to lower the ambient temperature by 10 to 12°C. Not only is milk production improved during the hot weather but the entire lactation is affected, with an increase in production over herdmates of 550 kg. of milk. The cooling increases feed intake and decreases postpartum body weight loss. The fertility rate is markedly improved in animals that are made comfortable during hot summer months (Stott and Wiersma 1974).

High temperature and humidity will not affect the production of milk if high-quality grass is being grazed (Dragovich 1979).

Corral Systems

In countries where freezing temperatures and snow are not problems, loose-housing systems usually are based on outside corrals or lots. In areas with excessive rainfall, a covered free-stall area, an exposed concrete feed alley or lot, and a feed bunk—with or without a cover—are common. A dirt outside lot is provided for exercise. In areas where rain is not a problem, outside dirt lots—sloped for drainage—with feed bunks along one end or the side are popular. Sun shades are provided to reduce heat stress. In certain cases, evaporative coolers are incorporated into shade structures to further reduce heat stress during hot weather. The number of cows per corral pen varies from 25 to 125, depending on the number of cows that can be put through the milking parlor. Cows should not be required to stand in the holding area for more than one hour per milking.

Veterinary Handling Facilities

Confining cows in free-stall and open drylot systems for diagnosis, breeding, and treatment requires considerable time. In large herds of 100 or more milking cows, the chores associated with the hospital area occupy a large segment of time. Since the demand to use these facilities can occur any time of the day or night, they must be conveniently located and easy to use. In free-stall or loose housing, these procedures are particularly difficult because an animal is not confined to a particular stall. The milking parlor is commonly used for the monthly herd health examination of cows but is not ideal. Cows may be reluctant to enter the parlor at nonmilking times, the parlor design may be undesirable for rectal examination of cows, and large quantities of manure accumulate during the examination of many cows. An ideal situation would include a hospital area consisting of box stalls for cows undergoing daily medical or surgical treatment and an area separate from the milking parlor for the examination of cows. On the day of the herd health visit, cows to be examined are identified and sorted out into a holding area as they leave the parlor. A chute system connected to the holding pen allows the movement of cows into a raceway and into an individual animal holding stanchion with easy access on all four sides for a detailed clinical examination if necessary.

Calf Housing

Infectious diseases of the respiratory tract are a major cause of economic loss in housed dairy calves, particularly during the winter months in the northern climates (Roe 1982). The economic losses are due to mortality and unthriftiness caused by acute and chronic enzootic calf pneumonia. Commonly observed epidemiologic determinants are crowded calf pens, inadequate ventilation, high relative humidity and dampness, and calves that are not well managed and fed. Often the calves are raised in close proximity to the adult cows, which promotes the spread of infection. Calves are often born in the same building that houses the milking herd, and the nonimmune calf is immediately exposed to viruses and bacteria that may be shed by older animals that may be immune carriers.

The important management principles for improved calf health include calf housing isolated from the adult herd, periodic depopulation of the calf barn or pens, sanitizing the calf nursery area, and, where weather permits, the use of low-cost calf-rearing portables such as the "calf hutch" (Turnbull 1980).

In the ideal situation, the calves are reared in a calf barn or area completely detached or separate from the main adult cow barn. The calves are born in a well-bedded calving box stall and are force-fed liberal amounts of colostrum within two hours after birth and left with the cow for two days. Following this, the calves are transferred to individual stalls where they remain until weaning, when they are mixed into groups. The ventilation needs can be calculated based on the outside ambient temperatures, the total volume of the calf barn, and the insulation values of the walls and ceilings. During the winter months, four air changes per hour are required; during the summer, 20 are recommended (Bates and Anderson 1979). During the winter months, supplemental heat is necessary to maintain the relative humidity at about 70% and the inside temperature at 40 to 50°F (7 to 10°C) (Anderson et al. 1978; Anderson and Bates 1979). In situations where calves are raised in the same building as older animals, the flow of air should always be from the younger toward the older animals (Anderson and Bates 1982a, 1982b). To conserve heat supplied by the animals or supplemental heat, it is imperative to remove winter exhaust air from near the floor. Air near the floor is six to 10 degrees cooler than air near the ceiling, so exhausting air from the lower level removes less heat but removes essentially the same amount of moisture. To accomplish this, a duct extending to within 15 inches of the floor is used around the continuous fan.

Ventilation for animal health is more than a thermodynamic process for moisture and temperature control. An essential but often overlooked function is dilution of aerosol contaminants. For dilution there should be a minimum continuous air exchange at the rate of four changes per hour and a spatial volume of five to seven cubic meters per animal. The rate of aerosol generation is more relative to the health of the calves than the number housed. One sick calf can produce many more pathogenic organisms than a large number that are healthy. Thus, recirculation of the air within the structure is undesirable. A volumetric air exchange to dilute aerosol contamination, independent of the number of animals occupying the structure, is essential.

The quality of air in a calf house is critical in the control of respiratory disease (Pritchard 1981). The installation of recirculating air filter units will result in a marked reduction in the concentration of airborne bacteria and a subsequent decrease in the incidence and severity of clinical and subclinical respiratory disease (Pritchard 1981). Marked changes occur in the concentration of airborne bacteria in a calf house following changes in the outside temperature and humidity (Jones and Webster 1981), and an air filter may be a very effective method of control.

Periodic Depopulation

The practice of periodic depopulation, cleaning, and disinfection, followed by leaving the area empty for a few days, is an effective method for the control of the common infectious diseases, especially of calves. As the occupation time increases—that is, over several weeks or a few months—without a clean-out, the contamination and infection rate increase. Calf barns in particular should be depopulated, cleaned, and disinfected at least twice yearly. It assumes even greater importance if infectious disease has been a problem in a particular group of calves.

Manure Storage and Disposal, and Sanitation in Dairy Barns

The efficient and economical production of clean milk requires clean cows, a clean milking parlor, and clean milkers. The cleanliness of cows' udders and flanks is an important factor in clean and efficient milk production. Dairy cows confined for several months of the year may become dirty unless the housing system operates efficiently to keep them clean. As herd size increases and more cows are confined, manure accumulation and disposal become major problems. A variety of systems of manure disposal have been developed, including elaborate systems that automatically wash the ventral body wall and udder of cows prior to entry into the milking parlor. Thus, cleanliness of cows is of prime importance.

A highly efficient, easily cleaned milking parlor is essential. Drainage systems must be excellent, supply of water must be adequate, and the milkers must enjoy their chores in the parlor.

The main concerns in waste disposal systems in dairy herds are as follows:

1. The ecological concern is to ensure that there is no pollution of surface and ground waters.

2. The manure handling system must be economical, labor-efficient, and safe for both man and animals.

3. Odor must be minimized. Manure gas poisoning must be prevented.

4. The manure must be handled in such a way as to control fly population.

5. The bedding used must not contribute to disease problems such as mastitis caused by sawdust contaminated with *Klebsiella* spp.

6. The manure handling system must be effective, in order to prevent slippery floors and keep cows clean. A high degree of animal cleanliness must be maintained.

7. There are certain health hazards associated with the handling of animal wastes. The handling of feces and urine as a liquid slurry (without bedding) that is spread on arable land or pasture may result in the spread of diseases such as salmonellosis, Johne's disease, leptospirosis, anthrax, and protozoal and helminth infections (Jones 1979). Salmonellae may be found in low numbers in slurries, but 90% die during the first two to four weeks when the material is stored and survive on grass for short periods only. The danger of disseminating salmonellosis by the use of a slurry system can be significantly reduced if the slurry is stored for at least one month before spreading on pasture and if pasture treated with stored slurry is not grazed for a similar period after spreading (Jones 1979).

Manure Handling Systems

There are several different dairy waste management systems (Forster 1980). The benefits and costs of alternative waste disposal systems are important determinants in selecting a dairy waste management system. There are at least five basic housing and waste handling systems: (1) confined free stall; (2) confinement stall; (3) free-stall open lot; (4) large-scale systems using year-round pasture or open lots with shade; and (5) large-scale systems using confined free stall with flushing. The first three basic systems are typical in cooler and humid regions. The last two are found in warmer and more arid regions.

In the confined free stall, the manure collects in the alleyways and must be scraped and spread daily. Only limited storage is available for those days when access to fields is limited. Excessive accumulation will result in slippery floors, dirty cows, unsanitary conditions, and the necessity for extra washing of cows at milking time. Free-stall systems with slotted-floor alleyways allow the waste to collect in storage pits, which are emptied as necessary.

Confinement stall systems usually have a gutter cleaner to collect and transport the waste to a spreader or storage pile. Stacking manure immediately outside the barn causes run-off and fly problems.

Free-stall open lot systems allow cows to move between the free-stall area and outside paved lot. Tractor scraping removes waste from the free-stall area and the lot. A system of collecting run-off is necessary, and may include a settling basin, a detention pond, and an irrigation system.

Unpaved open lots are large-scale systems found primarily in hot humid regions. Manure is scraped from the lot and stockpiled or transported directly to cropland. Run-off control is needed when rainstorms occur.

In the year-round pasture system, cattle are grazed on pasture but brought into a center for milking. The milking center is flushed, and the waste water is irrigated on surrounding pasture.

The confined free-stall waste-water irrigation system is common in large herds. Large volumes of water are sluiced along the alleyways, carrying waste off the lot. Some systems have solid/liquid separation devices at the end of the sluicing operation wherein solids are screened out for other uses such as bedding; the liquid portion is irrigated on crop land. In some cases, the liquid is diverted to a lagoon for further clarification, and the lagoon is used as a source of flush water (Yeck 1981).

Manure collected and stored in pits or tanks must usually be agitated prior to emptying. In addition to the manure (feces and urine), a pit will sometimes contain dirt, sand, straw, sawdust, and feed spilled onto the floor from feed bunks. The contents of the pit have various densities, resulting in some sedimentation and separation. Agitation is required to break up clumps, to get the settled-out solids into suspension for complete removal of solids, and to create a homogeneous slurry that can be handled by the pump, tank spreaders, and possibly an injector. During emptying of storage pits, manure gas—the result of anaerobic oxidation—may be released. Hydrogen sulfide is particularly toxic at certain levels and can kill people and animals in less than a few minutes.

An adequate force of mechanical ventilation is necessary from the level of the pit to remove these toxic gases.

Public pressure and regulatory requirements are placing demands on dairy operators to control barnyard run-off resulting from rainstorms and snow meet. Run-off can transport considerable solids and nutrients and can pollute the rivers, streams, and lakes it enters. Large herds and confined open-lot feeding of cattle have added to the seriousness of the situation, and control measures are needed. Systems for controlling run-off include a solids settling area, a porous dam, a detention pond for the liquids, and a disposal area.

The economics of dairy waste management systems have been examined, and some generalizations are apparent (Forster 1980). Waste management systems vary substantially with size. There are remarkable economies of size. The larger the herd, the less the cost of waste management, which can be considerable per cow per year. Confined dairy systems have higher waste management costs than open-lot systems. Storage of waste does not pay unless the waste is incorporated into the field by injection or plowdown.

Review Literature

Albright, J.L. and Allison, G.W. Effect of varying the environment upon the performance of dairy cattle. J. Anim. Sci., 32:566–577, 1971.

American Society of Agricultural Engineers. National Dairy Housing Conference. The Kellog Center for Continuing Education. Michigan State University. East Lansing, Michigan. Feb. 6–8, 1973, pp. 1–409.

American Society of Agricultural Engineers. Livestock Environment II. Proc. 2nd Int. Livestock Environ. Symp., Apr. 20–23, 1982, pp. 1–624.

American Society of Agricultural Engineers. Second National Dairy Housing Conference. Madison, Wis., Mar. 14–16, 1983.

Bickert, W.G. and Light, R.G. Housing systems. J. Dairy Sci., 65:502–508, 1982.

Cement and Concrete Association. Animal housing injuries due to floor surfaces. Proc. Symp. Cement and Concrete Assoc., Fulmer Grange, Sloughs, Berks, England, November 1978, pp. 1–177.

Clark, J.A. (Ed.). Environmental aspects of housing for animal production. Proc. 31st Nottingham Easter School in Agricultural Science. London, Butterworths, 1981.

Collier, R.J., Beede, D.K., Thatcher, W.W. et al. Influences of environment and its modification of dairy animal health and production. J. Dairy Sci., 65:2213–2227, 1982.

Hahn, G.L. Housing and management to reduce climatic impacts on livestock. J. Anim. Sci., 52:175–186, 1981.

Harry, E.G. Air pollution in farm buildings and methods of control. A review. Avian Pathol., 7:441–454, 1978.

Hoglund, C.R. and Albright, J.L. Economics of housing dairy cattle. A review. J. Dairy Sci., 53:1549–1559, 1970.

Kelly, M. Good dairy housing design—a form of preventive medicine? Vet. Rec., 113:582–586, 1983.

National Research Council. Effect of Environment on Nutrient Requirements of Domestic Animals. National Academy Press, Washington, D.C., 1981.

Nott, S.N., Kaufmann, D.E. and Speicher, J.A. Trends in the management of dairy farms since 1956. J. Dairy Sci., 64:1330–1343, 1981.

Roe, C.P. A review of the environmental factors influencing calf respiratory disease. Agric. Meteorol., 26: 127–144, 1982.

Sainsbury, D. and Sainsbury, P. Livestock health and housing. London, Baillière Tindall, 1979.

Turnbull, J.E. Housing and environment for dairy calves. Can. Vet. J., 21:85–90, 1980.

Wathes, C.M., Jones, C.D.R. and Webster, A.J.F. Ventilation, air hygiene and animal health. Vet. Rec., 113: 554–559, 1983.

Weaver, A.D., Anderson, L., DeLaistre Banting, A. et al. Review of disorders of the ruminant digit with proposal for anatomical and pathological terminology and recording. Vet. Rec., 108:117–120, 1981.

References

Anderson, J.F. and Bates, D.W. Influence of improved ventilation on health of confined cattle. J. Am. Vet. Med. Assoc., 174:577–580, 1979.

Anderson, J.F. and Bates, D.W. Interaction of environment and genetics. In: Livestock Environment II. Proc. 2nd Int. Livestock Environ. Symp., Apr. 20–23, 1982a, pp. 298–302.

Anderson, J.F. and Bates, D.W. Livestock environment perspectives for the 1980's—Veterinary medicine. In: Livestock Environment II. Proc. 2nd Int. Livestock Environ. Symp., Apr. 20–23, 1982b, pp. 601–604.

Anderson, L. and Lundstrom, K. The influence of breed, age, body weight and season on digital diseases and hoof size in dairy cows. Zbl. Vet. Med. A., 28:141–151, 1981.

Anderson, J.F., Bates, D.W. and Jordan, K.A. Medical and engineering factors relating to calf health as influenced by the environment. Trans. Am. Soc. Agric. Engin., 21:1169–1174, 1978.

Arave, C.W. and Albright, J.L. Cattle behavior. J. Dairy Sci., 64:1318–1329, 1981.

Arkins, S. Lameness in dairy cows. Irish Vet. J., 35:135–140, 1981.

Arkins, S. and Hannan, J. Studies on the prevention of digital diseases in Irish dairy cows. Proc. XII World Cong. Dis. Cattle, Netherlands, Sept. 7–10, 1982, Vol. II, pp. 801–804.

Baggott, D.G. and Russell, A.M. Lameness in cattle. Br. Vet. J., 137:112–132, 1981.

Bakken, G. A Survey of environment and management in Norwegian dairy herds with reference to udder diseases. Acta Agric. Scand., 31:49–69, 1981.

Barth, C.L. State-of-the-art for summer cooling for dairy cows. In: Livestock Environment II. Proc. 2nd Int. Livestock Environ. Symp., Apr. 20–23, 1982, pp. 52–61.

Bates, D.W. and Anderson, J.F. Calculation of ventilation needs for confined cattle. J. Am. Vet. Med. Assoc., 174:581–589, 1979.

Bickert, G.W. and Light, R.G. Housing systems. J. Dairy Sci., 65:502–508, 1982.

Blom, J.Y. Traumatic injuries and disease in dairy cows in different housing systems. In: Livestock Environment II. Proc. 2nd Int. Livestock Environ. Symp., Apr. 20–23, 1982, pp. 438–443.

Britt, J.H. Strategies for managing reproduction and controlling health problems in groups of cows. J. Dairy Sci., 60:1345–1353, 1977.

Collier, R.J., Beede, D.K., Thatcher, W.W. et al. Influences of environment and its modification on dairy animal health and production. J. Dairy Sci., 65:2213–2227, 1982.

Collis, K.A., Vagg, M.J., Gleed, P.T. et al. The effects of reducing manger space on dairy cow behavior and production. Vet. Rec., 107:197–198, 1980.

Davies, R.C. Effects of regular formalin footbaths on the incidence of foot lameness in dairy cattle. Vet. Rec., 111:394, 1982.

Dewes, H.F. Some aspects of lameness in dairy herds. N.Z. Vet. J., 26:147, 148, 157–159, 1978.

Dragovich, D. Effect of high temperature humidity conditions on milk production of dairy herds grazed on farms in pasture-based feeding system. Int. J. Biometeor., 23:15–20, 1979.

Eddy, R.G. and Scott, C.P. Some observations of the incidence of lameness in dairy cattle in Somerset. Vet. Rec., 106:140–144, 1980.

Ekesbo, I. Disease incidence in tied and loose housed dairy cattle. Acta Agric. Scand., Suppl. 15, 1966, pp. 1–74.

Forster, D.L. Economic comparisons of alternative waste management systems for swine and dairy cattle. J. Anim. Sci., 50:360–366, 1980.

Freeman, A.E. Genetic variation in nutrition of dairy cattle. In: The Effect of Genetic Variance on Nutritional Requirements of Animals. National Academy of Sciences. Washington, D.C., 1975, pp. 19–46.

Friend, T.H., Polan, C.E. and McGilliard, M.L. Free stall and feed bunk requirements relative to behavior, production and individual feed intake in dairy cows. J. Dairy Sci., 60:108–116, 1977

Gjestang, K.E. The effects of environmental factors, floor design and materials on foot and limb disorders in dairy cattle. In: Animal Housing Injuries Due to Floor Surfaces. Proc. Symp. Cement and Concrete Assoc., Fulmer Grange, Sloughs, Berks, England, November 1978, pp. 79–87.

Gjestang, K.E. Feeding table geometry in relation to dairy cow comfort. In: Livestock Environment II. Proc. 2nd Int. Livestock Environ. Symp., Apr. 20–23, 1982, pp. 433–437.

Glicken, A. and Kendrick, J.W. Hoof overgrowth in Holstein-Friesian dairy cattle. J. Hered., 68:386–390, 1977.

Hahn, G.L. Housing and management to reduce climatic impacts on livestock. J. Anim. Sci., 52:175–186, 1981.

Harper, A.D. Cow cubicles—20 years on. Report on a conference held at NAC, Stoneleigh, Feb. 1983. Farm Building Progress No. 72, pp. 5–9, 1983.

Hazen, T.E. Criteria needed to design animal quarters for comfort and productivity. J. Anim. Sci., 32:584–589, 1971.

Hedlund, L. and Rolls, J. Behavior of lactating dairy cows during total confinement. J. Dairy Sci., 50:1807–1812, 1977.

Hodges, J., Hiley, P.G. and Froese, J. Effects of total environment change on milk production. Can. J. Anim. Sci., 58:631–637, 1978.

Hoglund, C.R. and Albright, J.L. Economics of housing dairy cattle. A review. J. Dairy Sci., 53:1549–1559, 1970.

Hoover, N.W. Cow identification and recording systems. J. Dairy Sci., 61:1167–1180, 1978.

Jones, C.R. and Webster, A.J.F. Weather induced changes in airborne bacteria within a calf house. Vet. Rec., 109: 493–494, 1981.

Jones, P.W. Health hazards associated with the handling of animal wastes. Vet. Rec., 106:4–7, 1979.

Kammel, D.W., Cramer, C.O., Converse, J.C. et al. Thermal environment of insulated, naturally ventilated dairy barns. In: Livestock Environment II. Proc. 2nd Int. Livestock Environ. Symp., Apr. 20–23, 1982, pp. 62–71.

Koskiniemi, K. Observations on the incidence of teat injuries in different cowsheds. Nord. Vet. Med., 34:13–19, 1982.

Light, R.G. Engineered management for free stall systems. National Dairy Housing Conference, Feb. 6–8, 1973, pp. 82–91.

Little, W., Collis, K.A., Gleed, P.T. et al. Effect of reduced water intake by lactating dairy cows on behavior, milk yield and blood composition. Vet. Rec., 106:547–551, 1980.

Martig, J., Levenberger, W.P., Tschudi, P. et al. Causes of specific traumatic sole ulcerations in the cow. Zent. fur Vet. Med. A., 30:214–222, 1983.

Martin, R.O. Design and operations of a complete herd replacement facility. National Dairy Housing Conference, Feb. 6–8, 1973, pp. 321–335.

Martin, R.O. Dairy housing environment in northern climates for the 1980's. Livestock Environment II. Proc. 2nd Int. Livestock Environ. Symp., Apr. 20–23, 1982, pp. 605–613.

Nasi, M. and Saloniemi, H. Effect of environment change on injuries of udder and legs in dairy cows. Nord. Vet. Med., 33:185–193, 1981.

Natzke, R.P., Bray, D.R. and Everett, R.W. Cow preference for free stall surface material. J. Dairy Sci., 65: 146–153, 1982.

Newman, L.E. and Kowalski, J.J. Fresh sawdust bedding— A possible source of Klebsiella organisms. Am. J. Vet. Res., 34:979–980, 1973.

Norell, R.J. and Appelman, R.D. Change of milk production with housing system and herd expansion. J. Dairy Sci., 64:1749–55, 1981.

Nott, S.B., Kaufmann, D.E. and Speicher, J.A. Trends in the management of dairy farms since 1956. J. Dairy Sci., 64:1330–43, 1981.

Pollock, W.E. and Hurnik, J.R. Effect of two confinement systems on estrous and diestrous behaviour in dairy cows. Can. J. Anim. Sci., 59:799–803, 1979.

Prentice, D.E. Growth and wear rates of hoof horn in Ayrshire cattle. Res. Vet. Sci., 14: 285–290, 1973.

Pritchard, D.G., Carpenter, C.A., Morzaria, S.P. et al. Effect of air filtration on respiratory disease in intensively housed veal calves. Vet. Rec., 109:5–9, 1981.

Rebhun, W.C. Interdigital papillomatosis in dairy cattle. Proc. XII World Cong. Dis. of Cattle, Netherlands, Vol. II, 1982, pp. 833–837.

Roe, C.P. A review of the environmental factors influencing calf respiratory disease. Agric. Meteorol., 26:127–144, 1982.

Russell, A.M., Rowlands, G.J., Shaw, S.R. et al. Survey of lameness in British dairy cattle. Vet. Rec., 111:155–160, 1982.

St. Pierre, H., Baril, J., Bouvier, D. et al. Incidence au Quebec des diverses affections du pied chez la vache laitiere. Proc. XII World Cong. Dis. of Cattle, Netherlands, Vol. II, 1982, pp. 833–837.

Saloniemi, H. Udder diseases in dairy cows—Field observations in incidence, somatic and environmental factors, and control. J. Sci. Agric. Soc. Finland, 52:85–184, 1980.

Saloniemi, H. and Nasi, M. Effects of environmental change on udder health of dairy cows. Nord. Vet. Med., 33:178–184, 1981.

Stott, G.H. and Wiersma, F. Response of dairy cattle to an evaporative cooled environment. In: Proc. 1st Int. Livestock Environ. Symp., 1974, pp. 88–95.

Stott, G.H., Wiersma, F. and Woods, J.H. Reproductive health program for cattle subjected to high environmental temperature. J. Am. Vet. Med. Assoc., 161: 1339–1344, 1972.

Toussaint Raven, E. Lameness in cattle and foot care. Neth. J. Vet. Sci., 5:105–111, 1973.

Turnbull, J.E. Environmental requirements for mature dairy cows. National Dairy Housing Conference. Amer. Soc. Agric. Engin., 1973, pp. 142–153.

Turnbull, J.E. Housing and environment for dairy calves. Can. Vet. J., 21:85–90, 1980.

Weaver, A.D., Andersson, L., DeLaistre Banting, A. et al. Review of disorders of the ruminant digit with proposals for anatomical and pathological terminology and recording. Vet. Rec., 108:117–180, 1981.

Whitaker, D.A., Kelly, J.M. and Smith, E.J. Incidence of lameness in dairy cows. Vet. Rec., 113:60–62, 1983.

Yeck, R.G. Managing dairy wastes. J. Dairy Sci., 64:1358–1364, 1981.

Veterinary Aspects of Dairy Cattle Genetics, Breeding Programs, and Culling Practices

8

The major objective of a progressive breeding program in a dairy herd is to select superior sires and cows that will result in daughters producing high levels of milk economically. The identification and culling of cows with low milk yield is an important component of a breeding program in which genetic progress is being made.

Veterinarians have traditionally not been involved in decisions regarding the selection of sires and the evaluation of cows in dairy herds. However, they frequently make recommendations about the disposal of dairy cows that are affected with incurable infertility, mastitis, lameness, and other chronic illnesses. As part of a totally integrated dairy herd health system, veterinarians who take an interest in dairy cattle production can provide some useful advice on genetics, breeding programs, and culling practices. The fact that milk yield is dependent on both the genetic potential of the cow and the environmental effects makes it important that the veterinarian become acquainted with the breeding programs as well as the environmental factors.

Breeding programs should be relatively simple, particularly for large herds. Selection goals should stress traits that are directly related to or indirectly associated with economic returns to the dairyman. Major selection emphasis should be on milk and fat, using artificial insemination (AI) progeny-tested sires. Selection for conformation traits is also practiced if such traits are limiting or making production less efficient.

GENETIC INDICES USED IN SELECTION OF DAIRY COWS AND SIRES

The sire and dam contribute equally to the genetic makeup of each progeny. However, the sire has a much greater influence on the genetic merit of a herd because of the number of offspring he may have and the accuracy with which his true genetic merit can be predicted. With AI, the sire can be selected from among the outstanding sires in the entire country, whereas the cows selected must constitute the majority of those in a single herd (Stout 1983a).

To assure that superior herd replacements are purchased or that the best replacement heifers are developed, dairymen must have the knowledge and understanding of genetic measurements or indices available for evaluation of sires and cows.

In the last 25 years, the field of dairy cattle genetics has been tremendously productive. Genetic parameters have been established for most economically important traits, genetic evaluation of sires and dams has become a highly sophisticated and accurate science, availability of genetically superior breeding stock is widespread, selection index procedures for estimating pedigree value and trait combination scores have received wide acceptance and use, and the rate of genetic advance for economically important traits has accelerated (White et al. 1981) (Table 8-1).

Artificial insemination has been the focal point of genetic improvement of dairy cattle. The widespread use of bulls for the process of AI in many dairy herds has enabled development of an accurate evaluation system as a basis of selection of sires for use in the next generation (Miller 1981). Milk production of the average cow in the United States has more than doubled since the first AI organization began operation in 1938.

Evaluation of Sires

Measurements used in sire evaluation include Pedigree Index for young untested bulls and Predicted Differences (PD) for Milk, Fat, Dollars, and Type for bulls with daughter information (Stout 1983a). Repeatability, a measure of the reliability of the estimate of the transmitting ability of PD, is also used in selection.

Predicted Difference. The evaluation of a sire's performance is based on the performance of his daughters. The United States Department of Agriculture (USDA) provides estimates of genetic transmitting ability of dairy sires in the form of Predicted Differences for Milk, Fat, Dollars, and Type. The practical use of these indices is reviewed (Stout 1983a).

Repeatability. Repeatability (R) is a measure of the reliability of the estimate of the transmitting ability of PD. The repeatability of a sire's summary varies in magnitude, depending on the number of daughters, number of herds, distribution of daughters across herds, records per daughter, days in milk of records in progress, number of herdmates, and number of average R of sires of herdmates.

The addition of more daughters in one herd increases the R very little. The additional representation of more herds in the sire's summary results in a greater increase in R. This should be expected because more dairymen are involved, as are more feeding programs, milking systems, facilities, types of management, and sets of herdmates. Sire summary R will vary from 15 to 99%. At low levels there is some indication of the sire's true transmitting ability, whereas at the higher levels there is reasonable certainty that the summary has accurately evaluated the sire. Most AI centers will sufficiently sample a bull so that his early proof will have R values of 50% or higher.

Table 8-1. REPEATABILITY AND HERITABILITY OF YIELD AND COMPOSITION TRAITS

	Repeatability	Heritability
YIELDS		
Milk	0.50	0.25
Fat	0.50	0.25
Protein	0.55	0.20
Solids (not fat)	0.50	0.20
Total solids	0.50	0.20
Lactose and minerals	0.45	0.20
PERCENTAGES AND RATIOS		
Fat	0.75	0.50
Protein	0.70	0.40
Solids (not fat)	0.60	0.50
Total solids	0.75	0.55
Protein and fat	0.65	0.50

From White, J.M., Vinson, W.E. and Pearson, R.E. Dairy cattle improvement and genetics. J. Dairy Sci., 64:1305–1317, 1981.

Evaluation of Cows

Cows are evaluated on the basis of their own record, Pedigree Index, Estimated Producing Ability, and Estimated Average Transmitting Ability. Young animals are evaluated by Pedigree Index or Pedigree Estimate of Breeding Value (Stout 1983a). Breed associations also classify cows according to type.

To properly evaluate the producing ability of the cow, her performance record is adjusted according to the nongenetic factors that affect her production. These include the age of the cow, number of times milked per day, breed, length of lactation, and production compared with her herdmates.

Dairy Herd Improvement Association Programs

The Dairy Herd Improvement Association (DHIA) has had a major impact on dairy cattle improvement and genetics (Voekler 1981). In DHIA programs, once a month the milk production of each enrolled cow is weighed by an official supervisor at two consecutive milkings. Milk samples are taken for composition analyses. In addition, considerable data on individual cow and herd production are collected and processed through DHIA centers, and reports are mailed back to the farmer. Immediate processing and access to the data bank can be obtained through the use of computer terminals and printers located on the farm. These programs are available in Canada, the U.S., and other countries. They are usually financed by participating dairy farmers and are commonly subsidized by provincial or state governments.

There has been a remarkable growth in the use of the services provided by DHIA programs in the last 25 years (Sechrist 1983). In the U.S. in 1983, approximately 43% of all dairy cows were enrolled in the DHIA. In addition to the provision of the traditional information such as total milk and fat yield of each cow and herd summaries of production and reproductive performance, there are now available optional reports such as action sheets that indicate when certain events will occur or procedures should be done. Infrared analyzers are now used for butterfat and milk protein determinations. Individual monthly somatic cell counts are done on composite milk samples. A national DHIA Verified Identification Program (VIP), the first all-breed grade identification system, is now available. Certain DHIA programs also now offer optional services such as feed testing, soil testing, farm enterprise analysis, and progesterone analysis of milk for pregnancy diagnosis (Sechrist 1983).

The DHIA has become an information management system. The accomplishments of the DHIA include the following:
□ Improvement in management
□ Improved production
□ Excellent dairy extension program
□ The backbone for genetic evaluation systems
□ The artificial insemination success story. The DHIA provided the records system to determine genetic selection. The DHIA provided the central processing centers and the United States Department of Agriculture (USDA) provided the summaries of genetic information for sire selection. This allowed the AI industry to establish schemes to locate and develop the animals necessary for true genetic improvement. Genetic progress is the pride of the dairy industry.

The DHIA reports provide the dairy producer and the veterinarian with a monthly summary of individual cow and herd performance, including the costs of milk production, which must be monitored regularly. The reports also rank cows in the herd according to production, which provides a data base for the selection of cows and sires for breeding and for the culling of low-yielding cows.

An explanation and interpretation of the various reports provided by DHIA services has been reviewed (Stout 1978; Stout 1983c). An itemized summary of the reports with an indication of their significance is presented here.

1. *The Sample-Day and Lactation Report* is a monthly update of information for each cow in the herd.

(a) *Sample-Day Data* include the weight of milk, the per cent butterfat, and the grain mix fed on a sample day. The milk price of the day and the cost of feed is used to calculate the income over feed cost for each cow. A cow's grain needs are determined by calculating requirements for milk production, body maintenance, stage of gestation, and growth allowance. Nutrients supplied by the forage fed are subtracted from total requirements to determine the weight of grain mix needed at the protein and energy levels reportedly being fed.

(b) *The Lactation-to-Date* section is an accumulation of production data since calving. The total days of lactation are listed along with the totals of milk and butterfat calculated for those days based on the sample-day production. The butterfat percentage is a weighted average. The income over feed cost is the income accumulated after subtracting the cost of the previous dry period plus all feed consumed to date. This information will begin to tell a story about each cow. At approximately 120 days of lactation, a cow will have achieved 50% of her actual production for the lactation.

Breed Class Averages (BCAs) are indices of the cow's production expressed as percentages of the 305-day Breed Class Standard for all cows of the breed calving at the same age. For a cow that has been in milk for more than 45 days and less than 305 days, estimated BCAs based on current lactation totals are given. This estimate assumes that the cows will be in milk for a 305-day lactation. The deviation from herd average is the difference between the cow's BCA milk and fat index and the Rolling Herd Average BCA milk and fat of all cows completing lactations in the herd within the last 12 months.

Breed Class Averages are an evaluation of the production ability of a cow adjusted for age. They enable the dairyman to compare each cow's performance with that of other cows milking in the same herd under the same conditions. BCA values provide a reliable standard, through this deviation from the herd average, for use in culling low producers from the herd. Herd replacements should be kept from superior cows.

(c) *Annual Projections.* Each month the milk production accumulated for Lactation-to-Date is projected to a 305-2X-ME basis. This standardizes each cow's record to a 305-day lactation length, two daily milkings, and the same age mature equivalent. By projecting all records to a standard level, valid comparison can be made between cows. The comparison is listed as "Difference from Herdmates."

(d) *Management Data* include the remaining columns of the Sample-Day and Lactation Report. "Lactation Number" records the number of calvings, whereas "Days Dry" gives only the dry days for the previous dry period. The "Days Dry" column may give some indication of past breeding management. Cows should have 45 to 60 days dry.

The "Freshening Date" listed is the day of last calving, with the "Age" being the age at time of calving. An indication of calving interval can be determined by looking at Freshening Date and Due Date.

The "Due Date" column is updated with each breeding date. Cows may be reported open or pregnant on the subsequent barn sheets, following pregnancy testing. When reported open, the due date will clear and a (B) for breeding reminder will appear in the "Action Needed" column. Other Action Needed reminders are (D) for Dry at 42 or 60 days before due date, (F) for start increasing grain 14 days before calving, and (P) for pregnancy check 42 days following breeding.

Persistency is a percentage figure that tells how well the animal is holding up in production. It is the extended 305-2X-ME record for the lactation-to-date for this test shown as a percentage of the comparable figure for last month. Persistency tells how well a cow's production fits the average production curve.

All cows being above 100% persistency could indicate that better management conditions on the current sample day were more favorable to milk production than the previous month. A change in quality of feed, labor problems, milking equipment problems, and so on, which will affect the entire herd, will be quite obvious as the percentage in this column increases or decreases.

The "Condition Affecting Record" column lists any particular information that would affect the size or validity of the record being produced, e.g., diseases such as mastitis.

2. *The Herd Summary* provides the information of the monthly Sample-Day and Lactation Report and supplies running 365-day averages of all data for the herd.

(a) *The Reproductive Summary* lists reproductive performance in the herd according to the following: average days calving to conception interval; animals diagnosed as pregnant; number of animals not bred since calving; and average services per conception.

(b) *The Summary of Animals to Be Milking, Dry, or Calving* allows the dairyman and the veterinarian to plan ahead for drying off cows and for vaccination schedules.

(c) *The Feeding Summary* provides the complete feeding information for groups of cows on sample-day and annual averages for 365 days. The kind of ration being fed and the quality codes for each part are listed. On an annual basis, the amount of forage dry matter consumed should normally be about 2 kg./100 kg. body weight. With excellent-quality forage, the intake might reach 2.3 kg./100 kg. body weight without reducing milk production. Higher levels of dry matter intake would probably reduce total energy intake, causing loss of milk production.

(d) *The Cost and Return Summary* lists the feed costs, the value of the product, and income over feed costs. This information is calculated on a per cow and per herd basis for a sample day and for the previous 365-day average.

(e) *The Lactation Summary* provides data to compare the producing animals by lactation groups. First-lactation animals should be equal to or superior to later-lactation groups when replacements are properly reared and are sired by superior bulls. A low first-lactation average may indicate a need for better heifer management or improved sire selection.

(f) *The Production Summary* includes data for each sample date during the previous 365 days. Trends can be noted relative to herd size, turnover, per cent in milk, daily milk, and fat test. Herd averages for the 365-day period ending with each sample date can measure the herd production progress. Per cent cows in milk must always be considered when comparing test-interval daily milk averages. The daily milk average includes data with 80% in milk for all cows milking and dry.

Data Collection

Data regarding yield of milk and milk composition in North America are collected through local Dairy Herd Improvement (DHI) organizations and are processed through a dairy record center. The center usually calculates lactation yield and fat yield according to uniform national standards and also records other data. Estimated body weights, breeding dates, and monthly somatic cell counts in milk and protein or solids, but not fat content, are currently recordable by most of the computing centers. Uniform lactation milk and fat records are forwarded to the Animal Improvement Program Laboratory for sire and cow evaluation. This laboratory then calculates estimated transmitting abilities for all identified cows and sires.

Conformational traits are observed by trained classifiers, and results of these data are summarized by the respective breed-registry organizations. Each of the respective breed organizations uses different traits and carries out the program as it feels will be most useful to its members. Most of the data are collected on registered cows. In addition, many of the artificial insemination units collect data on daughters of their sires. Traits collected by these units vary greatly and include stature, milking ease, temperament, udder characteristics, and various type traits.

Dairy Cow Quality

Dairy cow quality means breeding to obtain the economically best cows, keeping these good cows healthy as long as possible so that they reach their genetic potential, culling low-yield cows, and constantly looking for better daughters.

The general requirements of a cow quality program include the following:

1. A successful breeding program that steadily improves the herd's genetic ability for high performance in the economically important traits as rapidly as possible.

2. Controlling diseases that cause premature culling of high-producing cows.

3. Successful culling programs based on accurate records of milk production and possibly other traits desired by the owner.

Two types of evaluation of cows are needed by the dairy industry: (1) the estimation of breeding values and (2) evaluation for culling. Cows to be dams of bulls for testing should be selected exclusively on their estimated genetic merit. The culling of females from the herd should be based on the past and current phenotype of the cow as a prediction of future net returns (Pearson and Miller 1978).

Estimating Breeding Values

Systematic estimation of the breeding values of cows in North America has been limited to milk and fat yield and an index of the two variables. For these traits, the estimation procedure is quite sophisticated. Currently, the cow index is used by the AI centers as the major selection criterion of bull dams.

Most of the economically important traits of dairy cattle are inherited in a quantitative manner, i.e., no new genes are made through selection; rather, herd genetic improvement is brought about by increasing the number of desirable genes and decreasing the number of undesirable genes in the herd.

The tools are now available to accurately identify genetically superior animals. Undesirable genes will still occur and result in poor performance and the necessity for culling.

Even though only 50% of the genes in the offspring come from the male parent, most of the genetic improvement in dairy cattle is the result of male selection. This is true because much more selection pressure is possible in the male, through the use of progeny testing (Philipsson et al. 1978). The accuracy of estimating a bull's genetic value is much higher than for a cow because bulls can have many more offspring than cows. With the use of artificial insemination, only one in thousands of males born is needed for breeding. In contrast, 70% or more of the females born are needed because they are the producing, as well as the reproducing, units of the herd. Fewer bulls are needed; thus more can be culled.

A logical procedure for the development of a profitable breeding program that will result in maximum or near maximum improvement in genetic ability for economically important characteristics of dairy cattle would include the following:

1. Identify and record the parentage of each animal in the herd.

2. Enroll the herd in a performance testing program like DHI (Dairy Health Improvement).

3. Define the goals or objectives for the individual.

4. Identify those traits that can or should be improved by selection.

5. Determine the current status of the herd in regard to these traits.

6. Minimize nongenetic female culling so that genetic culling can be maximized.

7. Evaluate the available sources of information to identify genetically superior animals.

8. Breed a high proportion (70 to 80%) of the herd females to sires with proven ability to transmit superior performance in the desired traits.

9. Breed a small proportion of the herd females to highly selected young sires.

10. Avoid breeding to bulls known to be carriers of genetic defects or abnormalities.

11. Ensure that nutrition, housing, and management are optimal in order to allow the animals to express their genetic potential.

12. Breed dairy heifers to dairy sires, not beef sires.

Selection of Cows in the Breeding Program

Milk Yield. The most important single trait possessed by foundation dairy cows in a herd is high milk yield. These cows are also characterized by a strong constitution, and they remain healthy and strong throughout the rigors of a long, productive life.

One economically important end result of a strong constitution is the capacity for longevity. The more lactations during which a cow remains profitable, the longer the period over which the dairyman can amortize the investment of the cow.

Each cow's first-lactation yield is of primary importance to her profitability. In addition, initial selection of sires is primarily on the basis of first-lactation yields of their daughters. Cows with higher first-lactation yield tend to have a longer productive life and higher lifetime yield than cows with lower first-lactation yields (Gill 1976). Positive phenotypic and genetic correlations exist between first-lactation yield and lifetime yield, so that selec-

tion primarily on the basis of first-lactation yield will result in cows with greater longevity.

The physiological basis for genetic improvement in dairy cattle is currently of interest (Blosser 1979; Kiddy 1979). About 25% of the variation in milk production is primarily due to genetic differences, but the number of actual genes involved is not known. The identification of specific genetically controlled mediators of physiological and biomedical activities would possibly allow the identification of genetically superior animals in the first few weeks or months of their lives.

Type Traits. The physical traits that appear to have the greatest economic value in cows are udder strength and good-quality feet and legs. In herds that sell breeding stock, dairy character and final classification score are important (Stout 1983b).

Body Size and Efficiency of Feed Utilization. High-yielding cows are usually larger in size than low-yielding cows, but large size does not necessarily result in high-producing cows. Thus, dairymen should select for high-producing cows rather than large cows, which may be inefficient and unprofitable.

Reproductive Efficiency. Dairymen should strive for a high rate of reproductive efficiency in the herd. The heritabilities of most reproductive characteristics of cows are relatively low and, in fact, a positive genetic relationship exists between breeding problems, level of yield, and longevity. Thus, an effective herd health program of diagnosis and treatment of reproductive problems is very important for maximum genetic progress. Without early diagnosis and corrective action if possible, reproductive problems can cause the loss of cows that would score high in selection index rankings and extend the generation interval, thereby decreasing the amount of genetic progress made in a given period of time. Such a program should also result in improvement in reproductive efficiency through genetic improvement of reproductive traits.

Mastitis and Milking Rate. The heritability of resistance to mastitis is low, probably around 0.10. This suggests that resistance to mastitis would respond to selection but at a slow rate.

Milking speed is also an economically important trait of dairy cows. Slow-milking cows require extra labor for the milking process, and efficiency of labor utilization is one of the most important factors of profitable management. However, there is no genetic correlation between yield and milking speed. Therefore, selection for higher yield can be independent of milking speed. Selection for rapid milking speed may be selecting for cows with increased susceptibility to mastitis.

Selection of Bulls in the Breeding Program

The greatest opportunity for genetic improvement in a herd is through the bulls that are selected for use in the breeding program. The selection differential within each herd can be much higher for bulls than for cows, because the bulls that are used by means of frozen semen can be selected from among the outstanding bulls in the entire country, whereas the cows selected must constitute the majority of those in the single herd.

The most important reason for the selection of high Predicted Difference (PD) bulls in a breeding program is that an important economic relationship exists between a bull's PD for milk yield and his daughters' Income Over Feed Cost (IOF). Future income can be increased substantially by breeding cows to sires that transmit superior levels of yield to their daughters. In addition to the extra income over feed cost, daughters of genetically superior bulls have been shown to have greater longevity, higher lactation yield of milk components, higher efficiency of feed utilization, and higher voluntary forage intake. All of these traits contribute to the greater relative profitability of the daughters of such bulls. The components of milk, such as butterfat, should also be considered when selecting bulls.

The USDA-DHIA Predicted Difference is the uniform standard of measuring the transmitting ability of dairy bulls in the United States. Its greatest value is as a device for ranking bulls on transmitting ability for yield. PD is an estimate and subject to change depending on the information that is available when the estimate is made. It is possible for the estimate to change with a different sample of information or at a later time when more data on more daughters are available. For this reason, the Repeatability is given along with the PD. As previously explained, Repeatability is a measure of the reliability of the estimate of transmitting ability. The proper interpretation of this reliability factor is very important in the intelligent use of PD for making genetic improvement.

Variation Among the Daughters of a Bull. The individual lactation records made by the daughters of a bull will vary greatly. Some of

the best bulls have some very low-producing daughters and vice versa. Thus, it is difficult to estimate the transmitting ability of a bull accurately from a small group of daughters.

Planning Mating for Maximum Genetic Improvement

The choice of bulls that are to be used in a herd's breeding program and the planning of individual matings to these bulls should be done according to the following five-step procedure:

1. Make a list of all available bulls with superior PD for yield and income.

2. Rate these bulls on their transmitting ability for other economically important traits.

3. Consider the price of each bull's semen and his breeding efficiency. The semen of certain bulls may be overpriced because of popular names or show ring winnings. One of the most important keys to genetic improvement and a profitable herd is to use bulls with high breeding efficiency. Bulls that have a low breeding efficiency in AI should be used with caution regardless of a high PD. The repeated use of bulls with a low conception rate may cause economic loss through additional AI costs and cows that are open and dry for unnecessarily long periods of time. Other causes of lowered breeding efficiency due to AI are poor insemination technique, poor laboratory techniques of freezing and storage of semen, and careless handling of frozen semen during transfer and shipment.

4. Select a group of bulls with high PD out of outstanding sires and dams with Repeatabilities below 50 or 60% for use on about 25% of the herd.

Plan individual matings for each cow in the herd with a specific bull. After the high-Repeatability bulls have been chosen for use on the majority of the herd and a group of very promising low-Repeatability bulls selected for about one fourth of the herd, individual matings should be planned as the final step. These pairings should take into consideration the strengths and weaknesses of each cow and of each bull. Then specific matings can be made that will result in maximum overall genetic progress by increasing yield while at the same time doing as much as possible to improve major faults that individual cows may transmit to their offspring.

The dairy industry does not have a single unified breeding program. Like other species of livestock, the breeding decisions are made by thousands of independent producers. Breeders who produce young bulls for sampling, the AI organizations that choose the young bulls to be sampled and select those to be retained after sampling, and all dairymen who choose the sires and dams of female replacements contribute to the breeding program of the dairy industry. The achievements of the current breeding program of the industry represent their joint efforts. The AI industry and milk-recording systems are the foundations of the current breeding program. In fact, the milk-recorded population of AI-bred cows is the foundation of the progeny testing program carried out by each center. The number of young bulls that can be sample each year by each AI unit is directly related to the size of this population. Theoretically, all cows that are AI-bred could be enrolled in a milk recording program. However, in Canada in 1980, only 37% of the dairy cattle population was milk-recorded and potentially available for progeny testing bulls. Since only about 85% of milk-recorded cows are bred artificially, it is estimated that only 31% of the total cow population is both milk-recorded and bred artificially. These cows are the basis of young sire sampling and progeny testing. Failure to increase milk-recording enrollments, particularly in the artificially bred population, greatly under-utilizes the available genetic resources. The success of the young sire sampling program of an AI center is dependent on the genetic superiority of the sires, the dams of those young sires, and the intensity of selection of young bulls based on completed progeny tests (McAllister 1980).

Determining the selection goal is the first step in an effective breeding program. The long genetic lead time makes it important to maintain a single consistent goal. The single most important path of genetic improvement is the choice of the sires of the young bulls.

Future breeding programs will continue to be based on AI and selection. As total dairy cow performance becomes more well defined, breeding goals will likely include more traits than milk yield, butterfat composition, and type conformation. If maximum genetic progress is to be achieved, many more young sires will need to be sampled in proportion to the size of the milk-recorded population. Only through continued use of superior proven bulls along with more intense selection of bull dams in producing future groups of young sires to be sampled will maximum rates of genetic progress through AI be achieved.

There is some indication that some of the economically important diseases of dairy cattle such as mastitis, ketosis, and milk fever show genetic variation (Philipsson 1980). There is inadequate information available, but it is suggested that disease frequency should be taken into account, together with other traits, especially in the selection of bull sires, provided progeny tests can be obtained on sufficiently large daughter groups. A reliable system would require a nationwide method for the recording of diseases in such a way that the data could be continuously evaluated for breeding purposes. In Sweden, a system exists for the continuous recording of diseases of all animals treated by veterinarians. All veterinary reports are continuously computerized, and various types of disease statistics have been produced. The recorded disease data have been combined with pedigree information from the milk-recording scheme and thus can now also be used for genetic analysis. Although the heritability of mastitis incidence in dairy cattle is low, field records are sufficiently accurate for progeny testing AI bulls, provided the progeny groups are large enough (Lindstrome 1978).

CULLING COWS

Intensity of selection in dairy cows is relatively low, because 70 to 75% of the females are retained to maintain herd size. The 25 to 30% culled annually can contribute significantly to the genetic improvement of the herd if they are culled for genetic reasons (low production because of lack of genetic ability). If, however, most or all of them are culled for nongenetic or management reasons (infertility, mastitis, lameness, or diseases of the digestive tract), less genetic progress is possible. The rate of culling can also be increased if the generation interval is shortened (heifers calving at 24 months of age rather than later), if reproductive efficiency is high (fewer cows culled as non-breeders and production of more calves), and if calf mortality is low. Genetic progress through female culling or selection therefore is affected by rate of culling, reason for culling, number of heifer calves born, heifer mortality, and age of heifers at first calving, as well as genetic ability of the herd replacements.

A theoretical analysis of culling and selection in dairy cattle on the basis of first-lactation yield indicates that mean yield of the herd is little affected by culling (Hill 1980). At the optimum of about 70% of cows retained, the annual increment in yield is about 1%, so it is likely to be more economical to bring fewer heifers into the herd and practice a minimum of culling. If a substantial genetic trend is incorporated and yield is to be maximized in later generations, the benefits of culling are greater, and fewer animals should be retained after first lactation. The greatest benefits from culling are obtained if it is practiced in midlactation. Genetic improvement in commercial herds is more cheaply obtained by selecting replacement calves only from the best cows rather than by retaining most of the heifer calves and culling the poorest after one lactation.

There is some indication that the marked increase in milk yield as a result of improved genetic selection has resulted in a parallel increase in health problems (Hansen et al. 1979a). The incidence of problems such as mastitis, reproductive failure, locomotor disorders, and digestive disturbances is higher and more costly in high-yield cows than in low-yield cows. The labor requirements are also higher. However, the extra annual income from the group with superior genetics for production will usually offset the additional costs of health care. There is also evidence that the season of the year, stage of lactation, year of parity, and the interaction between the season of the year and stage of lactation contribute to variability in many categories of health care labor and expense.

The summer season in the United States has a deleterious effect on health. The stage of lactation is the greatest source of variation, with the early stages being four times more variable than later stages. Increases from first to fifth and later lactations are threefold (Hansen et al. 1979b).

Diseases of dairy cattle that result in premature culling unassociated with low milk yield due to genetics have a major economic impact on the herd. A herd with an average life of 5.3 lactations will have 20% more earned income than a similar herd with an average productive life of 3.3 lactations (Renkema and Stelwagen 1979a, 1979b). This illustrates the economic importance of improved health, permitting a longer herd life. A mathematical model suggests that about 20% of heifers in their first lactation could be culled. The strongest selection should be made two to three months after calving, and those producing less than about 88 per cent of the herd average should be culled. Diseases such as mastitis, metritis, re-

tained placenta, and pneumonia are associated with culling, and besides the direct costs of treatment, the loss of potential income because of early culling and failure of the cow to reach her maximum milk yield is a major economic loss (Cobo-Abreu et al. 1979a, 1979b). This emphasizes the need for control of these diseases at the lowest economical level possible.

Ideally, cow culling decisions should be based on future net returns (Allaire and Cunningham 1980). Actual milk yield and composition, value of calves, feed costs, labor and facilities costs per day, individual cow care costs, and cow depreciation should be included in future net returns. Milk-producing ability of the cow will be the major contributor to the prediction. Adjustment for current reproductive status could substantially improve the prediction of net return during the remainder of the current lactation and the possible next lactation. Body weight may be another useful predictor, mainly because of its influence on the amount of feed for maintenance and salvage value. Age or lactation number may be useful and may be a predictor of cow depreciation and individual cow care costs. Projection of future net returns should be predicted from deviations from the herd mean for the various traits and should use parameters and prices supplied by the dairyman. This will help to remove some of the effects that are peculiar to a given herd. On a practical basis, most culling decisions for production are made during first lactation, and the remainder of the culling is to remove cows that have become less profitable.

The DHI computing centers usually provide some form of within-herd evaluation of current lactation each month. These include deviation from herdmates, a letter grade indicating the quartile of the herd in which the record falls, and a relative value expressing the record as a percentage of the herdmate or contemporary average. Estimated producing ability of the cow based on all her records is calculated either once or twice yearly by some centers. The calculation of income over feed cost on test day and totaled over the lactation to date, and the monetary value of milk expected in the 305-day lactation are also available in some DHI monthly reports. Additional culling aids provided to the dairymen through the DHI program include optional management lists of low-producing cows or potential culls based on various methods of predicting income from milk production, income over feed costs for the remainder of the current lactation, monthly somatic cell counts, and a calving-to-conception interval of 21 days over the dairyman's goal.

Culling Program

An important and rather neglected part of a dairy herd management plan is the system of culling cows. In general terms, cows are culled because of poor intrinsic milk production; susceptibility to or occurrence rate of disease, especially reproductive inefficiency and mastitis; and poor genetic quality, including both productivity and breed type parameters. In stud herds, part of the productivity of the herd is sale of surplus stock as producing animals. In commercial herds, this tends not to happen, and adult cows tend to be culled from the top of the herd as heifers become available as replacements, to the great financial disadvantage of the herd.

Culling Classification

Culled animals may be classified as follows:
1. *Emergency culls.* These include deaths and sale because of severe disease. These occur at any time and are emergencies because they have to be disposed of at the time.
2. *Failure to perform culls.* These are animals culled because of low production, which may result from inheritance of a characteristic or other nondisease cause of low production compared with peers; reproductive inefficiency; chronic mastitis; or other disease of a chronic debilitating nature. These animals are usually culled at the end of their current lactation.
3. *Excess to requirement culls.* These are cattle sold because the potential population increase by the herd exceeds the desired herd size. A computer simulation model of a herd enables a farmer to decide easily whether or not a particular heifer calf should be returned or should be culled and sold as a productive animal. Such a model is available for use under British conditions (Gartner 1981, 1982a, 1982b). The stage at which they are sold varies with the demand. In most circumstances, they are sold as breeding or calving heifers for replacement into other herds. Adult cows are placed on a list and sold off as they become the lowest producer in the herd.

Culling Guidelines

Herd size and herd composition are interrelated characteristics. The size of a herd is largely determined by a management decision in which a number of factors are taken into consideration, especially the size of the farm and the availabilities of family labor. Once that decision is made, it is then necessary to decide at which point the major culling pressure should be exerted. If the potential genetic gain is high because the sires are much higher producers than the dams, the selection pressure will be at the older end of the age group to make room at the bottom for the much better equipped heifers. However, if, as happens in more developed countries, the genetic gain from the sire is only marginal, it is usually more economical to select out the heifers early—at first calf—and keep older cows until they are at their peak of production in their fifth or sixth lactation.

The following discussion relates to modern practical situations in commercial herds. It is assumed that the 100-cow herd has a calving rate of 95%.

Loss of emergency culls up to 2 years of age	9
Of the surviving 86 calves, the heifers number	43
The standard culling rate (including 10% for all disease culls, 10% for low production, 2% deaths, and 3% miscellaneous) is 25%. Deduct	25
This leaves a surplus of heifers (over replacement needs) that are available for sale of	18

Genetic Gain

If the potential genetic gain is very high, it is possible to keep cows for only three lactations and replace them with their superior daughters. In the average situation, cows are kept for an average of four lactations, i.e., up to six years of age, and then culled for reasons of low production. If the genetic gain in the particular breeding program is marginal, then it could be financially more profitable to keep cows up to their 6th or 7th lactation.

Disease Control

If mastitis and reproductive efficiency can be significantly restrained, the culling rate for them can be greatly reduced, and genetic selection can be strengthened or the cows can be kept for longer lifetimes. This means that the herd will become larger or animals will have to be sold as productive units. In these circumstances, it is not unusual to have farmers identify such cows as culled for low production, when they are really useful cows but with a lower production than the program demands.

Disposals from 18 Friesian herds enrolled on the Melbread Dairy Herd Health Recording Scheme over three consecutive calving seasons revealed that the culling rate was approximately 20% of all cows calved (Gartner 1983). The reason given most frequently for culling was infertility, which represented 8.6% of all cows calved in the first year and declined to 6.6% in the third year. The percentages of cows culled for low yield, mastitis, and unclassified reasons were similar at approximately 3%. Death, injury, accident, lameness, old age, and behavioral faults each accounted for less than 2% of the cows culled. Culling for mastitis increased with lactation number. Several studies like this one have highlighted infertility as the predominant reason for culling in modern dairy herds (Martin et al. 1982; Dohoo et al. 1982, 1983). However, the per cent of culling due to infertility usually declines over a period of a few years if the herd is on a herd health program with a good recording system. The important implication of a reduction in culling for infertility is that it allows more culling for insufficient yield and other reasons, which may enhance the genetic merit and general health of the herd.

Competition for Pasture Space

When large numbers of heifers are retained for replacements, especially if they compete for available pasture land with the milking cows, the potential genetic gain is not usually enough to compensate for the loss in actual milk yield (Gartner and Herbert 1979).

A Culling Plan

It is not possible to specify a plan that will work for everybody. Much will depend on:
□ whether the herd size is to be static
□ the prevalence of mastitis and reproductive inefficiency, both of which are more damaging as cows get older
□ production shortfalls for nondisease reasons, which are most damaging in young cows
□ potential genetic gains available. For example, in herds that mate seasonally, it is common practice to bring in a bull to breed residual cows naturally, after AI has been used to achieve a 65% conception rate. The calves of the paddock bulls, which may represent 15 to 20% of the total calf drop, are always culled.
□ policy with respect to mastitis culls. A rigid policy of culling cows with more than three attacks of clinical mastitis in one lactation may drop the herd below approved size. A

choice must then be made to let them stay or to buy more heifers.
□ policy with respect to reproductive inefficiency culls
□ a rigid policy of excluding all cows that fail to conceive by 180 days after calving or that are not pregnant by 18 months of age. This may have the same effect as heavy culling for mastitis. The questions are whether to keep the damaged stock or to sell them and then whether or not to renew numbers by purchase or to wait for natural increase.

A reminder flow chart (Fig. 8–1) shows the major points of a culling program. Many of the decisions on the points in the plan are susceptible to variations between years and seasons and financial circumstances. The answer to the question about whether to cull a mastitis cow may be different if the atmosphere in the dairy industry is buoyant than if the indications are for a downturn in the market. The only way in which these questions can be answered satisfactorily at the particular time is to measure the effects of the various strategies under consideration in a computer simulation model.

However, in general terms, it is possible to make the following policy points in a culling program:
□ maintain the least possible replacement rate with an objective of seven lactations per cow
□ control mastitis and reproductive inefficiency severely to reduce culling for them to a minimum
□ dispose of excess to requirement culls at the earliest possible stage of their lives
□ subscribe to a locally developed simulation model, which will help to decide the optimum replacement rate for particular sets of circumstances

Composition of the Herd

The distribution of age groups within the herd is a very important indicator of its management efficiency. In herds where disease control is poor, the average herd age is lowered because of the higher prevalence of mastitis and reproductive inefficiency, especially in older age groups (Allaire et al. 1977), and the need to cull heavily for those conditions. Similarly, in herds where the genetic standard (cow quality) is poor and there is an opportunity to breed to high-quality bulls, the selection against the dams may be so high that again the average herd age will be lower.

There are two obvious circumstances in which the average herd age will be higher than normal. Herds in which culling for disease is

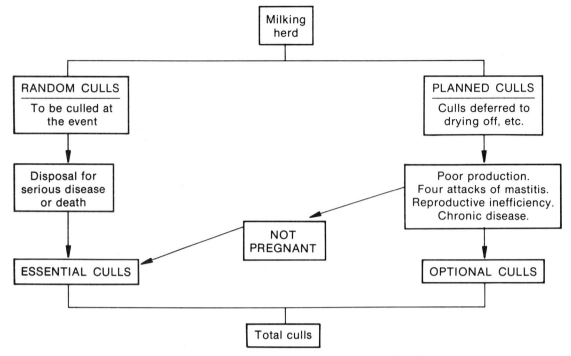

Figure 8-1. Outline of a culling program in a dairy herd.

low because the diseases are controlled may have an average herd age that is two years older than normal, and the profitability of each location may be 20% higher than in normal herds. The other circumstance in which average herd age is raised is when the herd is being increased in size.

References

Allaire, F.R. and Cunningham, E.P. Culling on low milk yield and its economic consequence for the dairy herd. Livestock Prod. Sci., 7:349-359, 1980.

Allaire, F.R., Sterwest, H.E. and Ludwick, T.M. Variations in removal seasons and culling rates with age for dairy females. J. Dairy Sci., 60:254-267, 1977.

Blosser, T.H. Physiological bases for genetic improvement in dairy cattle—introductory remarks. J. Dairy Sci., 62:813-824, 1979.

Cobo-Abreu, R., Martin, S.W. and Stone, J.B. The association between disease, production and culling in a university dairy herd. Can. Vet. J., 20:191-195, 1979a.

Cobo-Abreu, R., Martin, S.W., Stone, J.B. et al. The rates and patterns of survivorship and disease in a university dairy herd. Can. Vet. J., 20:177-183, 1979b.

Dohoo, I.R., Martin, W.S., Meek, A.H. et al. Disease, production and culling in Holstein-Friesian cows. 1. The data. Prev. Vet. Med., 1:321-334, 1982/1983.

Gartner, J.A. Replacement policy in dairy herds on farms where heifers compete with cows for grassland. I. Model construction and validation. Agricultural Systems, 7:289-318, 1981.

Gartner, J.A. Replacement policy in dairy herds on farms where heifers compete with cows for grassland. II. Experimentation. Agricultural Systems, 8:163-191, 1982a.

Gartner, J.A. Replacement policy in dairy herds on farms where heifers compete with cows for grassland. III. A revised hypothesis. Agricultural Systems, 8:249-272, 1982b.

Gartner, J.A. Dairy cow disposals from herds in the Melbread Dairy herd health recording scheme. Br. Vet. J., 139:513-521, 1983.

Gartner, J.A., and Herbert, W.A. A preliminary model to investigate culling and replacement policy in dairy herds. Agricultural Systems, 4:189-215, 1979.

Gill, G.S. and Allaire, F.R. Relationship of age at first calving, days open, days dry and herd life to a profit function for dairy cattle. J. Dairy Sci. 59:1131-1139, 1976.

Hansen, L.B., Young, C.W., Miller, K.P. et al. Health care requirements of dairy cattle. I. Response to milk yield selection. J. Dairy Sci., 62:1922-1931, 1979a.

Hansen, L.B., Touchberry, R.W., Young, C.W. et al. Health care requirements of dairy cattle. II. Nongenetic effects. J. Dairy Sci., 62:1932-1940, 1979b.

Hill, W.G. Theoretical aspects of culling and selection in dairy cattle. Livestock Prod. Sci., 7:213-224, 1980.

Kiddy, C.A. A review of research on genetic variation in physiological characteristics related to performance in dairy cattle. J. Dairy Sci., 62:818-824, 1979.

Lindstrome, U.B. and Syvajarui, J. Use of field records in breeding for mastitis resistance in dairy cattle. Livestock Prod. Sci., 5:29-44, 1978.

Martin, S.W., Aziz, S.A., Sandals, W.C.D. et al. The association between clinical disease, production and culling of Holstein-Friesian cows. Can. J. Anim. Sci., 62:633-640, 1982.

McAllister, A.J. Are today's dairy cattle breeding programs suitable for tomorrow's production requirements? Can. J. Anim. Sci., 60:253-264, 1980.

Miller, P.D. Artificial insemination organization. J. Dairy Sci., 64:1283-1287, 1981.

Pearson, R.E. and Miller, R.H. Cow evaluation in North America. Livestock Prod. Sci., 5:19–28, 1978.

Philipsson, J., Dommerholt, J., Fimland, E. et al. Problems in cow evaluation and current use of cow index. Report of a working group on cow evaluation. Livestock Prod. Sci., 5:3–18, 1978.

Philipsson, J., Thafuelin, B. and Hedebro-Velander, I. Genetic studies on disease recordings in first lactation cows of Swedish dairy breeds. Acta Agric. Scand., 30:327–335, 1980.

Renkema, J.A. and Stelwagen, J. Economic evaluation of replacement rates in dairy herds. I. Reduction of replacement rates through improved health. Livestock Prod. Sci., 6:15–27, 1979a.

Renkema, J.A. and Stelwagen, J. Economic evaluation of replacement rates in dairy herds. II. Selection of cows during the first lactation. Livestock Prod. Sci., 6:29–27, 1979a.

Renkema, J.A. and Stelwagen, J. Economic evaluation of replacement rates in dairy herds. II. Selection of cows during the first lactation. livestock Prod. Sci., 6:29–37, 1979b.

Sechrist, R.S. The value of DHIA to producers and to the industry. In: Dairy Science Handbook, Vol. 15. F.H. Baker (Ed.), International Stockmen's School Handbook, Westview Press, 1983, pp. 91–103.

Stout, J.D. The role of DHI records in herd health programs. Bovine Pract., 13:31–38, 1978.

Stout, J.D. Genetic indexes used in dairy cow and sire selection. In: Dairy Science Handbook, Vol. 15. F.H. Baker (Ed.), International Stockmen's School Handbook, Westview Press, 1983a, pp. 145–157.

Stout, J.D. Form and function of dairy cattle. In: Dairy Science Handbook, Vol. 15. F.H. Baker (Ed.), International Stockmen's School Handbook, Westview Press, 1983b, pp. 159–168.

Stout, J.D. Dairy cattle management by DHI objectives. In: Dairy Science Handbook, Vol. 15. F.H. Baker (Ed.), International Stockmen's School Handbook, Westview Press, 1983c, pp. 135–143.

Voekler, D.E. Dairy herd improvement associations. J. Dairy Sci., 64:1269–1277, 1981.

White, J.M., Vinson, W.E. and Pearson, R.E. Dairy cattle improvement and genetics. J. Dairy Sci., 64:1305–1317, 1981.

Planned Animal Health and Production in Beef Cattle Breeding Herds

9

INTRODUCTION

Beef cattle enterprises vary widely between countries and even within countries, and the definition of a practicable herd health program is difficult in anything other than the broadest terms. To do this involves taking a series of the most appropriate models at various phases along the spectrum of beef cattle farming, describing the various influences that determine their profitability, and indicating how best to superimpose a preventive veterinary program.

The cattle industry is one of man's most valuable renewable resources and provides farmers with the most efficient means of utilizing forages grown on millions of hectares of forests, rangelands, and pastures.

In the 25 years from 1958 to 1983, there was a tremendous development in the beef cattle industry in North America and elsewhere (Koch and Algeo 1983). Cattle numbers increased and beef consumption per capita increased from 28 kg. in 1958 to 43 kg. in 1976 and then declined to about 35 kg. A broad spectrum of economic, cultural, and technological factors brought about great changes in many segments of the industry. Consumer demand for lean yet tender tasty beef was a force for change. Genetic research stimulated the adoption of record of performance procedures as tools for improving economic traits of breeding herds. Cross-breeding was introduced and widely adopted to optimize average genetic merit and to utilize hybrid vigor. The importation of European breeds of cattle into North America greatly increased the genetic base available to beef producers. Important developments related to reproductive efficiency included estrus synchronization, nutrition requirements for reproduction, pregnancy diagnosis, superovulation, and embryo transfers.

The beef industry now faces a future that promises more change than in the past 25 years. Computer-assisted multidiscipline systems analysis of breeding and feeding operations will evaluate life cycle production with attention to matching genetic, nutritional, and managerial resources. The major emphasis will be on a technological revolution in reproductive performance (Dziuk and Bellows 1983). Reproductive efficiency will be enhanced by hormonal control and multiple births. Adaptation of the target weight concept for developing replacement heifers will become commonplace. Hormonal regimens or feed additives that will accelerate body and skeletal growth will become available and will be used to stimulate pelvic growth of the pregnant dam and, at the same time, retard fetal growth. In this way, problems of dystocia will be greatly reduced. With successful methods of ovulation control combined with conception rates exceeding 90%, calving seasons will be shortened. Induced calving will be incorporated into the calving season for additional concentration of labor and compression of the calving season. Nutritional regimens will be clearly defined for maintaining pregnant, prepartum, and lactating or nonlactating postpartum dams. Hormonal regimens will be developed that will shorten or eliminate the postpartum anestrous period and accelerate repair of the postpartum uterus so that the interval from calving to conception will not exceed 30 days. Breeding seasons of 60 days will be replaced by breeding periods of 12 hours, with pregnancy rates exceeding 90% being commonplace.

Effective techniques or treatments for production of multiple births will be developed. Pregnancy diagnosis will be made prior to 21 days. Nonpregnant females will be immediately recycled through an ovulation-control sequence or will be culled. Bull fertility will be evaluated by in vitro techniques. Breeding programs will be based on new selection criteria derived from blood and tissue components that can be used to predict genetic complements of the offspring and heterosis. Artificial insemination companies will offer cloned, parthenogenetic, sired embryos for production of single or twin births, and embryo transfer will gain a sizable portion of the AI market. Lifetime immunity against common infectious and reproductive diseases will be produced by a single treatment of the calf with new vaccines during the early postnatal period.

The above glimpse into the potential future of beef production is remarkable. The "space age" in beef production is upon us. However, along with this revolution will come extreme demands for correct management decisions. The role of the manager will not decrease but will increase. Professionalism will be the goal for managers, animal scientists, veterinarians, teachers, administrators, and others involved in this revolution.

Beef cattle farming is not a rigidly compartmentalized industry. It comprises a continuous range of more and more intensified farming activity, from the Australian rancher with 25,000 head of cattle on an arid-zone farm at one extreme, to the North American farmer-rancher with 50 to 500 breeding cows, to the Japanese farmer with three animals each being fed on their own individual diets in single loose boxes at the other end of the spectrum. There are at least five different phases of production in the spectrum. The commercial ones are the cow/calf or single suckling operations of commercial beef herds at varying levels of intensification. As a model, we have selected a 200- to 300-cow herd on improved or irrigated pasture and receiving supplementary feed in time of pasture shortage. This appears to be the common denominator of beef production, or is likely to be so in the foreseeable future. Some material on extensive ranch-style beef farming and purebred farms or studs that provide the seed stock to enable commercial herds to supplement their pool of genetic resources is provided at the end of the chapter. Feedlots and unweaned calf-rearing units are described in the section on feedlots. The European beef industry is generally conducted on the basis of much smaller herds and would require special consideration beyond the scope of this book.

The information provided assumes that the farms are stocked with Bos taurus—British breed-type beef cattle or their crosses. *Bos indicus*—Brahman-type cattle—are making a significant numerical impression on beef cattle populations in tropical areas, but overall their effect is small. They do have significant differences from *Bos taurus* cattle in terms of their productivity indices, and a small section on this subject is presented at the end of this chapter.

At the standard size of 200 to 300 breeder cows and with the lower occurrence of disease than in dairy cattle, the family-size beef farm is much easier to provide for in terms of herd health programs than its dairying counterpart. The cattle are commonly run in mating groups of about 50 head, and it is not difficult to remember or easily record all that happens to each group. In most instances, an expensive external data storage and analysis service to handle the information is not required.

CHARACTERISTICS OF THE BEEF CATTLE INDUSTRY THAT INFLUENCE THE TYPE OF ANIMAL HEALTH AND PRODUCTION SERVICE

In many countries, beef cattle producers operate on a low-input, low-realization basis. Their production operation is a way of life that has changed little in several generations and tends to resist change. During the breeding season, cows and bulls run in the hills or pastures with little attention. Calves are sold at auction when producers need money and, in their mind, little is gained by having a uniform calf crop with increased weaning weights. Improvement of the herd by input of good genetic material is of little interest. Thus, many beef cattle producers are not interested in artificial insemination and certainly not in controlled breeding efforts, which require financial outlay for drugs, semen, and improved facilities. They also do not want to increase their management effort in the operation.

It is necessary to decide whether or not it is financially desirable to add the costs of a herd health service to existing costs on a beef farm. First of all, it is assumed that emergency services are provided at a level that is mutually satisfactory to the farmer and to the veterinarian. In many such associations, there are added the standard components of preventive medicine relevant to the particular farm, including

testing for tuberculosis and brucellosis and control of these diseases, strain 19 vaccination, vaccination against clostridial and other diseases, drenching for worms, spraying for ectoparasites, pregnancy diagnosis, and so on. There is no attempt to accurately measure productivity of the herd, or if there is, the productivity index is not related to the intensity of disease control. Another form of preventive medical practice includes the provision of advice, usually arising out of existing disease problems but not off-the-cuff. It is advice by experts; such a system has been described in which several expert advisers together visit the farm each year so that conflicts between items of advice can be resolved on the spot. The problem, of course, is the cost of the advisers.

The ability of the veterinarian to provide the herd health and production advice is a major factor that limits the extent to which beef farmers will utilize the service. Most veterinarians engaged in beef cattle practice are also involved in general farm animal practice, and they are not always available to spend the time necessary to properly evaluate a beef herd. Also, because they are in general practice, they are unlikely to be beef cattle veterinary specialists. The animal health and health-related production problems of the various aspects of the food-producing animal industry will be best served by species or industry specialists, in this case a beef cattle veterinary specialist in private practice and not employed by a government agency. Another major factor that affects the practicability of a beef cattle herd health service is the seasonality of the work. It is extremely difficult for a veterinarian to provide a planned animal health service to many beef farmers at the same time of the year. Success depends on detailed organization, strict adherence to farm appointments, and exceptionally good cooperation on the part of the farmer.

The variable economic importance of the beef herd to different beef cattle farmers, the small size of most beef herds, the low level of disease occurrence, and the generally good management that they have make it difficult to plan and provide an economical beef herd health service. In grain-growing areas of the world, although beef cattle may be raised in large numbers, they are often considered as an enterprise secondary to grain production on the farm. The goals and values of these grain/cattle farmers are often not consistent with the goals and values of veterinarians and agrologists, which may be to optimize production. This places a severe strain on the practicability of providing a planned animal health service, and the veterinarian must then show the farmer, by an analysis of the disease and production records, that the service can be rewarding and profitable.

The addition of a purebred cattle enterprise would further increase the demand for a planned animal health service, because the value of the output is greater and the potential of greatest profitability needs to be protected as much as the actual interest capital.

The introduction of a beef herd health program can be encouraged by making farmers aware of the economic importance of measuring productivity. This is an era of measuring productivity by weight gain and selecting progeny for breeding replacements on that basis. Farmers can then see that their selection program can be valueless unless their heifers are selected based on genetically controlled weight gain and not on weight variations determined by *Ostertagia* spp. Once the farmer begins to record calving dates, weaning and yearling weights, and other critical production indices in the breeding herd, the data can be analyzed and compared with theoretical objectives or with similar anonymous data generated on farms in the same area. This sort of comparison among peers is a powerful persuader in encouraging farmers to utilize a complete herd health service.

The development of a data bank from many farms in a locality can also assist in answering production-type questions relating to a particular area. It is becoming more and more clear that questions about disease prevention and production practices that are indigenous to a certain area must be answered by accurate observation of what has occurred in previous years. This requires the development of an accurate data bank from many representative farms.

In summary, the practicability of providing a preventive medicine service for a beef cattle breeding herd will depend on the motivation of the farmer, the size and value of the herd and whether it warrants a herd health service, and the competence and interest of the veterinarian. Beef farmers ask, "What can a veterinarian do for my herd, what will it cost, and what will be the economic returns on time, labor, and the investment of veterinary fees, drugs, and vaccines?"

THE DEVELOPMENT OF A VIABLE HERD HEALTH PROGRAM FOR A BEEF CATTLE BREEDING HERD

The herd health program described in this chapter is based on beef herds that obtain a significant part or most of their annual income from the sale of weaned calves at six to eight months of age or fat cattle off grass at one to two years of age. The general recommendations may be utilized, with modifications for local differences, in commercial beef herds ranging in size from 50 to 10,000 breeding cows. The principles also apply to purebred herds that sell breeding stock.

There may be additional enterprises on the farm, including cereal grain or corn production, cash cropping, grass and seed production, hay production, and sheep production. These other enterprises often require that beef cattle work be done at selected times of the year rather than all the time, which creates problems for continuous surveillance and the need to confine some activities, e.g., calving, to predetermined time limits. The unit may be entirely pasture-dependent, including year-round grazing, with prepared feed supplementation when required; or in the temperate zones of the world, large amounts of hay must be prepared and fed for two to six months during the winter season. Regardless of which situation exists, beef farms are heavily dependent on climate and are limited in their location to areas that have a very good and dependable climate. Otherwise, there needs to be irrigation. The beef cattle management expertise on these farms and the records available will vary from excellent to unsatisfactory. Handling facilities will also vary from being excellent to poor, and the time spent doing physical diagnostic work, pregnancy diagnosis, and bull evaluation may be either very efficient and rewarding or inefficient, frustrating, and uneconomical.

The disease problems that exist on these farms will be varied, but the major epidemic diseases such as brucellosis, tuberculosis, and vibriosis are likely to have been reduced to a very low level or almost eradicated in the area. The major diseases and problems are likely to be inadequate animal identification, poor reproductive performance that is usually related to undernutrition and unsatisfactory breeding practices, a high incidence of dystocia, neonatal calf diarrhea, and pneumonia in the calves at weaning time. In some areas, other

Table 9–1. SHARED RESPONSIBILITIES FOR A SUCCESSFUL BEEF HERD HEALTH PROGRAM

Veterinary Responsibilities	Owners' Responsibilities	Uncontrollable Factors
Regular visits to herd	Desire to achieve optimum production	Weather, rain, food supply, sporadic diseases (i.e., anaplasmosis)
Prebreeding (bull and female evaluation)	Animal identification	Livestock prices
Summer—surveillance of disease records	Records	
Fall—pregnancy diagnosis, weaning procedures	Vaccination, drenching, and treatment of simple diseases	
Winter—nutritional surveillance	Closed herd and effective quarantine policy for imported animals	
Calving season:	Organization and management of the herd	
Provide advice on vaccination and other prophylactic schedules	Herd free of tuberculosis and brucellosis	
Collect and analyze data and prepare recommendations	Good animal and crop management (nutrition, genetics)	
Identify clinical and subclinical disease and provide advice	Willing to consider advice and make changes in management techniques	
	Financial management of the herd	

diseases will predominate such as bloat, ostertagiasis, fascioliasis, and nutritional deficiencies of phosphorus, selenium, copper, cobalt, and the like.

OBJECTIVES OF A BEEF CATTLE HERD HEALTH PROGRAM

The profitability of a beef calf production enterprise depends basically on the reproductive rate of the cow, the subsequent growth rate of the calf to weaning, and the overall efficiency of feed utilization (Trenkle and Willham 1977). These parameters are themselves subject to a wide range of genetic, nutritional, environmental, and managerial factors.

The major objective in a beef herd health program should be to assist the farmer or rancher in the production of one healthy weaned calf from each breeding female exposed to the bull per year (Wiltbank 1970, 1982, 1983). One weaned calf per cow per year is a theoretical objective that is unlikely to be achieved (Bellows et al. 1979). However, a weaned calf crop of 85 to 90% is practicable, and the degree to which the producer can reach this level of production will influence net income (Hanly and Mossman 1977; Mossman and Hanly, 1977). There may be a difference of 30% in profitability between a weaned calf crop of 75 and 90%.

The weaned calf crop is the number of calves weaned as a percentage of the total number of all females exposed to the bulls in the previous breeding season.

The calf crop weaned may be only 70 to 73 per cent because of the losses from breeding to weaning.

Factors That Affect the Weaned Calf Crop During the Production Cycle in A Cow/Calf Operation and Methods for Improvement (modified from Bellows et al. 1979)

Factors	Methods for Improvement
Failure of females (heifers and cows) to conceive (approx. 20%)	Restrict breeding season to 42 to 63 days. Breeding females must reach critical minimum weight at beginning of breeding season so that 90% will come into heat in the first 21 days of the breeding season. Breeding bulls must be of high fertility, high serving capacity
Abortion (approx. 1–2%)	No known method that will reduce this level of abortion
Perinatal mortality (approx. 2–5%)	Breeding bulls must sire calves that minimize the incidence of dystocia. Management of herd at calving time to minimize acute undifferentiated diarrhea of calves
Postnatal mortality	A preweaning program designed to minimize the effect of stress and incidence of respiratory disease

Requirements Necessary to Achieve Objectives

The general requirements necessary to achieve the objectives of the program are shown in Table 9–1. A successful herd health program in beef cattle herds is dependent on the cooperative combined efforts of the veterinarian and the owner or herdsman. There are also uncontrollable factors, such as undesirable weather, shortage of feed, unexpected sporadic disease, and a marked drop in livestock prices, that may nullify any positive economic gains made in a well-planned herd health program.

BASIC FORMAT FOR A BEEF HERD HEALTH PROGRAM

Selection of Farms

Veterinarians should select with care those herds to which they wish to offer a herd health service. There is not much point in attempting to work with farmers who are not interested in beef cattle improvement or who are not managerially or financially capable of utilizing and profiting by the program. The stricter the selectivity based on the following criteria, the fewer failures there will be. The recommended criteria are:

1. A breeding herd of cows that will generate sufficient work to be efficient and economical. In Canada, this may be a 100-cow herd and in Australia, a 200- to 300-cow herd.

2. Animal identification must be accurate and comprehensive. A system of metal and plastic ear tags, brisket tags, neck chains, branding, or electronic devices is necessary. An event diary must be maintained by the farmer.

3. The producer must be interested in beef cattle improvement using an effective breeding program (Fredeen 1983).

4. The farmer must be prepared to submit all dead animals for necropsy. Adult deaths are unlikely to be more than 2 to 3% per year, and necropsies can usually be done on the farm. Aborted fetuses and dead calves should be examined in a diagnostic laboratory if possible.

5. The herd should be a closed herd, and a quarantine system should be maintained to the point where introduced animals are segregated until they can be submitted to veterinary inspection.

6. Significant changes in management policy that are likely to affect health must be discussed between the farmer and the provider of herd health service before they are introduced.

7. The herd must be free of tuberculosis and brucellosis.

8. Response trials are often necessary to make a diagnosis or test a prevention technique, and the farmer must be prepared to conduct them.

9. The weighing or body condition scoring of animals is necessary to assist the objective selection of breeding replacements.

Initial Assessment of Productivity Status

There are two parts to this examination. One is to identify the farm and its characteristics and the aspirations and objectives of the owner. The other is to examine existing records or to create new ones, and compare them with the owner's objectives and those set up as theoretical standards. It is then possible to determine if a herd health program can provide a suitable guarantee of profitability.

To identify the farm's characteristics, a farm profile document is completed. An annual report may be prepared on the basis of existing data for the preceding year (Janzen 1983). However, very few farmers keep records that are adequate for this assessment, and it is usually necessary to develop this basic data. During this inaugural or surveillance year, no recommendation may be made on disease prevention or management except for emergency situations.

On the basis of the information provided in the herd profile and in either the annual report based on past data or on information accumulated in a surveillance year, it should be possible to determine whether a farm has a significant shortfall in performance compared either with that achieved by other farms in the area or with a theoretical objective. If a farmer achieves all the targets—and it is very rare for him to do so—he may opt to join the full program as insurance anyway. If not, he may join on a surveillance basis only. In this case, he provides all the data on the forms provided to him—the same ones as are used in the full service. The data analysis center then returns a full report on performance, and, provided the targets are achieved, no veterinary participation on the farm is required.

Starting the Herd Health Program

This step is a major one and includes a number of important facets, which follow.

The Herd Health Program Itself

This is a collection of the most recommended techniques for the particular area under consideration. Thus, the program can be devised in a general sense by a central organization, but it should be capable of modification by a local adviser. It will also be necessary for the local adviser, who will probably also fill the role of herd veterinarian, to assess each client individually and to modify the program—or to vary the intensity with which it is presented—to suit that particular client's managerial capacity, resources, objectives, and constraints. Veterinarians who wish to provide a beef herd health service must first gain the confidence of the producer, usually through the practice of individual animal medicine. Usually within a few years, it will become apparent to both the farmer and the veterinarian that certain planned veterinary services are desirable and economically justifiable. Initially, these would include pregnancy diagnosis, evaluation of the breeding soundness of bulls, and advice on vaccination schedules.

The Determination of Targets of Performance

If objectives are policy goals such as calving in the spring, targets of performance are the numerical and financial goals that are set up so that the level of efficiency can be assessed. Determination of these targets requires some experience in what the industry is capable of achieving, with some consideration being given to the constraints provided by local environmental and other circumstances. In an extensive service organization, it is soon possible to use the results of the big achievers in the service as the guidelines to optimal performance.

Failure to achieve predetermined targets, when all available information suggests that the program should have done so, requires a detailed analysis of the records to identify the cause.

It may be necessary to conduct the response trial in which—by either intuitive judgment or a proper experiment—a certain technique or treatment is tested and the results measured.

The Annual Cycle of Activities

This includes a decision on the number of visits that should be made each year, when they will be made, the work to be done at each visit, and the timing and content of reports on the work to be done. As much as possible, the visits must be coordinated with other activities on the farm to avoid unnecessary collection and examination of cattle. If the herd is being performance-tested by weighing, these activities need to be considered.

It is necessary to discuss the means of fitting programed beef herd health work into an annual work schedule in a practice and, where possible, avoiding the other busy seasons of the year. Beef cattle practitioners are usually busy with emergency work during the calving season, and very little planned veterinary service can be provided. During the prebreeding season, there is usually sufficient time to examine bulls for breeding soundness, to assess the reproductive potential of the female herd, and to discuss breeding plans, artificial insemination, estrus synchronization, and vaccination of the herd. However, the veterinarian must organize his farm visits efficiently in order to visit all subscribing herds within about a 60-day period. Similarly, pregnancy diagnosis visits should be organized so that all farms can be visited within a 60-day period. This is necessary to identify nonpregnant cows as early as possible and to determine their fate.

The development of multiple-person practices will allow veterinarians to specialize in beef cattle practice and to devote the time necessary to do the work, analyze the data, and prepare the reports.

The Collection, Storage, and Analysis of Data and the System of Reporting to the Farmer

An enormous amount of information may be collected from a beef farm. The secret of financial success in a beef herd health program, as with all the other species, is to know what kinds of information are essential to enable an accurate assessment of performance to be made. It is therefore first necessary to select critical indices of performance and then to devise ways of collecting the information without alienating the farmer with a flood of paper and without going to the farm so often that travel costs are prohibitive. Having collected the data, it is necessary to store it economically and efficiently so that it can be retrieved easily. Data from most beef herds can usually be handled easily manually. For larger herds that may generate a large volume of data, the use of a computer may be desirable and necessary.

The system of reporting to the farmer is important. Reports should follow visits to the farm and annual reports should be prepared and discussed with the owner and herdsman. These will be discussed later in the chapter.

Specific Components of a Beef Herd Health Program

The specific nature of a beef herd health program will vary widely, depending on the size of the herd, whether the herd is managed intensively (irrigated pastures) or extensively (semi-arid rangelands), and the production and financial goals of the owner. The number of scheduled herd health visits will vary from one to four or more per year.

For herds with one short breeding and one short calving period each year, at least two visits are recommended. These are for pregnancy diagnosis six to eight weeks after the last day the bull was with the females and for a prebreeding visit to examine the bulls for breeding soundness and to evaluate the breeding potential of the females. The principal target of any beef herd health program is the maintenance of a high level of fertility, and thus the two most important visits of the year are those just cited.

The details of activities that are recommended for each visit in Southern Australia are shown in Table 9–2 and for Canada in Table 9–3.

As mentioned above, the major emphasis in beef herds is the achievement of a high reproductive performance. The role of the veterinarian is to assist the farmer in the selection of bulls of high fertility and in the management of heifers and cows to ensure a high percentage of conception in a restricted breeding season.

Under Canadian conditions, beef cattle usually calve in late winter or early spring (February to April). The breeding period and summer pasture extend from June to August, and the calves are weaned from October to November, when they are six to eight months of age. The winter period during which the herd is fed on stored feed extends from about November to May.

In the Canadian beef herd, which is the model that will be used here, there are four important times during the year when the veterinarian has a vital role to play. The components of the veterinary service that can be provided at each of these visits will be presented along with a brief review of the factors that influence performance at critical points during the production cycle. The four strategic times are:

1. *Prebreeding visit* (examination of bulls and females)—April to May
2. *Pregnancy diagnosis and weaning of calves visit*—October to November

3. *Winter feeding and management visit*—December to April
4. *Precalving and calving visit*—March and April

The recommendations outlined here as a model can be modified to suit almost any beef herd where the major aim is to produce one weaned calf per cow per year.

The herd health visits should be coordinated with certain beef herd farming activities. The important policy is to anticipate problems before they occur or are likely to occur and to introduce economical disease control or prevention techniques well in advance of the expected occurrence.

Prebreeding Visit

At the prebreeding visit, at least one month before breeding, the bulls are examined and the state of the female herd is assessed.

Examination of All Bulls for Breeding Soundness. A complete examination of bulls for breeding soundness includes examination of the serving behavior and capacity of the bull (deBlockey 1978; Chenoweth 1983), a physical examination for the detection of abnormalities that may interfere with breeding (musculoskeletal injuries or defects, abnormalities of the penis and prepuce) (Chenoweth 1983), examination of the condition and size of the testicles, and examination of the quality of semen (Cates 1983).

Reproductive Efficiency and Male to Female Ratios. Recommendations for the bull to breeding female ratio (BFR) in a breeding beef herd have varied from 1:10 to 1:60 (Rupp et al. 1977). For limited breeding seasons, a BFR of 1:25 has been commonly utilized under range conditions in the western United States. The use of fewer bulls would improve the production from a breeding herd through better utilization of selected sires, provided conception was not delayed or decreased. Good reproductive efficiency can be obtained by using good bulls at ratios of 1:40 to 1:60. In multiple-sire mating, 70% or more of heifers may be bred by more than one bull at a given estrus. This overlap is inefficient because single-sire mating groups result in comparable pregnancy rates. However, in single-sire mating groups, some bulls are unable to breed large numbers of heifers. This indicates that the fertility, libido, and mating ability is more important than the breeding female ratio. Thus, a major problem for the veterinarian and the animal breeder is to devise methods that

Table 9–2. COORDINATION OF BEEF HERD FARMING AND BEEF HERD HEALTH ACTIVITIES IN SOUTHERN AUSTRALIA

Month (Applicable in Southern Australia)	Farm Activity	Herd Health Visit	Principal Activity at Herd Health Visit	Data-Recording Documents	Activity by Data-Recording Bureau
May–June–July	Mating/joining period of 8 to 10 weeks	—	—	Farmer provides Data Bureau with Farm Event Diary and Management Summaries monthly through year	Monthly updating of each cow's Lifetime Record (or Bull Record Card) and Annual Management Summary. Check errors with farmer
Sept.–Oct.	Weighing at 200 days (or corrected to 200 days) just before weaning	1st pregnancy diagnosis visit (PDX)	Pregnancy diagnosis test sampling empty cows. Discussion Report No. 1 and Bull Soundness Report Vaccinate Strain 19 *Br. abortus*.	Records. Essential to record the identity of females in each mating group, the bulls and their dates in and dates out and PD result or infertility exam	Prepare Report No. 2. An updated standard cow listing (cow's lifetime records) with P.D. results added and analysis of fertility index expressed as $\dfrac{\text{Cows pregnant}}{\text{Cows mated}} \times 100$. Analysis for herd and for individual bull mating group
December	Weaning at 240 days	—	—	Weights sent to Data Bureau	Prepare Report No. 3. Analysis of rate of gain performance (individual and progeny-of-bull groups). Best sent in combination with Report No. 2
January	Postweaning weighing	2nd pregnancy diagnosis visit	PDX doubtful or late cows and small heifers omitted at 1st PDX. Obtain 2nd test samples from empty cows. Check bulls going to autumn sales	As for PDX visit No. 1	If necessary send Report No. 2 modified by findings of the visit, i.e., Report No. 4
Feb.–March–April	Calving calf birth weights	—	—	—	At end of calving close books for the "beef year." Prepare Report No. 1 (standard cow listing including updated lifetime records of all cows).
April–May	Weigh heifers at 400 days prior to joining at 450 days	Bull examination visit	Examine bulls for breeding soundness	Bull Examination Record. Bull Record Card	Urgent recommendations about bulls or females to farmer before joining begins.

210

Table 9-3. COORDINATION OF BEEF HERD FARMING AND HERD HEALTH ACTIVITIES IN CANADA

Time of Year	Farm Activity	Herd Health Activity	Data Recorded
April–May	Preparation of females and bulls for breeding	Vaccination for diseases that may cause fetal wastage (I.B.R., Campylobacter fetus). Weigh breeding females. Examine bulls for breeding soundness. Ensure freedom from brucellosis	Vaccines used. Weights of breeding females (have they reached suitable breeding weight)
June–July	Breeding season and early summer pasture	Vaccinate calves for clostridial diseases at about 2 months of age. Regular inspection of breeding herd	Dates of the beginning and end of breeding season. Female/bull ratio
August–September	Summer pasture	Preweaning program (decide on schedule of vaccination of calves for respiratory disease)	Date of vaccination and vaccines used
October–November	Weaning and weighing of calves. Culling cows. Treatment of warbles.	Pregnancy diagnosis. Selection of cows to be culled. Feed analysis and plan winter feeding	Total number of cows pregnant and classified according to stage of pregnancy; number of cows nonpregnant and whether normal or abnormal. Reasons for culling cows and bulls. Total number of calves and average weaning weight
December–January–February	Winter feeding	Check cows regularly for lice, loss of weight, abortion	Weight of representative cows regularly. Amount of feed used
March–April	Surveillance and management of calving herd	Provide necessary assistance at calving. Ensure calves receive colostrum within 2 hours after birth. Early treatment of sick calves. Identify cows that experience dystocia	Weight of cows before calving. Calving dates. Number of cows requiring assistance. Calf mortality

identify bulls with acceptable semen quality, libido, and mating ability.

It is important for its subsequent production as a cow that a heifer conceive early in its first mating season (Morris 1980a, 1980b). This is because an early calving heifer (1) weans a heavier first calf; (2) has a greater change of conception as a first-calf cow than a late calving heifer; and (3) has a greater chance of calving early at its second and subsequent calvings and thus weaning heavier calves over its lifetime than a late calving heifer. Furthermore, to maximize the chances of heifers conceiving early in their first mating season, they should be mated to bulls with high serving capacity. The first estrus conception rate is higher in heifers mated to bulls with high serving capacity than in heifers mated to bulls with medium serving capacity; thus, they will conceive earlier in the breeding period.

The Management of Reproduction in the Females in the Beef Herd. The target of reproductive performance in the beef herd is one weaned calf per female exposed in the breeding season. The role of the veterinarian in the reproductive management of the beef herd is to identify and correct those factors that interfere with achievement of the targets of performance.

Causes of Inferior Reproductive Performance. The two major problems in beef cattle reproduction are low net calf crop and long breeding seasons (and hence long calving seasons). The net calf crop is the number of calves weaned as a percentage of females exposed in the breeding season. Data from well-managed research station beef herds indicate that net calf crops are approximately 70% (Bellows et al. 1979). In these same herds, the major losses in calf crop have been identified and can be separated into four broad categories of the reproductive cycle.

Category of Reproductive Cycle	Per Cent Loss
Females not pregnant at the end of the breeding season	17.4
Perinatal calf deaths	6.4
Calf deaths birth to weaning	2.9
Fetal deaths during gestation	2.3

The components of reproductive wastage in commercial beef herds are as follows:

	Average (%)	Range (%)
Heifers and cows not in calf after 3½ to 4 months of the breeding period	10.0	0–50.0
Calves lost during gestation (between 3 to 8 months) —heifers 2%, cow 1%	1.0	0–2.0
Calves lost at birth		
Heifers	1.0	0–45.0
Cows	0.25	0–6.0
Normal live calves lost between 6 hours after birth and weaning		
Heifers	5.0	0–25.0

Some surveys of reproductive performance in commercial beef herds have shown that:

1. On average, 10% of cows bred do not become pregnant (range 0 to 50%). Approximately 20 to 50% of this group are second calvers.

2. An average of 10% of heifers bred do not become pregnant (range 0 to 40%).

3. An average of 10% of pregnant cows and heifers are late in calf (range 0 to 45%). These late calvers are often not pregnant in the subsequent year.

Breeding seasons of six months or longer are not uncommon and in many herds last at least 90 days (Janzen 1978). Long breeding seasons perpetuate lowered production in beef herds for three reasons: (1) At weaning, the calves from late-calving cows are lighter in body weight than calves born earlier; (2) factors such as nutrition, losses at calving, and calfhood diseases cannot be controlled adequately, and ranchers hope for success rather than planning effectively for it; and (3) the opportunity for individual cows to have calving intervals greater than 12 months is greater in long breeding seasons than in short breeding seasons.

These results show clearly that failure of females to become pregnant ranks first and perinatal calf losses rank second in their effects on net calf crop. In addition, long breeding seasons and long calving seasons reduce the body weight of calf weaned per cow per year. Both the net calf crop and the average weaning weight must be considered when evaluating the production efficiency of the beef breeding herd.

Methods to Improve and Maintain a High Level of Reproductive Performance. The best opportunities to achieve a high level of repro-

ductive performance in beef herds include (Wiltbank 1983):

1. Increase the percentage of females showing estrus during the first 21 days of the breeding season

2. Increase the conception rate at first service

3. Shorten the length of the breeding season to 60 days or less (45 to 60) from the traditional length of 90 days

4. Decrease the calf losses due to dystocia and neonatal diseases

1. INCREASE THE PERCENTAGE OF FEMALES SHOWING ESTRUS DURING THE FIRST 21 DAYS OF THE BREEDING SEASON. The factors determining the number of cows showing estrus early in the breeding season are as follows:

Time of Calving. The length of time between calving and the breeding season has a profound effect on the onset of estrus and conception rate on first service. The percentage of cows that show heat and become pregnant on first service is low before 50 days after calving. There is a marked increase in both factors from 60 to 90 days after calving. This postpartum anestrus in beef cows may also be due in part to the sucking of the calf. Removal of the calf for a period of 48 hours may stimulate the onset of estrus in cows calved at least 50 days (Beck et al. 1979). Also, young cows require more time to come into heat than other cows, a problem that can be minimized by the provision of an adequate energy intake before and after calving. Thus, late-calving cows will not show heat early in the breeding season, the conception rate to first service will be low, and the cows will always be late calvers. Beef producers have unwisely used long breeding seasons in an attempt to increase the pregnancy rate in late-calving cows. This is counterproductive because it results in females that calve later and later each year, with smaller and smaller calves at weaning time.

2. INCREASE THE CONCEPTION RATE AT FIRST SERVICE. The conception rate at first service can be maximized by having cows calved at least 50 days, in good body condition, and preferably on an increasing plane of nutrition. The use of bulls of known high fertility will also increase conception rate at first service.

Heifers being bred for the first time must have sufficient body weight at the beginning of the breeding period to concentrate their calving the first time. The *critical minimum weight* is the weight of those heifers, irrespective of breed, at which one can expect a minimum pregnancy rate of 85% over a 42- to 45-day period, bred at least three weeks ahead of the mixed-aged cows (Hanly and Mossman 1977; Mossman and Hanly 1977).

The estrus activity is affected by the previous management, and the weights are relative to the particular farm, but there are some general guidelines. The critical minimum weight must be determined for each farm. One method is as follows: Weigh the heifers three weeks before turning them out with the bull, on the day the bulls are turned in with them, and when the bulls have been with them for 20 days, 42 days, or 45 days. Check for pregnancy six weeks after withdrawal of the bull and relate the length of pregnancy, body weight, and approximate time of conception.

The farmer must identify the critical minimum weight he must achieve to undertake a short breeding period. Until this is achieved, it is impossible to get one calf per cow per year during its productive lifetime. Heifers with a high rate of pregnancy in their first breeding season will maintain a 95% pregnancy rate each year over a limited breeding period throughout a four-year herd lifetime.

3. SHORTEN THE LENGTH OF THE BREEDING SEASON. The breeding season should be no more than 60 days for cows and 45 days for heifers. If the cows have calves at least 50 to 60 days of age and are in good body condition, a high percentage (85%) will come into heat and become pregnant in a 45- to 60-day breeding season. Decreasing the breeding season from 150 days or even from 90 days to 60 days may present a cash-flow problem because of the culling of cows that is required, which reduces the total number of weaned calves available for sale. However, sometimes the breeding season can be shortened with only small losses in calf numbers the first year. At other times, rather drastic changes must be made. There are two possible methods: (a) development of a plan in which the breeding season is shortened by two to four weeks per year and in which heifers are bred for only 40 to 60 days; and (b) development of a plan in which cows are bred in the fall and spring programs. Forage supply must be carefully evaluated in the latter type of program. Results of shortening the breeding seasons indicate that net calf crop, the actual weaning weight, and the total weight of calf weaned per cow all increased.

4. DECREASE THE CALF LOSSES DUE TO DYSTOCIA AND NEONATAL DISEASES. Calf losses due to dystocia can be minimized by using bulls that will sire calves that will be born from heifers unassisted. The provision of surveillance and obstetrical assistance during the calving season will also decrease losses associated with dystocia (Hodge et al. 1982). The management of the herd at calving time to control acute diarrhea of calves is presented in a later section.

Breeding Management of Heifers and Cows. *In order to get one calf per cow per year over a three- to five-year lifetime in a commercial beef herd, it is necessary to restrict the breeding and calving periods to 42 to 63 days, to obtain a 95% in-calf rate, and to have as close to 100% weaning as possible each year* (Mossman and Hanly 1977).

Beef production involves continuity of performance in a concentrated breeding, management, and feeding system. A beef cow must not only produce a calf each year but must produce it at the correct time in relationship to the calving of all the other cows. If the calf is not produced at the correct time in relation to the average, it has less chance, over a limited breeding period, of getting pregnant as a replacement heifer two years later. The number of cows cycling when the breeding period begins determines the length of the calving season the following year. If the calving season is too long, there will be insufficient top-quality heifers to use as herd replacements two years later. Under optimum management and nutrition conditions, cows should be bred over a period of 42 to 60 days, preferably 42 days, and if they do not become pregnant in this period, the unit has not reached its maximum production potential.

The five time-related factors that have the greatest effect on herd performance and profitability are as follows (Hanly and Mossman 1977; Mossman and Hanly 1977):

1. The number of heifers in estrus on the first day of breeding, which is related to nutrition, body weight, management, and previous herd performance

2. The length of the interval from calving to first heat and conception, which is related to the time of calving and breeding, nutrition, and management

3. The length of gestation, which varies between breeds, e.g., Angus 273 to 279 days and Charolais 284 to 296 days

4. The percentage calving in the first 21 days of the calving season

5. The repeatability of herd performance within limited breeding systems over a three- to five-year period

The consequences of a long calving season include the following:

1. Prolonged calving, producing an uneven line of weaner calves and a decrease in market value

2. Increase in the percentage of late pregnancies and nonpregnancies due to late cycling and anestrus

3. Increased culling of first calvers as not pregnant

4. Increased supply of replacement heifers to maintain herd numbers

5. Poor yearling size and poorly grown replacements in some herds, with 20 to 50% of two-year-old replacements being unsatisfactory

6. Impossibility of effective feed budgeting

7. Decreased net profit per breeding cow

Mismanagement and misunderstanding of the breeding cow and heifer under adverse nutritional conditions are responsible for low pregnancy rates in 90% of herds. This includes lack of feed budgeting and saved pasture, and the impossibility of providing it owing to a prolonged calving period; breeding at the incorrect time; and the fallacies that more stock per acre means more profit per acre, that a late calf is better than no calf, and that decreasing feed intake before calving and at calving will decrease calf size, pelvic fat, and dystocia.

Nonpregnant cows and heifers mean a loss of capital stock, and the more late pregnant and nonpregnant cows, the less profit from the herd. When current returns are marginal for a 90% effective calving rate over 45 to 63 days, losses will result if 10 to 40% fail to produce a good weaned calf.

The theoretical basis for the achievement of a high rate of pregnancy in a herd of mixed-age cows and heifers is based on the following assumptions:

1. The average conception rate for each heat cycle is 60%

2. The per cent of first-calf heifers and mixed-aged cows that come into heat at certain intervals after calving under optimal nutritional and management conditions is as follows:

No. of Days After Calving	Per Cent in Heat
FIRST-CALF HEIFERS	
80	60–70
90	70–80
100	80–95
MIXED-AGE COWS	
80	80–89
90	90–94
100	95–100

3. Estrus will occur in at least 90% of yearling heifers in the first 21 days of the breeding season if they are at a critical minimum weight and good body condition at the beginning of the breeding season

4. Bulls of proven breeding soundness (semen quality, libido, serving capacity) are used

With this background, a theory of beef production proposed by Mossman and Hanly (1977) is reviewed here.

MATHEMATICAL MODEL I: HEIFER BREEDING MANAGEMENT. A herd of 100 well-grown cycling heifers in excellent body condition is mated to 3% proven bulls for 105 days. It is proposed that each 21 days, 60% will become pregnant. The theoretical conception rate in 100 heifers over 105 days is shown at the bottom of the page.

The total number of services required to get 100 beef heifers pregnant at a 60% conception rate is 164 services, i.e., 1.64 services per heifer. It will take 105 days to get 100% heifers pregnant. If breeding is terminated at day 42, 84% will be pregnant; at day 45, 85 to 86% will be pregnant. Another 60 days are required to get the remaining 14 to 16% in calf.

If it is assumed that it takes 100 days after calving for an average first-calf heifer to return to heat, then the time to the second breeding (second breeding year) is 380 days (280 + 100). When the heifer returns to heat, she will require 1.64 services on average. Therefore, to become pregnant again it requires another 0.64 of a service, or 0.64 of a 21-day cycle, i.e., 13.4 days. The time of the first conception to the second conception (the calving interval) is now 293.4 days (280 + 100 + 13.4). Therefore, the average heifer takes 393 days from first conception to second conception, which means that she is 28 days behind starting her lifetime production of one calf per cow per year. Thus, theoretically,

Days of Breeding	No. Bred	No. Conceiving	No. to be Rebred	No. of Services Each 21-day Cycle
21	100	60	40	100
42	40	24	16	40
63	16	10	6	16
84	6	4	2	6
105	2	2	2	2

the heifers should be bred 28 days ahead of the cows.

The theoretical heifer calving pattern for 105 days is:

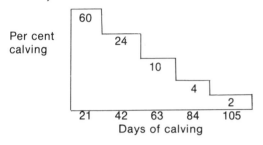

Per cent calving

Days of calving

Calving Index for 105-Day Second Breeding (see chart at the bottom of the page)

If the heifers are first bred at the same time as the cows, the average calving interval is 393 days. From the 100th day after calving, it will take *105 more days* to get *all* the heifers pregnant again, a period of 485 days (280 + 100 + 105). It is impossible to get pregnant again (within 365 days) heifers that were not pregnant by the 62nd day of their first breeding period, because the calving index is greater than 455 days. If a mating period of 63 days is planned for the herd, then heifers not pregnant by the 45th day of their breeding period will not become pregnant during the herd breeding period.

This theory for reproductive failure is the basis of a limited heifer mating (42 to 45 days) 28 days ahead of the herd, in which a minimum of 85% of heifers are pregnant and pregnancy-tested six to eight weeks after the end of the breeding period. The remaining 15% are the potential not-pregnant animals and could be culled and sent for slaughter. This would depend on current and predicted market prices and the availability and costs of feed.

The calving pattern for the remaining 85% of heifers from the 100 heifers that were examined for pregnancy six to eight weeks after mating is as follows:

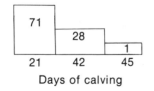

Per cent calving

Days of calving

With a concentrated breeding period, it is possible for heifers to calve in the spring on selected calving grounds with more control over feed intake before and after calving. This results in large savings in feed, which is virtually impossible with a 90-day breeding period. Another major economic advantage of concentrated calving is that the labor and surveillance that are required at calving time can be intensified and more effective. It is more economical and beneficial to be watching several animals calving through the night than it is to watch one animal every night or every other night for a period of 90 days.

MATHEMATICAL MODEL II: COW BREEDING MANAGEMENT. In a traditional cow/calf operation, cows may calve over a period of 105 to 120 days. Approximately 20% of the cows will calve each 21 days. This results in a wide range in weaning weights of calves at 200 days after the first cow calved. By improving the management and concentrating the breeding over a 63-day period, the weaner calf production from the cows can be increased.

Methods of shortening the breeding season of cows from three to six months, as it is on many beef farms, to 42 to 63 days include culling late calving cows and decreasing the breeding season by 10 days each year until all cows are calving in a 45-day period. The economic feasibility of each method can be calculated.

The nutrient requirements of a beef cow following calving will vary according to the nutritional status that existed through the previous winter in spring-calving cows, the size of the cow, and the management. In general, beef cows that are nursing calves on pasture should be maintaining body weight or making small weight gains for the 70 to 90 days following calving, so that a high percentage will come into heat within 45 days of the beginning of the breeding season. Cows with nursing calves are often turned onto pasture or rangelands, which are inadequate nutritionally, within a few weeks following calving. Unless these cows are supplemented with a supply of energy, they lose weight, have prolonged periods of anestrus—longer than that associated with suckling—and come into heat only after beginning

Gestation Length	100 Days After Calving	Cycle of Breeding	60% Conception	Calving Index
280	100	21	13	414
280	100	42	13	435
280	100	63	13	456
280	100	84	13	477
280	100	105	13	498

to gain weight early in the summer months when sufficient grass becomes available. Thus, the reason that cows are often left with the bulls for three to six months is because it takes that long for 95% of them to come into heat. If they were gaining a small amount of weight following calving, 95% of them would come into heat within 45 days of the breeding season. Cows must also be bred to bulls of high fertility and serving capacity.

A management system designed to improve reproductive performance in a cow herd must have the following prerequisites: (1) 45-day breeding season; (2) heifers calving earlier than the cow herd; (3) controlled levels of feed before and after calving; and (4) bulls with high fertility and serving capacity.

SUMMARY. To ensure a highly consistent reproductive program in a beef herd, 90 to 95% of the females must calve early each year and wean a calf. To accomplish this, the producer should follow these steps:

1. Feed heifers to reach a target weight consistent with their breed

2. Breed heifers in a 45-day period to a bull known to sire calves that will be born unassisted

3. Use a 60-day breeding season in the cow herd

4. Have cows in good to moderate body condition at calving time

5. Have cows gaining weight three weeks before breeding and during the breeding season

6. Remove calves for 48 hours at the start of the breeding season

7. Breed to fertile bulls

Prevention of Abortion. An abortion rate of about 2% is common and is usually of no medical concern; the cause is usually not determined. The common causes of infectious abortions in cattle include brucellosis, leptospirosis, and infectious bovine rhinotracheitis.

If leptospirosis and infectious bovine rhinotracheitis are endemic or a potential threat to the herd, the breeding females and males should be vaccinated at least three weeks before the breeding season. It is assumed that the herd is free of brucellosis.

Farmers should be encouraged to submit to the diagnostic laboratory all aborted fetuses, portions of placenta, and serum samples from cows that have aborted. The laboratory examination of portions of placenta will increase the diagnostic rate, which is normally as low as 30%.

Controlled Breeding and Artificial Insemination in Beef Herds. Artificial insemination (AI) has been widely practiced in dairy cattle; however, its use in beef cattle was not significant until it was used as an essential tool for rapid expansion of the newly introduced breeds. The extensive nature of beef herd management has complicated estrus detection. Sparse population and distances between herds made availability of trained AI technicians a problem. Also, most beef breed associations had very restrictive policies for registration under AI. In the last 25 years (1958 to 1983), innovative management of breeding herds, widespread training of cowboys in heat detection and inseminating techniques, use of teaser bulls, the necessity of AI for extensive use of semen from bulls of the newly introduced breeds, and less restrictive policies by breed associations have greatly increased the use of AI in beef herds. The use of AI is increasingly recognized as a tool for genetic improvement rather than a factor related to convenience. Although only approximately 5% of beef females are bred by AI in North America, there is evidence of a steady increase.

There is an enormous literature that deals with artificial insemination in beef cattle, which is available in other books. The introduction of the use of prostaglandins for controlled breeding shows considerable promise as a method of improving the genetic plasm in the herd. Manns (1983) has provided an excellent review of the subject. The use of prostaglandins to synchronize heat in a group of animals can allow producers to detect estrus more easily and thereby make artificial insemination a more accessible breeding tool.

There are currently two methods of controlled breeding that have been described.

METHOD 1—SINGLE-INJECTION PROGRAM. Beef cows should be a minimum of 50 days post partum and be in satisfactory body condition. The steps in the program are as follows:

Days of Program	Action
1–5	Detect estrus and breed
6	Inject cows not previously bred
7–12	Detect estrus and breed
13+	Continue to detect estrus or turn in with bulls

METHOD 2—TWO-INJECTION PROGRAM. In this method, cycling cows are given two injections of prostaglandins 10 to 12 days apart, followed

by a fixed-time insemination 75 to 80 hours after the second injection of the prostaglandin. Two inseminations may be used, spaced 24 hours apart, with the first one coming 68 to 72 hours and the second 92 to 96 hours after the prostaglandin injection.

As of 1983, the level of fertility achieved with such controlled breeding programs has not been satisfactory, providing a pregnancy rate ranging from 40 to 50%. One of the principal problems with this procedure has been the high proportion of noncycling cows. It is quite common to find 25% noncyclic cows within a group of animals that are all beyond 50 days post partum. This is an important area for research and future development.

Pregnancy Diagnosis and Weaning of Calves Visit

Pregnancy Diagnosis. Pregnancy diagnosis by rectal palpation should ideally be done as early as eight to 10 weeks after the bulls have been removed from the breeding pasture. However, because of the difficulties of gathering up beef cattle from large pastures and rangelands, pregnancy diagnosis is commonly not done until four months following breeding. For example, in Canada, it is not commonly done until October or November, which also coincides with weaning time, the onset of winter feeding and management, and the time when the cows are usually four to six months pregnant. This time also coincides with the onset of cold weather and snow, which makes the work of pregnancy diagnosis unpleasant and is a source of stress for the weaner calves.

Good and efficient handling facilities and personnel for pregnancy diagnosis should be encouraged. Excellent facilities based on research have been described (Grandin 1979).

All females are examined by rectal examination and are identified and sorted into one of the following groups: (a) early pregnancy, (b) late pregnancy, (c) not pregnant, and (d) abnormalities of the reproductive tract whether pregnant or not.

Those cows that are not pregnant can be held and fed separately until the market prices are attractive or sold immediately if feed is not readily available and economical. Culled cows placed in a feedlot will usually make economical gains (Graham and Price 1982; Price and Berg 1981). Whether the nonpregnant cows are culled or retained, they should be brought back into the yards at the end of the visit and submitted to more intensive examination to determine the cause of infertility. The kinds of examinations will depend on the common causes of infertility in that herd or in the local area. Tests may include those for vibriosis, leptospirosis, brucellosis, copper deficiency, phosphorus deficiency, and other nutritional deficiencies. An investigation of a high percentage of nonpregnant cows would also include a retrospective examination of the bull/cow ratio used during the breeding seasons, the nutritional status and body condition score of the females immediately before the breeding season, and the breeding soundness of the bulls.

Those cows that are late-in-calf can also be identified and culled if deemed necessary. If the percentage of these is higher than expected, the breeding program must be examined.

At this same time, cows can be culled for lameness, chronic mastitis, squamous cell carcinoma of the eye, low-weight calves, and undesirable conformation. Cows with "bottle-shaped" teats measuring more than 35 mm. in diameter should be culled (Fusch 1982). The mortality rate in calves born to these cows is higher than in calves born to cows without such teat defects. Subclinical mastitis in beef cows can account for a significant decrease in weaning weight of calves compared with calves sucking noninfected cows (Haggard et al. 1983).

Assessment of Reproductive Performance. This is an opportune time to collect all available breeding records. The reproductive performance of the herd should be assessed at the time of pregnancy diagnosis and weaning. Every animal should be accounted for according to the following evaluation:

1. *Pregnancy rate =*

$$\frac{\text{No. of females pregnant}}{\text{No. of females exposed at breeding}} \times 100$$

2. *Per cent of females not pregnant*
3. *Per cent of females late-in-calf*
4. *Per cent of females with physical abnormalities* of any body system. The number and nature of the abnormalities should be recorded
5. *The weaning weight of each calf and the average weaning weight*
6. The number of bulls used in each breeding group during the breeding season

7. The length of the breeding season

8. The body condition scores of the cows and heifers at the time of weaning

9. The average body weights of the yearling heifers at the beginning of the breeding season

This information may provide an explanation for a low pregnancy rate in the heifers

This data should be examined, and recommendations for changes in management should be made in a written report to the producer.

Weaning of Calves and Preimmunization and Preconditioning Programs. Beef calves are usually weaned at six to eight months of age. They may be weaned at three months of age and placed on supplemental feed, but this may be uneconomical. Weaning at 90 days of age may result in an increase in the pregnancy rate of cows (Pimentel and Deschamps 1979). Experimentally, calves can be weaned at six to eight weeks of age and reared efficiently to an acceptable weight at normal weaning age with a minimum of labor (Lusby et al. 1981). Early weaning before the breeding season will also permit high conception rates in first-calf heifers too thin to nurse a calf and still be bred at an adequate rate. In grassland countries, they may not be weaned until 10 to 12 months later and may even be left on pasture until market weight at 18 to 25 months of age.

All beef calves should be weighed at the time of weaning and the information recorded. Weaning weights are influenced by the breed and age of the cow, the age and sex of the calf, and the amount of milk produced by the cow (Butson et al. 1980). The association between weaning weight and milk yield is so significant that the introduction of dairy breeding into the dam line to increase milk yield and subsequent weaning weight may be a viable consideration for a breeding program in cow/calf operation. Weaning weights may be increased by the use of growth-stimulating implants (Ralgro) or by the use of creep-feed while on pasture. Growth-stimulating hormone implants are often economical, but creep-feed may be uneconomical.

In Canada and the U.S., beef calves are weaned at six to eight months of age in the fall of the year (September to November). The calves may remain on the home farm and be fed stored forage and grains throughout the winter and then placed on pasture the next spring or may be sold as feeder cattle for the feedlot. Some are usually kept as herd replacements. A large proportion of weaned beef calves are; however, sold directly or indirectly through public·livestock sale yards, at six to eight months of age, to feedlots. In the feedlots, they are grown out and finished to a market

weight of 500 kg. at 12 to 18 months of age, depending on the breeds used.

One of the major disease problems with calves weaned at six to eight months of age in North America is acute respiratory disease, especially pneumonic pasteurellosis or "shipping fever pneumonia," which occurs most commonly from seven to 10 days after weaning or after arrival in a feedlot.

Although it is not well documented, the epidemiologic evidence suggests that acute respiratory disease is associated with the stresses that occur because of weaning or with those environmental stresses that coincide with the time of weaning. The stressors include weaning itself, inclement weather in the fall of the year, temporary starvation and deprivation of water for a few days following weaning, transportation from the farm over long distances (up to 4000 km.) to the feedlot, comingling in public livestock sales yards for up to several days, and processing on arrival at the feedlot (castration, dehorning, branding, vaccination, hormone implants, injections, or prophylactic antibiotics).

Successful control begins with good management techniques when the calves are still on the range and continues with care in handling and transportation and the judicious use of vaccines where applicable.

Because of the common occurrence of the disease at the time of shipment from the range to the feedlot, much attention has been given to reducing its incidence at this time. This has led to the development of the concept of preconditioning in North America.

PRECONDITIONING AND PREIMMUNIZATION. The objective of preconditioning is to prepare the weaned calf for the feedlot environment by subjecting it to the stress of weaning, vaccination, and other common processing procedures well in advance of its entering the feedlot. Properly done, preconditioning includes:

1. Castration, dehorning, and branding at least three weeks or more before weaning

2. Treatment with a systemic insecticide for warbles and lice. In certain areas it may be desirable to deworm calves at this time

3. The administration of all vaccines at least two weeks before weaning

4. Holding calves for a period of three to four weeks after weaning until they have become accustomed to dry feed and drinking out of water tanks before offering them for sale

5. In some situations, producers may elect to creep-feed the calves for at least one month or so before calving

With these procedures done three to six

weeks before weaning, the only stress the calves will be subjected to at weaning time will be separation from their dams.

The practice of preconditioning calves began in the early 1960s in Iowa, largely due to the efforts of J. Herrick. By 1969, the first year of a state-wide program, 61,000 calves were enrolled. By 1979, there were 400,000 calves in the program. A preconditioning program was started in Alberta in 1980 and is called the "Alberta Certified Preconditioned Feeder Program" (Church et al. 1981). Under the Alberta program, calves must be owned by the producer at least 60 days prior to certification by a veterinarian and be at least four months old before vaccination. The program allows for either a preimmunization program or a full preconditioning program. Calves are vaccinated against the clostridial diseases, infectious bovine rhinotracheitis, and parainfluenza-3 (PI-3) virus infection at least three weeks prior to certification. Calves on the full preconditioning program are weaned at least 30 days prior to certification. Calves meeting the above requirements are identified by different colored tags indicating either preimmunization or preconditioning. Certificates signed by a veterinarian accompany the calves to the calf sale yard.

The preconditioning program will be successful only if both the calf producer and the feedlot operator benefit. There is general agreement that preconditioning reduces the incidence of shipping fever and chronic pneumonia. What is uncertain is whether the producer can recover the extra costs involved in preconditioning.

Cow-calf producers could benefit in the following ways:

□ Weaned calves should be able to gain 0.68 to 0.91 kg. (1.5 to 2.0 lb.) per day on a hay-grain ration or silage-grain ration to sale date
□ Weaned calves should shrink less in transit to sale
□ Net sale price for preconditioned and preimmunized calves should be higher
□ Producers using these programs should be able to develop a reputation for good calves
□ Cows from which calves are weaned earlier have a chance to develop better body condition before winter, which should lower winter feed requirements
□ Where calves are weaned earlier than has been traditional, pastures should have an increased carrying capacity for dry cows

The feedlot operator should derive the following benefits:

□ Knowing the history of the calves, the operator should be able to do a better job of managing them
□ Reduced vaccination and processing costs
□ Preconditioned calves should begin to eat and drink earlier on arrival and should therefore begin to gain weight sooner
□ Both preconditioned and preimmunized calves should require fewer treatments. Relapses and deaths due to respiratory diseases should be reduced.

There is no definitive information available on the economics of preconditioning or preimmunization of beef calves. There is considerable anecdotal information available, which is sometimes contradictory and unreliable. The concept is biologically sound, but it must be economical for the producer and the feedlot operator before widespread adoption of the practice will occur.

SOME ADDITIONAL COMMENTS ABOUT PRECONDITIONING OF CALVES. During transportation, adequate bedding must be provided. Calves should not be without feed and water for more than 8 to 12 hours and should be offered hay and water every 24 hours during long trips. This will minimize the considerable loss of body weight due to shrinkage and the effects of temporary starvation.

The vaccines used in a preconditioning or preimmunization program will depend on the occurrence of the disease in the herd or in the area. In some areas, calves may be vaccinated for *Hemophilus somnus* infection, *Leptospira* spp., bacterial bovine virus diarrhea, and other infections.

Providing creep-feed for several weeks prior to weaning has been successful in producing thrifty healthy calves but may not always be economical. A diet containing a mixture of cereal grains, a protein supplement, and the necessary vitamins and minerals is provided for the calves in a creep arrangement to which the dams do not have access. At weaning time, the cows are removed from the calves, and the stress on the calves is minimal. This program has been very successful in purebred herds where it may be economical, but in commercial herds it is only economical when the market value of the calves warrants it.

In the transfer of cattle from one owner to another, the ideal situation would be to avoid public sale yards and move the cattle directly from the ranch to the feedlot. This avoids the stress of handling, overcrowding, temporary starvation, exposure to infection from other cattle, and the unnecessary delays associated with buying and selling. However, large intensified feedlots are unable to buy cattle directly from ranchers according to their needs at a particular time. Inevitably, they purchase large groups of cattle of different backgrounds. This has led to the development of processing procedures in which, after arrival, cattle are individually identified; injected with a mixture of vitamins A, D, and E; treated with a residual insecticide; perhaps given an anthelmintic; injected with a long-acting penicillin; and vaccinated for clostridial and respiratory diseases. The subject of conditioning and processing calves after arrival in the feedlot is presented in Chapter 10. Bacterins and viral vaccines have been used extensively in an attempt to control pneumonic pasteurellosis in cattle but with limited or no success thus far. The pasteurella bacterins may have been inefficient because they did not contain the serotype most prevalent in the area, or they may not have been suitably antigenic and protective. The technology of producing a bacterin that contains the antigens necessary to stimulate the appropriate protective antibodies has not yet been developed. Recent work has shown that weaned beef calves that possess high levels of antibody to *Pasteurella hemolytica* are resistant to the experimental disease. This suggests that a major effort should be directed toward the development of a pasteurella vaccine that will stimulate the protective immunity against infection of the lung.

Based on the observation that prior infection of the respiratory tract with either infectious bovine rhinotracheitis (IBR) or parainfluenza-3 virus may lead to pneumonic pasteurellosis, the vaccination of beef calves two to three weeks before weaning and of older feeder cattle two weeks before shipment to a feedlot has been recommended as part of a preconditioning program. The results have been variable, but vaccination of young calves with an intranasal modified live virus vaccine containing the IBR and PI-3 viruses has provided immunity against experimental challenge with *Pasteurella hemolytica*.

It is important to vaccinate the calves at least two weeks before they are weaned, stressed, or transported to a feedlot. Vaccination immediately after arrival in a feedlot, although commonly done, is not reliable because there is insufficient time for antibodies to develop before the animals are exposed to the infectious agents in the feedlot. Such vaccination of newly arrived cattle against respiratory disease is contrary to the principles of immunology. The animals are vaccinated when they are under stress and then mixed in with other cattle

that may be carriers of the infectious agents. Under these conditions, there is insufficient time for immunity to develop, and respiratory disease is the net result.

However, in spite of all the recommendations for the vaccination of calves in a preconditioning program, there is almost no scientific evidence that any of the available vaccines is efficacious for the control and/or prevention of acute respiratory disease in recently weaned or shipped calves (Martin 1983). There has been a lack of well-designed field trials that include adequate controls.

MANAGEMENT OF DISEASE IN WEANED BEEF CALVES. Infectious diseases will occur in beef calves within a few days or longer after weaning regardless of a preimmunization or preconditioning program. Infectious diseases of the respiratory system and of the digestive tract are most common, and regular surveillance by visual inspection at least twice daily is necessary to detect and treat affected calves as early as possible. A morbidity rate of up to 10% can usually be managed successfully by identification and treatment of individual animals. When the morbidity rate exceeds 10%, the use of mass medication with antimicrobials or chemotherapeutics in the feed and/or water may be considered. Mass medication by injection of all in-contact animals may also be useful in the treatment of epidemics.

Winter Feeding Management Visit

Health and Management of the Pregnant Females. The management of animal health and production of the beef herd during the winter season involves consideration of the needs of the pregnant females, heifer replacements, feeder or stocker calves being held over the winter, and bulls. A health and nutritional management program should be developed for each group. These aspects of the beef herd have not received due consideration by veterinarians, perhaps because producers have not been able to appreciate tangible results from the monitoring of health and production of the herd during the winter months. It is an area of beef herd health that needs some field research to determine the extent of the losses that may be occurring.

In most countries, the winter feeding and management of the beef breeding herd coincides with the period of pregnancy in beef cattle. In grassland countries, pregnant beef cattle may have access to grass throughout most of pregnancy and calve out on green pasture. In other situations, pregnant cattle may be expected to use dormant range throughout the winter, supplemented with energy and protein using grain-protein concentrate mixtures to maintain a high level of reproductive performance. In Canada, where grazing forage is available for only 150 to 180 days each year, depending on geographical location, pregnant beef cattle are fed a variety of roughages (hay, straw), with or without supplemental grain, and vitamins and minerals throughout the winter months, which vary from 50 to 180 days. In some areas, cattle continue to graze on range into the early winter months and are fed on hay for only 50 days, then are placed on range in the early spring. In most other situations, the winter feeding period is about six months long, and feed accounts for 50 to 70% of producing a weaned calf under these conditions.

The major emphasis for the pregnant non-lactating beef cow during the winter months is on nutrition. The role of the veterinarian is to assist the farmer in planning an economic feeding program that results in optimum reproductive performance.

There is general agreement that the nutrition of the pregnant beef cow, particularly the first-calf heifer, can have a marked influence on the subsequent reproductive performance of the cow and the viability and health of the calf from birth to weaning. Undernutrition during pregnancy in first-calf heifers commonly results in an increased incidence of dystocia because of lack of weight and size (Makarechian et al. 1982; Wiltbank and Remmenga 1982), weakness at the time of parturition, insufficient colostrum, weak calves at birth, and a high percentage of prolonged postpartum anestrus, which results in a high percentage of nonpregnant animals that may have to be culled. If they are left in the breeding pasture to be bred over a period of three to six months, a high percentage will ultimately conceive, but they will be late calvers in the next season. The high rate of culling of nonpregnant animals and late calvers among young beef heifers and cows is a major cause of economic loss in beef breeding herds. The effects of undernutrition on reproductive performance are greater in first- and second-calf heifers and cows than in older cows. Thus, pregnant heifers should be fed and managed separate from cows and on a higher plan of nutrition than cows.

The effect of winter weight loss in beef cows on subsequent reproductive performance has been well documented. Excessive weight loss in two- and three-year old cows results in

delayed onset of estrus after calving and an increase in the percentage of nonpregnant animals and late calvers. Mature cows may reproduce satisfactorily on diets that are unsatisfactory for the younger cows. Thus, young cows respond favorably when fed a diet higher in energy than that fed to cows (Davis et al. 1977).

Dystocia in beef heifers is an important cause of perinatal calf loss. In primiparous heifers, dystocia is primarily a function of two factors: weight of the calf and weight and size of the dam (Makarechian et al. 1982). The weight of the calf is a function of genetic and environmental factors. Genetic factors include sex, length of gestation, breed, heterosis, inbreeding, and genotype. Nongenetic factors include age and parity of the dam as well as nutrition of the dam during various phases of gestation.

The ability to predict or reduce dystocia in light of present knowledge is far from adequate (Price and Wiltbank 1978). Bulls of certain breeds are known to sire heavy calves, whereas bulls of other breeds sire light calves. This is probably the best control of calf size currently available. However, within breed of sire and breed of dam, variation is still large and very unpredictable, and therefore calf size cannot be controlled. A few bulls within some breeds have been identified that sire calves in which the incidence of dystocia is low. The use of measurement of pelvic area to decrease the incidence of dystocia without utilizing some method of controlling or predicting calf size would be ineffective. However, a combination of culling heifers with small pelvic areas and using bulls that sire calves with small birth weights might reduce dystocia significantly (Makarechian and Berg 1983).

Dystocia rates in beef heifers cannot be reduced significantly by nutritional restriction during late pregnancy. In controlled feeding trials, the restriction of energy intake in the bovine female to a level that maintains maternal body weight has little influence on the development of the fetus, even though maternal metabolism may be altered considerably by the level of energy intake (Prior et al. 1979).

Within certain limits, experimentally, the level of material dietary energy does not influence fetal weight or composition (Prior and Laster 1979). However, the loss of 0.5 kg./day during the last trimester of pregnancy in beef heifers is associated with weak labor, increased dystocia rates, increased perinatal mortality, reduced calf growth rate, prolonged postpartum anestrus, and a reduced pregnancy rate (Kroker and Cummins 1979). These are not evident in heifers that are maintaining or gaining weight at a moderate rate during late pregnancy. It is recommended that heifers be fed to allow modest rates of body weight gain (0.5 kg./day) during late pregnancy.

The effect of winter body weight loss in beef cows on calf birth weight and subsequent performance of the calf to weaning is not clear. Some results indicate that an average Hereford cow winter body weight loss of 60 kg. to calving reduces birth weight by approximately 2 kg. (Jones et al. 1979) and even up to 20% (Tudor 1972), whereas other observations report that a 50-kg. loss in cow weight had no effect on calf birth weight (Jordan et al. 1968). These differences may be due to the body condition of the cows (degree of fatness, body score) at the beginning of winter. The effect of cow body weight loss during the winter months on calf performance from birth to weaning and weaning weight is also variable. Some studies indicate no significant effect of winter weight loss on the average daily gain or weaning weight of the calf (Jones et al. 1979), whereas other reports indicate that weaning weights increase with amounts of winter feed provided to the dam. Undernutrition of beef cattle during late pregnancy may result in a marked decrease in body weight of the cows, which is regained within several months after calving (Hight 1966). However, the percentage calf crop at weaning is markedly reduced, and the weaning weight of calves born to underfed cows is also much lower.

The level of energy intake can markedly alter reproductive performance in two-year-old heifers nursing their first calves. Pregnancy rates 120 days after calving are directly related to the postcalving energy intake level (Dunn et al. 1969).

Protein malnutrition in late pregnancy may be a factor contributing to neonatal mortality in beef calves. Beef cows fed 0.37 kg. crude protein/day during the last four months of pregnancy had a decreased gestation period of 274 days versus 282 days and decreased weight gains compared to controls fed 0.96 kg. (Waldhalm et al. 1979). Calf mortality in the low-protein group was due to dystocia or prematurity. Cow weight and weight loss is a function of the interactions within a herd. Genetic background, breed of cow, management, amount and quality of feed, and degree of shelter provided during cold and windy weather all have a part to play in weight loss.

The challenge is to provide an adequate and economical diet to pregnant cattle during the winter months that will *minimize weight loss*, produce *healthy vigorous calves* that receive adequate levels of colostrum, and result in a high pregnancy rate during a restricted breeding season. This may be accomplished by a plan that includes the following:

1. Cows should not lose excessive weight in the fall of the year. Cows going into the winter months in good body condition can lose more weight without deleterious effects on reproductive performance than cows that are in poor body condition at the beginning of winter.

2. First-calf heifers and young and mature cows should be divided into groups for the winter feeding program.

3. A random sample (10%) of each group of cows should be weighed three times during the winter—beginning, mid-way, and a few weeks before calving. This will serve as a monitoring system of cow weights and allow economical adjustments in the diet depending on weight loss or gain.

4. First-calf heifers should be fed separately from mature cows because the effect of an energy deficiency is much greater in heifers than in cows.

5. The wintering diet of pregnant cattle should provide the nutritional requirements for maintenance and pregnancy. Cow weight losses should not exceed the weight of the fetus and its fluids. In countries where the winter months are cold, the maintenance requirements for energy will increase from 15 to 65%, depending on the body condition of the cow and whether shelter from cold winds is provided.

In areas where specific mineral and vitamin deficiencies are known to occur, supplementation with the necessary nutrients is necessary; the details can be obtained from standard feeding guides.

Veterinarians should encourage farmers to assess their available feed supplies at the beginning of winter, submit samples from new batches of feed for analyses, and formulate the diet that will provide optimal results and yet be economical. The goal is to use the most inexpensive feed or combination of feeds that will provide the nutrient requirements necessary for continued optimum reproductive performance. This means that a cow must deliver a viable calf, return to heat, and conceive by 80 days following calving, and wean a calf that is heavy enough to provide above average net returns.

The alternative method of feeding pregnant beef cows is to practice the old adage "The eye of the master feeds his cattle." In fact, most beef farmers monitor body condition of their cows by visual evaluation and increase or decrease the quantity and quality of feed as necessary. The cows are fed to satisfy a certain level of body condition that by previous experience of the farmer has been associated with satisfactory performance. This, of course, leads to a wide variation in results because of the inherent inaccuracies in visual appraisal of animals that are being examined every day by the same attendant.

Parasite Control. Where applicable, the entire herd should be treated for warbles, *Hypoderma* sp., after the first killing frost with a suitable systemic insecticide. If the herd is confined throughout the winter months, all cattle should be examined regularly for evidence of louse infestation and treated accordingly. Suitable control for other indigenous parasites is indicated.

Wintering Grounds. In countries with cold winter climates, where beef cattle are confined and fed in small holding areas, there should be adequate bedding to prevent excessive build-up of manure, and a shelter break from wind should be provided. The wintering grounds should be easily accessible for the transportation of feed. The pregnant females should be divided into two or more different groups for winter feeding. The young mature cows in good condition need the least amount of daily surveillance and will usually do well on a diet that provides the needs for maintenance and pregnancy. Pregnant heifers need more surveillance and their nutritional requirements are greater because they are still in the stages of early growth. Older cows cannot compete with more aggressive mature cows in better condition and may need additional feed to minimize losses in body weight and in some cases to prevent starvation. Also, the wintering grounds should be separate from the calving grounds. The cattle should be moved from their wintering grounds about one month before calving. This separation of wintering grounds from the calving area will minimize the degree of contamination from the build-up of manure and ensure that calves are born in a clean environment. The management of the herd during the calving season to minimize neonatal mortality is discussed in the next section under the calving visit.

Diseases of Pregnant Beef Cattle. The diseases that occur in pregnant beef cattle will depend on the diseases that occur in the area, and control will depend on the expected incidence of each disease. Specific control measures are usually not indicated for sporadic diseases such as foot rot, actinobacillosis, and pinkeye. These diseases are treated as they occur.

Other diseases that may occur in outbreak form in pregnant beef cattle include hypocalcemia and hypophosphatemia, hypomagnesemia, starvation, pregnancy toxemia, and abomasal impaction. These are nutritionally related diseases and can be controlled satisfactorily by the provision of an adequate diet throughout the winter months.

Health and Management of Heifer Replacements and Breeding Bulls During the Winter Season

HEIFER REPLACEMENTS. In order to optimize lifetime production, calving heifers at two years of age has become a widely accepted practice among beef producers. If a heifer is to calve at 24 months of age, she must be cycling and fertile at 15 months of age. However, many 15-month-old heifers have not reached puberty. Puberty in heifers is influenced by age, growth rate, breed, and level of nutrition. Age at puberty, date of conception, and conception rate are largely determined by management of heifers during the winter period immediately after weaning. Reproductive performance is enhanced if heifer calf replacements are fed to gain weight at a rate of at least 0.5 kg./day from weaning to breeding. Thus, replacements should gain approximately 100 kg. from weaning to breeding. The winter weight gains may be more beneficial than the gains during the breeding season (Leminager et al. 1980).

Aborted fetuses, samples of placenta, and serum samples from cows that abort should be submitted to a diagnostic laboratory. Abortion should not exceed 2% of all pregnant heifers and cows. Abortion rates above this require detailed epidemiologic and laboratory examinations.

A management system for replacement heifers from weaning through to breeding includes the following:

1. For each 100 heifer replacements required, place about 150 heifers in the wintering grounds and before breeding select for retention those that become pregnant in a six- to eight-week period.

2. Feed heifers from weaning through to breeding to gain 0.5 kg./day. They should continue to gain weight throughout the breeding season.

3. Vaccinate heifer replacements for those diseases that can cause abortion—infectious

bovine rhinotracheitis, vibriosis, and lepto-spirosis—depending on the occurrence of these diseases in the area.

4. Provide suitable permanent identification.

5. Weigh heifers three weeks before breeding to determine the critical minimum weight.

BREEDING BULLS. Breeding bulls may be raised on the farm or bought as service-age bulls directly from another herd or from farm bull sales. Some bulls offered at sales have been evaluated for superior growth rate at test stations. The evaluation of bulls for breeding soundness has been described earlier.

Bull calves destined to become breeding bulls should be fed for maximum growth throughout the winter months. A complete vitamin and mineral-salt mixture should be included in the diet at recommended levels. Yearling bulls are susceptible to nutritional osteodystrophy and degenerative joint disease, which may be made worse by marginal deficiencies of calcium and phosphorus. Offering the vitamins and minerals ad libitum is not reliable, and these ingredients should be incorporated in the diet.

Service-age bulls that have been used for one or more breeding seasons require little specific attention throughout the winter months. They should be kept on a maintenance diet and should not be fattened. Two months prior to the breeding season, supplemental feed should be increased to condition the animal for breeding. Breeding bulls should be vaccinated for those diseases that may cause abortion in the cow herd. All bulls should be subjected to an examination for breeding soundness each year. In cold climates, freezing of the testicles may have occurred, which will result in poor semen quality.

Precalving and Calving Visit

The precalving and calving visits consist of the provision of advice on the management of the beef herd before and during the calving period. The emphasis is on reduction of perinatal and neonatal calf mortality. The two major concerns are (a) *getting a live calf* and (b) *keeping the calf alive* during the first week of life when calf mortality is usually high. Because the body condition and nutritional status of the heifers and cows before and after calving has a major influence on subsequent reproductive performance during the breeding season that follows, the veterinarian must incorporate these findings with those related to calf health. Unless he is a resident vet-erinarian, it is unlikely that he will visit the farm herd more than once or twice during the calving season. Several emergency visits may be made to attend to dystocia, but it is difficult to give meaningful advice while in a hurry. However, the veterinarian should make a scheduled visit to the herd about one month before the first calf is expected, to examine the nutritional status of the herd, the calving grounds, the facilities available for handling dystocias and weak and orphaned calves, and the plans for handling cow/calf pairs after calving. Thus, the role of the veterinarian here is to provide advice based on examination of the herd and the facilities. The role of the farmer is to consider the advice, introduce as much of it as is practical and economical, and keep adequate records on abortions, calving dates, number and nature of dystocias, and calf mortality. The farmer must be encouraged to consult with the veterinarian regularly throughout the calving season. Plans for calving grounds, calving facilities, and nursery pastures (pastures for cow/calf pairs) should be made during the previous year. This is especially true in countries with cold, snow-covered winters of several months' duration. Unless plans and construction are carried out during the summer months, it is usually not possible to adequately construct calving pad-docks and nursery pastures during the middle of the winter, when the frozen ground is covered by considerable snow. In grassland countries where snow cover is not a problem and calving occurs on open pasture, the problem of perinatal and neonatal calf mortality due to cold exposure and acute undif-ferentiated neonatal diarrhea may not be as critical as in countries where calving occurs in late winter and early spring.

Management of the Beef Herd at Calving to Minimize Perinatal Mortality Due to Dystocia and Abnormal Maternal Behavior. Dystocia, stillbirths, weak calves, and maternally ne-glected calves are major causes of perinatal mortality. The mortality rate is much higher in calves born to first-calf heifers than in calves born to mature cows. Thus, much more surveillance, obstetrical assistance, and care of the newborn calves must be provided for the heifers and their calves.

In Western Canada, the management cycle of most beef herds follows a typical pattern. First-calf heifers and cows with spring-born calves are dispersed onto summer pasture or range areas in April and May for breeding in June and July and remain there until the calves are weaned, usually in October or November. The pregnant females are fed winter roughage, usually mixed hay or straw plus some grain, or silage for a variable length of time from November to May, depending on the amount of snowfall and the availability of feed. Calving begins as early as January in some herds and may continue into May and June; however, peak calving rates occur in March and April.

The distribution of time of normal parturition in beef cows is relatively uniform over a 24-hour period (Yarney et al. 1982). There may be an uneven distribution of the time of abnormal parturition, with the highest incidence occurring from 1100 hours to 1500 hours and the lowest from 2300 hours to 0300 hours. There is some indication that the distribution of calvings between day and night can be altered by time of feeding. Feeding at 2200 hours may result in 79% of cows calving between 0600 hours and 2200 hours (Lowman et al. 1981).

The system described here will deal with the principles of management of beef herd calving in late winter and early spring as is done in Canada, but the general principles are applicable to the management of the beef herd at calving time regardless of the region. The major objectives are to get a live calf and to keep it healthy during the first few weeks of life when it is most vulnerable to infectious diseases (Radostits and Acres 1983).

The prerequisites of the system are:

1. *The calving grounds are separate from the wintering grounds.* The calving grounds should be scraped free of snow if possible, well-drained, and bedded with straw or wood shavings if available, to minimize the exposure rate of newborn calves to infectious agents.

2. *The first-calf heifers are calved separate from the cows.* Heifers need more intensive surveillance and obstetrical assistance than cows.

3. *In large herds, the heifer herd, particularly, is divided into small subgroups of 40 to 50 animals for more effective surveillance and early detection of animals that need obstetrical assistance.*

4. *The dam and its calf are moved out of the calving area to a nursery pasture 24 hours after the birth of the calf.* They are kept and fed there until calving is finished; then the herd is moved out to summer pasture.

5. *Surveillance and obstetrical assistance are provided on a 24-hour basis if possible.* With a restricted breeding season of 42 to 60 days, it becomes economical in large herds to employ the assistance necessary to provide continuous surveillance over a short period of time.

Detailed features of the system for calving heifers on a large commercial beef cattle ranch are summarized here (Church and Janzen 1978). Some of the practices may be applicable to other beef herds.

The calving-maternity unit is close to other relevant facilities consisting of working corrals, scales, and feeding pens. The main feature of the unit is a maternity barn with 55 8- × 10-foot box stalls. The floor of the pens and center alleyway is compacted porous sand. The calving area is a preparation, storage, and observation room. The entire calving-maternity unit operates on a continuous through-put basis.

Two to three weeks before the beginning of the calving season, the pregnant heifers are moved from the winter feeding area to a large precalving holding area. Each day, or every second day, heifers that appear to be within a few days of calving are identified visually and moved to one of two observation pens. In the observation pens, the heifers are mechanically fed hay in fence-line feed bunks. The pens are bedded with wood shavings and have overhead lights to facilitate 25 hours surveillance by the animal attendants. The smallest observation pen can be continuously observed through windows in the preparation room of the calving section. Heifers that are expected to calve within 24 hours are placed in the small observation pen to allow easier observation during darkness. The large observation pen is scrutinized by riders on horseback.

Often, the first sign of parturition is the passing of the cervical seal, which shows as thick, tenacious mucus clinging to the vulva or tail. Heifers may begin parturition anywhere from two hours to two or three days after passing the cervical mucus. Frequently, the heifers will pass vaginal secretions from the vulva when lying down that often resemble the cervical seal. The stage of relaxation begins about one to three hours before the beginning of the first stage of labor. During relaxation, the heifers are usually noticed to be carrying their tails elevated and to be slowly walking around the resting area sniffing the ground. Occasionally, they will turn their heads toward the flank and switch their tails. This behavior appears to be a reliable indication of imminent parturition. As the heifers progress into the second stage of parturition, abdominal contractions become evident, and the chorioallantoic membrane usually protrudes from the vulva in 30 to 60 minutes. During this stage, the heifers are frequently very restless and may get up and change position several times. During this period of restlessness, the chorioallantoic membrane usually ruptures, and fluid is expelled. Abdominal contractions become more forceful, and protrusion of feet—encased in the amnion—from the vulva is frequently seen in five to 30 minutes. Heifers normally expel the fetus within 30 to 60 minutes after the chorioallantoic membrane has ruptured. Heifers that are observed not to be making any progress or that have gone over 60 minutes of hard labor without expulsion of the fetus are brought into the working area for assistance.

Heifers that have been in hard labor without progress for about one hour will frequently tire, cease laboring, get up, and start to walk around and enter a stage of inertia. Occasionally, attendants may provide light hand assistance in observation pens to heifers that remain recumbent when approached. These guidelines for assistance have been established in order to ensure as high a percentage of strong viable calves as possible.

Calves born without assistance are left in the observation pens and observed to be certain that they suck and that the heifer accepts or "mothers" them. Usually, after 12 to 24 hours, when the newborn calf and dam have "paired off" well, they are moved to a nursery pasture. Those that do not nurse and heifers that do not accept their calves are moved into the maternity unit for special assistance. Heifers requiring assistance are brought into the restraining chute, and examined, and obstetrical assistance is provided if necessary.

Calves born with assistance should be evaluated immediately for evidence of hypoxemia and given appropriate assistance. Calves that are weak or handicapped with an edematous tongue or that are injured during the birth process should be given colostrum, preferably milked from its dam immediately after birth. This can be given by gravity flow using a plastic bag and stomach tube.

Assisted heifers and their calves are placed in clean, well-bedded box stalls in the maternity barn so that a bank of stalls is occupied at one time while another bank is being cleaned and scraped and allowed to dry. While in the maternity barn, the calves and heifers are regularly observed for nursing, mothering, expulsion of placenta, neonatal diarrhea, or other problems. A daily record for each heifer and calf is kept up to date. When calves are nursing strongly and paired with their dam, they are moved from the barn to the first postcalving holding area, usually after 24 hours in the barn. Any calves encountering difficulty are kept in longer until they are ready to go out with the heifer.

Heifers and calves in the first holding area have access to an automatic waterer and are mechanically fed loose hay on the ground. They are observed frequently for mothering, nursing, and health problems. After several days in the first holding meadow, they are all paired up and moved to a second holding meadow where they remain for several more days. Finally, they are moved to a third large meadow where they will remain until they are moved out to spring pasture. All holding pastures are regularly observed, and any animals with problems are moved back to nearby pens at the maternity unit for necessary attention.

Confinement of Hereford heifers in a pen during parturition may result in a marked increase in the incidence of dystocia and stillbirths when compared with animals left to calve in either a paddock or a large yard (Duffy 1981). Also, the continued presence of an observer during second-stage labor may be associated with an increase in both calving problems and assisted parturitions.

Maternal neglect of calves requires constant surveillance. Every calf that is born is closely monitored to be certain it is nursing and the heifer accepts it. Heifers that refuse to mother their calves are confined to box stalls and are tied up twice a day, if necessary, to allow the calf to nurse. If the calf is too weak to nurse or refuses to suckle, the heifer is milked and the calf fed by stomach tube. Calves that are born weak or that suffer from exposure are placed in incubators with heat lamps and are bottle-fed or fed with a stomach tube. Frequently, heifers that produce weak calves and those with prolonged or difficult births are liable to neglect their calves.

The attendants supervising the newborn/dam pairs in the postcalving holding pastures continually watch for abandoned calves or those that have been attacked by predators. Coyotes, ravens, magpies, and eagles are common predators and will quickly attack weak or neglected newborn calves.

The mixed-aged cows are calved on calving grounds separate from the heifers. Surveillance and obstetrical assistance is usually provided only during daylight hours. Both cows and calves are observed visually during the day for any evidence of maternal neglect, orphaned calves, and illness of the cow or calf.

Induction of Parturition with Corticosteroids. Parturition may be induced before full term using synthetic corticosteroids (MacDiarmid 1983a, 1983b). Reasons include to synchronize the calving period with the seasonal availability of feed supplies; to ensure that calving coincides with the availability of labor; to facilitate observation and management of calving; to overcome the inconvenience caused by late-calving cows; and to avoid or minimize dystocia problems.

In large breeding herds, toward the end of the calving period it may be desirable to induce parturition two to three weeks before full term in those animals that are late calvers. This will accelerate the completion of calving in the herd and make it possible to move the herd out to the summer pastures.

When it is desirable to induce parturition within the last two to three weeks of pregnancy, single injections of short-acting corticosteroids such as dexamethasone, betamethasone, and flumethasone are reliable and predictable. In most cases, calving will occur within two to three days. Earlier in pregnancy, the short-acting corticosteroids are less effective, and long-acting formulations are most reliable. However, the response time tends to be variable and unpredictable, a problem that can be overcome by use of an initial priming dose of long-acting steroid followed several days later by an injection of a short-acting formulation.

The problems associated with the induction of parturition include stillbirths, neonatal mortality due to prematurity, retained fetal membranes, metritis, and subsequent lowered reproductive performance in the cow.

Induction of parturition in the last two to three weeks of pregnancy with short-acting corticosteroids is usually successful. The ability to absorb colostral immunoglobulins is not impaired in calves born following the use of short-acting compounds. In contrast, calves born earlier following the use of long-acting steroids are lethargic, slow to stand and suck properly, and do not absorb immunoglobulins normally because of prolonged effects of the corticosteroid. Calves born prematurely, 14 to 32 days before term, may grow slower than calves born closer to term, and the effect of growth rate may last for up to six months.

The incidence of retained fetal membranes is greater in cattle in which parturition has been induced than in animals calving at full term (MacDiarmid 1983b). The literature indicates that the incidence in induced animals varies from 8 to 93%, whereas in naturally calving animals, the incidence varies from 0 to 20%. The effect of the retained fetal membranes on subsequent fertility is not clear. Some field trials indicate a subsequent delay in conception, whereas in others there was no significant effect. Most cows with retained fetal membranes lasting longer than 24 hours will develop varying degrees of metritis and delayed uterine involution.

In pasture-bred beef cattle in which the exact breeding dates are unknown, the induction of parturition should be limited to those animals that are due to calve in two to three weeks. This requires that the herdsman visually examine each animal in the group and select those that appear to be close to calving. Those that appear to be more than three weeks from term should not be induced unless deemed necessary. In large herds, the number of animals induced should be limited to a size that the animal attendants can ably supervise and provide with obstetrical assistance and care for the newborn calves. The birth of a large number of calves during a period of a few days can result in a heavy workload, maternal neglect by two-year-old heifers presumably because of the confusion created by all the births, and an increase in neonatal mortality due to exposure to cold, predation, septicemia, and acute undifferentiated diarrhea.

Control of Acute Undifferentiated Infectious Diarrhea and Other Infections of Newborn Beef Calves. A major cause of neonatal mortality of beef calves from one to 20 days of age is acute diarrhea due to one or a combination of the following: enterotoxigenic K99[+] *E. coli*, rotavirus, coronavirus, and *Cryptosporidia* sp. Epidemiologic observations indicate that herd epidemics occur commonly and may affect 30 to 50% of all calves born; the case fatality rate can vary from 10 to 30%.

Many herd problems with calf diarrhea are initiated because cows are crowded during the winter season (Radostits and Acres 1983). As the degree or duration of confinement in the winter feeding area increases, the risk of transmission of enteropathogens from carrier cows to other cows and heifers in the herd also increases. Hence, a large portion of cows may be shedding enteropathogens in their feces or have contaminated udders and underbellies when they are moved to the calving area. When this occurs, calving grounds that were relatively "clean" can become heavily contaminated very quickly. A similar pattern of events may occur even when cows are not confined during the winter period but are crowded into a relatively small area for calving. Even worse, winter feeding and calving may be done in the same area.

Newborn calves that are confined to the calving area further increase the population density, which not only increases the transmission of infectious agents but also increases stress and reduces transfer of passive immunity. Calves born into a highly contaminated environment may become infected during or shortly after birth and remain clinically normal but shed enteropathogens, thereby contributing further to environmental contamination. Diarrheic calves become a primary source of infection not only for other calves but also for adult animals and the environment. Hence, management of the beef herd throughout the winter and spring should be aimed at breaking the cycle of transmission of enteropathogens from carrier animals to the environment and eventually to newborn calves. This can be done by increasing resistance and decreasing the risk of infection of both cows and newborn calves. The management techniques used for prevention and control of epidemics of diarrhea are similar. However, preventive management provides many more options, because it involves integrating a variety of procedures into the herd management program throughout the year. In contrast, when faced with trying to control an epidemic that is already under way, producers are restricted to using far fewer management procedures. They must deal with an immediate problem and therefore can use only those procedures that can be adapted and applied quickly. Alteration of management during spring calving is made even more difficult because resources such as labor, feed, and bedding are limited, or their application is restricted by inclement weather or shortage of facilities.

Proper management implies several things. It implies the ability to recognize a potentially dangerous situation and to adjust management procedures to remove the potential hazards. For example, a heavy snowfall creates a potentially dangerous situation for several reasons. Herds are often confined, causing a build-up of contamination in the wintering area and on the cows. When the snow starts to melt, usually after some calves are already on the ground,

the ground surface becomes wet and muddy. Under these conditions, a potential exists for severe outbreaks. Steps should be taken before calving starts, to decrease this potential. Cows should not be wintered and calved on the same ground. The proposed calving area should be kept relatively free of snow, and the herd should be moved onto this area shortly before the onset of calving.

Proper management also implies the ability to recognize and correct the conditions that are causing a problem. No one can predict and avoid all of the potential dangers that will arise, and epidemics will still occur in spite of apparent good management in some herds. However, the duration and severity of many outbreaks can be limited by altering or modifying management programs as soon as problems arise. For example, a farmer may have calved his herd of 100 cows in a 12-acre field for the past two years and not had any diarrheic calves. However, this year he has increased the number of calving cows to 120, and early spring storms have made the ground surface much wetter than it was during the past two years. About 50% of the calves have diarrhea. He should recognize that the transmission distance between animals is reduced, since there are fewer square feet per cow/calf pair this year, because more cows are calving within the same total area. Also, if the ground surface is wet, the level of contamination with infectious agents is likely to be higher. He should allow each cow/calf pair more space, perhaps by dividing the herd into two groups of 60 or by moving to a larger area. He should also supply more clean, dry bedding than in previous years.

It is not possible to outline one management system that is suitable for all herds under all circumstances. There are at least five basic management principles for the prevention and control of calf diarrhea, each of which can be adapted in individual herds to a greater or lesser degree. The five principles are:

1. Reduction of the infection pressure on the calf
2. Remove the calf from the contaminated environment
3. Establish a high level of colostral immunity in the calf
4. Increase the specific immunity of the calf
5. Reduce stress

REDUCTION OF THE INFECTION PRESSURE ON THE CALF. It is not possible to completely remove the infectious agents that cause diarrhea from the calf's environment, but the infection pressure can be minimized. Some enteropathogens are carried by the cow and are transmitted to the calf during or shortly after calving. It is also likely that some bacterial and viral pathogens can survive for long periods in manure, contaminated bedding, and perhaps soil. Excess surface water, which is often a problem in calving grounds during the spring thaw, may be another source of contamination. Calving inside during the winter and spring can be particularly dangerous, because contamination builds up quickly in poorly ventilated, damp areas that are not exposed to sunlight. After treating or handling diarrheic calves, people also become a primary source of contamination.

The major objective is to keep the level of environmental contamination low so that the calf's natural defense mechanisms are not overwhelmed, particularly before it ingests colostrum. The following recommendations will assist in reducing and controlling the level of contamination:

- Avoid confining the herd as much as possible during the winter feeding period. Rotate feeding and bedding areas so that cows and heifers are not forced to remain in a contaminated environment. This will help to reduce the number of infected "carrier" cows that shed enteropathogens in their manure. Udders and underbellies will also be less contaminated, reducing the risk that cows and heifers will be a primary source of contamination when they are moved into the calving area.
- Do not calve cows and heifers in the same location where they were held during the winter months.
- Move cows and heifers into the calving area one to two weeks prior to the onset of calving. This will prevent the excessive accumulation of manure and contaminated bedding in the calving area.
- Do not allow cows and heifers to become "overconfined" during calving. The herd, particularly the heifers, must be observed during calving. However, they should not be restricted to small areas, particularly muddy corrals or small paddocks. Even animals calved on large areas can become confined by excessive snow or by restricting the placement of feed or bedding to the same area.
- Allow animals plenty of space at calving. If the ground surface is muddy or wet, allow more square feet per cow/calf pair. If the calving herd cannot be turned out because of excessive snow, plow or scrape strips on sidehills and hilltops so they have sufficient space to disperse. Change the location of feeding and bedding ground every few days to encourage the herd to migrate within the calving area.
- Do not calve in the same location year after year, particularly if diarrhea has been a problem in that area previously. Attempt to rotate calving grounds from year to year.
- Locate calving grounds to take advantage of natural shelter and where the soil type and the contour of the land allow natural drainage of surface water.
- Calving areas should be cleaned up and left vacant through the hot, dry summer months. All manure and excess bedding should be removed so that fresh, underlying soil is exposed.

Once an outbreak has started, it is very difficult to remove the source of contamination from the calving area. Even if diarrheic calves are isolated, infectious agents may survive for a period of weeks or months in contaminated barns or sheds, in bedding, soil, and ground surface water. Livestockmen who handle and treat sick calves also become a common and potent source of transfer of enteropathogens from calf to calf. If movement away from a contaminated calving area is not possible, provide as much clean, dry bedding as possible and attempt to disperse animals by spreading out bedding in the lounging areas. If possible, the person treating sick calves should not have any direct contact with newborn healthy calves.

REMOVE CALVES FROM THE CONTAMINATED ENVIRONMENT. The incidence of diarrhea is higher in calves born and kept in confinement than in calves born on open range. This is because as the number of square feet available per cow/calf pair in the calving area decreases, several things happen:

1. The calving area becomes more contaminated.

2. The transmission distance between animals decreases, thereby increasing the rate of passage of infectious agents from animal to animal.

3. The transfer of passive immunity from cow to calf may be impaired because of crowding.

4. Stress may increase.

Therefore, the potential for an outbreak of calf diarrhea is high when the entire pregnant herd is allowed to calve out in the same area and the calves are allowed to accumulate in the same location until all the calves are born.

Avoid Calving in Areas in Which the Level of Contamination with Infectious Agents is Likely to be High. These areas include:

1. Barns and sheds—the level of contamination builds up rapidly during the winter because effective cleaning and disinfection are difficult. In addition, ventilation and sunlight are restricted so that infectious agents survive for long periods. Therefore, avoid using barns or sheds that have been used to house or treat affected calves

2. Corrals and paddocks in which there is an excess of mud and manure or in which the animal population density is high

3. Local areas within the calving ground such as restricted feeding, watering, and bedding areas and low-lying areas with poor drainage.

4. Areas that have been contaminated by diarrheic calves

Attempt to calve in a clean, dry area where animals are not restricted in their movements. If calving has to be done in a confined area, try to remove the cow and calf to a new area as soon after birth as possible as described next.

PREVENT CROWDING IN THE CALVING AREA. A management system based on the dual principals of (1) dividing the calving herd into smaller subgroups and (2) dispersing newborn calves soon after birth will help prevent crowding and will also increase the ease of providing surveillance and assistance to those cows that need attention. Two such systems that have been used in Western Canada are outlined in Figure 9–1.

The herd of pregnant females is divided into smaller subgroups, which are calved in separate areas. In addition, the dam and the calf are moved out of the main calving area into a nursery area within one day of birth of each calf. This system helps to overcome the problems of crowding, mismothering, failure of calves to suck colostrum early enough, and calf diarrhea. By moving the cow/calf pairs out of the main calving area as the calves are born, the job of observing the remaining calving cows is also made much easier.

The following recommendations were suggested for the use of the divided calving areas:

1. The calving area is sheltered by trees or a wind-break fence (8 feet high, 20% porosity). A shelter and handling facilities may be included for difficult calvings. Nursery pastures each contain two calf shelters with a wind-break fence at each end. The calf shelters are 24 feet long, 10 feet deep, and 8 feet high in front and are easily moveable on skids. They are used primarily as creep areas, bedded for use of calves only.

2. The calf shelters are bedded with straw and made comfortable for the calves.

3. The water supply to the calving and nursery areas is provided by a winter water line and tank with an electric heater. If necessary, water troughs may be kept open by using propane or coal heaters, or water may be hauled by truck for short periods.

4. It is preferable to have an extra area (corral, barn) for chronically sick animals, weak calves that are sure to be a problem, and cows with no milk.

5. The pregnant cows are moved to the calving area approximately two weeks before calving. The bedding should be as clean and dry as possible, especially when calving starts.

6. Within one day after calving, the dam and calf are moved to one of the nursery areas.

7. The nursery areas are filled to maximum density of 35 to 40 cows for each 10- to 12-acre area.

8. The cow/calf pairs are kept in the nursery areas for approximately four weeks and then moved to the summer pastures when the youngest calf is about three weeks old.

9. In small herds, it may be possible to calve and maintain the herd in a corral until calving is complete, but it is not recommended.

10. With herds larger than 150 cows, the system can be duplicated. Alternately, older cows may be allowed to calve on the range, and heifers and other cows of particular concern (exotics, purebreds, known problem calvers) can be managed as described.

11. The calving and nursery areas are harrowed two or three times after use and left vacant until grass is re-established. They may be grazed over the summer as required, harrowed again in the fall, and left vacant for as long as possible over the winter months.

It is difficult to specify the ideal population density in each area because it will vary, depending on weather and ground surface conditions, the level of environmental contamination, and herd immunity. As a general rule, provide as much space per cow as possible. The system described here was originally designed so that 70 cows would calve in 16-acre pastures; however, the entire area is not always available to the cows because of heavy snowfall. Some advantages of this system are:

1. It is easier to examine the pregnant cows and heifers as one group and the cows that have already calved as another group.

2. Dams and calves are together with their own kind and find one another more readily.

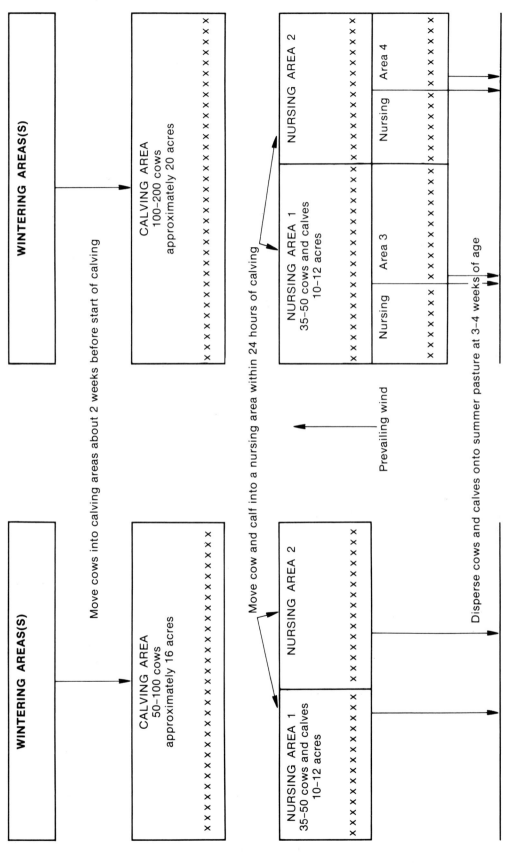

Figure 9-1. Lacombe-type beef herd calving management system for groups of 50–100 or 100–200 cows. xxx = 20% porosity fence

231

They are not disturbed by females that are close to calving claiming another's calf.

3. There is a more relaxed environment for the calf, less movement in the herd, and less likelihood of being trampled.

4. Calves of approximately the same age are grouped together, which facilitates movement to large pastures according to age and for branding and castrating schedules.

5. The herd is already divided if an outbreak of diarrhea develops.

Disadvantages include:

1. The initial cost of construction. This should be more than compensated for by reduced expenditures on medication and calf losses.

2. Increased time and labor for snow removal, feeding, bedding, and observing multiple groups. Reduced time spent on treating sick calves should compensate for these added inputs.

These recommendations can also be applied during an outbreak. Cows that have not yet calved should be removed from the contaminated calving area to a "clean" location, and one of the systems described above for reducing population density should be started. Most cases of *E. coli* diarrhea are initiated during the first 24 hours of life, so handling of calves during the first day should be avoided if possible. In order to break the cycle of infection, it may be necessary for livestockmen to take special precautions to avoid contaminating their hands, clothing, and boots. In some cases, it may be beneficial to wear disposable rubber gloves and clean coveralls if it is necessary to handle newborn calves when moving them from the calving grounds to holding areas or postcalving areas. Foot baths may also be used by workers moving from one pen to another. A fence line is normally sufficient to control spread.

ESTABLISH A HIGH LEVEL OF COLOSTRAL IMMUNITY IN THE CALF. The newborn calf must ingest colostrum within a few hours after birth. The antibodies in the colostrum are absorbed with maximum efficiency during the first six hours after birth; thereafter, the efficiency of absorption is reduced quickly and very little occurs after 24 hours.

If calves ingest liberal quantities of colostrum within 12 hours after birth, they will usually attain serum immunoglobulin levels high enough to prevent bacteremia, septicemia, and death from diarrheal dehydration. The minimum amount of colostrum that calves should ingest during the first 12 hours to attain satisfactory serum immunoglobulin levels is 50 ml./kg. of body weight (5% body weight). Therefore, a 40-kg. calf should get about 2 L. as soon as possible after birth.

Colostral immunoglobulin concentration is a major factor in the total amount of immunoglobulin absorbed from colostrum when it is fed to newborn calves (Stott and Fellah 1983). The greater the concentration of immunoglobulin in the colostrum, the greater is the total amount absorbed. However, the factors that influence the concentration of immunoglobulin in the colostrum of beef cattle have not been reported.

The amount of colostrum ingested by the calf within a few hours after birth is dependent on three factors:

1. *The amount of colostrum available from the dam*, which will depend on the maturity of the cow and adequacy of the nutrition throughout the winter. Based on a survey on one Hereford ranch, 50% of the two-year-old heifers had only 500 ml. or less of colostrum immediately after calving, 75% had only 750 ml. or less, and only 6% had between 1000 and 2000 ml. This suggests that under some conditions, heifers may not have sufficient colostrum. This shortage of colostrum is due to a combination of inheritance, lack of maturity, and inadequate nutrition. (Petrie et al. 1984).

2. *The maternal behavior of the dam and whether or not she lets the calf suck.* Maternal neglect may occur in up to 20% of two-year-old heifers. They make no effort to establish a dam/calf relationship and abandon their calves or do not allow them to suck. Some of these heifers can be encouraged to accept their calves. The heifer is restrained in a head gate and her hind legs hobbled so she can't kick. The calf is held up to the teats and encouraged to suck. Confinement of the heifer with the calf in a small pen for a few days will often result in acceptance of the calf. When the dam/calf relationship has been established (when the calf is sucking and is encouraged by the mother to suck), the cow and calf should be moved out of the main calving area to a nursery area or pasture. This will prevent overcrowding, which is a common predisposing cause of calf diarrhea.

3. *The vigor of the calf and whether or not it can suck the cow.* The vigor of the calf and its desire and ability to stand, "seek the teat," and suck the necessary amount of colostrum will depend on the health of the calf and the environment. Newborn calves may be weak at birth because of congenital defects and infec-

tion or because of a difficult and prolonged birth. The cause of the "weak calf syndrome" is still uncertain, but in utero infection of the fetus in late gestation is a possibility. Prolonged difficult dystocia may cause intrapartum hypoxia; edema of the soft tissues of the head, including the tongue; and inability of the calf to suck early enough. All of these calves must be given colostrum as soon as possible either by nipple bottle or force feeding using a stomach tube. Calves that are born in deep snow or are exposed to very cold and windy weather may become hypothermic, weak, and unable to stand or suck within one hour. These calves must be detected early, fed quantities of colostrum, and placed in a dry, weather-protected area until they have regained their strength.

INCREASE THE SPECIFIC IMMUNITY OF THE CALF. The degree of immunity to specific enteropathogens in each animal (individual immunity) and within herds (herd immunity) varies, depending on previous exposure to the infectious agents.

Most strains of *E. coli* known to cause diarrhea in calves possess the K99 antigen, which helps the bacteria to colonize the calf's small intestine (Bellamy and Acres 1979). The K99 antigen is a filamentous structure found on the surface of most enterotoxigenic *E. coli* (ETEC) regardless of serotype. Colostral antibodies against the K99 antigen will prevent diarrhea caused by K99 + ETEC (Acres et al. 1979). Under natural conditions, the colostrum of less than 10% of beef cows contains K99 antibody; therefore, many calves remain susceptible to *E. coli* diarrhea during the first few days of life even though they ingest colostrum soon after birth. Immunity to the K99 antigen can be induced by immunizing pregnant cows during the third trimester of gestation. Bacterins prepared from a K99 + strain of *E. coli* (*VICOGEN*—Connaught Laboratory, *COLIGEN*, Fort Dodge Laboratories) are available for administration to cows twice, the first time six weeks before calving and the second time about three weeks later. In the event of an outbreak, some beneficial immunity may develop within three weeks following the first injection. Cows that calve up to 45 to 60 days after the second injection have protective colostral antibody titers.

In contrast to the above, individual as well as herd immunity to rotavirus is high in beef herds in Western Canada. In a survey of 10 cows from each of 20 herds, 146 cows (73%) and 19 of 20 herds (95%) were positive for rotavirus anti-body (Mohammed et al. 1978). Therefore, over 70% of beef cows appear to have colostral levels of rotavirus antibody high enough to prevent diarrhea during the first five to seven days of life. However, colostral antibody levels decline rapidly after calving, and many calves probably become susceptible to rotavirus diarrhea by one week of age because antibody levels in the milk reaching the lumen of the small intestine are not high enough to prevent infection and multiplication of the virus (Saif and Smith 1983). Also, because of this decline in antibody levels, outbreaks of rotavirus diarrhea can occur year after year regardless of the presence of colostral antibody in most of the cows at calving.

When herd immunity is low, outbreaks of rotavirus diarrhea can occur in younger calves, but this appears to be the exception rather than the rule. Sporadic cases will also occur in younger calves if they do not ingest colostrum or when the volume of colostrum ingested is low (i.e., heifers).

A modified live virus vaccine that contains both rota- and coronaviruses can be administered to the cow prior to parturition. However, the differences in antibody titers in colostrum and whey between vaccinated heifers is not significantly different (Myers and Snodgrass 1982).

There is not, nor is there likely to be in the near future, a vaccine that is effective against all enteropathogens causing diarrhea in calves. Multiple-component vaccines that provide protection against several enteropathogens appear to be technically feasible and may become available within the foreseeable future. Although neither manufacturer of the above vaccines has recommended that both be administered together, there does not appear to be any reason at this time why they should not be administered at the same time, but by separate injection. This type of approach should be most beneficial in herds where infection with K99 + ETEC and rota- or coronavirus exists. Colostrum from vaccinated cows can also be frozen, stored, and fed to weak or neglected calves, or used for treatment of sick calves.

Apparent failure of the vaccines under field conditions may occur for a variety of reasons. Other enteropathogens, such as Cryptosporidia, *Salmonella* sp., and other viruses that are not related to the antigens in the vaccines, may be present. There may be strains of ETEC that colonize the small intestine by some mechanism other than K99 antigen and against which K99 antibody will not be protective. Such strains have not yet been identified. There is also increasing evidence that there are different strains of bovine rotavirus that could be immunologically distinct. If so, a viral vaccine prepared from one strain of virus might not protect against all other strains of the virus that occur in the field. Also, in herds where animals are crowded within the calving area or where the level of environmental contamination is high, the protective level of colostrum may be overwhelmed by infection pressure. Individual calves may also fail to ingest colostrum for a variety of reasons.

The decision to vaccinate the pregnant dams will depend on consideration of the risk factors in the herd. They are as follows:

1. Has the enteropathogen been isolated from diarrheic calves in previous years?

2. Is the disease considered to be economically important in the herd? Vaccination must be cost-effective.

3. What are the characteristics of the calving grounds? Is there sufficient area per calving animal; is the ground surface well drained; is there adequate protection from cold winds, and is it easy to move animals from one place to another?

4. What is the nutritional status of the pregnant animals? Will they have a sufficient amount of colostrum? A major factor in the efficacy of the vaccine is the amount of colostrum ingested by the calf.

5. What is the level of management? Vaccination is not a replacement for inadequate management. The recommendation to use any of the available vaccines for the control of diarrhea in calves in herds that are poorly managed may give the owner a false sense of hope; the results may be poor, and the reputation of the vaccine may be unjustifiably questioned.

THE REDUCTION OF STRESS. Stress is the reaction by which the animal body adapts to environmental conditions. The ability of newborn animals to adapt to changes in the environment is limited, and conditions that appear to have no effect on mature animals may be detrimental to the newborn calf. It has been recognized for many years that stress is a contributing factor in many individual cases and in outbreaks of calf diarrhea. However, because many different environmental conditions can cause stress and because stress is difficult to measure, it has not been possible to identify all of the factors that contribute to the problem. Also, some conditions such as overcrowding, which cause psychological and physical stress, also lead to increased levels of contamination and exposure to infectious agents.

The results of a questionnaire about the epidemiology of calf diarrhea sent to the ranchers in Alberta and Saskatchewan have helped to identify some of the factors that contribute to stress (Acres 1976).

1. *Inclement weather:* Many outbreaks occurred within 48 hours following snowstorms when the weather was classified as cold and changeable. Later in the spring, rain will also precipitate epidemics.

2. *Poor ground surface conditions:* Ground surface conditions preceding outbreaks were classified as "wet" by 81% of ranchers. Excess surface water and cold, wet bedding makes it difficult for calves to find a comfortable place to sleep and leads to the build-up and spread of contamination. Locate calving areas to take advantage of natural drainage away from surface water. Use clean, dry straw for bedding. Increase the amount and depth of bedding as ground surface conditions become wet or muddy.

3. *Crowding:* Crowding can cause stress and increase exposure to infectious agents. These two effects are difficult to separate; however, as the number of square feet per cow/calf pair decreases, the incidence of diarrhea increases.

During the first two weeks of life, calves spend most of their time sleeping or sucking. Under crowded conditions, their resting and feeding patterns may be altered. This stress, added to increased exposure to infectious agents, may result in a higher incidence of diarrhea. Every effort should be made to ensure that calves have a clean, dry, sheltered area in which nursing and resting are not disturbed.

Records of Calving. The following data is necessary to evaluate calving and calf health.

1. *Calving dates:* The date of first calving and the daily number of calvings until the last calf is born are necessary to evaluate the effectiveness of the breeding program. With an effective limited breeding season, 60 to 70% of the heifers and cows will calve within the first three weeks of the calving period, and 95% will calve within the first six weeks.

2. *Abortions:* Abortions that occur in late pregnancy are usually seen by the farmer; these should be recorded and should not exceed 2%.

3. *Number of dystocias:* Each dystocia should be recorded. The type and degree of obstetrical assistance should also be recorded,

i.e., manual assistance, fetal extractor, and the magnitude of the pull required. Cesareans are also noted and suitably identified for possible culling at weaning time. The theoretical objective is to have no dystocias. However, this is highly unlikely. The dystocia rate in first-calf heifers under the best conditions may be up to 15% and in the cow herd up to 2%.

    4. *Calf viability and statistics:*
      (a) Number of calves born alive
      (b) Number of calves born dead
        (i) Stillbirths; died just before birth; results of necropsy
        (ii) Died during or immediately after birth due to prolonged birth; results of necropsy
      (c) Number of calves that became ill in the first week of life and between the second and fourth weeks of life; reasons for illness (diarrhea, septicemia, navel-ill), number of deaths, and results of necropsy; treatments used and success rate
      (d) Number of calves mismothered by first-calf heifers and by cows; number of calves successfully re-mothered and number unsuccessful following attempts to encourage dam to accept the calf and allow it to suck
      (e) Number of calves with congenital defects
      (f) Number of calves lost or unaccountable

In a beef herd, most calf losses occur at or shortly after birth, and the losses range from 5 to 14%. Most losses occur in first-calf heifers, and 50% of the calves lost at birth can be saved by improved management, which includes continuous surveillance and the provision of prudent obstetrical assistance when necessary.

Following the losses that occur at birth, the next most common calf losses are those that are associated with infectious diseases, such as acute undifferentiated diarrhea, and those associated with exposure to inclement weather (cold climate, sudden unexpected snowstorms, and excessive heat).

Management of Calves From Two Months of Age to Weaning. Following the calving season, the herd is turned out to summer pasture until weaning. Health care management of the calves during this period is minimal except for routine branding and identification, routine vaccinations, prophylactic injections for specific nutritional deficiencies (vitamin E, selenium, and copper), and the treatment of clinical disease. In areas where clostridial diseases are endemic, calves should be vaccinated with the appropriate clostridial bacterins or toxoids. Calfhood vaccination for brucellosis may be indicated in areas in the early stages of an eradication program. Calves with clinical pinkeye should be caught and treated accordingly. All dead calves should be submitted for necropsy if feasible. Dates of vaccination, treatment of clinical disease, and number of dead calves should be recorded.

Advice That May Be Given at Any Visit

At each visit to the beef farm, there are a number of items that can be discussed and for which advice may be given. All observations and advice given should be recorded and submitted to the farmer in the form of a written report.

Vaccinations. The vaccines and vaccination schedules used will vary, depending on the location of the herd and the diseases that are considered endemic in the area. On most beef farms, calves are vaccinated against the clostridial diseases at the appropriate times. Although the most commonly used clostridial vaccine is the two-way vaccine containing *Clostridium chauvoei* and *Cl. septicum*, in some areas there may be a need for the multiple-antigen bacterin that contains *Cl. chauvoei, Cl. septicum, Cl. novyi types B and D, Cl. perfringens type D toxoid, Cl. tetani, and Cl. perfringens types B and C.*

Vaccination of the breeding herd against abortion due to the infectious bovine rhinotracheitis virus may be indicated if the disease is endemic.

An *E. coli* vaccine containing the K99+ antigen and used with the rotavirus and coronavirus vaccines may be indicated for herds with a problem of acute undifferentiated diarrhea in the newborn calves.

Other vaccines that may be indicated in a beef herd include *Leptospira* spp., *Vibrio* sp., bovine virus diarrhea, and *Brucella abortus*—strain 19.

Vaccination recommendations given by the veterinarian should be in the form of a written report that outlines specifically which vaccines are recommended, when they should be given, and the frequency of administration.

Disease Incidence. The diseases that have occurred since the last visit should be identified from the farm records. The morbidity and case fatality rates should be considered to determine any unusual trends. The methods of treatment used by the farmer and the results obtained should be discussed and new advice given in a written report. The results of necropsy examinations should be explained and any necessary action taken.

Management Changes. Any changes since the last visit by the veterinarian should be reported by the farmer. Changes in herd management that may profoundly affect the performance of the herd and that the veterinarian should be aware of include change of pasture, the introduction of new breeding animals, changes in weaning procedures, and changes in the nutrition of the cow herd during the winter months.

Nutritional Advice. The economical feeding of the beef herd is one of the most important factors that determine the magnitude of the profit or loss in a beef herd. Therefore, it is incumbent upon the veterinarian to monitor the nutrition of the herd to ensure that it is adequate to achieve optimal reproductive performance each year. The veterinarian should encourage the producer to assess the feeds available on the farm, have certain feeds analyzed by a feed testing laboratory, and assist the producer in formulating the most economical diet for the different age groups in the herd. The general feeding plans may not vary significantly from year to year, but often the details of the diet will change because of yearly variations in climate, growth of crops, and the availability of purchased feeds.

The most common nutritional deficiency in beef herds is a lack of sufficient feed containing sufficient energy to meet the demands of growth in young animals and the demands of reproductive performance and lactation. These deficiencies are easily recognizable but not always easily corrected because of economics. Mineral deficiencies are also common in beef cattle because they are not being hand-fed a balanced diet.

On certain farms that have experienced specific nutritional deficiencies, such as copper and selenium deficiencies, the strategies for provision of the nutrients must be determined.

Conduct of Trials Specific to Each Farm. There may be trials in which the response of animals to the administration of a nutritional supplement is measured. At a scheduled visit, the treatment and control groups can be selected and identified, the treatment applied, and the animals weighed. Subsequent weighings can be done by the farmer.

Surveillance Tests for Laboratory Examination. Blood samples should be taken from all cows that have aborted since the last visit and submitted for brucellosis and leptospirosis

testing. If specific nutritional diseases such as copper deficiency are suspected, blood samples may be taken from 10 to 25% of each age group. Feces may be collected if intestinal helminths are suspected. On farms with specific nutritional deficiencies, it may be desirable to obtain feed and soil samples in addition to blood samples at least twice annually in order to monitor the changes that are occurring following supplementation with the specific nutrient.

Introduced Cattle. All animals introduced to a herd should be kept isolated until the next subsequent visit and then examined. All should have a physical examination of the genital tract and, if possible, of the feet and legs, especially while walking, and of the mouth to ensure that the teeth and their apposition are satisfactory. A full clinical examination of all body systems may be appropriate for a single high-priced quiet animal but is unlikely to be very productive for the common run of young herd bulls or replacement heifers. All introduced cattle should have been tested and certified negative for brucellosis, tuberculosis, and leukosis. The vaccination history must be obtained and cattle not vaccinated for the common endemic diseases such as blackleg and perhaps infectious bovine rhinotracheitis should be vaccinated as soon as possible after arrival. All introduced cattle must be suitably identified and the information entered into the herd records with date of arrival and other pertinent data.

Advice on Genetics and Breeding Plans. In general, veterinarians have not been active in the provision of advice on applied genetics and breeding programs for beef cattle. However, they could be. Most beef farmers have used breeding plans and made the selection of breeding stock with little outside assistance. Selection of breeding stock for improvement of performance requires an understanding of the applied aspects of the science of heredity and an appreciation of the economically important heritable traits. Veterinarians engaged in beef herd health and production management can assist the farmer along with the animal geneticist in planning effective breeding programs that will result in continuous progress in performance. Breeding programs for commercial beef cow/calf herds have been described (Fredeen 1983).

Preparation of Reports. After each visit, a report should be prepared and sent to the farmer. It is essential that the results set out in each report be discussed with the farmer. On the basis of the discussion, it should be possible for the farmer to make management decisions on the length of the breeding seasons, the size of the breeding groups, vaccination schedules, anthelmintic administration, and the provision of specific nutrients such as copper and selenium. From the veterinarian's point of view, these discussions are profitable in bringing together all the laboratory findings, the history, the clinical findings, and the environmental and management factors so that the best diagnosis is made and the most appropriate action taken. Producers will respond and take notice of a written report that contains observations and recommendations, whereas the same recommendations given verbally are often not considered because they do not have the same impact as the written word.

Assessment of Performance in the Beef Cow/Calf Herd

Collection and Storage of Data. As set out in the first part of this book, it is essential that only critical data be collected. *The amassing of enormous amounts of data is uneconomical,* particularly to the beef producer who is accustomed to relatively little book work and only at isolated times during the year. Masses of paper are counterproductive. As in the dairy herd health system, the difficult question to decide is whether to allow farmers to record events as they happen—whether they will be relevant or not—or whether to have them record events in a structured diary that requires them to comment on a number of management and environmental matters on which information is specifically required. As in the dairy system, we compromise in our program by using both.

The documents used for recording the data include the Farmer's Event Diary, a Monthly Management Summary, and the Farm Information Report. They are discussed here.

FARMER EVENT DIARY. This is an unstructured diary, preferably self-carboned on one page so that at the end of each month the farmer can pull out the completed pages and forward them to the Data Analysis Bureau. In it he is requested to record daily events in the following categories: disease events—including deaths, illnesses, and treatments; reproductive events—including bulls in and bulls out, identities of bulls and cows in each breeding group, and births; climate—including rainfall and exposure to inclement weather; feed supply—including pasture, amounts and types of supplementary feeds fed to whom and for how long; feed supplementation and other practices used for health reasons; health materials used, e.g., worm drenches and louse sprayings; the detail of man-hours used in these events; and the purchase price or estimated value of materials used.

VETERINARIAN'S RECORD. The veterinarian is asked to record all of his observations and activities in the diary. These should include diagnoses, treatments, and special examinations, e.g., bull evaluations. The veterinarian must keep a record of all observations and examinations made during visits to the herd.

MONTHLY MANAGEMENT SUMMARY. Because it is essential to make a record of some matters every month, the diary is supplemented by a Monthly Management Summary, which the farmer is asked to send in together with his diary sheets at the end of each month. In this summary, the farmer comments on whether or not there has been rain during the month, what the climate was like, the status of the feed supply, and whether he had drenched, vaccinated, hand-fed, dosed with magnesium, or introduced a bloat-preventing mechanism.

It is important that information be provided that will permit the following matters to be determined: *Have cattle introduced to the herd been vaccinated against resident disease, checked for breeding soundness, treated for worms, lice, and so on?* Of the deaths that occurred, which of them were diagnosed only by the farmer and which *by a field veterinarian or by a laboratory?* Of those diseases that were identifiable by laboratory diagnosis, what proportion of them were in fact so diagnosed? *Is selection in the herd aimed at culling cows and bulls that produce calves with congenital defects?* Does selection for production in the herd include selection of animals who produce calves with high birth weight or high body weight at weaning? In the best of all possible circumstances, each of the questions will be answered by an "in diary" entry.

FARM INFORMATION REPORT. The two documents just mentioned are the principal methods of collecting information, but they are limited to collecting factual information on events as they happen. The annual updating of the Farm Information Report by the owner represents the only mechanism for recording the owner's overall management policy and general resources, including acreage, fertility, climate, and labor.

Result Reporting. The reporting of results can only derive from the data that has been collected, stored, and analyzed. In addition to the numerical results derived from that analysis and the financial estimates that flow on from them, there must be an assessment of the quality of that performance by the farm and recommendations on how any inadequacies should be corrected. As has been pointed out in previous chapters, the recording and analysis can be performed by a nonveterinarian, but the value judgments and medical recommendations are matters that must be dealt with by the veterinarian.

A decision on whether the performance in any of the productivity indices is abnormal will depend initially on whether it is outside the range of theoretical targets. As local data become available, it will become possible to substitute means and standard deviations from one's own results for these arbitrary targets. Part of the reason for the establishment of the data bank described earlier is to provide these locally-based answers. The answers will be so much better if they include a partial budgeting assessment of net losses incurred by shortfalls from targets. Ideally, recommendations for change should include the cost of and estimated returns from recommended changes.

Assessment of Annual Performance in the Beef Cow/Calf Herd. The following information should be collected as it becomes available throughout the production cycle of the herd.

BREEDING SEASON RECORD
1. Number of yearling heifers exposed to bulls
2. Number of bulls bred to yearling heifers
3. Dates of breeding heifers
4. Body weights of heifers three weeks before and at beginning of breeding season
5. Number of mixed-age cows exposed to bulls
6. Number of bulls exposed to mixed-age cows
7. Dates of breeding cows
8. Body condition scores of cows at beginning of breeding
9. Record of evaluation of bulls
10. Pregnancy rates:

(a) $$\frac{\text{Number of yearling heifers pregnant at pregnancy diagnosis}}{\text{Number of yearling heifers exposed to bulls}} \times 100$$

(b) $$\frac{\text{Number of mixed-aged cows pregnant at pregnancy diagnosis}}{\text{Number of mixed-age cows exposed to bulls}} \times 100$$

(c) Number of yearling heifers to be culled at time of pregnancy diagnosis and reasons
(d) Number of mixed-age cows to be culled at time of pregnancy diagnosis and reasons

WEANED CALF RECORD
1. Net calf crop is

$$\frac{\text{Number of calves weaned}}{\text{Number of females exposed to bulls}} \times 100$$

2. Average weaning weight: Individual calf weights range from lowest to highest; frequency distribution of calf weights

POSTWEANING RECORD. Postweaning average daily gain; yearling weight

CALVING RECORD
1. Abortion rate is

$$\frac{\text{Number of abortions}}{\text{Number of females pregnant at time of pregnancy diagnosis}} \times 100$$

2. Calving percentage is

$$\frac{\text{Number of females that deliver live calf}}{\text{Number of females diagnosed pregnant at time of pregnancy diagnosis}} \times 100$$

3. Distribution of calving is the daily frequency of calvings and the cumulative distribution of calvings throughout the period. The total number of calvings on each day is recorded. With an effective breeding program, 90% of the calvings will occur between 42 and 60 days after the beginning of the calving season.

4. Dystocia rate is

$$\frac{\text{Number of calvings requiring obstetrical assistance}}{\text{Number of calvings}} \times 100$$

5. Stillbirth rate is

$$\frac{\text{Number of calves born dead at term}}{\text{Number of calvings}} \times 100$$

The stillbirth rate includes calves that are born dead at term unassisted and those that die within a few minutes after an assisted birth associated with dystocia. Both groups may be due to intrapartum hypoxemia and/or injuries associated with dystocia. However, they may also be due to illness of the fetus at term.

6. Birth weight of calves: Born alive and unassisted; born alive and assisted; born dead and unassisted

7. Postnatal calf mortality: Birth to 10 days; 10 days to 30 days; one month to weaning

ANIMAL HEALTH. Dates and diagnoses of illnesses in any animal; include treatments used and outcome; include dates and diagnoses of all mortalities; include results of necropsies

NUTRITION RECORD. Record feeds used on each group of animals throughout the year; record results of all feed analyses; record body condition score of pregnant females

Targets of Performance. The performance indices of the herd must be evaluated against targets of performance that are practical and possible in commercial herds. They are as follows:

1. Pregnancy rate (42- to 60-day breeding period): Yearling heifers—95%; mixed-age cows—100%
2. Per cent females culled for infertility at time of pregnancy diagnosis (42- to 60-day breeding period): Yearling heifers—not to exceed 5%; mixed-age cows—not to exceed 15%
3. Calving record:
   (a) Abortion rate: Not to exceed 2% of all pregnant females
   (b) Calving percentage: 96%
   (c) Distribution of calving: 90% of calves should be born within a 42- to 60-day period
   (d) Dystocia rate: Two-year-old heifers—not to exceed 15%; mixed-age cows—not to exceed 5%
   (e) Stillbirth rate: Not to exceed 2%
   (f) Postnatal calf mortality: Birth to 10 days of age—not to exceed 5%; 10 days to 30 days of age—not to exceed 2%; one month to weaning—not to exceed 1%
4. Weaned calf record: Net weaned calf crop—85%; weaning weight (as percentage of cow weight)—60%
5. Growth rate of heifer replacements from weaning to breeding: 100 kg.
6. Cow mortality: Not to exceed 2% annually

Purebred Pedigree (Stud) Beef Herds

The policies relevant to preventive medicine and pedigree beef herds resemble those applied to dairy herds rather than to commercial beef herds. When newborn calves are worth $500 to $1000 rather than $50 to $100, the economic pressures to ensure that the reproductive and survival indices are maintained are greatly increased. The expenditure to protect this capital investment is correspondingly expanded. Monthly visits are more commonly the practice than two to three seasonal visits used for commercial herds. A suggested program follows. It is designed for a spring calving period in the northern hemisphere and can be adjusted for other circumstances simply by changing the months.

January–February

1. Check that first-calf and second-calf heifers are on a sufficiently good level of nutrition, preferably by weighing, to ensure good calf weights without causing overfatness and dystocia and to provide a good basis for rapid return to estrus after calving. *Adult cows are dealt with in the same way, but they are not so much at risk as the heifers.*

2. Any maternal vaccinations aimed at creating high levels of antibodies in colostrum and hence a passive immunization of calves should be carried out. Enteric colibacillosis is an example.

3. Ensure that supplies and facilities are available for calves starting to appear next month.

March–April

This is the calving season, and preparations should be made early for all the activities that will occur. There must be intensive surveillance of calving groups, especially heifers, not only to assist with calving difficulties but also to ensure that calves are properly identified and mothered, to identify whether or not they are born alive, and—if they are born alive—that they can in fact stand and drink colostrum; a minimum intake of a pint in the first 2 hours is essential.

Each calf should be identified by tag and checked for congenital defects, especially of the teeth, heart, nervous system, and external genitalia. When necessary, the following injections should be given: vitamins A, D, and E, and selenium and copper.

All cows that are subject to dystocia or retained placenta or that have a vaginal or uterine discharge should be examined and treated if necessary and identified for future reference. The treatments should be continued until the discharge ceases.

The treatment of calves for the prevention of individual diseases is presented under diseases of dairy calves.

May

Arrange prebreeding weighing of heifers to

determine if feed supplementation is necessary. Intensively examine all bulls for breeding soundness. All cows that are to be bred are examined to determine whether there has been satisfactory involution of the uterus.

Other tasks include castration and dehorning, vaccination at two months of age for infectious bovine rhinotracheitis, bovine virus diarrhea, parainfluenza-3 virus, and the clostridial diseases, and leptospirosis if necessary. If vaccination against vibriosis is indicated, this should be done now. Heifers commencing their breeding life should be vaccinated twice, the injections being six weeks apart and the booster being given 10 days before breeding. Older animals receive one vaccination each year at this time.

June–July

This is the breeding period. Postnatal examinations of cows to assess uterine involution or prebreeding examinations of uteruses, especially in cows that have had retained placenta or dystocia, are recommended. Arrange dietary supplementation of females to provide extra energy and encourage greater fertility. *This is also a season of greatest risk of hypomagnesemia, and either energy or magnesium or both should be provided in the diet for animals outside.* Establish adequate surveillance of breeding activity of bred females to ensure that the fertility level of each bull is being maintained. Animals still on the farm and at pasture at 15 months of age need to be treated for ostertagiasis at this time. Where fascioliasis is enzootic, all animals should be treated now.

The bulls are turned into the breeding pastures for six to eight weeks. The heifers are usually given two weeks extra, the bulls being put in earlier and taken out at the same time as the cows. Some purebred herds breed singly by hand-mating with a bull or by artificial insemination. Heat detection becomes very important in these circumstances. Accurate identification of the sire is essential.

Creep-feeding may be instituted at this time.

September–October

Weaning of calves, pregnancy diagnosis, and culling of nonproductive animals take place at this time. A pre-immunization or preconditioning program for the calves to be weaned is done at this time. Calves are vaccinated and placed on a weaning ration at least two weeks before weaning.

All females that are not pregnant are separated and possibly reexamined, and a decision is made about immediate culling and slaughter.

Females with significant clinical abnormalities are likewise identified and a decision made about disposition.

Reasons for culling include chronic incurable lameness, advanced squamous cell carcinoma, chronic clinical mastitis, unthriftiness of unknown etiology, and any chronic incurable disease that interferes with production.

November–December

The available feed supplies and nutrient requirements for the herd throughout the winter months should be evaluated.

OTHER ACTIVITIES. Most owners of purebred herds find it worthwhile to conduct annual tests for brucellosis and tuberculosis and to maintain a status of official accreditation of freedom from these diseases. If all aborted fetuses are examined in a laboratory and nonpregnant cows routinely sampled and examined for brucellosis or venereal disease, it is reasonable to assume freedom from these diseases. All animals over six months of age should be tested for tuberculosis, and all cattle over 15 months of age should be tested for brucellosis.

All purchased animals introduced to the herd should be known to be free, by history or by test, from the diseases such as salmonellosis, brucellosis, leukosis, and tuberculosis, that are likely to be introduced in this way. All animals that die should be submitted for necropsy examination.

Herd Health Programs for Extensively Grazed Ranch-Type Beef Herds

Having worked on very large ranches in northern Australia, it is difficult to imagine a herd health program that would go much beyond satisfying the criterion of percentage survival. Under extensive conditions, which are essentially exploitative, farming is so much at the mercy of the environment that disease control retires to a relatively minor position. The provision of superphosphate, the introduction of special pasture plants, and the provision of fences and water supply are the procedures that lift an extensive beef program from subsistence to profitability. This is not to say that disease is unimportant, but when contagious bovine pleuropneumonia, babesiasis, tick worry, foot and mouth disease, rinderpest, and anthrax are under control and the supplementation of diets with phosphorus, copper, and cobalt is a practical reality, there does not seem to be much more that one can specifically recommend. The program recommended for small herds can obviously be expanded to include much larger herds. It would seem to be inevitable that the program would have to be diluted as the herds become larger and the cows further apart. But it is not a matter of size alone. Certainly, very large herds of up to 10,000 breeding females are handled in extensive herd health programs, provided they are managed intensively agriculturally. And the same causes of poor production occur on the extensively-run farms as on the intensive one (Donaldson 1968), but control measures are more difficult and expensive to apply.

Data available on extensively-run ranch properties indicate that reproductive inefficiency is a major cause of loss. The *experience in northern Australia is that less than half of the heifers calve at two years of age and of these, more than half do not conceive and calve again until they are four years old.* A common pattern is to calve only in alternate years (Donaldson 1968). Year-round mating is the rule, with two mating seasons of three months each being practiced on the better farms. Experience in New Zealand (Young 1967) and Australia (Osborne 1960; Lamond 1969) also indicates poor reproductive performance, partly due to poor nutrition and partly due to dystocia. Supplementary feeding of the heifers and cows and early weaning of the calves at six months of age can cause dramatic improvement in fertility (Armstrong et al. 1968).

Special Consideration of Bos indicus Cattle

Bos indicus cattle, including the Brahmans of Asia and the Afrikanders of South Africa, have achieved great popularity in the western world during the past 50 years, but they still represent only a small proportion of the total beef population. A list of their virtues indicates their good performance in subtropical countries, especially when their supervision is close and personal. Their disadvantages are related principally to their high-strung and nervous temperaments, which can make them almost unmanageable if management is hustling and boisterous. A large part of their efficiency in subtropical climates is related to their hides—which have a very large surface area per unit of body weight and a very sleek hair coat, both of which promote efficient cooling—and greater thickness and mobility due to *well-developed panniculus muscles, making them more repellent to insects.* On the other hand, British breeds of cattle fare indifferently in hot countries, specifically when the average annual isotherm exceeds 65°F (18.3°C). The tropical

degeneration that occurs beyond this point is characterized by stunted growth and a marked drop in fertility (Bonsma 1967).

The popularity of Brahman cattle has led to a plethora of crossbreed derived Taurindicus cattle, including the Santa Gertrudis, Brangus, Brayford, and Droughtmaster in the U.S. and the Bonsmara in Africa. The objectives are obvious, and the principal rules have been to have at least 50% of Brahman blood, and usually ⅝, and to avoid any inclusion of white skin.

Brahman females have a very low incidence of dystocia, but matings of Brahman bulls to non-Brahman cows usually have a high level of calving difficulty.

Brahman cattle are shy breeders, and are reputed to breed only at night. Their overall fertility in conditions of climate and feed suited to British breeds is generally considered to be low. But in the tropics, where British breeds do not do well, cross-bred Brahmans may be as much as 20% better than their parents. The evidence on the poor fertility of Brahmans and Afrikanders is conflicting (Donaldson 1971; Warnick 1967), but there seems little doubt that puberty occurs late, probably averaging about 20 months compared with 12 months for British breeds, and the intercalving period is longer, averaging 410 days as compared with 375 days for British breeds. The important observation seems to be that there is a great deal of variability between individual Brahman animals in their reproductive efficiency. *This suggests that strict culling for fertility could achieve good results quickly.* The great popularity of these cattle has probably discouraged selection pressure for fertility, and the effect of strong culling in individual herds may have contributed to the conflicting results mentioned above. Calf survival is reported to be good (Francis 1972).

Compared with British breeds, Brahman cattle and their crosses are better at maintaining their weight in the dry season and gaining weight in the wet season in the tropics. Their growth rate is midway between British breeds and exotic European breeds. The cows have a medium milk supply. In terms of meat economy, Brahmans are in the middle third. They have a medium fat cover and carcass conformation and yield of saleable meat.

Brahmans have a noticeable resistance to tick infestations so that losses due to tick worry and babesiasis are low compared with all other breeds.

In general, it can be said that Brahman crosses with British breeds have notable merits in heat tolerance, tick resistance, helminth tolerance, and general immunity to pathogens of most kinds. All of these characteristics confer low mortality and morbidity and good growth rates on young animals, and well-being and productivity in adults. In addition, there are attributes in feed utilization and metabolism that help them cope with periods of restricted availability of pasture feed. However, these cattle have shortcomings, especially in reproductive efficiency, behavior, and temperament, that can be crucial to management and may even be fatal to it, especially under conditions of extensive grazing. It so happens that Afrikanders are excellent in these areas and can be considered to be comprehensively complementary to Brahman crosses (Turner 1972; Andrews 1972).

Review Literature

Dziuk, P.J. and Bellow. R.A. Management of reproduction of beef cattle, sheep and pigs. J. Anim. Sci., 57:(Suppl. 2), 355–379, 1983.

Koch, R.M. and Algeo, J.W. The beef cattle industry: Changes and challenges. J. Anim. Sci., 57:(Suppl. 2), 28–43, 1983.

Ministry of Agriculture, Fisheries and Food. An approach to improving the fertility of dairy and beef herds in Great Britain. A working group's report to the chief veterinary officer, 1977, p. 30.

Radostits, O.M. (Ed.) Symposium on Herd Health Management—Cow-Calf and Feedlot. Vet. Clin. North Am. [Large Anim. Pract.], (5)1:1–209, 1983.

Trenkle, A. and Willham, R.L. Beef production efficiency. Science, 198:1009–1015, 1977.

References

Acres, S.D. The epidemiology of acute undifferentiated neonatal diarrhea of beef calves in Western Canada. Ph.D. Thesis. University of Saskatchewan, 1976.

Acres, S.D., Isaacson, R.E., Babiuk, L.A. et al. Immunization of calves against enterotoxigenic colibacillosis by vaccinating dams with purified K99 antigen and whole cell bacterins. Infect. Immun., 25:121–126, 1979.

Andrews, L.G. The major non-infectious causes of reproductive wastage in beef cattle in the Northern Territory. Aust. Vet. J., 48:41–46, 1972.

Armstrong, J., Henderson, A.G., Lang, D.R. et al. Preliminary observations on the productivity of female cattle in the Kimberley region of north western Australia. Aust. Vet. J., 44:357–363, 1968.

Beck, T.W., Wetteman, R.P., Turman, E.J. et al. Influence of 48 hour calf separation on milk production and calf growth in range cows. Theriogenology, 11:367–373, 1979.

Bellamy, J.E.C. and Acres, S.D. Enterotoxigenic colibacillosis in colostrum-fed calves: Pathologic changes. Am. J. Vet. Res., 40:1391–1397, 1979.

Bellows, R.A., Short, R.E. and Staigmiller, R.B. Research areas in beef cattle reproduction. Beltsville Symp. in Agric. Res. Anim. Prod., pp. 3–18, 1979.

Bonsma, J.C. In: Factors Affecting the Calf Crop. T.J. Cunha, A.C. Warnick and M. Koger (Eds.). Univ. of Florida Press, Gainesville, Florida, pp. 44–59, 1967.

Butson, S., Berg, R.T. and Hardin, R.T. Factors influencing weaning weights of range beef and dairy-beef calves. Can. J. Anim. Sci., 60:727–742, 1980.

Cates, W.F. Examination of the bull for breeding soundness. Symposium on Herd Health Management—Cow-Calf and Feedlot. Vet. Clin. North Am. [Large Anim. Pract.], (5)1:157–167, 1983.

Chenoweth, P.J. Examination of bulls for libido and breeding ability. Symposium on Herd Health Management—Cow-Calf and Feedlot. Vet. Clin. North Am. [Large Anim. Pract.], (5)1:59–74, 1983.

Church, T. and Karren, D. Alberta Certified Preconditioned Feeder Program, 1981, Alberta Dept. of Agric., Edmonton, Alberta.

Church, T.L. and Janzen, E.D. A system for calving heifers on a large commercial ranch. Bovine Pract., 13:40–44, 1978.

Davis, D., Schalles, R.R., Kiracofe, G.H. et al. Influence of winter nutrition on beef cow reproduction. J. Anim. Sci., 46:430–437, 1977.

deBlockey, M.A. The influence of serving capacity of bulls on herd fertility. J. Anim. Sci., 45:589–595, 1978.

Donaldson, L.E. Investigations into the fertility of Brahman crossbred female cattle in Queensland. Aust. Vet. J., 47:264–267, 1971.

Donaldson, L.E. The pattern of pregnancies and life-time productivity of cows in a northern Queensland beef cattle herd. Aust. Vet. J., 44:493–495, 1968.

Duffy, J.H. Influence of various degrees of confinement and supervision on the incidence of dystocia and stillbirths in Hereford heifers. N.Z. Vet. J., 29:44–48, 1981.

Dunn, T.G., Ingalls, J.E., Zimmerman, D.R. et al. Reproductive performance of 2-year-old Hereford and Angus heifers as influenced by pre- and post-calving energy intake. J. Anim. Sci., 29:719–736, 1969.

Dziuk, P.J. and Bellows, R.A. Management of reproduction of beef cattle, sheep and pigs. J. Anim. Sci., 57: (Suppl. 2), 355–379, 1983.

Francis, J. Reproductive efficiency of Bos indicus and derived taurindicus cattle in Queensland. Aust. Vet. J., 48:577, 1972.

Fredeen, H.T. Breeding program for a commercial cow-calf herd. Symposium on Herd Health Management—Cow-Calf and Feedlot. Vet. Clin. North Am. [Large Anim. Pract.], (5)1:103–117, 1983.

Fusch, J.E. The use of teat-size measurements or calf weaning weights as an aid to selection against teat defects. Anim. Prod., 32:127–133, 1982.

Graham, W.C. and Price, M.A. Feedlot performance and carcass composition of cull cows of different ages. Can. J. Anim. Sci., 62:845–854, 1982.

Grandin, T. Handling livestock. Vet. Med./Small Anim. Clin., 74:697–706, 1979.

Haggard, D.L., Farnsworth, R.J. and Springer, J.A. Subclinical mastitis of beef cows. J. Am. Vet. Med. Assoc., 182:604–606, 1983.

Hanly, G.F. and Mossman, D.H. Commercial beef production on hill country. N.Z. Vet. J., 25:3–7, 1977.

Hight, G.K. The effects of undernutrition in late pregnancy on beef cattle production. N.Z. J. Agr., 9:479–490, 1966.

Hodge, P.B., Wood, S.J., Newman, R.D. et al. Effect of calving supervision upon calving performance of Hereford heifers. Aust. Vet. J., 58:97–100, 1982.

Janzen, E.D. Some observations on reproductive performance in beef cattle in Western Canada. Can. Vet. J., 19:335–339, 1978.

Janzen, E.D. Health and production records for the beef

herd. Symposium on Herd Health Management—Cow-Calf and Feedlot. Vet. Clin. North Am. [Large Anim. Pract.], (5)1:15–28, 1983.

Jones, S.D.M., Price, M.A. and Berg, R.T. Effect of winter weight loss in Hereford cows on subsequent calf performance to weaning. Can. J. Anim. Sci., 59:635–637, 1979.

Jordan, W.A., Lister, E.E. and Rowlands, G.J. Effect of varying planes of nutrition of beef cows on calf performance to weaning. Can. J. Anim. Sci., 45:151–161, 1968.

Koch, R.M. and Algeo, J.W. The beef cattle industry—changes and challenges. J. Anim. Sci., 57:(Suppl. 2), 28–43, 1983.

Kroker, G.A. and Cummins, L.J. The effect of nutritional restriction on Hereford heifers in late pregnancy. Aust. Vet. J., 55:467–474, 1979.

Lamond, D.R. Sources of variation in reproductive performance in selected herds of beef cattle in northeast Australia. Aust. Vet. J., 45:50–58, 1969.

Leminager, R.P., Smith, W.H., Martin, T.G. et al. Effects of winter and summer energy levels on heifer growth and reproductive performance. J. Anim. Sci., 51:837–842, 1980.

Lowman, B.G., Hankey, M.S., Scott, N.A. et al. Influence of time of feeding on time of parturition in beef cows. Vet. Rec., 109:557–559, 1981.

Lusby, K.S., Wetteman, R.P. and Turman, E.J. Effects of early weaning calves from first-calf heifers on calf and heifer performance. J. Anim. Sci., 53:1193–1197, 1981.

MacDiarmid, S.C. Induction of parturition in cattle using corticosteroids: A review. Part 2. Effects of induction, mechanisms of induction, and preparations used. Anim. Breed. Abstr., 51:403–419, 1983a.

MacDiarmid, S.C. Induction of parturition in cattle using corticosteroids: A review. Part 2. Effects of induced calving on the calf and cow. Anim. Breed. Abstr., 51:499–508, 1983b.

Makarechian, M. and Berg, R.T. A study of some of the factors influencing ease of calving in range beef heifers. Can. J. Anim. Sci., 63:255–262, 1983.

Makarechian, M., Berg, R.T. and Weingardt, R. Factors influencing calving performance in range beef cattle. Can. J. Anim. Sci., 62:345–352, 1982.

Manns, J.G. The use of prostaglandins for regulation of estrus cycle and as an abortifacient in cattle. Symposium on Herd Health Management—Cow-Calf and Feedlot. Vet. Clin. North Am. [Large Anim. Pract.], (5)1:169–181, 1983.

Martin, S.W. Vaccination: Is it effective in preventing respiratory disease in feedlot calves? Can. Vet. J., 24:10–19, 1983.

Mohammed, K., Babiuk, L.A., Saunders, J.R. et al. Rotavirus diagnosis: Comparison of various antigens and serological tests. Vet. Microbiol. 3:115–127, 1978.

Morris, C.A. A review of relationships between aspects of reproduction in beef heifers and their lifetime production. 1. Association with fertility in the first joining season and with age at first joining. Anim. Breed. Abstr., 48:655–676, 1980a.

Morris, C.A. A review of relationships between aspects of reproduction in beef heifers and their lifetime production. 2. Association with relative calving date and with dystocia. Anim. Breed. Abstr., 48:753–767, 1980b.

Mossman, D.H. and Hanly, G.J. A theory of beef production. N.Z. Vet. J., 25:96–100, 1977.

Myers, L.L. and Snodgrass, D.R. Colostral and milk antibody titers in cows vaccinated with a modified live rotavirus coronavirus vaccine. J. Am. Vet. Med. Assoc., 181:486–488, 1982.

Osborne, H.G. The investigations of infertility syndromes in beef herds. Aust. Vet. J., 36:164–171, 1960.

Petrie, L., Acres, S.D. and McCartney, D.H. The yield of colostrum and colostral immunoglobulins in beef cows and the absorption of colostral gammaglobulins by beef calves. Can. Vet. J., 25:273–279, 1984.

Pimentel, C.A. and Dechamps, J.C. Effects of early weaning on reproductive efficiency in beef cows. Theriogenol., 11:421–427, 1979.

Price, M.A. and Berg, R.T. On the consequences and economics of feeding grain ad libitum to culled beef cows. Can. J. Anim. Sci., 61:105–111, 1981.

Price, T.D. and Wiltbank, J.N. Dystocia in cattle. A review and implications. Theriogenol., 9:195–219, 1978.

Prior, R.L. and Laster, D.B. Development of the bovine fetus. J. Anim. Sci., 48:1546–1553, 1979.

Prior, R.L., Scott, R.A., Laster, D.B. et al. Maternal energy status and development of liver and muscle in the bovine fetus. J. Anim. Sci., 48:1538–1545, 1979.

Radostits, O.M. and Acres, S.D. The control of acute undifferentiated diarrhea of newborn beef calves. Symposium on Herd Health Management—Cow-Calf and Feedlot. Vet. Clin. North Am. [Large Anim. Pract.], (5)1:143–155, 1983.

Rupp, G.P., Ball, L., Shoop, M.C. et al. Reproductive efficiency of bulls in natural service: Effects of male to female ratio and single versus multiple-sire breeding groups. J. Am. Vet. Med. Assoc., 171:639–642, 1977.

Saif, L.J. and Smith, K.L. A review of rotavirus immunization of cows and passive protection in calves. Proc. Fourth International Symposium on Neonatal Diarrhea. Veterinary Infectious Disease Organization. Oct. 3–5, 1983. University of Saskatchewan, Saskatoon.

Stott, G.H. and Feelah, A. Colostral immunoglobulin absorption linearly related to concentration for calves. J. Dairy Sci., 66:1319–1328, 1983.

Trenkle, A. and Willham, R.L. Beef production efficiency. Science, 198:1009–1015, 1977.

Tudor, G.D. The effect of pre- and post-natal nutrition on the growth of beef cattle. 1. The effect of nutrition and parity of the dam on calf birth weight. Aust. J. Agric. Res., 23:389–395, 1972.

Turner, H.G. Selection of beef cattle for tropical Australia. Aust. Vet. J., 48:162–166, 1972.

Waldhalm, D.G., Hall, R.F., DeLong, W.J. et al. Restricted dietary protein in pregnant beef cows. 1. The effect on length of gestation and calfhood mortality. Theriogenol., 12:61–68, 1979.

Warnick, A.C. Reproduction of Brahmans in Florida. In: Factors Affecting the Calf Crop. T.J. Cunha. A.C. Warnick and M. Koger (Eds.). Univ. of Florida Press, Gainesville, Florida, pp. 260–267, 1967.

Wiltbank, J.N. Maintenance of a high level of reproductive performance in the beef cow herd. Symposium on Herd Health Management—Cow-Calf and Feedlot. Vet. Clin. North Am. [Large Anim. Pract.], (5)1:41–57, 1983.

Wiltbank, J.N. More calves in the 80's. Mod. Vet. Pract., 63:16–20, 1982.

Wiltbank, J.N. Research needs in beef cattle reproduction. J. Anim. Sci., 31:755–762, 1970.

Wiltbank, J.N. and Remmenga, E.E. Calving difficulty and calf survival in beef cows fed two energy levels. Theriogenol., 17:587–602, 1982.

Yarney, R.A., Rahnefeld, G.W., Parker, R.J. et al. Hourly distribution of time on parturition in beef cows. Can. J. Anim. Sci., 62:597–605, 1982.

Young, J.S. Some observations on reproductive performance in selected commercial beef herds. N.Z. Vet. J., 15:167–173, 1967.

Health and Production Management in Beef Feedlots

10

INTRODUCTION

A beef feedlot is a place where young growing cattle are fed a high-energy diet for the purpose of producing marketable beef at the lowest cost and in the shortest time possible. Depending on the starting body weight and age of the cattle, the period of confinement and feeding will vary from 60 days to 12 months. Beef feedlots have evolved from small family farm lots in which 25 to 100 head of cattle were finished annually, into large, capital-intensive enterprises that market thousands of finished cattle annually. In the family farm feedlot, the calves were born and reared on the home farm, weaned at six to eight months of age, fed a growing ration until they were one year of age, and then finished on a high-energy ration, usually grains, until they reached marketable weight at 18 to 24 months of age. The health and production problems were minimal, and expansion of this kind of enterprise was limited only by the capital investment and the desire, knowledge, and labor necessary for expansion. In North America, expansion of these farm feedlots was limited, compared with the proliferation of the capital-intensive enterprises that fed and marketed thousands of cattle annually. In North America, beginning in the 1950s, "cheap land, cheap cattle, cheap feed, and cheap money" led to the development of a very large feedlot industry. Cattle are obtained either as calves weaned at six to eight months of age or as yearlings at 12 to 14 months of age, placed in the feedlot, and fed for periods ranging from 60 days to 12 months, depending on initial age and weight. The animals are obtained and transported long distances from many different genetic, nutritional, and geographical backgrounds and co-mingled in the feedlot. Net profit in these intensive feedlots has depended not only on good animal management and animal health but also in a large part on the purchase and selling prices of the cattle. It is a creed among feedlot owners that *if cattle are bought right, you can make money.* However, in recent years, the steady consumer demand for beef; the competition by feedlots to purchase cattle; and the high cost of land, grain, labor, feedlot facilities, transportation, and interest on borrowed money has considerably narrowed the profit margin to the point where it is often more economical to invest capital elsewhere. In some cases, the occurrence of disease has a major economic impact on net profit in the feedlot, whereas at other times, if the selling price of cattle increases markedly during the finishing period, disease may play only a minor role in net profit. Unexpected fluctuation in the prices of feed and cattle can result in large financial losses.

In North American feedlots, the male castrate (steer) is the predominant animal, but heifers, cull cows, and bulls are also fed for beef production.

The energy crisis has caused an introspective view of energy use in agriculture in general and of beef production in particular. It is now recognized that the much-boasted efficiency of American agriculture, by which one farmer feeds 50 or more people, has been achieved via the substitution of fossil fuels for the labor of man and horses. Total energy used in the various steps of the beef production system under conditions of cow/calf production on the range in Colorado with yearling steers fed a high concentrate diet is as follows (Ward 1980):

Distribution of Energy Consumption in Average Beef Production

	Per Cent
Cow/calf production	21.2
Stocker (180 to 320 kg.)	16.0
Feedlot (320 to 500 kg.)	62.8
	100
Feed production	86.4
Feed processing	3.5
Feed operation	10.1
	100

Cow/calf production includes support of cows, including their winter feed. Transport of personnel and supplies to the pastures represents the largest single energy input. The feedlot phase represents 60% of the total energy use, of which more than 80% is allocated for feed production. Despite heavy mechanization, feed processing and feedlot operation constitute a small percentage of the total. The fact that so much of the energy input is in the form of feed means that growth promotants that increase feed efficiency make an important contribution to energy conservation. Since 63% of the energy is used in the feedlot phase of beef production, it seems obvious that an important means of energy conservation would be a reduction or elimination of the use of heavy concentrate feeding in the feedlot and an increase in the use of forage only. However, forage finishing requires more time and a higher percentage of feed intake for maintenance. In addition, because cattle would be older when they reach market weight, beef quality characteristics would be less desirable. Nevertheless, the most significant energy savings in beef production can probably be obtained by a reduction in the amount of grain fed to heavy feedlot cattle. This often can be achieved by an elimination of an additional two weeks of feeding, a current practice commonly employed to increase the percentage of cattle grading choice. Ten per cent of the total energy for finishing an animal is used in these two weeks to produce an additional 1 kg. of protein along with about 4 kg. of largely undesirable fat. Cattle can be fed for shorter periods and slaughtered with a lower percentage of fat, and they will still provide beef of acceptable quality. The realization of this type of energy conservation, however, will require changes in attitude toward grading and marketing of beef.

Energy conservation can also be achieved by reducing the practice of feeding calves instead of yearlings, a practice exercised in periods of tight supplies that promotes inefficient use of energy.

The extensive use of hormone implants and feed additives as growth promotants and to improve feed efficiency has been economical but has not had a major impact on reducing the high costs of feeding high-level grain diets.

Because of the high cost of grain, there has been considerable research activity, on a global basis, to find inexpensive alternative feeds for feedlot cattle. The alkali treatment of cereal straw to improve its energy availability shows considerable promise as a method of economical utilization of a roughage to replace a portion of the grains in growing cattle diets (Lesoing et al. 1980a, 1980b).

There has also been considerable activity in the assessment of feeds for beef cattle other than the traditional grains and roughages. Potato processing residue can replace barley as an energy source for finishing beef cattle (Stanhope et al. 1980).

Major changes have occurred in the beef cattle feedlot industry in the 25 years from 1958 to 1983 (Koch and Algeo 1983). In the 1960s, the commercial and custom cattle feeding industry in the United States underwent a dramatic shift in numbers, geographical location, and technological handling of cattle and commodities. Large-scale custom feeding operations developed in which the operators of the feedlot do not own the cattle but only feed and handle them on consignment for absentee owners. Large-scale modern abattoirs were built in the beef-producing areas. Growth promotants came into general usage and have been an economic benefit to the industry. Research into

grain processing led to increased efficiencies in feed utilization, and many changes occurred in the marketing and processing of beef cattle.

In the 25 years from 1958 to 1983, there has been a major drive in the beef cattle industry to produce the superior carcass (Berg and Walters 1983). This carcass is characterized by a high proportion of muscle, a low proportion of bone, and an optimal level of fatness. The major changes that have occurred have been a decrease in fatness at an acceptable slaughter weight and an increase in growth rate accompanied by larger mature sizes. Changes in body form have accompanied the changes in the growth rate and composition. All of this has led to major changes in the grading systems for beef in North America (Bredenstein and Carpenter 1983).

It is clear that the efficiency of beef production has been steadily improved by applying new knowledge of nutrition and breeding (Trenkle and Willham 1977).

The beef feedlot industry in the United States and Canada developed as a result of the surplus of grains and the demand for beef from the North American public. In Europe, where land and feed is expensive, intensive beef feedlots are rare, and dual-purpose cattle are customary. In most European countries, beef and veal production is a by-product of milk production, and consequently the production levels are dependent mainly on changes in dairy cow numbers one to two years earlier (Allen et al. 1982).

ECONOMICS OF THE FEEDLOT

There are two important economical factors that determine the profitability of a feedlot operation.

1. The cattle increase in weight, and the cost of the gain in weight must be less than the value of the weight. This seems an obvious comment, but it is not a sufficient factor in itself because it is often not possible to make a sufficient profit out of a simple gain in weight.

2. The quality of the entire animal is changed so that the whole carcass increases in value per kg. of body weight, and this "margin" is the basis of profitability for the feedlot system. The margin is always small because the demand of the available feeder cattle is great so that prices for them remain high. What makes the system work is the demand for a continuous supply of meat of guaranteed and

uniform quality and tenderness at all times of the year.

The principal factors that affect the cost of growth and the finishing of cattle in the feedlot are the capital cost of using the lot, the cost of labor, and the cost of feed. The longer the animal remains in the lot to make a specified gain in weight, the less economically efficient the system becomes. Accordingly, there is an incentive to feed out cattle quickly. On the other hand, very heavy feeding may go beyond the point of optimum conversion, so weight gain per day and feed conversion efficiency must both be kept in view as criteria of efficiency because they tend to operate in opposite directions. The rate of gain per day increases as the proportion of grain in the diet increases, but the efficiency of conversion decreases at the same time. Increasing the intake of roughage in general has the opposite effect so that a decision on the optimum proportion of grain and roughage is critical to profitability. The decision must also take into account the relative costs of grain and roughage. There are also limitations on the amount of grain that can be fed safely. One of the most dreaded diseases in feedlot management is carbohydrate engorgement, which can affect an entire pen of cattle in a very short period of time.

Daily rate of gain in body weight and feed conversion efficiency are both strongly inherited, and the purchase of appropriate animals, especially if their carcasses are likely to have a low peripheral fat content, can make a considerable contribution to profitability. The exotic European breeds have attracted considerable attention because of their high-quality performance in this area.

Another important factor in determining profitability is disease. The failure to adequately control disease at an economical level can result in complete loss of profitability and also in the loss of part or all of the asset invested in the cattle. The spectrum of diseases that occur will vary considerably, depending on the management system and the geographical location of the lot. These diseases will be discussed in a later section on the causes of economic loss in the feedlot.

Another management factor of great importance in maximizing the profitability of a feedlot is the number of throughputs that can be managed in a year. The capital investment is often such that it is uneconomical to confine cattle and not have them on a short introductory feeding phase followed by an intensive

heavy feeding period of about 120 days, i.e., 2 to 2.5 throughputs per year.

EFFECTS OF GENETICS ON BEEF PRODUCTION IN THE FEEDLOT

Increasing the efficiency of beef production systems by genetic methods primarily involves two procedures: (1) selection within breeds to enhance critical characters and (2) selection among and combinations of breeds to produce individuals that better fit production conditions and resources (Long 1980). Cross-breeding for beef production has become a generally recommended and accepted practice (Gregory and Cundliff 1980). The current recommendations for cross-breeding can be explained in terms of heterosis for traits usually considered desirable in terms of profitability. Beef production may be considered to be composed of two phases: (1) the cow herd phase, in which reproduction or increasing numbers is of primary importance and (2) the growth and fattening phase, in which weight production or increase is of primary importance. The characters critical in determining the efficiency during the growth and fattening phase include the postweaning average daily gain, yearling weight, postyearling weight, feed conversion, and carcass characters. Cross-breeding improves each one of these characters to varying degrees. The effects of management must be considered when assessing the economic impact of cross-breeding (Long 1980).

Much higher levels of heterosis have been observed involving crosses of *Bos indicus* and *Bos taurus* cattle than between crosses of breeds of *Bos taurus*. Much of this higher level of heterosis may be the result of a low level of climatic adaptability and thus of poor purebred performance of the *Bos taurus* breeds and perhaps of low beef production response capability of the *Bos indicus* breed in a moderately intensive beef production environment. The cross-breed is a genetic intermediate that may be better adapted than the parental pure breeds both to the climatic environment and for meeting beef production requirements in moderately intensive beef production systems.

VETERINARY MEDICINE IN THE FEEDLOT

It is only in recent years that the role of the veterinarian in the feedlot has become clear. The veterinarian must be a competent gross pathologist, a highly accurate clinical diagnostician, an epidemiologist, and have an applied knowledge of feedlot production and nutrition, economics and marketing, and computer-based record keeping.

The role of the veterinarian in the feedlot has changed from the traditional emphasis on the diagnosis and treatment of individual sick animals to one of a professional adviser. Advice on animal health and how it affects performance of the animals is based on the clinical and pathological examination of animals and on the records of animal health and performance. The details of these procedures will be presented later.

Compared with other specialties in veterinary medicine, e.g., small animal practice and dairy herd health, feedlot veterinary medicine has not yet become a recognized specialty with a reliable body of knowledge and a cadre of recognized veterinarians who conduct research in the field and publish the results of their work.

There is an urgent need for the development of a reliable body of knowledge in feedlot animal health that can be put to use successfully and economically by a veterinarian working in a feedlot. This body of knowledge must be able to maintain animal health at a level that will yield the optimum level of feedlot beef cattle performance.

TYPES OF FEEDLOTS

The end product of all feedlots is beef. The major variations between feedlots are the types of cattle that are fed, the feeds used, and the length of the feeding period. A brief description of the characteristics of the common feedlots follows.

North American Permanent Feedlots

The primary objective in the North American permanent type of feedlot is to control the nutritional environment and produce a standard product that exactly fits the specification of the consumer market. This is practiced to the ultimate degree at some feedlots in the United States where the owners of the feedlot also own an abattoir, usually located right next door. As the immediate market for the beef moves in one direction or another, the rations are varied, and the types and weights of cattle purchased may vary depending on the market. Every action is conducted in such a way as to achieve the best financial advantage.

The cattle and the facilities may be totally owned by the owner of the feedlot, who buys and sells the cattle and assumes total responsibility for the management of the production and health of the cattle. In "custom" feedlots, the cattle are owned by someone else, who makes a contract with the owner of the feedlot, who also assumes total responsibility for the management of the production and health of the cattle for a predetermined fee. The owner of the feedlot does not participate directly in the profit or loss of the cattle.

The modern feedlot in North America has become a highly mechanized, well-organized, highly financed enterprise. Capacities range from 1000 to 50,000 head and higher with at least two throughputs per year. Feed processing and feeding systems are highly mechanized, automated, and even computerized, and rations can be changed on short notice by on-site feed mills. Specialized personnel process the feed, pen-checkers monitor the animals regularly for illness, and a treatment crew is responsible for treatment of sick animals and the processing of cattle on arrival. Certain pens are allocated for new arrivals, and hospital pens are available for the segregation of sick animals. Detailed records are kept of morbidity, mortality, treatments given, and production performance. Detailed financial records are kept of each item of production so that aberrant variations can be examined and corrected if possible.

There must be a variety of options in the manner in which feedlots are operated, depending on local conditions of availability of cattle and feed; these may vary in the one locality from time to time. But the final stage in any beef feedlot operation is a period of intensive feeding on a carbohydrate-rich diet to finish the cattle with a light cover of fat on the carcass and deposition of fat in the muscle tissue itself.

The traditional permanent feedlot has a number of options. Cattle are bought at various ages, and the economics of the various situations are different. Young cattle may be bought at six months of age immediately after weaning when they may weigh 400 to 500 lb. (180 to 225 kg.) and are either fed intensively until they weigh 600 lb. (275 kg.) at nine to 10 months, or they may be fed roughage at slightly above maintenance levels until they are about 18 months old and weigh 900 lb. (400 kg.), when they are put onto heavy grain feeding. In the latter system, the feeding regimen is economical, but the capital invested in the cattle and the feedlot is not being used intensively enough to provide a good return. If they can be grown on pasture, the system is more economic.

In the heavy grain feeding programs, the special disease problems are those related to abnormal digestion, especially lactic acid indigestion and bloat. Very careful feeding management is necessary to avoid what can be very severe losses from these diseases and from polioencephalomalacia.

When older cattle are brought in—usually yearlings weighing 600 to 700 lb. (275 to 325 kg.) at 15 to 18 months of age—they are fed lightly for four to five months until they are 900 lb. (400 kg.) and then put onto full feed and marketed a month later at 1000 lb. (455 kg.). Because of disease problems with this method and the economic losses associated with prolonged stay in the lot, it is becoming increasingly common to buy only cattle that weigh up to 900 lb. (400 kg.) at entry that can be fed out in three months after an introductory period of 20 to 30 days. The objective in the heavy feeding part of the program is to achieve a growth rate of 2.0 to 3.0 lb./day (0.9 to 1.4 kg./day), which will add 300 lb. (135 kg.) of body weight in 150 days, 100 lb. (45 kg.) of it in the last 30 days. In terms of feed, the objective is to put on these weights using 1.5 to 2 lb. (0.7 to 0.9 kg.) of grain/100 lb. (45 kg.) body weight/day and 5 to 10 lb. (2.2 to 4.4 kg.) hay or 15 to 30 lb. (7 to 14 kg.) of ensilage/day.

The secret of managerial success in feedlot feeding is being able to get cattle onto full feed quickly without causing losses due to lactic acid indigestion. Details of recommended feeding programs are given later in the section on disease prevention. Because of the pressure to improve the economy of lot feeding, there is a constant search for low-priced, carbohydrate-rich feeds. In most cases it is unsuccessful, because the supply is not constant, and handling and spoilage are problems. One exception is potatoes and potato peelings that are rejected from the potato chip and canning industries. Another highly successful procedure is the feeding of sugar beet pulp from the sugar industry. A similar situation exists in Cuba, where the feeding of molasses, urea, and bagasse, the fibrous residue from sugar cane pressing, has created a revolution (agricultural variety). Junk roughage, such as lucerne stalks collected after seed harvesting, may be of some use when grain is very cheap, but usually the cost of chopping and supplementing with more nutritious feed, the variability of supply, and the risk of omasal—or even abomasal—impaction make them an unsatisfactory invest-ment as a rule. Fungal spoilage and poisoning are major problems with wet feeds such as pea vine ensilage. Dried pea vines can cause mania when infested with fungi, as they often are.

Australian Back-up Feedlots

A variation of the American type of "permanent" feedlot is the stop-and-go "back-up" feedlot, which has been developed in recent years in Australia. They are most valuable in areas where both grain and cattle are raised. The lots are usually small and are owned by the cattle breeder and raiser, providing the enormous advantage of avoiding profit sharing. Because the yards are used only occasionally, usually one year in three, capitalization is reduced to an absolute minimum. In good grass years when cattle can be fattened at pasture, the yards may not be used at all. In a bad year when, without a lot, the steers have to be held over for an additional year, they are packed into the yards and finished on grain.

In general, the steers are put into the yards at about 18 months of age and weighing only 550 to 600 lb. (250 to 275 kg.). The objective is to feed them for 100 days at the rate of gain of 2.5 lb. (1.15 kg.)/day in the lot. With an introductory period of 20 days, there is a gain of 250 lb. (115 kg.) in 120 days and a finishing weight of 800 to 900 lb. (360 to 400 kg.). A feed conversion efficiency of 7.1 is the objective.

The usual technique is to feed grain at a level of 80 to 90% of weight of the ration. Lactic acid indigestion is not uncommon as a result, and a common problem is a high rejection rate primarily of livers, but also of kidneys, at the slaughter point. Other offal, e.g., tripe, may be similar disadvantages. In Australia, where this method of feeding is expanding, the grains are often low in protein and can vary from 13% crude protein down to 3%. A nitrogen content estimation is desirable in these and other circumstances if there is any doubt about the adequacy of the protein supply. Another characteristic of Australian lot feeding is the lighter weights of finished cattle, due largely to the dislike of the consumer for overfat meat.

Because of the need to keep the capital costs low, these lots are temporary, lightweight construction intended to house cattle for only three months in any one year and only in some years. The fences are usually wooden posts with stretched wires between. These are not highly resistant to "rushing," and occasionally a set of yards will be flattened when the cattle suddenly take fright, usually about dusk when they are inclined to be frisky anyway. Troughing is a major cost in a feedlot, and the Australian system includes a specially designed, cheap, concrete feed trough that has minimum maintenance problems.

"Barley-Beef" Units in the United Kingdom

In this British system, cattle are introduced to the units when they are three months old and weigh 200 to 220 lb. (90 to 100 kg.). The objective is to market them at 800 and 900 lb. (360 to 400 kg.) before they are 12 months old. The capitalization per place in the unit is very small. Most of the buildings are old and have been converted cheaply—often badly—to a loose housing, dry litter system. In new installations, the buildings are flimsy iron on frame over slats. Because they are small and house relatively few animals, about 50 to 100 head, little money is spent on sophisticated machinery for milling or feeding out. These are provided by private feed supply companies which have grown enormously in the United Kingdom in the last two decades. They provide ready-mixed, custom-mixed rations. The cost of feed is therefore a much bigger item than in the United States. The other noticeable difference between the "barley-beef" and the American "permanent" feedlots is the need in the latter to push animals through an intensive feeding period quickly to utilize each highly capitalized cattle space to the fullest. Therefore, in these lots there is an average of 2.5 throughputs, whereas in a "barley-beef" unit, where the pressure of capitalization is not nearly as great, one throughput per year is the average.

A very similar system is common throughout eastern and western Europe and in Japan. The number of animals in an individual unit is usually quite small, and the intensity of the feeding program is usually inversely proportional to the number. Male castrates of the local indigenous, dual-purpose breeds are used and allowed to grow as big as 1500 lb. (680 kg.) on very heavy grain rations, supplemented with a great variety of additional growth stimulants, including beer. Particular emphasis is placed on maximizing the amount of lean meat in the carcass. The animals are maintained indoors in small groups for the feeding period, with manure and urine being disposed of through slatted floor or via a deep litter system (Allen et al. 1982).

European Vealer Units

These units take in calves that are a few days old and fatten them, basically on an artificial milk (milk replacer) diet, so that they are 260 to 300 lb. (115 to 135 kg.) body weight at 10 to 12 weeks of age. The milk replacer solves storage problems and effects the necessary economies compared with whole milk to make the system a viable one economically. The calves are kept in groups in small pens on litter or slats, or in individual crates on slats, in subdued light. The only really successful units are those that are fully enclosed, have control of temperature and humidity within certain limits, and are completely free of drafts. In addition, if the calf houses are divided into units, holding about 40 calves each, it is possible to follow an all-in-all-out policy, and disease losses are kept low. It is necessary to ensure that the calves have had sufficient colostrum for the first three to four days of life.

The main feeding problem in these units is dietetic diarrhea caused by overfeeding or by improper mixing or feeding of the milk replacer. The usual corrective procedure is to remove the feed for two to three feedings and offer oral electrolytes and water. It is essential to ensure that colibacillosis or salmonellosis is not the cause. The milk replacer used is basically skim milk powder with added vegetable fat, minerals, and vitamins. There must be adequate iron and magnesium in the milk replacer because two of the problems in the early days of vealer units, and also in other calf-rearing units where the diet is restricted to whole milk and straw, are hypomagnesemia and a poorly-described anemia.

The disease that determines whether a calf unit is profitable or not is enzootic pneumonia caused by the PI-3 virus plus various bacteria. Environmental control is essential to keep the effects of the disease at an acceptable level.

Other Feeding Systems

A Semi-Intensive Modification of the Standard "Barley-Beef" Unit

This has been devised to utilize the finishing capacity of the grain feeding period with the good growth effect of growing young stock on intensively managed grasslands. Autumn-born calves spend their first winter indoors in a growing unit. In spring, they go out to this highly intensive pasture and are kept there at the rate of three to four animals per acre. The next autumn, the cattle go into the "barley-beef" lot, are fed heavily on grain, and are sold the next spring at 18 months of age and at 900 to 1000 lb. (400 to 450 kg.).

The system is particularly adapted to utilization of grass and grain as fattening resources. It reduces the time spent in the expensive indoor unit and reduces the risk of pneumonia, laminitis, and lactic acid indigestion; however, these are replaced by the pasture-dependent diseases of lungworm, intestinal parasitism, and occasionally hypomagnesemia.

The Cuban Molasses-Urea-Bagasse System

This system is reputed to be much more economical than selling sugar on the world market. It has obvious advantages because of the ready availability of two of the feed products. (Preston and Willis 1974). A very high incidence of polioencephalomalacia is recorded as a disadvantage of the system (Loew 1975).

Intensive Calf-Rearing Units

One of the important but poorly recognized by-products of the dairying industry is the intensive calf-rearing unit, which takes calves at 24 to 72 hours of age and rears them on milk replacer until weaning, when they are directed toward "barley-beef" units. If they are heifers and there is a suitable market, they may find themselves back in the dairy as herd replacements. They are an alternative to vealer units, with the emphasis on growing the calves rather than fattening them.

These units are widespread but poorly documented in terms of disease risk, management, and economy. Possibly this is because they have been essentially one-man operations run as a part-time occupation. But in recent years there has been the development of very large commercial operations, which may accommodate as many as 300 calves.

The management of units reflects what happens in a regular dairy unit except that it is multiplied in size a number of times. The disease situation is different in that it is usually much more serious. The calves come from many origins and bring many infections together in the one place. They enter at an age when they are very susceptible to stress, and unless exceptional care is taken, many of them will be agammaglobulinemic because they have not received colostrum and it is now too late for absorption of colostral immunoglobulins. The capitalization is often meager, and poor ventilation, dampness, inadequate troughing, and poor hygiene contribute to a high incidence of infection and epidemics of disease. When the calves are housed indoors, virus pneumonia, secondary bacterial pneumonia, and enteritis due to *Escherichia coli*, *Salmonella* spp., and viruses—including rotavirus and coronaviruses—are the important causes of loss.

It is not intended to deal with the diseases here because they are presented in the chapters on dairying, and a herd health program similar to the one recommended there should be applicable.

OBJECTIVES OF A HEALTH MANAGEMENT AND PRODUCTION PROGRAM IN THE FEEDLOT

The general objectives of a planned animal health and production program in a feedlot include the following (Church 1980):

1. Rapid growth rate, minimal fat at an acceptable slaughter weight, and large mature sizes
2. Maximization of feed conversion efficiency
3. The reduction of morbidity, mortality, and culling rates
4. The optimal expenditures for biologicals and antimicrobials used for the control and treatment of disease
5. The maintenance of employee motivation to provide good animal management and the early detection and treatment of sick animals
6. A profit commensurate with other investment opportunities
7. The production of wholesome beef free of chemical residues

STANDARDS OF HEALTH AND PRODUCTION PERFORMANCE IN THE FEEDLOT

The major factors that influence profit or loss in the feedlot are the price of the purchased cattle, the total costs per unit of body weight gain, and the selling price of the finished cattle. The costs of production continue to rise each year. There are minor fluctuations in the costs of feed, which may increase net profit. However, major fluctuations in the costs of feeder cattle and the selling price of finished cattle result in major changes in profit and loss. The individual feedlot operator has no direct control of the price of cattle, and net profit depends on a gross margin large enough to offset costs. A decrease in the selling price of cattle can result in major economic losses; under these conditions the very best health and management program cannot result in a profit, but it can reduce the magnitude of the losses. Conversely, a marked increase in the selling price of cattle will usually result in large increases in net profit in spite of an unusually high incidence of disease and mortality in a particular group of cattle. In such cases, disease appears to be insignificant. In fact, in most well-managed feedlots, the wastage due to disease appears to be relatively small compared with other causes of economic loss. Some of the factors that affect the occurrence of disease and profit are presented in the discussion on the epidemiology of diseases of feedlot cattle (p. 252). These factors are in general well known to feedlot managers and are kept under reasonable control. As a consequence, the veterinarian's role can be relatively slim and may be reduced to an advisory capacity on the treatment and control of disease. Because management, nutrition, environment, and economics have such a close interrelationship with disease, the veterinary consultant to a feedlot must be familiar with these sciences. If the veterinarian becomes involved to a large degree, he may find himself fitted for the role of manager. This has in fact happened in some of the very large feedlots and gives some credence to the view that the veterinarian has had, in many ways, the most suitable training for this sort of work. The most important factor governing the efficiency and success of a feedlot herd health program is the *depth of knowledge* of its veterinarian of the managerial matters that form the basis of good health for the cattle that use it.

Other factors that affect the herd health service include not only the efficiency of the people riding in the pens and looking for sick animals but also the intensity to which their enthusiasm can be motivated by the management and the veterinarian. Good identification of animals as groups and identification when they are treated—preferably by colored ear tag—of the form of treatment being administered is important. Keeping the cattle together as groups so that their subsequent performance can be traced back to their origin and to their handling during the conditioning period is also important. Proper hospital yards and chutes are needed to permit adequate handling for prophylactic and therapeutic injections.

Production and Disease Targets in the Feedlot

There is a limited amount of published, documented information available on the standards of health and performance that should be expected and aimed for in a well-managed commercial beef feedlot. Most feedlots record the details of their cattle on a group or pen basis. The data usually include the following: the total weight and costs of cattle going into the pen, the total amount and costs of the feed consumed, the total number of animals—live and dead, the total costs of prophylaxis and treatment, and the total weight and selling price of cattle leaving the pen for market. From these records, it is possible to assess the health and production performance. The standards that are set out below are guidelines that need to be modified according to the prevailing conditions in each feedlot.

a. Assessment of General Efficiency

Average daily gain =

$$\frac{\text{Total weight gained by group (kg.)}}{\text{Number of cattle} \times \text{days on feed}}$$

$$= \text{not less than 1 kg./day}$$

Efficiency of feed conversion =

$$\frac{\text{kg. of feed to group}}{\text{kg. of body weight gained by group}}$$

$$= \text{less than 6}$$

Costs per kg. of body weight gain = variable

b. Assessment of Herd Health Efficiency

Morbidity rate = number of animals that were pulled from the pen and required treatment for an illness

Case fatality rate = per cent of treated animals that died. Should not exceed 5%

Population mortality rate = per cent of entire population in the feedlot that died during the year. A common standard is 0.75% or less. A feasible target is 0.50%, and 0.25% is excellent. Some feedlots report losses of 1.0 to 1.5% annually. However, the losses depend primarily on the age and kind of cattle that are purchased and fed. Annual population mortality rates may reach 5% when feeder calves at six to eight months of age, weighing an average of 225 kg., are placed in the feedlot. The population mortality rate for yearling cattle placed in the feedlot, weighing an average of 375 kg., is as low as 1.5%.

Culling rate = percentage of animals culled because of chronic illness or inferior performance before the fattening period was completed. Less than 3%.

Health and disease costs = the total costs of health and disease, including the value of dead animals and the costs of prophylaxis and treatment. The total costs are expressed as a percentage of the total costs per unit of body weight gain per day.

CAUSES OF ECONOMIC LOSS IN THE FEEDLOT

The causes of economic loss in the feedlot have not been well documented. However, the major factors that influence the achievement of optimum production and that must result in economic loss when unsatisfactory include the following:

1. *Nutrition:* The quality and adequacy of the feeds and feeding systems used has a major impact on growth rate and feed efficiency.

2. *Types of cattle fed:* The genetic background and the sex of the animals fed will influence growth rate, feed efficiency, and carcass quality.

3. *Environmental effects:* Because feedlot cattle are usually kept in confinement, often with a high stocking density, the effects of environment may interfere with optimum production.

4. *Management expertise:* As in any livestock enterprise, the level of management is important. Most of the success of a herd health program depends on the people feeding the cattle, identifying and treating sick cattle early, and keeping accurate records of the daily activities. In large modern feedlots, the management of personnel becomes one of the highest priorities.

5. *Disease incidence:* Disease may cause economic loss through mortality, the costs of treatment, or the effects on productivity. The impact of clinical and subclinical disease on productive efficiency and economic returns may be greater than the losses associated with mortality.

There have been very few studies of the economic value of production loss caused by disease in feedlots. In general, the population mortality rate is about 1% annually. Production losses in cattle fed intensively and semi-intensively vary from approximately 1 to 3% (Thomas et al. 1978). Acute infectious respiratory disease accounts for more than one half of the production losses and for the majority of losses from fatal disease (Church and Radostits 1981). The production losses are most marked during the early growth period. Compensatory growth occurs in animals that have recovered from diseases such as pneumonia, enteritis, and pinkeye (Thomas et al. 1978).

The bacterial and viral infections that cause acute bovine respiratory disease constitute the main threat to cost-effectiveness in most beef feedlots. The components of the loss include shrink, poor feed utilization, inefficiency of gain, one to two per population mortality, and the treatment costs (Pierson 1968).

In any feedlot, at any point in time, there is a background level of disease, a degree of inadequate management, some variation in the adequacy of the diet, some cattle that are genetically inferior in growth rate, and some alteration in the environment or management, which singly or collectively interfere with optimal production and cause economic loss.

The major diseases of yearling feedlot cattle in Colorado over a one-year period were as follows (Jensen et al. 1976a).

	Per Cent
Pneumonia	48
Diphtheria	6
Brisket disease	6
Hemorrhagic colitis	5
Riding injury	4
Bloat	3
Urinary calculi	2
Endocarditis	2
Abomasal ulcer	2
Bovine viral diarrhea	2
Embolic pulmonary aneurysm	1
Pulmonary edema	1

The morbidity was 5.1%, the case fatality rate 18.9%, and the population mortality 1.0%. Both morbidity and mortality were higher during fall and winter than during spring and summer.

The diseases that may occur in epidemics in feedlots and that are considered to be economically most important are listed here:

Respiratory Tract
Pneumonic pasteurellosis (shipping fever)
Pleuritis and pulmonary abscesses (complications of pneumonia)
Infectious bovine rhinotracheitis
Necrotic laryngitis
Atypical interstitial pneumonia
Alimentary Tract
Carbohydrate engorgement (rumen overload, D–lactic acidosis)

Hepatic necrobacillosis
Ruminal tympany (bloat)
Bovine virus diarrhea
Salmonellosis
Bovine malignant catarrh
Nervous System and Eyes
Polioencephalomalacia
Hemophilus meningoencephalitis
Hypovitaminosis A
Infectious keratoconjunctivitis (pinkeye)
Genitourinary System
Obstructive urolithiasis
Postcastrational infection
Diseases Caused by Clostridia spp.
Blackleg
Malignant edema
Bacillary hemoglobinuria
Infectious hepatitis
Tetanus
Poisonings
Monensin
Salt
Urea
Nitrate
Organophosphate insecticide
Physical
Trauma
Electrocution
Drowning
Traumatic anovulvitis
Musculoskeletal System
Enzootic nutritional musculodystrophy
Laminitis
Mycoplasma arthritis
Skin
Foot rot
Ergotism
Mange
Parasitic Diseases
Intestinal helminthiasis
Pediculosis
Warbles (*Hypoderma* sp.)
Sarcosporidiosis
Miscellaneous
Riders and bullers due to excessive dose of
hormone implant
Anaplasmosis
Leptospirosis

EPIDEMIOLOGY OF DISEASES IN FEEDLOT CATTLE

In its broadest terms, a study of the epidemiology of diseases of feedlot cattle would include a description of disease statistics such as morbidity rate, case fatality and population mortality rates, the prevalence of the major diseases, the age and seasonal incidence of the economically important diseases, and the epidemiologic determinants such as the characteristics of the host, the environment, and the causative agent of the disease that leads to subclinical or clinical disease. The economical losses associated with feedlot disease include the losses from deaths, treatment of animals with clinical disease, and suboptimal performance due to subclinical disease.

There is an urgent need to know more about the frequency, epidemiologic determinants, and economics of feedlot disease in order to develop animal health management programs that are geared to working on the most economically important diseases.

The morbidity rate, case fatality rate, and population mortality rate associated with disease of feedlot cattle will vary between feedlots and depend on several factors. The mortality rates are higher in beef calves six to eight months of age (5 to 8%) than in yearling cattle (1 to 2%). Morbidity and mortality rates are highest during the first 45 days after arrival in the feedlot compared with the later part of the feeding period when the cattle have become adjusted to the feedlot.

The commonly occurring economically important diseases of feedlot cattle are the infectious diseases and those associated with intensive feeding on high-energy diets. There are several epidemiologic determinants that are usually associated with diseases of feedlot cattle. The animals are usually young, from two to 10 months of age, and often have originated from several different sources and thus have unequal acquired resistance to infectious disease. The stress of long transportation during inclement weather is considered a major predisposing factor in the pathogenesis of respiratory disease. Marked fluctuations in ambient temperature, snowstorms, and heavy rainfalls often precipitate outbreaks of respiratory disease and infectious foot rot. The incidence of respiratory disease is much higher in feedlot cattle raised indoors with inadequate ventilation than in cattle raised outdoors. The stress of crowding, co-mingling, and the use of prophylactic vaccines and drugs, and other processing procedures following arrival in the feedlot, combined with an increased opportunity for spread of infectious agents from animal to animal, often result in epidemics of infectious disease (Martin et al. 1980). Rapid changes in the composition of feeds and in feeding systems and errors in the mixing and distribution of feeds often result in outbreaks of digestive tract disease. The condition of the ground surface of the feedlot will influence the prevalence of foot rot. A wet, soggy, poorly drained surface with inadequate bedding may be associated with frequent outbreaks of foot rot.

There is only a small amount of documented information available on the epidemiology of feedlot diseases. Infectious diseases of the respiratory tract account for up to 75% of the illnesses and up to 65% of the population mortality in large feedlots, which annually feed and market 100 to 400 thousand head of cattle (Jensen et al. 1976a). Pneumonia is the major disease of feedlot cattle in North America and the United Kingdom and may account for more economic losses than all other diseases combined. Approximately 75% of all cases of shipping fever pneumonia occur during the first 45 days of the feeding period. This emphasizes the importance of stresses, such as shipping, exposure to feedlot pathogens, inhalation of feedlot dust, and adaptation to diets as possible factors in the complex etiology and pathogenesis of shipping fever pneumonia (Jensen et al. 1976b).

Other minor diseases of the respiratory tract that occur in feedlot cattle include atypical interstitial pneumonia in yearling cattle (Jensen et al. 1976c), bronchiectasis in yearling cattle (Jensen et al. 1976d), brisket disease in yearling cattle that had previously grazed on mountain ranges (Jensen et al. 1976e), and embolic pulmonary aneurysms in yearling cattle (Jensen et al. 1976f).

Bulling among steers, an abnormal behavioral trait, is a common health and economic problem in feedlot operations. Riders simulate males and bullers simulate females. Bullers sexually attract the riders, which repeatedly mount and physically injure the bullers. Although this behavior may continue until the bullers become exhausted, collapse, and die, the main economic loss results from physical injury, stress to both bull and rider, and the necessity of early isolation of the affected animals. The frequency rate may approximate 3% per annum (Pierson et al. 1976).

COMPONENTS OF A HEALTH MANAGEMENT AND PRODUCTION PROGRAM IN A FEEDLOT

The continued profitable success of a modern feedlot is dependent on the right combination of good management, a favorable economic climate, and relative freedom from unfortunate occurrences such as epidemics of disease or unexpected increases in the costs of inputs such as feed or decreases in the price received for the final product. Success is heavily dependent on each person in the team, including the cattle buyer, the animal attendants, the nutritional consultant, the veterinarian, and the manager of the feedlot, assuming his responsibility and doing the best work possible. Until recently, the part played by the veterinarian has not been clear. However, progress has been made, and feedlot veterinary medicine is becoming a specialty science that the profession can offer to the feedlot industry.

Veterinary medicine has been slow to meet the challenge of the feedlot industry. One major reason has been our preoccupation with the diagnosis and treatment of individual sick animals. As feedlots became larger and more sophisticated, it became obvious that knowledgeable animal attendants could successfully and economically diagnose and treat the common diseases of feedlot cattle. Veterinarians were thus used less and less on a routine basis and were called only when alarming epidemics of disease occurred that were not responding to the usual treatment procedures or in which the feedlot personnel could not make a diagnosis. This has now changed, and feedlots recognize the value of *constant surveillance* by a veterinarian who has specialized in feedlot veterinary medicine.

The successful feedlot veterinarian will deal with a broad concept of disease in the feedlot and not restrict the definition to simply sick animals. The concept of disease should be broadened to include all of the identifiable factors that result in suboptimal performance, which include inadequacies in the feeds and feeding systems, the purchase of undesirable types of cattle, and clinical and subclinical disease in the clinical sense.

The Relationship Between the Veterinarian and the Feedlot Personnel

The respective roles of management, animal attendants, and the veterinarian must be understood.

The Responsibilities of the Feedlot Manager and the Animal Health Technician

The responsibility of the feedlot manager is to coordinate the animal health and production activities of the feedlot, using advice obtained from the veterinarian, the nutritional consultant, and any other advisory service deemed necessary. The manager must supervise the animal health technicians, whose major responsibilities include the identification and treatment of sick animals and the processing of new arrivals.

Very close surveillance of all animals in the lot twice, or in recently introduced animals three times daily must be maintained in order to detect illness in the earliest stage possible, when therapy is highly successful. Without efficiency in this activity, the remainder of the program is largely pointless. The probability is that the people who work all day in the lot and know the cattle, and who are paid a high premium for efficiency and are good cattlemen and cattle watchers, will be more efficient at identifying sick animals than even a veterinarian.

Segregation and treatment of the animals selected as being sick is necessary. The number of diseases likely to be seen in any one feedlot is relatively few, and many of them can be easily identified by a watchful cattleman, especially if he has been carefully briefed by the veterinarian. The manager must be aware of an unusual increase in the incidence or behavior of a disease.

Management must supervise the feeding procedures to be used throughout the feeding cycle, especially in the induction period of three weeks after the cattle come into the lot, which is directed at preventing disease.

The recording of all animal health and production performance data is also the combined responsibility of the animal health technicians and the feedlot manager.

The manager is also responsible for the supervision of the buying and selling of the cattle, the purchase and processing of feeds, and the purchase of drugs, vaccines, and other necessary supplies.

Most importantly, the manager must communicate effectively with the animal health technicians, the veterinarian, and any other consultants. An effective communication atmosphere will go a long way toward solving problems.

The Responsibilities of the Veterinarian

The veterinarian should be responsible for the maintenance of optimal animal health through the following activities:

1. Make regularly scheduled visits to the feedlot, be punctual, and stay as long as is required for adequate consultation.

2. Be available for emergency visits to the feedlot when disease epidemics occur unexpectedly.

3. Perform necropsies on as many dead animals as possible.

4. Examine sick animals with the treatment crew to ensure that reasonably accurate diagnoses are being made and rational therapy given.

5. On a regular basis, examine, analyze, and interpret animal health and production data and make recommendations by a written report.

6. Discuss overall animal health and production performance with the feedlot manager and other consultants.

7. Take an interest in all aspects of the feedlot operation and be aware of new developments in the feedlot industry.

The Program in Action
Constant Surveillance

Constant surveillance by the feedlot personnel and the veterinarian is required. The frequency of regular visits by the veterinarian to the feedlot will vary from daily to once weekly or once monthly depending on the size of the lot, the management capabilities, the type of cattle fed, and the nature and prevalence of diseases encountered. There are several components of a feedlot health and management service that a veterinarian can provide; the details of each of these will be described.

Regular Inspection

Regular inspection of all areas of the feedlot for possible sources or causes of health problems should be included in a feedlot health service. Errors in animal husbandry should be noted and recorded for discussion with the personnel. Attention should be given to the delivery of feed and water, the general well-being of cattle, and any unusual characteristics of each feeding pen. Many feedlot health problems can be attributed to errors in management.

Disease Surveillance

Continual disease surveillance through regular necropsy examination and regular observations of sick cattle is necessary. Ideally, a necropsy should be done by the veterinarian on all dead cattle. However, this is usually not possible because the veterinarian may not visit the lot on each day an animal dies, which may be almost every day of the year in a large feedlot. In the areas with colder climates, during the winter months the carcasses may freeze solid before the veterinarian is available, or conversely, during the hot seasons of the year the carcass may decompose beyond usefulness. Some feedlot owners need to be encouraged to employ a veterinarian to conduct regular necropsies. Advantages include the identification of diseases that are occurring; confirmation of the clinical diagnosis; evaluation of the effectiveness of the various personnel involved with the health of the cattle, such as the buyer, truck driver, processing crew, pen checkers, treatment crew, feeders, manager, and veterinarian; evaluation of the effectiveness of the treatment protocol; and evaluation of the effectiveness of specific disease prevention programs and any changes that may be necessary.

A focal point in management of disease in the feedlot is fast, accurate diagnosis. This necessitates a good surveillance system, a careful full-time search for sick animals, appropriate facilities for examination and treatment of sick animals, accurate identification of animals, and first-class laboratory facilities, especially a necropsy service. A typical flow pattern in a feedlot is illustrated in Figure 10–1.

The training and supervision of feedlot employees in the detection and early treatment of sick cattle should be emphasized. Employees should be given regular sessions that illustrate the clinical signs of the common diseases. It is the veterinarian's responsibility to ensure that adequate personnel are available to thoroughly inspect each pen of cattle at least once daily and preferably twice daily.

Surveillance Method. The feeding pens must be under surveillance every day and on at least two occasions per day. When certain epidemics of disease occur, such as hemophilus meningoencephalitis, it is necessary to check the animals as often as every six hours on a 24-hour basis for a period of 10 days in order to detect new cases as early as possible, when they will respond to treatment. The surveillance can be done from horseback or by walking through the pens, but it is essential to be up close and to be able to move the cattle apart, but slowly and with the least possible harassment. Pen checking is an art that requires constant practice and attention to small details.

How to Check a Pen of Cattle. Once he knows what signs to look for, a pen checker needs a system for finding sick cattle, and he

must look at all the cattle in the pen. Feedlot men know that sick cattle tend to drift away from well animals, and a "loner" deserves some special attention. As they separate, sick cattle often can be found around the outside edges of the pen. To spot those cattle, start checking before you go into the pen. Figure 10–2A shows how the pen checker can start to identify sick cattle. The most common mistake among pen checkers is to recognize a few sick cattle on the edges and, instead of marking those animals immediately, the checker goes directly to the center of the pen to stir up the other cattle. As a result, the sick and well cattle are all mixed, and the poor checker usually loses the sick cattle that were on the outside edges. It happens as shown in Figure 10–2B.

The best method of working through the pen is shown in Figure 10–2C. Note that this gives the pen checker a chance to quietly mark or pull the sick cattle on the outside edges when he first enters the pen. Then, he can go on to check the rest of the cattle. The pattern in Figure 10–2C gives the checker an opportunity to see all of the cattle, from both sides. It also allows him to check the waterers and the feed bunks and any other potential problems. His list ought to include the following:

▫ Brand or ear-tag identification on cattle in the pen. Are there strays? Have cattle been mixed?

▫ Conditions in the pen. Are there mudholes that need filling? Is the pen so bad the cattle can't lie down?

▫ Conditions at the feed bunk. Are feed trucks overrunning high-energy diets at the end of a bunk so green cattle in the next pen can get to it? What is the condition of the feed in the bunk? Does the bunk need cleaning? Are the water tanks full and operative? Has feed been spilled? Has feed been mixed and the wrong ration fed to the cattle?

On the subject of diets, a pen checker ought to learn to recognize every diet coming out of the feed mill by sight.

Here are some other bits of advice about finding sick cattle that ought to be followed by pen checkers:

▫ The "loner" animal deserves special attention. However, in certain cases, the sick animal may not be a loner. In nervous diseases, when the affected animal starts to lose its eyesight, it will actually seek the security of being close to the bodies and sounds of its penmates.

▫ Gaunt, "hollow" animals that are not "filled up" are abnormal. The animal that is not

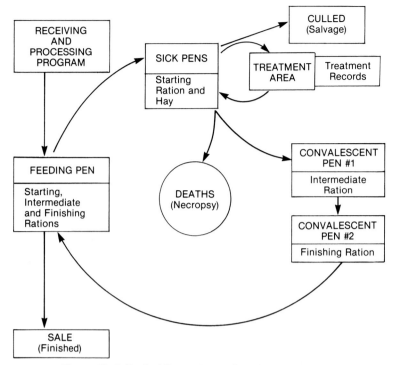

Figure 10-1. Typical flow pattern of cattle in feedlots.

gaining or keeping up with its penmates and the animal lacking appetite need to be pulled. Observe the left flank for fullness.

□ Pen checking assignments ought to be fixed. Each checker should be assigned pens with the sole responsibility to check those pens every day. In this way, he will be familiar with the history of the cattle and will learn the habits of those cattle.

Fixed assignments help management too. The death loss from certain pens and response of cattle to treatment allows management to identify the efficient pen checker and points up individuals that may need extra training.

□ Black cattle need extra attention. Their normally dark color often masks fine gradations of color that are a real tip-off in light-colored cattle. Bloody diarrhea is more difficult to spot on the black animal, especially if the animal is wet. Eye inflammations and tear staining of the face is more difficult to see on black cattle.

□ Study the ground. As we mentioned, droppings can tell you a lot. Close observation of the rumps on cattle will help identify the afflicted cattle. If you still have problems, study the fine hairs on the underside of the tail, or check pens at more frequent intervals to spot the sick cattle.

□ Get the cattle up. The animal that rises, stretches, and defecates is normal, but normal cattle also may skip that routine. You positively cannot identify lame or crippled cattle or cattle with foot rot while they are lying down; you also cannot spot coordination problems.

□ Use other senses in addition to sight. Listen. Can you hear labored breathing? Groaning, grunting, snoring, sniffling, and coughing all tell you something. Also, use your nose to detect abnormal conditions.

□ Observe cattle from a distance. When working a pen, look at the cattle in the pen behind you or ahead of you. The cattle will be undisturbed and quiet, and sick animals will often stand out more from a distance.

□ Work cattle slowly. Excitement can elevate temperatures 3 to 4°F, giving the treatment crew an abnormally high reading.

□ If you are in doubt, mild exercise of the animal may exaggerate symptoms enough to remove the doubt.

□ When cattle are found dead in the pens, have the pen checkers observe the necropsies and have the veterinarian review the fundamentals.

The selection of pen checkers is very important. They need to be very observant, very knowledgeable, and very trustworthy and must have sharp eyes if early diagnosis is to be

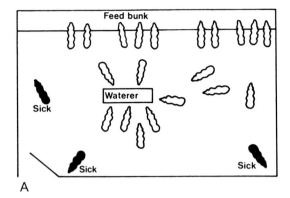

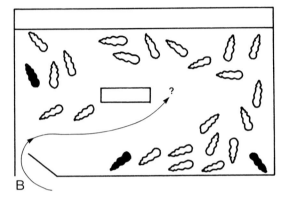

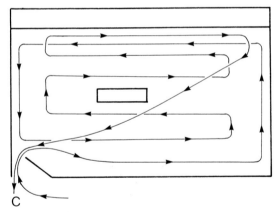

Figure 10-2. How to walk a pen. *A,* A typical pen. *B,* The wrong approach. *C,* A better method. (From Dull, R.O. Pen-checking is an art. Cattlemen. The Beef Magazine, September, 1980, pp. 30, 32, 34. Winnipeg, Manitoba.)

2. Reluctance to rise or move; to be lame or have other abnormal gait, such as knuckling of the fetlocks or dragging of the toes
3. Crusted muzzle, sunken eyes, and rough, dry-looking coat
4. Diarrhea (blood and mucus in the feces)
5. Coughing, nasal discharge, and rapid respirations
6. Straining to urinate with grunting and tail switching
7. Drooped head and ears; arched back
8. Failure to gain weight normally

Cattle showing these or other obvious signs of illness are examined more closely in the hospital area, and if treatment is appropriate, it is administered—in most cases, once daily for three days. After a convalescent period of a further three days, recovered animals are put back into their original pens. A decision, of course, rests on the nature of the disease, but most animals that do not recover or that relapse after the first treatment are re-treated. The criteria on which further decisions are based are obscure. Obviously, there comes a time when the expenditure of more money on an animal that is going to be an uneconomical proposition is unwarranted. A decision on what course to take depends on whether or not the animal's life is in danger or whether it is a matter of doing poorly. If the animal's life is at risk there is the potential loss of capital invested, and all efforts are directed toward avoiding this. If the animal can still be sold and chances of recovery are slim, it is usual to cull it after two courses of treatment. This rule of thumb depends on the fact that it costs a great deal more, in terms of labor, to keep an animal in the hospital than in the feeding yards, and sick animals should either be returned quickly to their own yards or be slaughtered. In some feedlots, it is the practice to make up a pen of slow gainers, but these can be an awful nuisance and in most cases do not provide the income per day required to finance the capital invested in the feedlot.

An important technique is to have especially close surveillance of the pens from which sick animals are taken. It is imperative that a potential epidemic be identified early so that mass medication in the feed or water or by injection of all animals can be considered.

Laboratory tests are conducted as required, and it is not proposed to detail these here. However, it should be a policy to conduct a necropsy on every animal that dies. A feedlot veterinarian needs to have a good pathology background and be as adept at interpreting

made. One such pen rider can maintain surveillance over 10,000 head of cattle. If the lot is large enough, it is most economical if the riders work in threes, permitting one to cut out and drive to the hospital yards.

The signs of ill health that are used to determine the presence of illness are:
1. Animals observed to be not coming up to the feed trough or to have less than normal gut fill, that is, to have a gaunt look

gross postmortem lesions as he is at interpreting clinical signs and lesions. The key to successful veterinary preventive medical service to a feedlot is prompt, accurate diagnosis, and the use of all available economical laboratory aids is to be encouraged.

Treatment Protocols

The veterinarian must specify procedures for the clinical management of sick cattle and provide a standard protocol that outlines specific treatments for disease syndromes, dosages, treatment intervals, routes of administration, and withdrawal times. The effectiveness of the treatment protocol should be regularly evaluated by determining the response rates for the various treatment regimens. The failure of feedlots to use regular competent veterinary supervision and analysis of treatment protocols often leads to the use of many different drugs indiscriminately, which results in an overexpenditure for treatment and often an increase in the case fatality rate.

Feedlot Records

Records are essential to monitor the incidence of disease, the response to treatment, and production performance. The records must be regularly analyzed by the veterinarian and feedlot manager. There are many variations of record systems for feedlots, but they should include the following information (Church 1980). The veterinarian must collect as much of this data as possible on a regular basis, analyze and interpret it, and submit a written report of recommendations to the feedlot manager. Some feedlots now have this data computerized, and regular summaries of health and production information and, most importantly, the costs of each component of feedlot production are made available.

1. **Daily Morbidity and Mortality Statistics** (Fig. 10–3). This data should be kept in a central location and updated daily by the pen checkers. It simply records the number of sick and/or dead cattle by pen or lot number and the date. It provides both the manager and the veterinarian with a rapid assessment of the location of disease problems in the feedlot.

2. **Daily Treatment Record** (Fig. 10–4). Each animal treated should be positively identified and recorded on the treatment card. The treatment personnel should record feeding pen, lot number, body temperature, disease suspected, treatment given, and disposition of the animal following treatment. The severity of the illness should be assessed in

order to properly evaluate treatment. Late treatment in advanced stages of disease, particularly respiratory disease, is a major cause of failure to respond in spite of the use of antibiotics of choice. A card is made out for each animal that becomes ill initially, and all subsequent illnesses are recorded on the same card. The cards are filed and retrieved for animals that relapse or die. The cumulative information on the card can be used to decide if an animal should be culled for chronic or recurring illnesses that are refractory to treatment, to decide on alternate treatments, to explain reasons for death and, of major importance, to evaluate the effectiveness of the treatments recommended.
of 2

3. **Morbidity and Treatment Analysis** (Fig. 10–5). Treatment data should be summarized and interpreted on at least a monthly basis. The analysis should include the diseases treated, treatments used, outcome of treatments, average days treated, and case fatality rates. The accuracy of the treatment analysis may be improved by correlating the clinical response rate with the results of necropsies and drug sensitivity testing of bacteria isolated from affected animals (Martin et al. 1983).

4. **Mortality Analysis** (Fig. 10–6). The causes of death determined by necropsy should be summarized on a regular basis. An analysis of the epidemiology of mortality rates would include total number of days the animal was in the feedlot, any premonitory signs that were observed, and treatment of the animal (with what drug, in what dosage, and at what stage of the disease). The location of the mortality in the feedlot and unexpected occurrences of mortality should also be recorded.

The mortalities may be classified into preventable and nonpreventable categories. Preventable mortalities are those that are considered to be due to inadequacies in management or in the techniques of feedlot personnel. In a large commercial feedlot that purchases cattle from a variety of sources, the personnel that may contribute to feedlot mortalities include the veterinarian, pen checkers, the feedlot manager, the treatment crew, the processing crew, feed mill and feeding system personnel, the truck driver who delivered the cattle, and the commissioned livestock buyer who bought the cattle. A regular summary of the possible relationship between mortality and the feedlot personnel will allow the manager to institute any necessary changes in management. For example, unexpected high mortality due to pneumonia in recently arrived

PULLS
DEADS

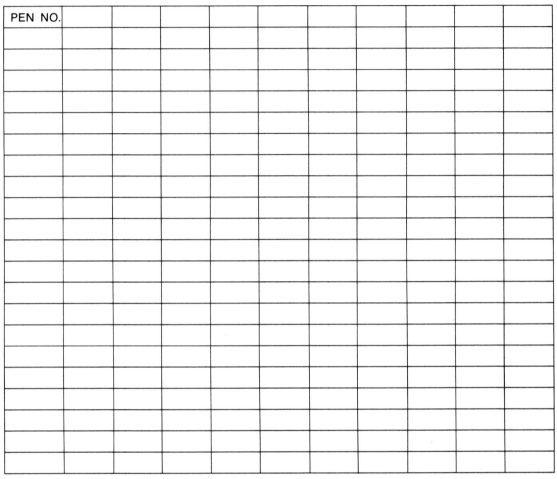

PEN NO.										

Figure 10-3. Daily pull and dead record.

cattle may be associated by the buyer with the purchase of animals that were affected with acute or chronic respiratory disease at the time of purchase.

5. **Monthly Disease Summary** (Fig. 10-7). This summarizes the relevant information on the morbidity and mortality on a monthly basis and is cumulative for annual analysis. The following information is included:

□ Total number of cattle received during each month

□ Total number and per cent morbidity of cattle received during the month (including causes of illness)

□ Average number of days each animal was treated

□ Case fatality rate (per cent)

□ Response to each treatment of major groups of diseases (per cent)

□ Total number and per cent morbidity of cattle resident in the feedlot for more than 30 days (including causes of illness)

□ Total number and per cent mortality of cattle received during last month (including causes of mortality)

□ Total number and per cent mortality of cattle resident in the feedlot for more than 30 days (including causes of mortality)

6. **Feedlot Performance Summary** (Fig. 10-8). Most feedlots complete a close-out summary for each group of cattle that have been finished and shipped to market. Important data include average daily gain in body weight, total feed consumption, feed conversion ratios and cost per unit of body weight gain, morbidity and mortality rates, culling rate, treatment costs per head, and disease prevention costs per head (i.e., vaccines). This

DATE	TEMP.	DEGREE ILLNESS	WEIGHT	PEN.	TET.	SULF.	MEDICATIONS OTHER	OTHER	DIAGNOSIS/ DISPOSITION

PEN _____ LOT _____ SEX _____ TAG. NO. _____

Figure 10–4. Daily treatment record.

MONTH_____	ALL CATTLE		RELAPSES		DEATHS	
	NO.	%	NO.	%	NO.	%
NUMBER HEAD						
Steers						
Heifers						
DISPOSITION						
Recovered						
Chronics						
Culled						
Dead						
DISEASES						
Shipping Fever						
Respiratory-Other						
Foot & Leg						
Digestive						
Urinary						
Nervous						
Other						
TREATMENTS						
Tetracycline						
Penicillin						
Sulfonamides						
Other						
Other						
Average Days Treated						
RESPONSE RATES						
Tetracycline						
Penicillin						
Other						
Other						

Figure 10-5. Morbidity and treatment analysis.

information can be used to correlate disease occurrence with type of cattle, season, origin of cattle, and certain disease prevention procedures that may have been applied to the particular pen of animals. An example of a lot report in a feedlot is shown in Figure 10-9.

THE LOT REPORT. The lot report gives the financial summary of the performance of that lot. The profit or loss on an individual lot basis can be estimated to evaluate the performance of different types of animals in relation to the entire feedlot. Begin the lot report when cattle enter the lot, update it throughout the feeding period, and complete it when the animals are sold.

When calculating the interest on the calf, the value can be the market value—if you bought the calf—or the production costs—if you have

(Text continued on page 268)

MONTH _____ 19___

DATE NO.	LOT NO.	DATE OF ARRIVAL	DIAGNOSIS	MANAGEMENT FACTOR RESPONSIBLE FOR DEATH	CODE	RECOMMENDATION TO PREVENT FUTURE LOSSES

CODE: 1. Veterinarian, 2. Checkers, 3. Treatment, 4. Processing, 5. Feeder, 6. Management, 7. Trucker, 8. Buyer, 9. Unavoidable.

Figure 10-6. Mortality analysis.

SUMMARY DEATH LOSS ANALYSIS

	JAN	FEB	MAR	APR	MAY	JUN	JUL	AUG	SEPT	OCT	NOV	DEC	TOTAL
TOTAL DEATHS													
UNAVOIDABLE DEATHS													
PREVENTABLE DEATHS													

SUMMARY DEATH LOSS BY ERROR AND MONTH

ERROR SOURCES	JAN	FEB	MAR	APR	MAY	JUN	JUL	AUG	SEPT	OCT	NOV	DEC	TOTAL
1. VETERINARIAN													
2. PEN CHECKERS													
3. TREATMENT													
4. PROCESSING													
5. FEEDER													
6. MANAGEMENT													
7. TRUCKER													
8. BUYER													
9. UNKNOWN & MISC.													
10. NOT EXAMINED													
TOTALS													

Figure 10-7. Summary death loss analysis.

	JAN.	FEB.	MAR.	APR.	MAY	JUN.	JUL.	AUG.	SEPT.	OCT.	NOV.	DEC.	TOTAL
NUMBER OF VISITS													
NUMBER CATTLE REC'D													
MORTALITY													
Total Deaths, No.													
Pen Deaths %													
Preventable Deaths %													
Cattle on Feed, %													
Closed-out Cattle %													
Respiratory %													
Foot & Leg %													
Digestive %													
Other													

MORBIDITY

Total Treated, No.												
Pull Rate Current %												
Pulls Closed-out %												
Respiratory %												
Foot & Leg %												
Digestive %												
Other %												
Ave. Days Treated												
Death Loss Treated %												

RESPONSE RATES

Tetracycline %				
Penicillin %				
Other				

Figure 10–8. Monthly herd health summary.

Lot No._____   Pen No._____

Feed and Weight Data:

Opening date_____Closing date_____Days on feed_____

Head in_____Head out_____Death loss_____head

Weight in_____lb. Weight out_____lb. Gain_____lb.

Total feed consumed_____/pen_____/head

Weight gain/head/day_____lb.

Feed consumption/head/day_____lb.

Feed consumption/lb. of gain_____

Cost Data

Yardage _____ /head

Milling _____ /head

Bedding _____ /head

Chute charge _____ /head

Feed cost_____ /head

Vet. and med. _____ /head

Marketing costs _____ /head

Interest on cash costs:

$$= \frac{\text{Bedding + Chute + Feed + Vet. costs}}{2} \times \frac{\text{Interest rate} \times \text{Feeding period}}{365 \text{ days}}$$

= _____/head

$$\text{Interest on calf} = Value \times \frac{\text{Interest rate} \times \text{Feeding period}}{365 \text{ days}} = \underline{\hspace{3cm}} /head$$

Total cost _____ /head

Total cost/lb. of gain _____ /head

Total revenue _____ /head

Total cost _____ /head

Profit or loss _____ /head

Figure 10-9. A lot report (to calculate cost data, refer to Figure 10-10 to determine yardage, milling and bedding costs, and chute charges). (From Finishing Cattle on the Family Farm, pp. 36-37. Animal Industry Branch Saskatchewan Agriculture Regina 1980.)

raised the calf at home. Use the current operating loan interest rate as the interest rate in the formulas.

CALCULATING FEEDLOT COSTS (Fig. 10-10)

Yardage. This includes labor costs (except chute labor), interest on operating money, investment cost, maintenance, and operation of all facilities.

Calculate the cost of labor by estimating the amount of time spent working on the feeder enterprise in relation to the total farm operation and charging the same portion of the annual wage to the feedlot. Multiply the number of days the feedlot is operated by the

the straw. The amount used is highly variable, number of head fed out annually. Divide this answer into the cost of labor. This will provide a per head per day cost of labor for the feedlot. Calculate the cost of hired labor in the same manner.

Calculate investment cost by using the appropriate amortization factor multiplied by the replacement cost of the facility.

Milling Charges. These include all operating, maintenance, and investment costs associated with all farm equipment used in the feedlot and are calculated on a per ton basis.

Bedding. Calculate bedding costs in cents

per pound based on the actual market value of depending mostly on weather. A very rough guideline would be three pounds per head per day.

Chute Cost. As cattle enter a feedlot, several procedures must be done: dehorning; branding; tagging; vaccinations and treatment for parasites; implanting; injection of vitamins A, D and E; and weighing. Calculate the cost of performing each of these and add them together as a miscellaneous or chute charge.

Vaccination Protocols

An important component of feedlot health programs is the planning of vaccination programs. The vaccines and the vaccination schedule will vary from area to area, depending on the prevalence of disease in the feedlot area and in the area from which the cattle originated. There is a tendency for feedlots to use too many vaccines in the hope that the common infectious diseases will be controlled at a low level. This usually results in overex-

penditures and less than satisfactory disease control. The kinds of vaccines used and the vaccination schedule should be based on the expected prevalence of the diseases, which in turn are based on sound statistical epidemiologic data obtained from the disease records generated by the feedlot.

Nutritional Advice

Large feedlots frequently consult a qualified nutritionist to assist in the formulation of least-cost diets. The veterinarian should establish effective regular communication with the nutritionist and be aware of the composition of the diets and any changes that are being planned. In other situations, the feedlot veterinarian may be in a position to provide regular nutritional advice as part of a complete service. Because feed is the major portion of the cost per unit of body weight gain, it is imperative that the diet be least-cost and at the same time provide the nutrients that will allow optimum growth and finishing. Most of the emphasis in

---

A. *Yardage*
  1. Labor cost
    Hired and owner labor (except chute labor):

$$\frac{\text{Total cost of labor}}{\text{No. of head} \times \text{No. of days}} = \underline{\hspace{3cm}}/\text{head/day}$$

  2. Facility cost
    (a) Operating cost:

$$\frac{\text{Annual maintenance and repairs}}{\text{No. of head} \times \text{No. of days (normally 365)}} = \underline{\hspace{3cm}}\text{head/day}$$

    (b) Investment cost:

$$\frac{\text{Replacement cost} \times \text{Amortization factor (20 years)}}{\text{No. of head} \times \text{No. of days}} = \underline{\hspace{3cm}}\text{head/day}$$

  3. *Total yardage cost*
    On a per head per day basis:
    Labor cost (1) + Facility cost (2a + 2b) = \underline{\hspace{3cm}}head/day

B. *Milling*
  1. Operating and maintaining equipment:

$$\frac{\text{Total fuel, oil and repairs}}{\text{No. of tons processed/year}} = \underline{\hspace{3cm}}/\text{ton}$$

  2. Investment cost of machinery:

$$\frac{\text{Replacement value of all machinery used in feedlot}}{\text{No. of tons processed/year}} \times \frac{\text{Amortization}}{\text{factor (10)}} = \underline{\hspace{3cm}}/\text{ton}$$

  3. Total milling cost per ton

$$\frac{\text{Operating and}}{\text{maintaining equipment}}^{(1)} + \frac{\text{Investment cost}}{\text{of machinery}}^{(2)} = \underline{\hspace{3cm}}/\text{ton}$$

C. *Bedding*
  Market value of straw per ton ÷ 2000 lb = \underline{\hspace{3cm}}/pound

D. *Chute charges*
  Chute charges or processing fees are a flat charge/head = \underline{\hspace{2cm}}/head

Figure 10–10. Cost calculation guide (the guide shown here is for feedlot costs associated with producing slaughter animals).

feedlot nutrition has been on developing least-cost diets that will support a maximum growth rate without any deleterious effects. There is considerable information available on the nutrient requirements for feedlot cattle and on the feeds and feeding systems used.

Nutritional deficiency diseases are uncommon in feedlot cattle because they usually receive a diet formulated to contain the nutrient requirements for maintenance and to promote rapid growth. Diets prepared according to the Nutrient Requirements of Beef Cattle should meet all the requirements under most practical conditions.

Specific nutrient deficiencies are extremely rare because diets are prepared every few days or daily, and it would be highly unusual for a feedlot to use a feedstuff deficient in a specific nutrient for a prolonged period. Such a situation may occur in a small farm feedlot that prepares its own feedlot diet with little or no attention to the necessity for supplementation of homegrown feeds.

The nutritionally related diseases of well-managed feedlot cattle are few but may be the cause of large economic losses when they occur. They include:

□ carbohydrate engorgement (grain overload or D-lactic acidosis)
□ ruminal tympany or feedlot bloat
□ feeding errors, i.e., accidental incorporation of an excessive amount of a feed additive such as monensin, or the sudden unintended changes in the ingredient composition of the diet

Investigation and Clinical Management of Epidemics of Disease

In spite of good management, unexpected epidemics of disease occur in feedlot cattle. With feeding accidents, many animals are affected suddenly, within one or two days. In outbreaks of acute infectious diseases like infectious bovine rhinotracheitis, pneumonic pasteurellosis, or hemophilus meningoencephalitis, the first few cases will be followed by a steady rise in the morbidity rate for several days and then a decline as the outbreak subsides in 10 days to two weeks after the index case.

In some cases, the diagnosis may be obvious, e.g., carbohydrate engorgement due to a feeding error. With infectious diseases of the respiratory tract, the etiological diagnosis may not be readily obvious and may require a detailed epidemiologic, clinical, and laboratory investigation. A complete investigation may require involvement of specialists in several disciplines. Every economical effort should be made to make a specific etiological diagnosis because it not only improves the efficacy of treatment and control but usually generates new knowledge about the disease, which may be applicable for future outbreaks.

With most outbreaks of disease in feedlot cattle, there is usually more than one method available for the clinical management of the problem, and the veterinarian is faced with making decisions that have major economic consequences. It seems logical that the best decision will be made when the most information is available. The details of the treatment of the specific diseases are described elsewhere, but the general principles for the investigation and clinical management of outbreaks of disease are discussed here.

The objectives of an investigation are to determine the specific etiology and the extent of the disease and then to take immediate corrective actions and make recommendations to prevent recurrences (Kahrs 1978). These objectives are best achieved by systematically delineating the characteristics of affected and unaffected animals within the study population and observing, recording, and analyzing the distribution of the disease with respect to time, place, and a variety of exposure factors and environmental influences. This analysis must be correlated with thorough physical examination and necropsy findings from representative patients.

A complete history should be outlined. This includes details on the first case (index case), the index date, the total number of sick animals, the treatments given, the case fatality rate, the population mortality rate, and the vaccination history. The origin of the cattle should be determined if possible, and the length of time the cattle have been in the lot may give some clues to a diagnosis. The composition of the feed and the nature of any recent changes in feeding practices should be determined. A sample of feed consumed by the affected animals should be obtained and analyzed or stored for future analysis.

A complete clinical examination should be done on several representative affected animals. Some normal in-contact animals should also be examined clinically. Frequently, there is evidence of the early stages of the disease in animals that appear normal on a distant examination. In the case of infectious disease, the appropriate samples, such as nasal swabs, blood, cerebrospinal fluid, and feces, should be taken from affected animals and submitted to the laboratory. Necropsies should be done on dead animals as soon as possible after death, before postmortem decomposition makes diagnosis difficult. If the diagnosis is not obvious on necropsy of animals that have died naturally, euthanasia and immediate necropsy of a few representative affected animals is recommended.

When the diagnosis is determined, the rationale for treatment is then outlined. Emergency slaughter for salvage may be the most economical method for the clinical management of diseases such as grain overload. Cattle affected with the common infectious diseases, such as pneumonic pasteurellosis or hemophilus meningoencephalitis, cannot be slaughtered for salvage, and treatment is necessary. Affected cattle should be suitably identified with an ear tag or back tag and the nature of the treatment recorded. Isolation and separation of affected animals from the normal population until recovery is apparent is the ideal situation.

When outbreaks of infectious disease are encountered, the intensity of surveillance must be increased in order to detect new cases in the early stages of the disease when the response to treatment is usually good. The detection of clinically affected cattle in the early stages of disease is difficult and requires considerable dedication by the pen checkers. Approximately 50% of the cattle that die from pneumonic pasteurellosis are found dead without any premonitory clinical signs. This occurs even in well-managed feedlots.

Mass medication of the feed and water supplies of all in-contact animals in an outbreak of infectious disease has received considerable attention. The antimicrobial agent of choice is placed in the feed or water as an aid in attempting to medicate animals in the early subclinical stages of the disease. The objective is to *abort* the outbreak. However, it is often difficult to assess the results, and few controlled clinical trials have been done to assess efficacy. The practice will probably continue on an empirical basis.

The injection of antimicrobials into all in-contact animals when the daily morbidity rate reaches 5 to 10% has been recommended. Long-acting oxytetracycline given intramuscularly to all in-contact animals may decrease the daily incidence of new cases (Janzen and McManus 1980).

Regardless of which mass medication system is used, none is totally reliable, and increased surveillance is usually necessary to detect new cases.

As much comfort as is economically feasible should be provided to clinically affected cattle. The amount of bedding should be increased, and protection from snow, rain, or excessive sunshine should be provided. In feeding accidents, the energy level of the feed should be reduced to a level similar to the starting ration. Following successful therapy, the cattle may be reintroduced to the high-energy rations.

All of the details of the outbreak should be listed in chronological order and then analyzed and interpreted. Correlations can be made between exposure factors and the occurrence of new cases during the course of the outbreak. Often epidemiologic determinants can be identified that explain why the disease occurred. This information can be used to control future occurrences. A detailed report of the outbreak, outlining the conclusions and recommendations, should be prepared and submitted by the veterinarian to the owner.

THE CONTROL AND PREVENTION OF DISEASES OF FEEDLOT CATTLE

The successful and economical control and prevention of diseases of feedlot cattle will depend on the right combination of purchasing healthy animals, a transportation system that minimizes stress, a feedlot pen environment that is comfortable, an adequate feeding system, a good surveillance system, and the judicious use of vaccines, growth promotants, and antimicrobial agents when necessary.

The Adequacy of Feedlot Facilities

Large commercial feedlots that purchase and market large numbers of cattle will have the usual facilities for unloading and loading and for weighing and sorting cattle. Some feedlots have starting or introductory pens that are equipped to observe and remove sick cattle easily. The cattle are fed in these pens until they have adjusted and been processed; then they are sorted and grouped according to size and condition and placed in finishing pens. However, in other feedlots, there are no introductory pens, and the finishing pens are filled to capacity as the cattle arrive. Adequate treatment facilities and hospital pens should be provided. Only severely ill animals that need daily treatment for several days should be removed from their original pens and confined in the hospital pen until they have recovered or are culled. The pens and alleyways should be well drained and easily accessible for scraping the ground surface as necessary. Good drainage requires a 6% slope. To avoid overstocking, each animal should be provided with 18 m.^{2} of space in well-drained land and 9 m.^{2} in a paved lot.

Cattle and feed need protection from wind, rain, snow, excessive heat, and sunshine. Make snow fences with 20% openings and locate them so that snowdrifts accumulate outside the pens and alleyways. Plant trees as windbreaks and place buildings and fences so that the wind is not deflected into feeding areas or sheds. An open-front shed over part of the feedlot provides protection for cattle from winter storms and hot summer sun. Each animal needs about 1 to 1.5 m.^{2} of cover. The shed should be open to the south or southeast. The front should be high enough so that the sun strikes the ground at the back on the shortest day of the winter. The back of the shed should be at least 2.5 m. high. A covered feed bunk protects feed from weather damage and affords cattle added comfort when eating. Feed remains dry and palatable, and waste is reduced.

Feedlots and Environmental Pollution

During the early days of development of feedlots, there was little to worry the operator other than feed costs and the ravages of disease. There was always the minor problem of locating the lot where drainage was good in order to avoid soft feet and a predisposition to foot rot. Recently, other more difficult problems have become apparent.

In keeping with a rise in most esthetic values, it is now necessary to prevent cattle from becoming too muddy. If they are too disreputable, slaughterhouse workers are likely to refuse to handle them. Then, there is the matter of environmental pollution via waterways, by dust, by smell, and by providing a breeding ground for flies. Anti-pollution campaigners find feedlots a particularly tasty prize because they offend so obviously and in so many ways. Manure disposal can no longer be effected by tipping it into a river, and a great deal of ingenuity has gone into ways of disposing of it. One of the most satisfactory ones is its conversion into a high-quality compost of protein-rich food by a process of continuous aerobic fermentation. To do this requires that the cattle be under roofs, on deep litter and earthen floors. The speed of the process—14 days—makes it economical. It completely avoids water pollution, there is absolutely no smell, and pathogens are destroyed by the heat generated in the fermentation process. It is necessary to do something of this sort because leakage of any sewage into a local waterway represents a breach of so many municipal regulations.

The control of flies is also becoming a major concern in many communities; this is largely a problem of controlling smell and generating enough heat to kill larvae. Anyone who has seen the dust cloud rising from a large feedlot in the dusk of a hot summer day will know that dust is another one of the main threats to the continuation of the feedlot system. A great deal of money now needs to be spent keeping yards scraped clean of dusty soil and spraying them with water from a boom spray every afternoon. There is no reasonable way of stopping the cattle from having their late afternoon stirring and playing.

Another important factor that is tending to act as a brake on productivity is animal welfare—a brake in the sense that it may result in reduced economic efficiency of production rather than being an embarrassment to progress. Those groups of people who look upon animal welfare as their responsibility tend to regard open yards as unkind and demand shelter from either the hot sun or from the cold.

Transportation of Cattle to the Feedlot

Transportation is considered to be one of the most important stresses associated with the acute respiratory disease complex in feedlot cattle. Even with the appropriate rest stops for unloading and feeding and watering, there may be major economic losses due to deaths or illness in feeder calves transported over long distances (2000 to 3000 km.). Severe outbreaks of pneumonic pasteurellosis may occur in feeder calves during these long trips, and upon reaching their destination, 2 to 3% may be dead and up to 25% may be clinically affected with acute pneumonia.

The producer or buyer should select the best method of transportation available. The most important principle in transportation of feeder cattle is to accomplish it in the shortest time possible. It will normally be either truck or rail transportation or a combination of the two, whichever is best suited to the particular situation. The transportation facility should be given sufficient notice, including special needs, in advance of shipment so that cars or trucks will be available, properly prepared, and ready for loading at the designated time. Extreme weather conditions should be avoided.

Cattle should be handled with a minimum of excitement. This is particularly important for newly weaned calves. Careless handling and transportation of weaned calves can negate any effort the producer may have made to produce healthy preconditioned calves.

There is considerable loss of weight in cattle within the first 24 to 48 hours following weaning, during shipment, and following deprivation of feed and water. The loss in body weight is known as *shrink*. It will vary from a minimum of 4% in cattle deprived of feed and water for 24 hours up to 9% in animals that are transported long distances over a period of two to four days. Some of the shrink is due to the normal loss of fluids and electrolytes from the digestive tract without normal replenishment. Excitement during handling and transportation increases the total amount of shrink. Most of the fluid and electrolyte shrink can be restored within a few days if the animals begin to eat and drink normally. Cattle subjected to long transportation or excessive handling for a few days will also be affected by tissue shrink. The total loss in body weight may not be restored for up to three weeks.

The transportation equipment and facilities should meet local standards and be prepared to transport cattle comfortably regardless of the season of the year. An adequate carrier will include a complete cover to protect the animals from the hot sun in the summer, rain and snow, and extreme cold in the winter. Modern carriers are now equipped with ventilators. Adequate footing or bedding should be provided to prevent slipping and falling. In cold weather, additional bedding such as straw should be provided.

When long trips of over 800 km. or 24 hours are necessary, calves should be unloaded, fed some good-quality dry hay, allowed to drink water, and rested for several hours before continuing the trip. In some countries, legislation prohibits the transportation of cattle over a certain length of time without unloading for rest, feed, and water. The optimum number of cattle that should be loaded per rail car or truck will depend on the size of the animals, the size of the vehicle, and local practices. On arrival at their destination, the cattle should be examined carefully for evidence of clinical disease. The provision of fresh hay and water will help to detect those that are anorexic and that should be examined more closely. This is particularly important if unexpected delays in transportation have occurred that will increase the level of stress in the animals.

The Purchase of Cattle and Their Introduction to a Feedlot

The purchase of cattle and their introduction to a feedlot has been a controversial issue in beef production ever since the development of commercial feedlots. Commercial feedlots attempt to purchase the most inexpensive cattle that will perform the best and provide maximum economic returns. However, infectious diseases of the respiratory tract, particularly "shipping fever" pneumonia due to *Pasteurella* spp., are major causes of morbidity and mortality during the first 30 to 45 days after arrival in the feedlot. Digestive diseases—especially carbohydrate engorgement—in cattle being placed on a high-energy diet within 30 days after arrival in the feedlot, although a major potential threat, can be controlled. The acute respiratory disease complex is much more difficult to control in feedlot cattle, even under good management conditions.

Epidemiologic observations over many years indicate that several determinants cause stress, which contributes to the pathogenesis of acute respiratory disease complex in feedlot cattle. The routine process of weaning beef calves at six to eight months of age in North America is often followed by respiratory disease. Any factor that causes additional stress at weaning time will result in an increased incidence of disease. Transportation over long distances without adequate rest and feeding periods will often be followed by a herd problem. Rapid changes in weather and unexpected snowstorms at the time of shipping may result in outbreaks of shipping fever. The placement of recently weaned beef calves, at six to eight months of age, into the feedlot is associated with much higher morbidity and mortality rates than older yearling cattle. Presumably, this is due to the higher level of acquired immunity in the older cattle. The stress of handling recently weaned beef calves is considered to be a major factor contributing to shipping fever pneumonia. Cattle are often vaccinated, dehorned, castrated, branded, implanted, and injected with vitamins and antibiotics within a few days after their arrival in the feedlot. Veterinarians have usually recommended that recently arrived cattle should not be processed for 10 days to two weeks or until the animals have become adjusted to the feedlot. However, many feedlot operators claim that delaying the processing until up to two weeks after arrival or until the cattle become adjusted does not result in a lower incidence of disease and is not economical. Carefully controlled trials to compare the different approaches have not been done. In fact, it may be difficult to duplicate the realistic commercial feedlot system in which cattle from many different sources are being introduced and mixed with other recently arrived cattle that may or may not be in the early stages of acute respiratory disease. The epidemiologic principles do not exist to control disease satisfactorily under these conditions. The acute respiratory disease complex may remain a major source of economic loss in the feedlot industry if it continues the common practice of introducing stressed cattle from different sources, with different immunological backgrounds, into populations of cattle in which disease is endemic.

This section will outline and describe the methods that are available to obtain cattle and introduce them into the feedlot and attempt to minimize the economically important diseases.

The major objective is to get the cattle onto a high-energy diet—which will result in rapid growth—as soon as possible, usually within 21 days, and at the same time to minimize the morbidity and mortality associated with acute respiratory disease, some other common infections such as hemophilus septicemia, and digestive diseases associated with adjustments to high-energy diets. A major consideration is to achieve all of these objectives most economically.

Origin and Purchase of Cattle

This is a very important phase of feedlot operations. A decision on what kind of cattle to buy and where to buy them is largely a matter of risk aversion. How much risk is the feedlot operator willing to take? It is possible to buy groups of uniform feeder calves or yearling cattle that come from one source and in which the disease incidence will be very low. However, these cattle cost more, and the gross margin is smaller than for cattle originating from several sources and accumulated and sold through public auction sales yards. The incidence of disease is much higher in weaned beef calves than in yearling cattle. In very young dairy calves being reared for barley-beef units,

the incidence of enteric colibacillosis and salmonellosis can cause high mortality rates.

The principles that need to be considered when purchasing cattle and introducing them to a highly intensive, heavy feeding environment are as follows:

1. Purchase healthy cattle.

2. Obtain cattle directly from the farm of origin if possible.

3. The disease incidence is lower in yearling cattle than in feeder calves.

4. Adopt the all-in–all-out principle. The cattle are purchased as a group, fed as the same group, and sold as a group. This would tend to break the chain of infection from one group to another. A corollary to this principle is to avoid the mixing of recently arrived cattle with cattle already resident in the feedlot. Because of fluctuations in the supply of cattle that may occur, feedlots will often continue to assemble and make up groups of cattle over a period of several days or a few weeks. As recently arrived cattle are added to existing groups, new outbreaks of disease occur, which may be perpetuated for several weeks.

5. Purchase preimmunized or preconditioned cattle if possible and if economical.

6. Transport the cattle to the feedlot in the shortest time that is economically feasible.

7. Develop a reporting system that regularly informs the cattle buyer of the condition of the cattle received and their subsequent performance. This will assist the buyer in the purchase of healthy cattle, avoiding unhealthy cattle and ensuring that they are transported by the most economical and least stressful method of transportation.

In the simplest system, a cow/calf producer weans the calves at six to eight months of age and places them in the home farm feedlot. The calves are gradually brought onto a growing and then a finishing diet and marketed at 12 months of age. Alternatively, the calves may be kept on a maintenance and growth diet until they become yearlings, at which time they are placed in the farm feedlot or sold to a commercial feedlot. These calves would usually be vaccinated for the clostridial diseases. They may also be vaccinated for infectious bovine rhinotracheitis and other common infectious agents associated with respiratory disease. If these cattle are kept in their original groups until market, the morbidity and mortality may be very low and insignificant. However, unexpected outbreaks of diseases such as hemophilus meningoencephalitis may occur under the best of management.

Preimmunization and Preconditioning

The large economic losses associated with the high morbidity and mortality due to acute respiratory disease in weaned beef calves shipped from the ranch, within a few days after weaning, to sales yards and then to feedlots led to the development of the concept of preconditioning. Preconditioning is based in part on immunological and nutritional principles. The first is that effective immunity against infectious diseases of the respiratory tract can be achieved only if the animals are vaccinated in sufficient time before natural exposure occurs after arrival in the feedlot. Preimmunization, or simply vaccination of calves two to three weeks before shipment from the ranch to the feedlot, against the common infectious agents associated with acute respiratory disease was the beginning of the practice of preconditioning (Hoerlein 1973). Vaccination prior to shipment did not appear to provide sufficient protection against disease in calves after arrival in the feedlot. However, calves were still being stressed during transportation and by salesyard procedures, and this led to a broader concept of preconditioning. In addition to vaccination, the newer efforts were increasingly directed to management procedures on the ranch that would assist the calf in making an easier transition to the feedlot.

Preconditioning of beef calves now includes the following (Church and Karren 1981):

1. The calves are weaned at least 30 days before shipment from the ranch.

2. The calves are individually identified, preferably with an ear tag applied by a licensed veterinarian.

3. The calves are castrated and dehorned at least two weeks before shipment so that adequate healing will occur.

4. The calves are vaccinated as necessary, under the supervision of the veterinarian, at least three weeks before shipment. The vaccines used and the vaccination schedule will vary from one area to another, depending on the prevalence of the disease.

5. Insecticides are applied; anthelmintics, as necessary, are given at least two weeks before shipment.

6. The calves are accustomed to eating from a feed trough and drinking from a water receptacle.

7. The calves are shipped directly to the feedlot by the most efficient means possible.

When these preconditioned calves are placed in a feedlot, they usually begin to eat and drink on arrival, and if not subjected to unusual stressors, the incidence of disease will be minimal. Surveillance on a daily basis is still necessary to identify cases of illness.

The proper preconditioning of calves involves cost to the primary producer. The rancher must gather and handle the calves early to vaccinate them, and after weaning he must provide an adequate diet until shipment. The loss of weight following weaning must be made up before the sale. If the producer is to engage in these practices, he must be adequately compensated. In Alberta, in 1981, the net returns were increased by $7.85 for preimmunized calves and $24.15 for preconditioned calves. The primary producer has shown considerable interest in delivering a quality calf to the feedlot but is understandably reluctant to add extra expense unless the returns are greater than the costs. The future of preconditioning will depend in large part on whether the livestock industry becomes convinced of its value. A major deterrent to the acceptance of preconditioning has been the lack of uniform procedures and certification by an impartial third party. The American Association of Bovine Practitioners has sponsored a standardized program that gives documented assurance to the feedlot that certain desirable procedures have actually been carried out.

Backgrounding

Backgrounding is a variation of preconditioning in which recently weaned calves are grown to yearling feeder cattle weight in a feedlot. The principal objective is to prepare yearling cattle to adjust to a high-energy finishing ration in a feedlot with minimal problems. This is achieved by feeding the calves a growing diet that yields rapid, efficient body weight gains without fattening. Maximum use is made of roughage type rations. The spectrum of diseases that occur in backgrounding operations during the first 45 days after arrival of the calves will depend on whether the calves were preimmunized, preconditioned, or obtained from several different sources with no preconditioning. The mortality rate may reach 10% in feeder calves with no preimmunization or preconditioning prior to arrival in a backgrounding feedlot. The infectious diseases of the respiratory tract (pneumonic pasteurellosis) and of the digestive tract (coccidiosis) may account for most of the losses. Cattle that have been through a backgrounding program usually go onto a high-energy finishing diet in a different feedlot with a minimum of problems. The ideal situation is to maintain the groups as they were formed in the backgrounding feedlot.

Processing of Nonpreconditioned Cattle on Arrival

The preconditioning concept is a valid one; however, it deals with only one segment of feedlot replacements. Ranch calves moving directly to the feedlot are only one source of replacements available to the large feedlots. Large commercial feedlots must rely on public sales yards, where cattle are offered for sale by public auction, and backgrounding feedlots as well as calves raised on a ranch. Cattle marketed through sales yards may or may not receive the benefit of good animal husbandry practices. These cattle usually originate from a variety of areas. After arrival at the sales yard, co-mingling of the animals is common, and they are subjected to strange environments, different feeds and watering systems, perhaps long periods without feed and water, excessive handling, weighing, blood sampling and disease testing for interstate travel, and mixing into uniform groups to meet the requirements of commissioned buyers who have specific orders for feedlots. In addition, some cattle moving through the sales yards may be subjected to the stressors of castration, dehorning, vaccination, and other processing procedures. All of these factors, coupled with exposure to the multiplicity of infectious agents, would provide ideal conditions for these cattle to require respiratory disase. The cattle are then transported to the feedlot. The trip may require only a few hours or may take up to 48 hours or more. During this time, the cattle may be deprived of palatable feed and water, inclement weather may occur, and on arrival at the feedlot the animals are highly susceptible to acute respiratory disease. The mortality rate in sales-yard cattle is approximately 75% greater than the mortality in cattle originating directly from ranches or from backgrounding feedlots (Braddy 1973).

The processing of cattle with unknown backgrounds, that have been subjected to the stresses of sales yards and transportation and that arrive at the feedlot at unexpected times of the day, in large numbers, often on a daily basis during peak buying periods, is a challenge for the veterinarian and his assistants. Cattle may arrive during off-hours because of problems in transportation. During peak periods, it may not be possible to process all cattle for several days, during which time an outbreak of acute

respiratory disease may occur in the animals waiting to be processed. Unexpected shortages in personnel, snowstorms, rainstorms, and accidental problems anywhere else in the feedlot all contribute to the vulnerability of cattle that have recently arrived in the feedlot. There will be wide variations in the nutritional status, genetic potential, vaccination history, and colostral immunity; some cattle will have been castrated and dehorned, and the age at which they were castrated and the completeness of the castration will vary considerably; some will have come from feedlots and others from range; others will have come from geographical areas where the incidence of siliceous urinary calculi is high, and some will have been implanted with anabolic steroids. Feedlot heifers may have been fed melengesterol acetate (MGA) to suppress estrus, whereas other heifers may be pregnant. These cattle must be conditioned during the first two to three weeks in the feedlot.

There is general agreement in the feedlot industry that recently arrived cattle of unknown backgrounds require extra surveillance and care during the first two to three weeks after arrival. There is also agreement that most of these cattle must be vaccinated as necessary and that some need to be castrated, perhaps dehorned, and given growth promotant implants. However, the most contentious issue is how soon after arrival the processing should be done. Another unsettled issue is the nature of the feed that should be offered to recently arrived cattle. Veterinarians have traditionally adopted the approach that non-preconditioned stressed cattle of unknown backgrounds should be allowed to adjust to their new surroundings for up to three weeks after arrival. During this adjustment period, the cattle are fed good-quality roughage, ensured of an adequate water supply, and provided with adequate bedding—especially during the first few days—so that they may rest. The cattle are checked carefully at least three times daily for evidence of illness, and sick cattle are identified and treated easily. After the cattle have adjusted and are eating an amount equivalent to 2% of their body weight, they are then processed as required. This system will provide good results, but the feedlot industry claims that it is uneconomical. The provision of only good-quality roughage for the first two or three weeks has been considered as a logical practice. However, controlled field trials in feeder calves subjected to marketing and shipping stresses indicate that increasing the concentrate or energy level in the starting diet up to about 72% improves performance compared with lower levels (Lofgreen et al. 1975). Increasing the concentrate level to 90% in the starting diet is undesirable during the first week after arrival, but after the first week it may be satisfactory.

Large commercial feedlots, with experienced personnel, may challenge recently arrived cattle with high-energy diets within two weeks after arrival. This is done in an attempt to get them on full feed as soon as possible, and economics is the motivating force. The system is like walking a tightrope—most of the time it is successful, but occasionally it is catastrophic. Over the long term, in large feedlots with a large turnover, it may be economical. In small farm feedlots with less experienced personnel, the conservative approach is recommended.

The major objectives of the feeding program during the introductory period are to get the animals eating, to avoid outbreaks of carbohydrate engorgement, and to avoid outbreaks of indigestion during the period when the cattle are most susceptible to acute respiratory disease. The conservative approach is to provide a highly palatable roughage or silage for the adjustment period. Following this starter diet, and when the animals are healthy and the common infectious diseases are not a problem, the animals can then be fed the growing and finishing diets.

In the Bruce County Project in Canada in 1978, 1979, and 1980, in which feeder calves were shipped from western Canada to Bruce County in Ontario and placed in small farm feedlots, usually on a one-time basis for the year, the results indicated that highest mortality rates were associated with the feeding of corn silage compared with hay and with the processing of cattle on arrival (Martin et al. 1980, 1981, 1982). The use of vaccines against respiratory disease, administered on arrival, also appeared to increase the risk of mortality. As a result of three consecutive years of epidemiologic observation in the Bruce County Project, the following recommendations for the handling of feeder cattle after arrival in the feedlot can be considered:

1. Feeder calves from different sources or arriving at the feedlot at different times should be kept separate for three to four weeks.

2. Feeder calves should be kept in groups of less than 100 for at least three weeks. This will facilitate early identification of sick calves and will minimize the possible spread of infectious agents.

3. Feeder calves should be fed dry, good-quality hay for at least one month. Hay should form the major component of the roughage during this period.

4. Silage should be introduced very gradually and should not become the major roughage during the first month after arrival. It is preferable to withhold silage until the initial upsurge of treatments for illness is over.

5. Start feeder calves on some barley-oats mixture, or equivalent energy density feed, one week prior to the introduction of silage.

6. The use of antimicrobials in the water supply within two to three weeks after arrival as prophylaxis against respiratory disease is not recommended because it may be associated with increased mortality (Martin et al. 1982; Hutchings and Martin 1983).

7. Feeder calves should not be processed on arrival; any processing should be limited to identification with ear tags or branding and, if necessary, anthelmintics and insecticides.

8. Vaccination on or shortly after arrival is unnecessary and probably harmful. Vaccination for the common diseases of feedlot cattle should be delayed for at least three weeks.

9. Feedlots should purchase fully preconditioned feeder calves.

10. Regular surveillance is necessary to detect and treat sick calves in the earliest stage of the disease.

11. Handling facilities should be designed to minimize the stress associated with all of the processing procedures to which feeder calves are subjected.

Limited observations in the southern United States indicate that during the four weeks after arrival of feeder calves in the feedlot, a delay in processing resulted in lower feed consumption, lower rates of gain, and inferior feed conversion compared with calves that are processed either at the point of origin or on arrival at the final destination. These differences persisted for a feeding period lasting up to 342 days (Lofgreen et al. 1978).

Studies by Lofgreen (1975, 1980) of the energy level of the diets offered to stressed feeder calves after arrival in the feedlot indicate that the diets containing 50 to 75% concentrate promote more rapid recovery of purchase weight than diets containing 25% concentrate. Diets containing levels higher than 75% are, however, detrimental and increase morbidity and mortality rates from respiratory disease (Lofgreen 1983).

In summary, there is insufficient documented information available to recommend whether non-preconditioned cattle, as they are currently being introduced into commercial feedlots, should be processed within a few days after arrival or two to three weeks later, when the cattle have become accustomed to the lot and have overcome the effects of the previous stressors. It will be necessary to conduct a large-scale epidemiologic investigation of several feedlots under different management systems over a few years to determine which system is most economical. However, even if definitive information were available that one system is more economical than the other, it would not preclude the veterinarian and the feedlot manager from modifying the time of processing because of necessity. Any one or more of several factors already discussed may indicate that processing should be delayed.

Regardless of the system used, immediately upon arrival the cattle should be weighed and examined for evidence of illness and treated if necessary. A veterinary diagnosis should be sought at the earliest possible time. Close examination and surveillance are desirable for groups of cattle with a history of unusual stress. The youngest and smallest cattle often need special attention, and it may be necessary to separate them from older cattle. All of the available history on each group of cattle should be obtained if possible. A reliable history of vaccination, vitamin injections, implants, and anthelmintic administration is obviously useful. The major objective during the first few days should be to avoid unnecessary deaths due to diseases that normally respond well to treatment. Depending on the condition of the cattle, during the first few days after arrival it may be difficult to easily distinguish sick cattle from healthy cattle, and careful clinical surveillance every few hours may be necessary. Observations at the time of feeding will often reveal anorexic animals that should be pulled from the pen and examined.

Specific Processing Procedures

Each processing procedure applied to non-preconditioned feeder cattle after arrival in the feedlot will be presented and discussed briefly.

Identification and Body Weight. All cattle must be weighed and identified immediately after arrival. Methods of identification include branding, ear-tagging, and electronic implants.

Vaccination. The vaccination of feedlot cattle has been controversial ever since the introduction of the vaccines, particularly those intended for the control of acute respiratory disease. An excellent review of the literature by Martin (1983) examined the published evi-

dence for the claims that vaccination with the respiratory disease vaccines will actually prevent respiratory disease or influence weight gains in feedlot calves. In general, there is little published data to support the use of vaccines against respiratory disease under feedlot conditions. Treatment rates and weight gains usually did not differ between vaccinated and nonvaccinated groups. In fact, the use of live bovine virus diarrhea vaccines was associated with a significant subsequent increase in treatment rates.

The vaccines available for the clostridial diseases are highly efficacious. The number of antigens to be used (two-way or eight-way) will depend on the prevalence of the clostridial diseases in the area.

Feedlot cattle may be vaccinated for the following diseases:
- Infectious bovine rhinotracheitis
- Parainfluenza-3 virus infection
- Bovine virus diarrhea
- Pneumonic pasteurellosis
- Septicemia due to *Hemophilus somnus*
- Clostridial diseases:
  Blackleg—*Clostridium chauvoei*
  Malignant edema—*Clostridium septicum*
  Bacillary hemoglobinuria—*Clostridium novyi* Type D (*hemolyticum*)
  Infectious hepatitis—*Clostridium novyi* Type B
  Tetanus—*Clostridium tetani*
  Enterotoxemia—*Clostridium perfringens* Types B, C, and D
- Leptospirosis—Vaccines containing the serovars prevalent in the area.

Castration and Dehorning. Castration and dehorning may be done along with the other processing procedures or delayed for two to three weeks if there is a high incidence of infectious disease in the group. Hemorrhage following castration is common with conventional methods used in bulls arriving at feedlots. Under some conditions, castration by the elastrator-ligation method reduces hemorrhage and stress among recently arrived feeder calves. There is also less total illness and death loss and higher average daily gain among calves castrated one to two weeks later. Also, method compared with the open emasculation method (Zweiacher 1980). The average daily gain is significantly greater in calves castrated on the day of arrival in the feedlot than in calves castrated one to two weeks later. Also, calves that are purchased as steers gain faster and have less health problems than bulls castrated after arrival at the feedlot.

Termination of Pregnancy in Heifers. Heifers over eight months of age should be examined for pregnancy and given the appropriate treatment for the termination of pregnancy. A dose of 500 μg. of prostaglandin $F_{2\alpha}$, combined with 25 mg. dexamethasone, will abort pregnant feedlot heifers, regardless of the stage of pregnancy (Barth et al. 1981).

Prophylactic Medication of Feed and Water. The use of antimicrobial and chemotherapeutic agents in the feed and/or water supplies during the conditioning period has been advocated for many years as an aid in the reduction of the incidence of infectious diseases such as bacterial pneumonia, hemophilus meningoencephalitis, liver abscesses, coccidiosis, and intestinal helminthiasis. They are used most commonly for the control and prevention of the common bacterial diseases. It has been difficult to consistently duplicate in commercial feedlots the beneficial results that have been attributed to medicated feedlot starter rations fed to cattle on an experimental basis. There are several possible reasons for this, which include:

1. The origin of the cattle going into different feedlots varies considerably, and thus their immune status, nutritional status, and degree of stress varies widely.

2. The amount of medicated feed consumed by newly arrived cattle will depend on their previous experience and the type of feed offered.

3. The amount of water consumed daily may vary.

4. The accuracy of the diagnosis of the illnesses will vary from lot to lot.

5. The general management methods will vary considerably from one lot to another, and valid comparisons are difficult.

6. The drug sensitivity of the organism may vary from one feedlot to another and from one group of cattle to the next.

The following generalizations have been found to apply when antibiotics are administered prophylactically. When a single effective drug is used to avoid implantation of a specific pathogen or to eradicate it immediately or shortly after it has become established but not yet clinically evident, the chemoprophylaxis is, with uncommon exception, highly successful. If the aim of prophylaxis is to prevent colonization and/or infection by any and all pathogens that may be present in the internal or external environment of an animal, failure is the rule.

Mass medication of the feed and water is also used to provide follow-up therapy for those animals already treated individually. If mass medication were reliable and effective, it would save on the costs of handling and treatment of individual animals. However, it is not totally reliable. Animals in the early stages of the disease may not drink enough medicated water or eat enough medicated feed. In addition, medication of the feed or water for those cattle that would not normally become ill is uneconomical. Another problem is the provision of a uniform concentration of drug in the water supply, either through automatic water proportioners in the waterline or by placing the drug directly into the water tanks, both of which can be unreliable. With a reliable mixing facility, the most accurate concentrations of the drug are achieved in the feed supply.

The following recommendations are offered as guidelines for mass medication for the control of some diseases of feedlot cattle:

- Sulfamethazine: 100 mg./kg. B.W. in the drinking water for five to seven days beginning at the first sign of illness in the group. The dose may be reduced to 50 mg./kg. B.W. for the next five to seven days.

- Oxytetracycline: 3 to 5 mg./kg. B.W. in the feed for seven days beginning at the first sign of illness in the group. Bloat may occur in some animals during or following medication of the feed, and careful surveillance is necessary.

- A combination of chlortetracycline and sulfamethazine is available for incorporation in the feed for the first two to three weeks for the control of acute respiratory disease.

- Coccidiostats may be added to the feed or water during the first three weeks after arrival for the control of coccidiosis.

- In areas where siliceous urolithiasis is a problem, the voluntary intake of water may be increased by the incorporation of salt in the diet at the rate of 4% by weight.

- Growth promotants are now commonly incorporated into the feed according to the preference of the feedlot. A popular one is monensin sodium at 11 to 33 ppm, which also acts as an effective coccidiostat.

- Anthelmintics may also be included in the feed in areas where intestinal helminthiasis is considered endemic.

- Other feed additives for feedlot cattle include ethylenediamine dihydroiodide for the control of foot rot and melengestrol for the control of estrus in feedlot heifers.

Although antimicrobials have been used extensively on a prophylactic basis in the feed or water supplies in an attempt to prevent infection or to "abort" early subclinical disease in feedlot cattle, the results have been inconclusive. It is not possible to categorically recommend that the use of mass medication, by whatever route, will reliably control infectious disease in recently arrived feedlot cattle from several different origins. There are simply too many epidemiologic determinants that vary widely between each group of cattle. There must be a high level of surveillance during the first few days and weeks to detect clinically ill animals in the early stages of disease.

Antibiotic Injections. The intramuscular injection of antibiotics into recently arrived stressed cattle is a widespread practice. The rationale is that the antibiotics will be effective against subclinical disease and perhaps prevent or minimize the effects of new infections. Theoretically, the injection of an antibiotic at therapeutic levels in a large number of animals should be effective in preventing clinical disease in those animals that would normally become ill. On a practical basis, it is difficult to synchronize the injection of an antibiotic with the expected onset of pneumonia, which probably accounts for some of the failures.

A daily intramuscular injection of oxytetracycline for the first three days after arrival of stressed feeder calves may reduce the percentage of animals that need treatment (Lofgreen et al. 1980). Long-acting oxytetracycline at the rate of 20 mg./kg. B.W. given once intramuscularly may be used as mass medication of all in-contact cattle in a group of cattle in which new cases of acute respiratory disease are occurring at the rate of 5 to 10% daily (Janzen and McManus 1980). However, it is still necessary to provide surveillance at least twice daily during the first three weeks after arrival to detect sick cattle.

Anthelmintics and Insecticides. Anthelmintics and insecticides are administered according to local conditions. The feedlot operator and veterinarian should be informed about feeder calves or yearling cattle that have originated from farm situations or areas where intestinal parasitism is likely. Young cattle raised on small farms where the stocking rate on pasture is high may be harboring a burden of helminths (Armour 1980). Young cattle may also be affected with chronic verminous pneumonia due to *Dictyocaulus viviparus*.

Injectable Anabolic Agents. The efficacy of anabolic agents in increasing live-weight gain has been shown in many different growth trials

under different husbandry and feeding systems. The best results are obtained in steers and veal calves treated with combined preparations of an androgen and an estrogen and in heifers treated with an androgen. Although the scientific evidence of efficacy is equivocal, it is an increasingly common practice to implant anabolic agents more than once during the growth of beef cattle. Anabolic agents are effective in calves as well as yearlings, and repeat implantation extends the period of their effect on growth (Reynolds 1980). The anabolic agents that have been used include trenbolone acetate, zeranol (Ralgro), hexoestrol, Synovex-S® (200 mg. progesterone and 20 mg. estradiol benzoate) and Synovex-H® (200 mg. testosterone and 20 mg. estradiol benzoate).

Ralgro implants are used in male and female nursing calves, grazing cattle, and cattle on finishing rations. The active ingredient is a cornmold derivative called zeranol. Implants may be given at birth and repeated at three months of age and every 60 days thereafter until 65 days before slaughter. Both average daily gain and feed efficiency are improved. The implants are administered to cattle soon after arrival in the feedlot as part of the processing procedures.

Synovex implants are available in two forms. Each formula is specific; Synovex-S® for steers and Synovex-H® for heifers. Cattle may be implanted on arrival and reimplanted 90 days later, but no later than 70 days before slaughter.

The possible hazards associated with anabolic agents result from their hormonal and possibly carcinogenic properties. Long-acting anabolic steroids should not be implanted into animals intended as breeding stock. Changes in behavior after implantation can also be a problem. The incidence of mounting and riding in steers implanted in feedlots has been increasing with the increased use of anabolic agents. Tissues from animals implanted with anabolic agents may contain residues of that agent plus their metabolites. At the end of the withdrawal period, up to 10% of the initial dose may still be found at the site of implantation. It is therefore most important that all implantation be done at the base of the ear, beneath the loose skin overlying the conchal cartilage. This area is traditionally discarded at slaughter.

Growth-Promotant Feed Additives. Several growth-promoting feed additives are available for incorporation into feedlot rations. The economic advantages include improved average live-weight gains, improved feed efficiency, and, in some cases, control of certain diseases. Monensin sodium may be used from the beginning of the feeding period until slaughter. It improves feed efficiency by about 10% and when used during the first 28 days of the feeding period will assist in the control of coccidiosis.

Chlortetracycline and oxytetracycline at levels of 10 g./ton of feed may be fed to feedlot cattle as growth promotants in some countries. The development of drug-resistant strains of bacteria in cattle fed the drug for long periods is a concern that must be monitored.

Vitamin Injections. A common processing practice is to inject each animal with a mixture of vitamins A, D, and E intramuscularly. This is to prevent any possible occurrence of hypovitaminosis A, which may be present in cattle that have originated from a dry carotene-deficient pasture or diet. However, the vitamins may be supplied in the feed at high levels during the conditioning period to increase liver levels.

The Problem of Drug Residues in Beef. A large number of feed additives, growth stimulants, and antibiotics are now fed to cattle in feedlots to improve the efficiency of their feed conversion. Synthetic steroid hormones, especially diethylstilbestrol, are notable examples. Most pure food legislation now restricts the levels at which these compounds can occur in food. The levels are very low, and the penalties for exceeding them are generally very high, so that the feedlot operator is presented with the problem of withdrawing the feed supplement from the ration in sufficient time to permit residues to disappear or deleting their use altogether.

Culling. Culling may be done at any point between examination of the cattle on arrival and a few weeks later, before they are placed on a high-energy diet. The basis for culling is to detect those animals affected with disease that will not respond economically to treatment or special diets. Some of the diseases that justify culling include chronic unthriftiness and inappetence of undetermined etiology, chronic laminitis, chronic lameness due to foot rot, chronic bloaters, chronic pneumonia, acute and chronic pulmonary abscess, and bovine virus diarrhea. Each of these diseases results in unthriftiness, and a clinical examination is necessary to make a diagnosis. If the diagnosis is not obvious, the affected animals should be weighed, confined and fed in a separate pen, and monitored for up to three weeks. Re-examination and reweighing in three weeks may assist in determining which animals should be slaughtered for salvage and which may be returned to a finishing pen.

Feeding Procedures. In general, there are three phases in feeding feedlot cattle; the *starting, growing,* and *finishing* phases. During the first few days after arrival and until the cattle are introduced to full feed, the traditional general recommendation has been to provide a good-quality roughage. The critical factor is to get the new animals to eat, so that ruminal flora and function are restored. Preconditioned feeder calves and backgrounded cattle will usually start eating and drinking with a minimum of difficulty. Feeding twice daily or more often is recommended during the adjustment period, so that cattle that do not eat can be identified and examined more closely. The use of self-feeders during the adjustment period makes it difficult to detect animals that are anorexic because they may eat at any time.

Failure to eat normally during the first few days may be encountered with feeder calves that are not preconditioned and feeder cattle that have been stressed by transportation and sales yards. The provision of a complete mixed starter ration, containing 72% concentrates, to newly arrived stressed feeder calves is now considered to be superior to rations containing less concentrates. Calves fed the higher-energy ration recover their purchase weights more rapidly and gain more economically during the first month in the feedlot than calves that are fed lower-energy rations (Lofgreen et al. 1975). Daily surveillance of the cattle and the consistency of their feces during the starting period is necessary to detect any evidence of dietary diarrhea due to indigestion.

When the cattle have become adjusted to the starting ration and when there is no evidence of acute respiratory disease or other major infections, the animals may be started on the high-energy growing and finishing rations. A widely accepted and successful practice is to use a complex mixed ration consisting of grain, chopped roughage, protein supplement if necessary, and the necessary vitamins and minerals. The level of grain is increased and the level of roughage decreased every few days until the predetermined levels are reached for the growing or finishing rations. Using this method, feeder calves can be adjusted to a growing ration and yearlings to a finishing ration in 15 to 20 days, usually without carbohydrate engorgement or bloat. In large feedlots, with many pens of cattle at different phases of the feeding program, outbreaks of carbohydrate engorgement occur when cattle are accidentally fed a finishing ration when they are adjusted only to the lower-energy rations. A high level of accuracy is necessary in the feed mill and by the personnel delivering the feed to the respective pens. Complete and thorough mixing of the feed must be ensured at all times.

BENEFITS OF A HEALTH MANAGEMENT PROGRAM FOR THE FEEDLOT

Feedlot operators who engage veterinarians for programed preventive medicine appear to be willing to invest money for this service because the veterinarian saves them money in the process. The economic losses due to respiratory diseases alone in feedlot cattle have been estimated at $10 to $20 per animal. This loss is derived from shrink, poor feed utilization, inefficiency of gain, 1 to 2% death loss, and the treatment cost of sick animals. In a recent study of diseases of 407,000 yearling feedlot cattle in Colorado, the morbidity was 5.1%, with a case fatality rate of 18.9% and a population mortality of 1%. Respiratory tract diseases were the most common and accounted for 75% of the illness and 64% of the deaths. From this limited data, it would appear that significant economic benefits from herd health programs are possible in feedlot cattle operations.

Review Literature

Agriculture Canada Publication 1591. Feedlot Finishing of Cattle. Information Division, Ottawa, 1976.

Berg, R.T. and Walters, L.E. The meat animal: Changes and challenges. J. Anim. Sci., 57(Suppl. 2):133–146, 1983.

Bredenstein, B.C. and Carpenter, Z.L. The red meat industry: Product and consumerism. J. Anim. Sci., 57(Suppl. 2):119–132, 1983.

Church, T. Preventive medicine in the feedlot. Symposium on Herd Health Management—Cow-Calf and Feedlot. Vet. Clin. North Am. [Large Anim. Pract.], (5)1: 29–39, 1983.

Hjerpe, C. Clinical management of respiratory disease in feedlot cattle. Symposium on Herd Health Management—Cow-Calf and Feedlot. Vet. Clin. North Am. [Large Anim. Pract.], (5)1:119–142, 1983.

Koch, R.M. and Algeo, J.W. The beef cattle industry: Changes and challenges. J. Anim. Sci., 57(Suppl. 2): 28–43, 1983.

Lofgreen, G.P. Nutrition and management of stressed beef calves. Symposium on Herd Health Management—Cow-Calf and Feedlot. Vet. Clin. North Am. [Large Anim. Pract.], (5)1:87–101, 1983.

Martin, S.W. Factors influencing morbidity and mortality in feedlot calves in Ontario. Symposium on Herd Health Management—Cow-Calf and Feedlot. Vet. Clin. North Am. [Large Anim. Pract.] (5)1:75–86, 1983.

Seideman, S.C., Cross, H.R., Oltjen, R.R. et al. Utilization of the intact male for red meat production: A review. J. Anim. Sci., 55:826, 1982.

Yates, W.D.G. A review of infectious bovine rhinotracheitis, shipping fever pneumonia and viral-bacterial synergism in respiratory disease of cattle. Can. J. Comp. Med., 46:225–263, 1982.

References

Allen, D.M., Bougler, J., Christensen, L.G. et al. Livestock production in Europe. Perspectives and prospects. III. Cattle. Livestock Prod. Sci., 9:89–126, 1982.

Armour, J. The epidemiology of helminth disease in farm animals. Vet. Parasitol., 6:7–46, 1980.

Barth, A., Adams, W.M. Manns, J.G. et al. Induction of abortion in feedlot heifers with a combination of cloprostenol and dexamethasone. Can. Vet. J., 22: 62–64, 1981.

Berg, R.T. and Walters, L.E. The meat animal: Changes and challenges. J. Anim. Sci., 57(Suppl. 2):133–146, 1983.

Braddy, P.M. Comments on preconditioning of beef cattle. J. Am. Vet. Med. Assoc., 163:827, 1973.

Bredenstein, B.C. and Carpenter, Z.L. The red meat industry: product and consumerism. J. Anim. Sci., 57(Suppl)119–132, 1983.

Church, T.L. Preventive medicine and management in beef feedlots. Can. Vet. J., 21:214–218, 1980.

Church, T.L. and Karren, D. Alberta certified preconditioned feeder program. Alberta Agriculture, Edmonton, Alberta, 1981, pp. 1–23.

Church, T.L. and Radostits, O.M. A retrospective survey of diseases of feedlot cattle in Alberta. Can. Vet.J., 22:27–30, 1981.

Gregory, K.E. and Cundliff, L.V. Crossbreeding in beef cattle: Evaluation of systems. J. Anim. Sci., 57:1224–1242, 1980.

Hoerlein, A.B. Preconditioning of beef cattle. J. Am. Vet. Med. Assoc., 163:825–827, 1973.

Hutchings, D.L. and Martin, S.W. A mail survey of factors associated with morbidity and mortality in feedlot calves in southwestern Ontario. Can. J. Comp. Med., 47:101–107, 1983.

Janzen, E.D. and McManus, R.F. Observations on the use of a long-acting oxytetracycline for in-contact prophylaxis of undifferentiated bovine respiratory disease in feedlot steers under Canadian conditions. Bovine Pract., 15:87–90, 1980.

Jensen, R., Pierson, R.E., Braddy, P.M. et al. Diseases of yearling feedlot cattle in Colorado. J. Am. Vet. Med. Assoc., 169:497–499, 1976a.

Jensen, R., Pierson, R.E., Braddy, P.M., et al. Shipping fever pneumonia in yearling feedlot cattle. J. Am. Vet. Med. Assoc. 169:500–506, 1976b.

Jensen, R., Pierson, R.E., Braddy, P.M., et al. Atypical interstitial pneumonia in yearling feedlot cattle. J. Am. Vet. Med. Assoc., 169:507–510, 1976c.

Jensen, R., Pierson, R.E., Braddy, P.M. et al. Bronchiectasis in yearling feedlot cattle. J. Am. Vet. Med. Assoc. 169:511–514, 1976d.

Jensen, R., Pierson, R.E., Braddy, P.M. et al. Brisket disease in yearling feedlot cattle. J. Am. Vet. Med. Assoc., 169:515–517, 1976e.

Jensen, R., Pierson, R.E., Braddy, P.M. et al. Embolic pulmonary aneurysms in yearling feedlot cattle. J. Am. Vet. Med. Assoc., 169:518–520, 1976f.

Kahrs, R.F. Techniques for investigating outbreaks of livestock disease. J. Am. Vet. Med. Assoc., 173:101–103, 1978.

Koch, R.M. and Algeo, J.W. The beef cattle industry: Changes and challenges. J. Anim. Sci., 57(Suppl. 2): 28–43, 1983.

Lesoing G., Rush, I. and Klopfenstein T. Wheat straw in growing cattle diets. J. Anim. Sci., 51:257–262, 1980a.

Lesoing, G., Klopfenstein T. and Rush, I. Chemical treatment of wheat straw. J. Anim. Sci., 51:263–269, 1980b.

Loew, F.M. A thiamin-responsive polioencephalomalacia in tropical and nontropical livestock production systems. World Rev. Nutr. and Diet, 20:168–183, 1975.

Lofgreen, G.P. Nutrition and management of stressed beef calves. Symposium on Herd Health Management— Cow-Calf and Feedlot. Vet. Clin. North Am. [Large Anim. Pract.], (5)1:87–101, 1983.

Lofgreen, G.P., Addis, D.G., Dunbar, J.R. et al. Time of processing calves subjected to marketing and shipping stress. J. Anim. Sci., 47:1324–1328, 1978.

Lofgreen, G.P., Dunbar, J.R., Addis, D.G. et al. Energy level in starting rations for calves subjected to marketing and shipping stress. J. Anim. Sci., 41:1256–1265, 1975.

Lofgreen, G.P., Stinocher, L.H. and Kiesling, H.E. Effects of dietary energy, free choice alfalfa hay and mass medication on calves subjected to marketing and shipping stress. J. Anim. Sci., 50:590–596, 1980.

Long, C.R. Crossbreeding for beef production: Experimental results. J. Anim. Sci., 51:1197–1223, 1980.

Martin, S.W. Vaccination: Is it effective in preventing respiratory disease or influencing weight gains in feedlot calves? Can. Vet. J., 24:10–19, 1983.

Martin, S.W., Meek, A.H. and Curtis, R.A. Antimicrobial use in feedlot calves: Its association with culture rates and antimicrobial susceptibility. Can. J. Comp. Med., 47:6–10, 1983.

Martin, S.W., Meek, A.H., Davis, D.G. et al. Factors associated with mortality in feedlot calves: The Bruce County Beef Cattle Project. Can. J. Comp. Med., 44:1–10, 1980.

Martin, S.W., Meek, A.H., Davis, D.G. et al. Factors associated with morbidity and mortality in feedlot calves: The Bruce County Beef Project, Year Two. Can. J. Comp. Med., 45:103–112, 1981.

Martin, S.W., Meek, A.H., Davis, D.G. et al. Factors associated with mortality and treatment costs in feedlot calves: The Bruce County Beef Project, Years 1978, 1979, 1980. Can. J. Comp. Med., 46:341–349, 1982.

Pierson, R.E. Control and management of respiratory diseases in feedlot cattle. J. Am. Vet. Med. Assoc., 152:920–923, 1968.

Pierson, R.E., Jensen, R., Braddy, P.M. et al. Bulling among yearling feedlot steers. J. Am. Vet. Med. Assoc., 169: 521–523, 1976.

Preston, T.R. and Willis, M.B. Intensive Beef Production. Second Edition. Pergamon Press, Oxford, 1974.

Reynolds, I.P. Correct use of anabolic agents in ruminants. Vet. Rec., 107:367–369, 1980.

Stanhope, D.L., Hinman, D.D., Everson, D.O. et al. Digestibility of potato processing residue in beef cattle finishing diets. J. Anim. Sci., 51:257–262, 1980.

Thomas, L.W., Wood, P.D.P. and Longlard, J.M. The influence of disease on the performance of beef cattle. Br. Vet. J., 134:152–161, 1978.

Trenkle, A. and Willham, R.L. Beef production efficiency. Science, 198:1009–1015, 1977.

Ward, G.M. Energy, land and feed constraints on beef production in the 80's. J. Anim. Sci., 51:1051–1064, 1980.

Zweiacher, E.R., Durham, R.M. Boren, B.D. et al. Effects of method and time of castration of feeder calves. J. Anim. Sci., 49:5–9, 1980.

Planned Animal Health and Production in Swine Herds

INTRODUCTION

The swine industry has grown from a small farmyard source of pork for the family farm to an intensified, highly mechanized, and capitalized production- and profit-oriented enterprise. As recently as 25 years ago, a few sows and their litters were reared in extensive conditions each year, whereas today farrow-to-finish operations with 100 to 1000 sows under intensive conditions and total confinement, and marketing 15 to 20 pigs per sow per year are commonplace.

This chapter outlines the general methods used in providing a planned animal health and production service to swine herds.

HISTORICAL ASPECTS OF THE SWINE INDUSTRY

In the last 25 years (1959 to 1983), remarkable changes have occurred in the swine industry in North America, the United Kingdom, and more recently Australia. These changes are well documented by Fredeen and Harmon (1983) and are presented here by way of introduction to the chapter on pigs. These rapid changes represent an example of the economic pressures that were placed on agriculture and how it responded with remarkable improved efficiency. However, and perhaps more important, the new technology of swine production created a number of animal health and production problems for which there are no simple solutions. Thus, a brief review of the recent history of swine

production will be beneficial in understanding the problems that exist today.

Some remarkable changes have occurred in the swine industry since World War II. Consolidation, specialization, intensification, and mechanization were the central features in the evolution of agriculture. The predominant theme was improved labor efficiency, and the means to this end lay in the substitution of machines for horses and manual labor. Agriculture evolved swiftly from a way of life to a business and, as competition for the labor force intensified, producers moved to larger and still larger equipment to replace the traditional sources of farm help. The resulting escalation of the capital investment required could be offset only by increasing the scale and intensity of individual operations. Increasing farm size was accompanied by consolidation of the hog industry—a marked decline in the number of production units and an increase in the number of pigs marketed per producer and total annual marketing. Specialization in the hog industry in North America began in about 1950 and has continued until the 1980s.

The search for improved labor efficiency initiated the advent of mechanization in the piggery, which, in turn, initiated trends toward large facilities and larger herds because the traditional low-cost, low-density housing practices were not amenable to the effective use of labor-saving equipment. This proved to be an endless cycle; each advance fed an upward spiral of capital costs, and producers responded by increasing the scale and intensity of production to amortize their increased capitalization; thus was born the perceived need for even bigger and potentially more efficient equipment and facilities.

This growth process was highly innovative, with leaders in the industry initiating practical experimentation to devise both housing and equipment to suit their needs. The problems they encountered ranged from the systems required for feeding, ventilation, and manure disposal to interior design and choice of construction materials. Gravitational ventilation systems with manual controls proved inadequate, and through trial and error the industry gradually evolved forced draft systems with complex controls sensitive to both humidity and temperature. Waste removal systems that involved separate handling of solids and liquids were replaced by deep-gutter and slatted floor designs that utilized gravity to move effluent into cisterns and lagoons. Mechanical systems for delivering metered amounts of feed—either dry or as a slurry—to individual pens were devised to minimize the labor involved in feeding. Pen size and shape, and even the location of equipment within pens, received increasing attention as producers sought to maximize housing density and improve the operational efficiency of automated equipment.

Hog finishing feedlot operations were the initial target of these evolutionary changes, but during the mid-1960s, producers turned their attention to methods for improving the traditional practices for breeding herd management. From early experiences with extensive farrowing and nursing facilities came an appreciation of the value of a fully controlled environment that buffered the sows from climatic stress, minimized competition among breeding females, and protected the nursing piglets from physical damage and disease exposure. These concerns for the well-being of the pigs led to the replacement of loose housing management of pregnant sows with single pen or tethering systems that eliminated fighting, improved sanitation, and permitted individual attention to the nutritional and other needs of each female. Farrowing facilities evolved from pens or stalls designed to protect piglets from injury by the sow to crates with slatted or metal mesh floors that greatly enhanced sanitation and disease control. The increased capital investment associated with this evaluation in sow housing proved a compelling motivation for adopting early weaning to reduce the interval between farrowing and rebreeding and thereby increase the annual litter production from each sow in the herd. This led to the introduction of environmentally controlled nurseries equipped with flat decks or cages that were designed to ensure a high level of sanitation.

One of the features of this whole evolutionary period was the fact that each change was followed by, not led by, research. The innovators were the producers, and it was their successes and failures that identified research needs. The producers themselves did most of the research, using a process of trial and error that led more than one operator to identify the jackhammer as their most vital piece of equipment.

Another feature of the period was the large number of subindustries that developed to meet the demand for buildings and equipment of improved design. With few exceptions, the basic designs were developed, tested, and proven by individual producers. Their interest lay in upgrading their own operations, not merchandizing the innovations, but their production successes fostered a viable and expanding market for specialized equipment. Equipment manufacturers were swift to capitalize on this potential, and today there are many suppliers of design packages and sophisticated equipment to meet the highly varied needs of an industry that encompasses all of the climatic and environmental conditions found in North America and elsewhere.

Twenty-five years ago the lament of agricultural researchers was the long lag time in the transfer of technology from the research station to the farm. Leading producers had an insatiable appetite for new knowledge, but they were in the minority, and research results generally seemed to have a low level of acceptance. This situation changed rapidly as the industry entered the era of specialization. Increasing capital costs had to be offset by increasing production efficiency, and the most successful producers were those who recognized this economic reality. Some producers have not updated their pre-1958 practices of nutrition, breeding, and management, and the performance of their pigs has lagged behind. Other producers who embraced the modern technology of nutrition, reproductive physiology, breeding, sanitation, physical environment, and management have forged ahead as illustrated by the Reese family in Georgia, who were honored by the National Pork Producers Council in 1982. During the two years before receipt of this award, the Reese farm averaged 21.4 pigs marketed per sow annually, with an average feed conversion of 2.88 for feedlot pigs and 3.46 for the entire operation, including feed for the breeding herd. These feed requirements are well below the industry averages recorded in the recent Illinois survey of 161 feeder operations (3.84) and 828 farrow to finish operations (3.96). These industry averages are inferior, and the Reese results superior, to the conversion ratio of 3.25 reported for the feedlot diets recommended for use 25 years ago.

Advances in Breeding and Genetics

From 1937 to 1957, a wealth of scientific knowledge about swine breeding and genetics was documented by researchers. However, there was little evidence of cohesive industry application. Some strong-minded breeders did achieve genuine genetic change as shown by the emergence during this period of meat-type strains from local populations of the historic lard breeds, but the great divergence of opinion on the criteria of merit to be applied ensured that the national averages for economic merit of commercial pigs remained virtually unchanged. The role of the show ring as the outstanding classroom for the assimilation, coordination, and dissemination of information in the art and science of animal husbandry continued to be stoutly defended, but its disruptive influence of continually changing ideals on cohesive selection programs was not appreciated. Another problem of the era was the inadequacy of techniques for objectively appraising potential carcass merit of the living animal. This limitation was finally overcome with the development of the backfat probe, which opened the door for the performance testing programs that have now largely replaced progeny testing throughout the world.

Advances in Health Control

In the era around 1957, when extensive management conditions prevailed in the swine industry, disease control was achieved largely by medication of the affected individuals. Veterinarians in general farm animal practice provided service to mixed farms, which produced grains, cattle, pigs, and sometimes other species of animals. The veterinarians were called to attend to the individual farrowing sow affected with dystocia, the individual sick sow or boar, or small groups of sick feeder pigs. Certain epidemic diseases like erysipelas or hog cholera were handled by vaccination or

the slaughter policy, depending on the disease control regulations of the country. The introduction of antibiotics allowed the treatment and limited control of certain diseases such as bacterial pneumonia. Veterinary service was ad hoc, the farm calling the veterinarian when a disease problem occurred—usually when pigs were found dead. The emphasis was certainly on clinical disease. There was little if any planned animal health and production. There was no precise regular surveillance of actual performance and comparisons with targets of performance. The farmer knew "intuitively" how well his pigs were doing.

Enzootic pneumonia and atrophic rhinitis were two diseases that received considerable laboratory and field research attention in the 1950s and 1960s. The recognition that the causative pathogens were transmitted from the sow directly to the piglet led to the development of programs utilizing SPF (specific pathogen-free) or MD (minimal disease) techniques. The piglets were taken from the sow by hysterectomy or cesarean section and reared in isolation facilities until old enough to be transferred to the farm, where they became the seed breeding stock to establish a new swine herd free of enzootic pneumonia and atrophic rhinitis. The techniques were effective, but producers quickly learned that reinfection was inevitable unless special precautions were taken to maintain the herd in complete isolation. From experience came a new appreciation of the importance of animal-to-animal contact and recognition of the merits of closed herd operations. The extreme measures required for maximum health security (e.g., hysterectomy-derived breeding stock, closed herd operations, closure of premises) were not economically feasible for most producers; conversely, the large operators, particularly those who ventured into costly large-scale seed stock production, had no alternative but to impose stringent health controls. For producers who did not adopt the SPF approach, management systems of all-in-all-out production separated by a period for thorough disinfection were devised to break disease cycles. Modern buildings featuring compartmentalized farrowing and nursery quarters are designed to facilitate applications of this management approach.

Although the SPF approach may have controlled enzootic pneumonia and atrophic rhinitis and some other important infections, it did not eliminate the common causes of neonatal mortality of piglets, such as crushing, starvation, chilling, and the infectious diarrheas. Nor did it control inferior reproductive performance, a major cause of economic loss in swine herds. As the swine industry consolidated and as intensification and specialization occurred, swine herds became larger and larger, and the economic losses due to poor sow productivity—due principally to inferior reproductive performance and high preweaning mortality—were correspondingly large, and many herds went bankrupt.

As herds became larger and as production became intensified, the value of animal health and production records became obvious, and it soon became clear that clinical disease was not a major limiting factor in most swine herds. The major problem was a failure to achieve optimum reproductive performance on a continuous basis. The achievement of breeding and farrowing in groups to make maximum use of the facilities was a major challenge. Anestrus in pubertal gilts and recently weaned sows raised under total confinement was and still is a major problem that requires constant surveillance. These problems encouraged the development of a wide variety of record-keeping systems that can monitor production almost on a daily basis and can identify where shortfalls in production are occurring; a diagnosis can then be made and appropriate action taken. Veterinarians who specialized in swine practice quickly recognized the need to be production oriented and to be concerned about the whole herd rather than providing veterinary care to individual sick pigs, a need that has not declined in importance. The veterinarian involved in a modern swine practice must be knowledgeable about nutrition, reproduction, housing and ventilation, and genetics and breeding in addition to the diseases that may affect production.

Advances in Nutrition and Feeding

The steady advances in the science of animal nutrition that highlighted the first half of this century tended to be assimilated rather quickly by the industry. Although the pre-1958 period was highlighted by identification and establishment of most of the nutrients required by pigs, the past 25 years have seen the addition of only one item—selenium—to the list of required nutrients commonly added to swine diets. Much progress has been made in refining the requirements of nutrients already considered essential. Balance and relationships of nutrients has occupied much time and effort in

recent years. As appreciation for differences in metabolizable energy in common feedstuffs has increased, and the methods of formulation have shifted from nutrients as a percentage of the diet to the more accurate nutrients per calorie of diet. This development has been most pronounced in sow diets, where the need for increased calorie intake at breeding, late gestation, and lactation and for decreased calorie intake in early and mid-gestation has been underscored by research on the relationship between nutritional status and reproductive function.

The feeding and nutrition of young pigs has changed markedly during the past 25 years. At the start of the period, the practice of weaning pigs at three weeks was fraught with problems such as postweaning diarrhea. Today, pigs weaned at three weeks or less at weights averaging about 5.5 kg. are housed in modern nursery facilities where they will attain a weight of 22 kg. by nine weeks of age with a mortality of no more than 1%. Weaned pigs are now raised in double- and triple-deck pens in nurseries with controlled environments.

Many aspects of feeding technology received considerable research attention, such as the design of equipment for automatic feed delivery, the consequences of diet dilution or other methods for controlling feed intake, and processing techniques to enhance nutrient digestibility and nutrient density. Linear programing for formulating least-cost diets led to the development of modern-day computer programs that can formulate diets according to cost and the nutrient composition of the available dietary ingredients.

Performance Trends

In the same 25 years under consideration, dressing yield increased from 69.5 to 71.0%, and percentage yield of backfat decreased from 14.6 to 5.3%. In Canada, there has been a steady increase in the proportion of carcasses indexing above average (index 100), which is a measure of the anticipated yield of trimmed retail product. The reduction of backfat has also continued at an undiminished rate. Although there is no evidence in either the U.S. or Canada to indicate the relative contributions of genetics, nutrition, or management to these changes in carcass merit, the steady rate of change is highly suggestive of a substantial and continuous genetic component. The development of larger herds with a greater economic incentive to succeed may have also contributed to a gradual improvement in the average levels of most production components, including carcass merit.

There has not been much improvement in sow productivity in the last 20 years. The average number of pigs marketed per litter increased from 6.26 to 6.69. Surveys also reveal a substantial relationship between unit size and average litter size at birth, which were larger in large herds.

There have been two undesirable attributes in the performance trends of the emergence of problems of pork quality. One is the development of PSE (pale, soft, exudative pork) and the closely allied problems of PSS (porcine stress syndrome). The other is the general problem of structural soundness. All sections of the swine industry are now aware of the association between the PSE-PSS complex and type of hog and of the management and handling techniques appropriate for reducing stress and progress in being made in controlling these problems.

The incidence of inadequate structure of feet and legs was relatively low under extensive management. This increased incidence, although characteristic of all pig populations reared in confinement, was of particular concern to breeders who confined boars for purposes of performance. Prospective buyers, unaware of or unwilling to accept the evidence that structural soundness was a lowly heritable trait, tended to discriminate against the breeders whose young boars exhibited any structural deficiencies. Considerable research has been done to clarify this issue, and the accumulated evidence indicates that the important determinants are amount of exercise, type of flooring, and nutrition. Thus, it appears that this problem has come to the fore because of the changes in housing and management associated with increased production intensity.

TYPES OF SWINE PRODUCTION UNITS

There are several different kinds of swine production units, and the major characteristics of each are as follows:

Farrow-to-finish enterprises aim to market all or most of their pigs at approximately 100 kg. body weight at 160 to 170 days of age. They commonly produce a three-way cross pig for market.

Farrow-to-weaner enterprises produce pigs for sale at weaning age to commercial feeder operations, which feed the pig from weaning age (three to six weeks) to market weight at 100 kg. body weight.

Feeder operations purchase weanling pigs and feed them to market weight. The disease incidence is usually high because of the purchase of pigs from many different sources and the spread of disease after co-mingling occurs.

Purebred breeders produce breeding stock (gilts and boars) for sale to other purebred herds or to commercial farrow-to-finish enterprises that need purebred stock in their hybrid operations. These herds commonly participate in a record-of-performance testing program in which a litter group of pigs is fed at a central station from weaning to market. At slaughter, carcass measurements are made, and the average rate of gain, feed efficiency, and carcass quality of the test group are reported to the breeder.

Specific pathogen-free (SPF) herds are herds in which the pigs have originated by hysterectomy or cesarean section and are raised in isolation in a laboratory environment until they were ready to be placed in the herd, usually at about four to five weeks of age. The pigs are allowed to mature on the farm and serve as breeding stock to restock other farms. The initial pigs are colostrum-deprived, but succeeding generations are born naturally and colostrum-fed. The major objective of SPF-derived herds is to eradicate atrophic rhinitis due to *Bordetella bronchiseptica* and enzootic pneumonia due to *Mycoplasma* spp. These two infections are usually transferred from the sow to the piglet during the nursing period. Eradication of these two diseases may result in marked improvement in the feed efficiency and the growth rate of pigs from weaning to market. However, the pigs in these herds are just as susceptible to all of the other common infectious diseases, reproductive problems, and neonatal mortality due to environmental influences as are pigs raised in conventional herds.

Under ideal conditions, no pigs are imported into established SPF herds. New genes are introduced by artificial insemination using imported semen from superior boars in other herds. Strict visitor restrictions are necessary to prevent the introduction of pathogens that are not eradicable by sanitation and hygiene. Very few SPF herds have been able to maintain true SPF status for more than a few years.

CONTROL AND/OR ERADICATION OF DISEASE IN THE SWINE HERD

In general, the major problems confronting the swine industry are not the specific infectious diseases but rather the complex production problems, which may be due to a combination of infection, mismanagement, environmental influences, genetics, and problems with feeds or feeding systems (Muirhead 1978). Thus the term *disease* must encompass all identifiable abnormalities that interfere with the achievement of desirable levels of production.

Some specific infectious diseases caused by single infectious agents can be eradicated, for example, enzootic pneumonia caused by *Mycoplasm* spp. Other infectious diseases can be prevented or reduced to a very low incidence through vaccination programs, for example, erysipelas. Many other infectious diseases of swine can be controlled only by using management techniques such as sanitation, hygiene, and adequate housing and ventilation.

A wide variety of other problems, such as neonatal mortality due to crushing, chilling, and starvation, and prolonged anestrus in weaned sows, must be controlled using management techniques and the provision of adequate facilities.

The central objective for the veterinarian and the producer is to maintain high levels of production using a combination of good management, genetics, housing, nutrition, and selective vaccination programs, all of which minimize the number or the magnitude of problems and specific diseases that interfere with the achievement of production targets.

TARGETS OF PERFORMANCE AND CURRENT LEVELS OF PERFORMANCE

Modern swine producers are interested in achieving certain targets of performance that are economical and in identifying the causes of failure to achieve those targets. The targets will vary from herd to herd, depending on the nature of the enterprise.

Some basic production targets for a 100-sow farrow-to-finish unit are as follows:

1. No. of litters per sow per year 2.0
2. No. of pigs born alive per litter 10.0
3. No. of pigs weaned per litter 9.0
4. Preweaning mortality <10%
5. No. of pigs marketed per sow farrowed per year 18
6. Average age in days to market 150-160

Some other acceptable and unacceptable levels of production and disease in intensive-rearing swine operations are recommended in Table 11-1. These figures are based on levels consistently achieved in herds of 100 to 250 sows. The interference level is the point at which corrective management techniques should be initiated.

The targets of production and disease, interference levels in the swine herd weaning piglets at three to five weeks of age, and the common causes of interference and their methods of correction are summarized in Table 11-2.

Traditionally, pig production was a secondary income for farmers whose major occupation was another kind of primary production, such as grain farming. In the last 25 years in countries like Canada, the United States, the United Kingdom, and Australia, there has been a marked decline in the number of nonspecialist pig producers and a marked increase in the number of pigs produced, particularly by specialist producers who operate intensified

Table 11-1. STANDARDS OF PRODUCTION AND DISEASE FOR BREEDING SWINE HERD

On a 5-week Weaning Program	Target	Interference Level
Weaning to service (days)	7	9
Returns to service (%)	6.0	12.0
Abortions (%)	0.8	2.5
Infertile (%)	2	5
Farrowing rate (%) = $\frac{\text{No. farrowing}}{\text{No. services}} \times 100$	89	80
Sow deaths/year (%)	2.2	3
Live pigs/litter	10.9	10
Stillborn (%)	5	8
Mummified (%)	0.5	1
Pigs weaned/litter	9.6	9.0
Deaths to weaning (%)	8-12	12-18
Litters of less than 8 pigs (%)	10	18
Laid on (%)	5	7
Congenital defects (%)	0.5	1.5
Low viability (%)	1.5	3
Starvation (%)	1	3
Deaths from diarrhea (%)	0.5	2
Miscellaneous deaths (%)	3	5
Litters/sow/year	2.25	2.0
Pigs marketed per sow farrowed per year	21	19
Postweaning deaths (%)	2	3
Finishing deaths (%)	1.5	2.5
Sows culled/100 sows/month	3	

From Muirhead, M.R. Veterinary problems of intensive pig husbandry. Vet. Rec., 99:288-292, 1976.

Table 11-2. TARGETS OF PRODUCTION AND INTERFERENCE LEVELS IN THE SWINE HERD WEANING PIGLETS AT 3 TO 5 WEEKS OF AGE°

Management of Performance	Target	Interference Level	Common Causes of Interference	Methods for Correction
Average days weaning-to-service interval	7	9	Postweaning anestrus in sows due to failure to detect estrus or true anestrus due to inadequate nutrition or lack of presence of boar. Seasonal infertility	Improve surveillance of heat detection. Examine nutritional status. Increase presence of boar when estrus is expected
Average age at first service for gilts (months)	7	8	Pubertal anestrus. Failure to detect estrus. Lack of presence of boar. Inadequate nutrition	Increase presence of boar with gilts on a daily basis. Ensure adequate nutrition
Returns to service (per cent)	6	12	Excessive use of boar. Poor semen quality	Increase number of available boars. Examine breeding soundness of boar
Abortions (per cent)	0.8	2.5	Infection with parvovirus, *Leptospira* sp. Importation of infected breeding stock	Purchase breeding stock free of infection. Quarantine imported stock. Vaccinate
Infertile services (per cent)	2	5	Infertile boar. Excessive use of boar. Poor estrus detection. Thin-sow syndrome	Examine boar for breeding ability and semen quality. Examine nutritional status of sows
Farrowing rate (per cent) = $\dfrac{\text{No. services}}{\text{No. of farrowing}} \times 100$	89	80	Failure to conceive because of infection. Abortion	Ensure accurate diagnosis
Sow deaths (per cent)	2.2	3	Peracute mastitis. Acute intestinal accidents. Other sporadic diseases	Prevent and control of specific diseases if possible
Sow culling/100 sows/month	3 or 36 per year	3 or 36 per year	Small litters. Mastitis. Arthritis. Persistent anestrus	Improve reproductive performance. Cull sows before litter size declines
Piglets born alive (number)	10.9	10	Excessive use of boar. Inferior breeding soundness of boar. In utero infections. Excessive energy intake in early gestation	Ensure optimum boar power. Reduce energy intake in early gestation to minimize embryonic death
Piglets born dead (per cent)	5	8	Intrapartum asphyxia due to dystocia	Survey farrowing and assist if necessary
Mummified piglets (per cent)	0.5	1	Parvovirus infection	Avoid infected imported breeding stock. Vaccinate
Number weaned per litter	9.6	9.0	Litter size born alive below 10. Neonatal deaths due to crushing, chilling, starvation, infectious enteritis, and other diseases of neonatal pig	Improve design of farrowing crate. Ensure early colostrum intake. Control agalactia in sow. Ensure sanitation and hygiene. Provide heat lamps
Preweaning mortality (per cent)	8–12	12–18	Neonatal deaths as above	Control neonatal deaths as above
Litter scatter (per cent)	10	18	Excessive use of boar. Breeding at incorrect time. Embryonic mortality	Judicious use of boars. Double-mating. Correct time of breeding
Litters per sow per year	2.25	2.0	Inadequate detection of heat. Failure to establish and maintain batch-farrowing	Improve detection of heat. Establish and maintain batch-farrowing
Number pigs marketed per sow per year	21	19	Small litter size. Less than 2.0 litters per sow per year. High neonatal mortality	Increase number of pigs born alive per litter and number of litters per sow per year. Control neonatal mortality
Postweaning death (per cent)	2	3	Postweaning check. Coliform gastroenteritis. Streptococcal meningitis	Ensure pigs are eating adequate amount of dry feed before weaning
Mortality during growing and finishing period (per cent)	1.0	2.5	Enzootic pneumonia. *Hemophilus* pleuropneumonia. Swine dysentery	Prevent introduction of carrier pigs. Provide adequate ventilation, sanitation and hygiene
Average age in days to market	160	170	Diseases of finishing pigs, especially pneumonias and enterides	Same as above
Feed efficiency (kg. feed per kg. body weight gain) Market pigs / Breeding herd	3.0 / 3.5	3.5 / 4.0	Diseases of finishing pigs, especially pneumonias and enteritis	Same as above

°The common causes of interference and their methods of correction are summarized.

operations. The standards of production have steadily improved to where 18 to 20 pigs are weaned per sow per year, the top herds are weaning 22 pigs per sow per year, and the feed conversions have steadily improved and now approach 3.0 kg./kg. live-weight gain (Ridgeon 1982).

There is considerable variation between herds in the levels of production, which suggests that there is still considerable scope for improvement. The data in Table 11–3 give an indication of the efficiency that is now being achieved in herds in Victoria, Australia.

ECONOMICS OF PIG PRODUCTION AND THE MAJOR CAUSES OF ECONOMIC LOSS

The establishment of a complete farrow-to-finish enterprise is a major financial consideration. In 1984 terms, the cost of establishing a 250-sow unit ranges from $3000 to $3500 (U.S.) per sow, including the cost of the breeding stock. The producer investing this sum of money is faced with high interest rates, fluctuations in the price of market pigs because of the pig cycle, and cash flow requirements to operate the enterprise.

The level of profitability in pig production is largely determined by the relationship of feed and market hog prices. Feed prices have usually increased at a greater rate per year than the rise in pig prices; consequently, gross and net margins have usually been small.

The efficiency of feed conversion in the swine herd is dependent on:

1. Reproductive efficiency of the sow (whose maintenance represents a substantial portion of the total feed budget)

2. Disease control, including clinical and subclinical disease

3. Feed wastage

4. Energy-expensive excessive fat carried by market pigs

Pig producers have steadily increased production by increasing the number of pigs weaned per sow per year and by improvement in feed conversion (Thomas 1980). A major contribution to containing production costs, however, has been the forced reduction in labor costs. Economic conditions have forced the pig industry to dispose of any surplus labor, and those that remain employed have increased productivity (Ridgeon 1982).

In order to maintain financial viability, the enterprise must achieve certain production objectives (targets of performance) such as number of pigs per sow per year. The points in the production cycle that are most critical and vulnerable and that affect the number of pigs produced per sow per year and in turn cause major economic losses include the following:

1. *Reproductive performance.* A decrease in conception rate and farrowing rate and a drop in the number of pigs born alive can cause major economic losses because of lost opportunity of profit. *No pigs, no profit.* Every economical effort must be utilized to achieve and maintain the birth rate at between 10 and 11 pigs born alive per litter (Govier 1978).

2. *Neonatal mortality.* The greatest losses in pigs born alive occur during the first three days of life. Preweaning mortality often reaches 25 to 30% but can be reduced to below 10% with good management and adequate farrowing crate facilities.

3. *Number of pigs weaned per litter.* The number of pigs weaned per litter is a function of the number of pigs born alive per litter and

Table 11–3. FIVE MOST PROFITABLE HERDS COMPARED WITH THE GROUP AVERAGE AND RANGE OF 18 HERDS 1979/80

	Group Average	Five Most Profitable Herds	Range for Herds in Study
Average size of breeding herd	102	120	13–438
Average gross margin per sow ($)	477	746	172–1056
Gross receipts ($ per sow)	1176	1394	575–1864
Per $100 output[*]: feed costs	60.6	50.0	39.9–86.6
other cash costs	8.6	7.2	2.8–27.3
margin	30.8	42.8	25.3–57.5
Costs of feed (cents per kg.)	15.0	14.1	10.6–17.0
Average return (cents per kg. dw)	148.7	150.2	134.1–179.0
Percentage sold as baconers	70.1	85.8	0–99.2
Numbers of litters per sow	2.02	2.1	1.65–2.21
Numbers of pigs born alive/litter	9.5	9.9	8.4–12.0
Number of pigs weaned/sow/year	18.0	18.2	12.5–21.6
Kg. feed per kg. meat	5.7	5.1	4.4–7.7
Feed cost (cents per kg. meat)	85.2	71.2	58.0–111.0

[*]Output is defined as the total value of all pigs (including sales and inventory change).
From Gardner, J.A.A. and Stewart, M.C. Pig production in Australia. Pig News and Info., 3:283–287, 1982.

the preweaning mortality. Increasing the number weaned per litter from eight to nine in a 100-sow unit will mean 200 extra pigs marketed per year.

4. *Feed efficiency in pigs from weaning to market.* The major cause of economic loss during the growing and finishing periods is the inadequate level of feed efficiency. The presence of subclinical and clinical diseases such as enzootic pneumonia, *Hemophilus* pleuropneumonia, atrophic rhinitis, swine dysentery, and parasitism will affect feed efficiency. Suboptimal performance will also occur because of overstocking in feeder pens, inadequate ventilation, tail-biting, and situations in which large quantities of manure accumulate on floor surfaces.

5. *Specific infectious diseases.* The economic losses resulting from specific infectious diseases are due to mortality, the cost of treatment, and the loss of potential production. The magnitude of the economic losses associated with the common diseases of pigs has been estimated (Muirhead 1978a, 1978b).

On an industry-wide basis, the economic losses associated with losses in pig production include the cost of veterinary fees, laboratory diagnosis, and medicines; the cost of the resources incorporated in breeding and other pigs, which are not recovered; and the resources used unnecessarily in the course of production (Beynon 1978). An overall reduction in mortality would enable the present level of output to be achieved with a smaller breeding herd, and there would be substantial savings in feed costs.

The economic losses associated with condemnation of pig carcasses at slaughter because of the presence of disease that renders the meat unfit for human consumption is estimated at about 0.5% of all pig carcasses (Bolitho 1978).

MONITORING PRODUCTION AND DISEASE IN THE SWINE HERD

A successful swine herd health and production program is dependent on a simple reliable record-keeping system that can be used to monitor performance and the incidence of disease. A regular analysis and interpretation of the records combined with a regular clinical examination of the herd—including necropsy examination of pigs that die naturally or of selected sick pigs—allows the veterinarian to identify problems that are interfering with production and to institute corrective measures (Muirhead 1978b, 1980). Such a system is outlined in Figure 11-1. Records define the levels of achievement in the herd and thus motivate the need for change or improvement. It is essential, however, that the information recorded be such that meaningful information is constantly produced. From this it can be determined whether productivity is being maintained at a predetermined level or if fluctuations are occurring in any particular parameter over a period of time.

Records alone, however, are not enough to identify the problem, and a clinical examination of the herd is essential. Once established, the recording system and data analysis will indicate the actual performance in that herd, which can be compared with predetermined targets. These levels may be ultimate standards, which will not be improved with existing knowledge, or those defined at selected points in an improvement program.

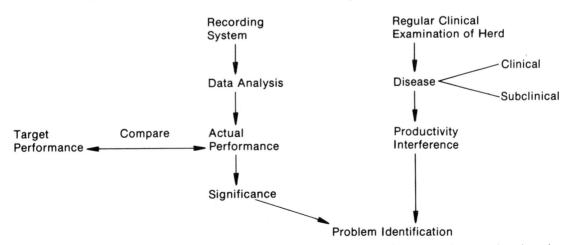

Figure 11-1. Pathways for identification and failure to achieve targets of performance using records and regular clinical examination. (From Muirhead, M.R.: The pig advisory visit in preventive medicine. Vet. Rec. *106*:170–173, 1980.)

Terms and Definitions

Animal production recording systems require a precise definition of the various classes of animal that are identified and the periods of time that are measured. There is no comprehensive list of the terms and definitions used in pig recording. Production recording systems have in the past relied on undefined terms and as a result, various classes of pigs are described in different ways. The following list of terms and definitions is recommended for use in manual recording systems and computer-based recording systems (Davies et al. 1983). (With the kind permission of the authors and the Ministry of Agriculture, Food and Fisheries.) Explanatory notes on the terms and definitions appear on pages 295 and 296.

A. The Breeding Herd

1. Sow

Any breeding female that has been served and is on the farm.

2. Maiden Gilt

A female transferred to the breeding herd but not yet mated.

3. Boar

A male pig over six months of age and intended for use in the breeding herd.

4. Sow Cull

Any live sow removed from the farm.

5. Boar/Sow Ratio

The ratio of boars to sows as defined in 1 and 3. Any definition must take into account the nonworking boar.

6. Herd Size

The average number of sows present in the herd as recorded on 12 or more equally spaced occasions during a year (365 days).

B. Fertility Data

7. (a) Service

One or more completed and recorded matings within the same estrus period.

(b) Date of Service

Date of first mating during any one estrus period (counted as day 0).

8. First Litter Sow

A female pig between the date of first effective service (a service that results in pregnancy) and the date of the next effective service following successful completion of pregnancy.

9. (a) Farrowing

Production of a litter of one or more live or dead pigs on or after the 110th day of pregnancy (day of service is day 0) (See Note i.)

(b) Farrowing Rate

The number of sows that farrow to a given number of services expressed as a percentage.

10. Induction

The use of a drug that is capable of inducing farrowing. Usually used from one to three days prior to the expected farrowing date to synchronize the farrowing of a number of sows on the same day.

11. Conception Rate

The number of sows that conceive to service expressed as a percentage of these services. Conception is assumed by nonreturn to estrus 21 days after service or identified by pregnancy diagnosis at about 30 days post service. These measures are not precise and the term *conception rate* is therefore of limited use.

12. Return to Service

A sow re-served after a return to service.

13. Regular Return

A return to service 18 to 24 days after the date of service. (See Note ii.)

14. Irregular Return

A return to service outside the period 18 to 24 days after the date of service. (See Note ii.)

15. Herd Farrowing Index

The number of farrowings taking place in 365 days divided by the average number of sows in the herd during that period as defined by 6.

16. Weaning Date (Sow)

The date on which a sow ceases to suckle piglets.

17. Weaning-to-Service Interval

The interval between date of weaning and the date of first service (date of weaning = day 0). (See Note iii.)

18. Empty Days

Empty days are average number of days between weaning (or gilts' first service) and effective service or removal from the breeding herd. (See Note ix.)

19. Abortion

The observed production of fetuses between service and up to and including the 109th day of pregnancy, and where none of the fetuses survive more than 24 hours. (See Note i.)

20. Premature Farrowing

The observed production of fetuses before the 110th day of pregnancy, but where some fetuses survive for more than 24 hours. (See Note i.)

21. Failure to Farrow

Sow not farrowed by 120 days after a presumed effective service.

C. Progeny: Preweaning Period

22. Litter

The production of a farrowing.

23. Number of Piglets per Litter

The total number of piglets born (including stillborn and mummified pigs) per litter.

24. Liveborn Piglets

Piglets that are born alive.

25. STILLBORN PIGLETS

Piglets found dead behind the sow farrowing (if necessary confirmed by postmortem examination to determine if the piglets have breathed).

26. MUMMIFIED PIGLETS

The number of dead piglets that are born degenerate (discolored and shriveled), i.e., they have died some time before farrowing.

27. PREMATURE PIGS

Piglets born alive (and surviving for more than 24 hours) before the 110th day of pregnancy. (See Note i.)

28. SMALL LITTER INDEX (SOMETIMES REFERRED TO AS LITTER SCATTER)

The percentage of litters born within any specified period in which the number of piglets in any litter (see 23) falls below x, where x is the nearest whole number lower than 1 standard deviation below the mean number of piglets per litter. (See Note iv.)

29. LIVE BIRTH WEIGHT OF LITTER

The total weight of piglets alive at birth or survived first 24 hours. (See Note v.)

30. SUCKLER

Piglet between birth and weaning.

31. SUCKLER (PREWEANING) MORTALITY

The percentage of liveborn piglets that die before weaning.

32. FOSTERING

The transferal of piglets from one litter to another for management purposes. Fostering-on is the introduction of extra piglets and fostering-off is the removal of pigs from a litter.

33. WEANING (PIGLETS)

The act of permanently removing piglets from the sow.

34. AGE AT WEANING

The number of days from farrowing to weaning (day of farrowing = day 0).

35. HERD WEANING AGE

The average number of days from farrowing to weaning for the herd.

D. Progeny: Postweaning Period

36. WEANER

A weaner is a pig between weaning and either the end of the stay in the weaner accommodation or 30 kg. if it is to remain in the same accommodation until slaughter. (As pigs are weaned at vastly differing ages, this definition can cover a wide age range.)

37. WEANER PIG MORTALITY

The number of weaners that die expressed as a percentage of the total number of weaners in that group initially.

38. FEEDER/FINISHER

Any pig in the stage of life between the end of the weaner period and slaughter weight or the time of transfer to the breeding herd.

39. PIGS MARKETED

Pigs marketed alive in any form or transferred to the breeding herd (NOT including sales from the breeding herd).

E. Feeder/Finisher Data

40. PORKER
41. CUTTER
42. BACONER
43. HEAVY HOGS

These are classes of finishing pigs that are categorized by weight. Different recording schemes and marketing systems use different weights. (See Note vi.)

44. LIVE-WEIGHT GAIN

The live-weight gain of the pig when sold less its birth weight. If the birth weight is not available, it is counted as 1 kg.

45. DAYS TO SLAUGHTER

The age of a pig at slaughter is the number of days from the date of birth of that pig (day 0) to the date of slaughter of that pig.

46. DAILY LIVE-WEIGHT GAIN

The live-weight gain of a pig divided by the number of days between two weighings.

47. FEED CONVERSION RATIO

The total weight of dry food consumed by a pig divided by its live-weight gain. (See Note viii.)

48. FEEDER/FINISHER PIG MORTALITY

The number of feeder/finishers that die in a group expressed as a percentage of the total numbers of feeder/finishers in that group initially.

49. AVERAGE DAYS TO SLAUGHTER

The average number of days to slaughter for a group of pigs, excluding those that die.

50. AVERAGE WEIGHT AT SLAUGHTER

The average live weight at slaughter. (See Note vii.)

51. TRANSIT DEATH

A pig dying in transit on the truck between the end of loading at the farm and the end of unloading at the abattoir or final disembarkation point.

52. LAIRAGE DEATH

A pig dying between the end of unloading at the abattoir and the point of slaughter.

53. CONDEMNATION

A carcass condemned wholly or in part.

54. CASUALTY/CULLS

Any pig for which payment is received that is slaughtered on welfare grounds or for persistent slow growth.

Explanatory Notes on the Terms and the Definitions

i. GESTATION LENGTH

This varies between herds according to

breed and other factors, but data held at Weybridge that relate to a large body of accumulated information from British herds give a mean figure ± 1 standard deviation (S.D.) of 114.5 ± 1.5 days. From this we can say that the 99% tolerance limits are 110 to 119 days.

ii. ESTRUS CYCLE LENGTH

A review of all available information suggested a mean estrus cycle length of 21 days ± 1.5 days (mean length ± S.D.), and this figure is widely accepted. These figures give 95% tolerance limits of 18 to 24 days, and this is the range that has been used for the calculation of regular and irregular returns (13 and 14).

iii. WEANING-TO-SERVICE INTERVAL

This depends on many factors, not the least of which is the length of lactation. Analysis of data from a variety of different sources suggests that for all practical purposes a mean figure of 7.5 ± 2.5 days (mean ± 1 S.D.) is acceptable. The interval is very variable because a wide range of factors affects it, e.g., the level of nutrition, disease status, management systems, and so on. But this figure is a satisfactory working guide in relation to weaning-to-service interval.

iv. TOTAL LITTER SIZE

It must be clearly recognized that litter size is also affected by a great many factors, including maternal age and breed, and disease status, and that it may vary from country to country. For the purpose of this book, it was felt that some figure that can be regarded as characteristic of the British situation and the variability that occurs between individuals should be given. For British herds the mean figure ± 1 S.D. for litter size is 10.75 ± 3.0 piglets. It is from this figure that the small litter index (28) is calculated, i.e., for the above figures the small litter index is the percentage of litters that contain less than seven pigs.

v. PIGLET BIRTH WEIGHT

Some indication of the mean and variability of normal piglet birth weights may be useful, and data obtained from Weybridge and other sources give the following:

Mean ± 1 S.D. = 1250 g. ± 250 g.

From this, the 95% tolerance limits are 750 to 1750 g.

vi. VALUES FOR SLAUGHTER PIGS

The Cambridge Pig Management Recording Scheme (Agricultural Economics Unit, Department of Land Economy, University of Cambridge), The Farmers Weekly, and the M.L.C. Economics Department use the following sets of values for slaughter pigs:

	Cambridge kg. (Live Weight)	F.W. kg. (Live Weight)	M.L.C. kg. (Dead Weight)
Porker	50–75	40–67	Up to 50
Cutter	75–105	68–82	50–81
Baconer	80–100	83–101	59–77
Heavy hog	105+	102+	82+

vii. HERD VALUES FOR SLAUGHTER PIGS

Many herds do not operate under a system of production that identifies individual slaughter pigs nor do they operate on a batch system. This precludes the use of the preceding definition. However, it is possible on a herd basis to estimate figures for the data given above, and the method used by the MLC in their pig herd recording scheme is shown at the top of the opposite page.

viii. FEED CONVERSION RATIO

On the farm, feed conversion ratio (FCR) estimates are required either for groups of pigs or for the whole finishing herd. If this is to be done accurately for any given period, it is necessary to record the weight of the food in stock at the beginning of the period, the weight of food entering stock during the period, and the weight of food in stock at the end of the period.

Similarly, it is necessary to know the weight of pigs in the group at the beginning and end of the period in question and the weight of pigs entering or leaving the group during the period. This means that all pigs entering and leaving the group need to be weighed and that all the pigs in the group also are weighed at the beginning and end of the recording period. This is a demanding task, and on most farms it is not attempted more than twice a year.

In assessing pig feed conversion efficiency as indicated by FCR, notes should be taken of the nutritive density of the diet.

ix. EMPTY DAYS

The number of empty days gives an indication of the regularity or rhythm of a herd's breeding performance and is independent of weaning age. The merit of this particular index is that it is easy to collect and gives a continuous indication of the regularity of breeding within the herd.

Information required is taken from the service book. A typical example in the simplest form contains the information shown at the bottom of the opposite page.

1. Average weight of pigs sold $= \dfrac{\text{Total wt. of sales} + \text{total wt. of transfers}}{\text{No. of sales} + \text{no. of transfers}}$

2. Average weight of pigs on entry $= \dfrac{\text{Total wt. of purchases} + \text{total wt. of transfers in}}{\text{No. of purchases} + \text{no. of transfers in}}$

3. Total weight gain $=$ Total wt. of sales $+$ total wt. of transfers out $+$ end of period total wt. $-$ (total wt. of purchases $+$ total wt. of transfer in $+$ start of period total wt.)

4. Per cent mortality $= \dfrac{\text{Deaths} \times 100}{\text{No. of sales} + \text{transfers out} + \text{deaths}}$

5. Feed conversion ratio $= \dfrac{\text{Total wt. of feed consumed}}{\text{Total wt. gain}}$

6. Daily live-weight gain $= \dfrac{\text{Av. wt. gain/pig}}{\text{Av. no. of days in herd}}$

7. Average weight gain $=$ Av. wt. of pigs sold $-$ av. wt. of pigs entering

8. Average days in herd $= \dfrac{\text{Av. no. of pigs in feeding herd} \times 30.4}{\text{Av. no. of sales and transfers out per month}}$

Statistical Note

Standard deviation (S.D.) is a measure of the scatter of individual readings about the mean (average). Where values are normally distributed, approximately 66% of values will fall between 1 S.D. either side of the mean, 95% within 2 S.D., and 99% within 3 S.D.

Identification of Pigs

Accurate identification of individual animals is essential for any comprehensive production recording system. Some form of permanent marking is required for performance assessment, herd security, disease surveillance, and quality control. Identification marks should be easy and painless to apply, legible at a distance, and tamperproof. At present, there is no single system that has all these attributes, the most common failing being the loss or illegibility of the identification mark well before the end of the animal's life in the herd. The methods commonly used include ear marking (notching, tattooing, or tagging) or body marking (slap marking). If animals destined for breeding purposes are to be correctly identified, experience suggests that the best system is ear tattooing early in life supplemented by a large flexible plastic tag inserted in each ear on entry into the breeding herd. Feeder pigs can be identified by ear tattoos that indicate the week of birth.

Sow's No.	Date Weaned (or Gilt's First Service)	Date Served (or Removed from Breeding Herd)	Boar Identity	Empty Days
G132	4/6	4/6	1 & 1	—
84	31/5	5/6	2 & 2	5
35	1/4	6/6	Removed	67
6	31/5	7/6	3 & 4	7
105	31/5	7/6	4 & 3	6
G98	21/5	12/6	1 & 1	22
18	7/6	12/6	2 & 2	5
65	7/6	13/6	3 & 3	6

Average no. of empty days $= \dfrac{\text{Total no. of empty days}}{\text{Total no. of sows served or gilts re-served}} = \dfrac{119}{7} = 17$

Data Recording on the Farm

The following events and animal identities are the basis of a pig recording system. The amount of data will vary from herd to herd and depends in part on the facilities available.

Data Recorded in the Breeding Herd

Sow identity
Birth date or date of entry
Service date and boar used
Boar identity (at service)
Failure to farrow
Abortion date
Farrowing date
Number born alive
Number born dead
Number mummified
Sex of piglets
Total litter weight at birth
Teat numbers (at three weeks of age)
Piglet identity
Piglet deaths (recorded as they occur)
Weaning date
Weight at weaning (total litter or individual pigs)
Weight of sow at weaning (or service)
Weaner deaths (as they occur)
Sow culling date
Feed consumed by breeding females in breeding barn and farrowing barn and piglets in nursery

Data Recorded in the Feeder/Finisher Barn

Identity of individual animals or pens
Date of entering feeder/finisher unit (or date at which 30 kg. live weight reached)
Weight at entry
Date sold off the farm
Weight at date of sale
Total amount of feed consumed per pig marketed to determine feed conversion ratio

Methods of Recording Data

These events and animal identities are recorded by the herdsman. He may use a notebook to jot down observations as he makes them, but these have to be transferred to some kind of record form. Record forms that are completed and kept in the piggery are called *barn records*. Record forms that are completed from notebook records or barn records but are kept in the farm office are called *office records*. Barn records or office records are used to calculate indices of performance. The calculations may be carried out manually, in which case it is important that the barn or office records be kept in such a way that calculation of indices requires the simplest possible manipulation of data. Calculations may also be carried out with the aid of computers. The calculation of indices is a simple task for the computer and allows for the calculation of far more sophisticated indices than is practicable with a manual system.

BARN RECORDS

Many different styles of barn records have been developed for use in the pig barn. The essential feature is that they allow the recording of the necessary data, which can then be extracted easily for the calculation of performance indices. Regardless of the system used, it should be simple and be readily accessible to each herdsman, the supervisor in the case of large herds, and the veterinarian. The records should be kept in a central location.

The minimum requirements for barn records include:

☐ a sow record card (Fig. 11–2)
☐ a daily diary (Fig. 11–3)
☐ a sow service card (Fig. 11–4)
☐ a daily record card (Fig. 11–5)

The Sow Record Card. It is essential that each sow has a record card that is kept with the animal (see Fig. 11–2). Normally these cards record events over one parity (weaning to weaning), although some sow records kept in the piggery contain a listing of events over the sow's adult lifetime. When the single parity record is complete, it can be stored in the office or can be used to complete a lifetime card (see Fig. 11–8). Sow cards may be clipped to the sow's stall and is moved when the sow is moved from the dry sow area to the farrowing barn and back again to the dry sow barn. Sow cards should be covered with a piece of removable transparent plastic because they become wet and soiled and difficult to read.

Daily Diary. The daily diary (see Fig. 11–3) is a useful technique for recording events throughout the day while the animal attendant is in the barn. The diary is pocket-sized and is self-duplicating, so that the duplicate copies may be collected regularly and the data posted directly into a computer bank.

Sow Service Card. The service card records all service events (see Fig. 11–4), including returns to service. The service card is ideal for bringing into the office for copying onto office records or for the direct calculation of indices.

Daily Record Card. This is essentially a register of events occurring over a 24-hour period (see Fig. 11–5). It should be completed at the same time each day and has two purposes:

		Sow card
SOW No.	DATE SERVED	BOAR No.
	2nd SERVICE	BOAR No.
DUE TO FARROW	FARROWED	
TOTAL BORN	BORN ALIVE	
PIGS FOSTERED OFF	PIGS FOSTERED ON	
DATE IRON	DATE CASTRATED	
No. PIGS WEANED	DATE WEANED	
REMARKS		

Figure 11–2. Sow record card.

1. It provides data for analysis by the veterinarian.

2. It provides the herdsman with a day-to-day summary of the productivity of the animals in the herd. Each card lasts one month and is kept on a clipboard. At the end of the month the card is passed to the office, where monthly totals are calculated and passed back to the herdsman. This toting-up procedure is the simplest possible way of keeping a monthly record of events and is far easier than making calculations from individual sow cards. In the early stages of a recording system, irrespective of the size of the unit, a weekly module rather than a monthly module may be desirable. With experience, this can be expanded to a 28-day system, but a weekly summary will give the manager more information as the system becomes established.

There is some overlap between the data recorded on sow cards, service cards, and daily event cards. This is inevitable; it can be avoided by having one record—for example, a sow service book (Fig. 11–6)—but it has the considerable advantage that the record cards provide data in an ideal form for manual computation of production indices. The three record cards described form a good all-purpose system, but the veterinarian and the herdsman may decide to use indices of productivity or fertility that are not easily computed from them. An example is a boar fertility record (Fig. 11–7). This is ideal for immediate identification of boars that are infertile.

PIGTALES		No.
DATE:	COMPLETED BY:	
IDENTITY	EVENT	DETAIL

PIGTALES		No.
DATE:	COMPLETED BY:	
IDENTITY	EVENT	DETAIL

Figure 11–3. Daily diary. (Courtesy of Pigtales Ltd.)

Month . . . .

SERVICES			SERVICES BT. FWD.		
DATE	Sow No.	Boar No.	DATE	Sow No.	Boar No.

SOWS AND GILTS NOT FARROWING TO ABOVE

DATE	SOW No.	REASON	REMARKS

R1 Return at 3 wks   AB—Aborted
R2 Return at 6 wks   N.I.P.—Found not in pig
R3 Return at 6 wks+   S.L.—Sold Lame

Figure 11-4. Sow service card.

Performance Records. Individual sow lifetime records (Fig. 11–8) are an extension of the single-parity record. The monthly herd performance record (Fig. 11–9) is an extension of the daily record. The herd performance report (Fig. 11–10) can be constructed with a mini-

mum of manual computation from the barn records (sow card, service card, and daily event record). The herd performance report provides a record of all the main indices of performance required, and it provides a ready comparison of present performance with the previous six-month average and also with a target figure set by the veterinarian. Targets introduce a discipline into management and enable problems to be identified. The report illustrated holds records for three months on the assumption that the veterinarian will be visiting every three months. If monthly visits are the rule, one "monthly" column is sufficient. This report provides the veterinarian with an ideal early warning system.

Visual Sow Charts and Wheels. Breeding wheels and wall calendar charts have been in common use on pig farms for many years. They usually take the form of a large disc or fixed board or chart. These visual display systems are a simple but effective method of providing immediate information on the present and future position of sows in the breeding herd. They are not in themselves a data-recording system, as they do not provide a permanent record, and are no substitute for accurate and complete barn and office records. They are management tools used on a daily basis to indicate to the herdsman the flow of breeding animals through the herd. The system will indicate to the herdsman when groups of sows are due to be moved from the gestation barn to the farrowing barn in sufficient time for adjustment to occur. This avoids sows farrowing in the gestation barn. It will also remind the herdsman to prepare for the weaning of a group of sows.

At a glance, on a daily basis, the sow breeding calendar wheel will indicate the following:

1. Expected date of farrowing of each sow, which allows the producer to transfer the sow to the farrowing crate several days before the expected farrowing date

2. Actual date of farrowing of each sow

3. Dates the pigs should be weaned and actual dates of weaning, which allows adequate preparation of nursery pens and weans most litters about the same time

4. Date each sow should come into heat after weaning her pigs

5. Actual dates of heat and breeding

6. Number of times sow was bred

7. The identity of the sows that have been diagnosed pregnant

Month

Days of Month	Litters	Pigs Born		Deaths		Pigs Weaned		Medication
		Alive	Dead	Pre weaning	Post weaning	No. of Litters	No. of Pigs	
1								
2								
3								
4								
5								
6								
7								
23								
24								
25								
26								
27								
28								
29								
30								
31								
TOTALS								

Figure 11-5. Daily record card.

Computer-Based Recording Systems

Some form of manual recording system is probably adequate for a small herd, but as the size of the herd increases, the limitations of such a system become obvious. A computer system is capable of storing extensive records of large numbers of animals, and it easily manipulates complex sets of data that would be impractical to handle manually (Pepper et al. 1977; Pepper and Taylor 1977).

A computer-based system may be more expensive than its manual counterpart, but the real cost of computer equipment (hardware) continues to decline as computer technology advances. The expensive part of a computer-based system is the program, or set of instructions (software), which may require several man-years to develop. However, many have now been developed, and their cost should not be a major limiting factor.

Most of the computer systems that are suitable for herd health and production recording were developed on large main-frame computers, which had the capacity to be connected to many distant points by way of telephone lines and terminals. Main-frame installations depend on the receipt and dispatch of data either by mail or by telephone lines using a terminal situated on the farm or in the veterinarian's office. Mail delays can impede the handling of the data, noise and interference on telephone lines can affect the transmission of signals and the quality of the report, and long-distance telephone charges may become a limiting factor. Also, because of multiple subscribers, the veterinarian or producer may be required to use the computer during inconvenient times of the day.

The future of computer-based systems for herd health probably lies in the use of mini- or

Sow ear No.	Date weaned	Parity	Boar ear No.	Service date	3 weeks time	Weaning to service interval	Date due	Date farrowed	No. born Alive	No. born Dead	Weaned No.	Weaned Date	Weaning age (days)

Figure 11-6. Sow service book.

Month	BOAR NO.		BOAR NO.		BOAR NO.		BOAR NO.	
	Sow No.		Sow No.		Sow No.		Sow No.	
1								
2								
3								
4								
5								
6								
7								
8								
9								
10								
11								
12								
13								
14								
15								
16								
17								
18								
19								
20								
21								
22								
23								
24								
25								
26								
27								
28								
29								
30								
31								

Figure 11-7. Boar fertility record card.

Identity		Litter No.	1	2	3	4	5	6
		Boar's identity						
		No. of services						
Genetic status		Service date						
Birth date		Farrowing date						
Arrival date		Induced (Yes/No)						
Entry date		Stillborn						
Leaving date		Mummified						
Culled/Died		Born live						
Dam's identity		Av. birth weight						
Sire's identity		Fosterings on						
		Fosterings off						
		Preweaning loss						
		No. weaned						
		Av. weaning weight						
		Weaning date						
		Litter tattoo						
		No. substandard						
		Problem 1						
		Problem 2						
		Problem 3						
		Problem 4						

Figure 11-8. Sow life record card.

microcomputers, which can be installed either on the farm or in the veterinarian's office (Kelly 1983). Minicomputers are essentially calculating machines with a built-in record storage capacity. The cost of the hardware depends to some extent on the size of the storage capability. It has been estimated that a standard floppy disc can store the data recorded for a 200-sow herd over at least a one-year period.

The first step in recording is similar in both manual and computer-based systems, that is, recording the initial observations. The initial observations are recorded on data capture sheets, which either are used to complete punch cards or are the basis for direct entry into the computer. However, this is labor-intensive, and each time data are handled or transferred from one sheet to another the number of errors increases. One way to minimize errors is to record the observations directly into some form of electronic notepad, which in turn reports directly to the computer. Developments in this type of recording and in

specific computer programs offer the promise of cheap and effective computer-based systems for the livestock industry.

Many organizations provide whole-herd recording systems, which depend on sending input to and receiving output from a mainframe computer through the mail. The emphasis in each system may be different. Some monitor the performance of the swine herd, and key factors such as farrowing index and feed conversion ratio are calculated on a six-month rolling average. Individual herd performance may be compared with that of several hundred other participating herds.

The outputs for a breeding herd may be as follows:

Average no. of sows and gilts in herd
Average no. of unserved gilts
Average no. of sows and gilts per boar
Average no. of litters per sow and gilt
Average no. of pigs born per litter
Average no. of pigs born alive per litter
Average no. of pigs reared per sow and gilt

Average no. of pigs reared per litter
Average weight of pigs reared (kg.)
Feed per pig reared (kg.)
Total feed cost per pigs reared
Total feed consumption per kg. pig produced
Total feed cost per kg. pig produced
Quantity of sow feed per sow and gilt
Cost of sow feed per sow and gilt
Quantity of pig feed per pig reared
Cost of pig feed per pig reared
Cost per cwt. of feed

Other computer-based systems are available that will monitor the physical and financial performance of the breeding and/or feeding unit every four weeks. Financial results are reported for each unit, and per pig and per sow if requested. Each report gives a summary of all data processed over the last year, which is useful in identifying trends.

Computer-based recording systems that are orientated toward health and production are available. The computer's store of records consists of a status file and a history file; an archive file is updated each week, and the status file is used for a series of printouts, some of which are produced weekly, whereas others are only provided on demand. These include:

1. A weekly inventory of breeding stock
2. A record of services showing the boar number, sow number, and number of days since weaning, and a list of sows with regular and irregular returns to estrus and sows due to farrow

The history file contains a record of each sow and boar in the herd. The file is used to compute herd productivity data when required. The archive file records sows and boars that have been culled.

A program to monitor reproductive effi-

Name: Month:

DRY SOWS, GILTS and BOARS	Sows	Gilts	Total
Total Servings	. . .	. . .	. . .
Returns to Service	. . .	. . .	. . .
Abortions	. . .	. . .	. . .
Hormone Inj.	. . .	. . .	. . .
Culls	. . .	. . .	. . .
Deaths and Emergency Slaughter	. . . Sows	. . . Gilts	. . . Boars
No. in Herd	. . . Sows	. . . Served Gilts	. . . Boars
		. . . Maiden Gilts	

FARROWING/REARING AREA No. Litters . . . . .   No. Live Births . . . . .   No. Stillborn . . . . .

No. Deaths . . . .   No. Litters Treated . . . . .   Drugs Used . . . .

. . . .   No. Sows Treated . . . . .

Drugs Used . . . .

WEANER POOL No. Litters Weaned . . . . . .   No. Pigs Weaned . . . . . .   No. Deaths . . . . . .

No. Pens Treated for Scour . . . . .   Drugs Used . . . .

No. Pens Treated Other Conditions . . . . .   Drugs Used . . . .

Preventive Medication . . . .

Age at Weaning (days) . . . . .   Average Weight at Weaning . . . .

Figure 11-9. Monthly herd record.

Data	Month	Month	Month	Six month average	Suggested target
No. of sows					
No. of gilts					
No. of board					
No. served to farrow					
No. farrowed					
Farrowing rate					
Pigs born alive					
Pigs born mummified					
% born dead					
% born mummified					
Total pigs born/sow					
Live pigs born/sow					
Piglet mortality					
Weaner mortality					
Fat pig mortality					
Pigs sold					
Pigs born/sow/year					
Pigs sold/sow/year					
	No. served farrow	No. now in pig			
1st month					
2nd month					
3rd month					
4th month					

Figure 11–10. Pig herd performance report.

ciency and weaner production using only one data recording sheet is available. The data sheet is sent to the computer center each month, and a monthly report is sent out that includes the following:

1. Production data—litters produced, numbers born and weaned, mortality rates, liveweight gain of piglets

2. Production efficiency—weaners produced per sow in the herd, feed used per weaner and per kg. of weaner produced

3. Reproductive efficiency—analysis of weaning-to-service intervals, farrowing intervals, returns to service, farrowing rates, boar data comprising numbers born and farrowing rates

4. Records of the lifetime performance of sows and culling rates

5. Finisher data—analysis of the live-weight gain and grading of bacon pigs

Any computer-based program should provide the following:

1. A period report. This is the most commonly used and is returned to the producer at the end of each reporting period.

2. Performance graphs. Simple graphs of several parameters are plotted, using the values for the last six reporting periods and comparing them with decision boundaries already set by the producer.

3. Interherd comparison. This analysis compares statistics from as many farms and as many periods as selected by the operator.

A word of caution. Computer-based recording systems are an aid to the veterinarian and the swine producer. Both parties must take the time when each printout is made available to analyze and interpret the results of the computer analysis, identify problem areas, investigate those areas clinically, take corrective action, and observe the results.

Interpretation of Animal Health and Production Data

The collection and analysis of health and production data is of little value unless the data are used to improve or maintain the efficiency and profitability of the swine enterprise. Whether the data are analyzed manually or with the use of a computer, the actual performance of the herd must be examined and interpreted.

The efficiency of the swine unit depends on maintaining a constant flow of pigs through the buildings to make most effective use of the available labor and facilities, which represent a considerable financial investment. One of the first tasks in planning production that can be achieved with the fixed resources of a swine unit is to set production targets. Subsequently, monitoring the herd's actual performance will reveal whether these initial targets are capable of being achieved. If they are not, they can be adjusted to more realistic levels, but the shortfalls may be due to disease or other problems interfering with the production cycle, and these have to be investigated and corrected. This process of setting targets, monitoring and assessing performance, investigating shortfalls, and revising targets is a continuous one and is dependent on comprehensive and accurate production records.

The best use of resources is achieved by aiming at a level output of pigs throughout the year. This usually means a weekly system of farrowing, the size of the group being appropriate to the size of the herd that can be sustained. It is important, in the early stages of planning, to decide on the size of herd; thus, the number of reproductive cycles can be predicted and the amount of accommodation for various phases of production calculated.

During the first 12 months after the establishment of a swine herd health program, the setting of targets of performance should be assessed at frequent intervals. The critical indices are the number of services and the number of farrowings per week. These indices provide a rough analysis of the production process and do not allow an investigation of the cause of shortfalls. A more comprehensive list of indices must be examined in detail to determine where losses are occurring.

Disease Recording

The records already described are only demographic (vital statistics). They do not, except by reference, describe clinical disease. The recording of specific disease incidents has not been a major feature of swine herd recording systems. Often a specific diagnosis of a sick pig is not made by the animal attendant, and the veterinarian is usually not called to examine and treat individual pigs. However, a daily diary should be kept of sick pigs and their location, the treatment given, the number of pigs that died with and without treatment, and the results of necropsies.

Herd Health Status

It is often desirable that some overall record of the health status of the herd be available. This can be of value in selling breeding stock and for admission to livestock shows and sales. It is also a guide to succeeding veterinary advisers. The report would consist of a list of production indices for the last six to 12 months and the status of the herd for the common infectious diseases such as atrophic rhinitis, enzootic pneumonia, transmissible gastroenteritis, swine dysentery, vomiting and wasting disease, parvovirus infections, sarcoptic mange, and erysipelas. The results of the examination of heads and lungs of pigs sent to slaughter within the last 12 months may also be included. The methods used to determine the disease status of the herd must accompany the report and be certified by the veterinarian. The report should also include a summary of the clinical observations made by the veterinarian over a period of 12 months.

COMPONENTS OF A PLANNED ANIMAL HEALTH AND PRODUCTION PROGRAM

The success of a swine herd health and production program depends on the enthusiasm and competency of the veterinarian and the willingness of the producer to maintain a high level of production through good management. This section will describe in general terms some of the methods commonly used to improve and maintain a high level of production and disease control in the swine herd.

The Regular Farm Visit

The veterinarian must make regularly scheduled visits to the swine herd. The frequency of the visits and the length of time actually spent on the farm will depend on the size of the herd and the current health and production status of the herd. In the initial stages of a program, the veterinarian may visit the herd once weekly for a few months in order to gain experience with the herd, to identify obvious problems, and to establish a recording system. Once the program is established, one visit per month to a 100-sow farrow-to-finish operation is often adequate. For larger operations, once-weekly operations may be desirable. Telephone consultations, emergency visits, and necropsy services may be provided between the regular farm visits.

The objective of the regular visit is to strive continually for increased productivity by managerial, environmental, and therapeutic control of disease in order to express maximum physiological function in that herd.

A procedure for routine visits to a swine herd is as follows:

1. *Previsit preparation.* Make an appointment with the producer at least one week in advance and be punctual at the appointed time of visit. Review and prepare the following:

Interpretation of previous production reports
   Laboratory results
   Ongoing investigations
   Special topic preparation

2. *Clinical and environmental examination.* In general terms, this includes the following:

Examination of summaries of production indices and disease incidence since last visit in order to identify problem areas
   Visual examination of each unit of the herd
   Clinical examination of selected sick pigs
   Necropsy examination when appropriate
   Collection of laboratory samples as necessary

Housing, ventilation, sanitation, hygiene, stocking density, comfort of animals
   Feeds and feeding systems

A series of checklists may be used to examine all aspects of each area of the herd. The clinical inspection is done along with the herdsman, and each item in the checklist identifies a possible problem and serves as a prompter for the herdsman to indicate the presence of a problem.

(a) *Reproduction and Service Area*
Boar/sow ratio
Boar fertility, service problems
Boar usage
Boar condition (mange, lameness, and other diseases)
Weaning-to-service intervals
Return rate and interval of returns to estrus
Farrowing rate
Sow stocking density
Sow body condition (trauma, stress, lameness)
Housing, environment, temperature
Nutritional levels
Estrus abnormalities
Uterine discharges
Treatments, hormones
Pregnancy diagnosis

(b) *Dry Sow Area*
Environment and temperature
Stocking densities/stall/tether problems
Feed levels, dung state
Body condition score
Udder line, chronic mastitis
Lameness
Estrus abnormalities
Vulvar discharges
Abortions
Sows not pregnant
Culls and reasons
Sudden death and results of necropsies
Parasite control
Treatments used and reasons

(c) *Farrowing and Nursery Area*
Sow body condition score
Sows not pregnant
Mastitis, metritis, agalactia
Farrowing fever
Parturition difficulties
Sudden deaths and results of necropsies
Litter size, litter scatter
Stillbirths, mummifications
Piglet viability, splay-leg, congenital defects
Neonatal diarrhea, starvation, trauma
Mortality levels
Piglet comfort (heat lamp)
Respiratory disease in nursing piglets (sneezing, ocular and nasal discharge, nasal deformity, coughing)
Sudden deaths
Diseases of the skin
Parasite control
Treatments used and reasons

(d) *Growing and Finishing Area*
Age at weaning, body weight, and variability in weight
Nutrition, water availability
Evenness of growth

Postweaning diarrhea

Housing, environment, and stocking densities

Insulation, temperature, and ventilation

Rhinitis, pneumonia

Skin conditions, mange

Vaccination programs

Sudden deaths and results of necropsies

Culls, lameness

Tail-biting, ear-chewing

Swine dysentery

Days to slaughter

Feed conversion rates

Other diseases

Parasite control

Treatments used and reasons

3. *Analysis and Discussion of the Results of the Visit*

Records of performance

Evaluation of diseases encountered

Epidemiologic discussions (what environmental, nutritional, managerial, or other factors are contributing to disease)

Remedial actions and recommendations

4. *Special Topics*

Each month a selected special topic may be investigated. These include:

a. Herd security

b. Stock introduction, herd replacement policies, gilt selection

c. Economic losses in the herd, feed costs and utilization

d. External/internal parasite control, vermin control, vaccination program

e. Fertility, boar management

f. Herd security check, diseases of the farrowing sow

g. Piglet problems

h. Diseases, mortality, and management of the weaned and finishing pigs

i. Housing utilization, alterations, associated diseases

j. Labor management and productivity

k. Slaughterhouse monitoring and pathological tests

l. Twelve-month appraisal and analysis

5. *General Problems* (i.e., flow of pigs through the entire enterprise)

6. *Preparation for Next Visit*

Arrange date and special problems to be investigated

Arrange for possible consultation with other specialists (i.e., genetics, nutritionist, agricultural engineer)

7. *Preparation of the Report*

Usually done in the veterinarian's office and sent to the producer within two days after farm visit

Emergency Farm Visit

Outbreaks of infectious disease may occur sporadically, and these should be investigated by the veterinarian. Prescriptions for mass medication of the feed or water supplies may be necessary, and it may be legally necessary to examine the pigs. Producers should be encouraged to notify the veterinarian of an unusually high incidence of mortality, dystocia, coughing, agalactia, and the like, which should be investigated immediately rather than left until the next monthly visit.

Nutritional Advice

Veterinarians involved in preventive medicine in swine herds should become well informed about the nutrient requirements of the different age groups of pigs.

Since feed constitutes from 60 to 80% of the cost of producing a market pig, every economical effort must be made to increase the efficiency of feed utilization. The trend is to use complete feeds formulated by feed company nutritionists who are familiar with the nutrient composition of local feedstuffs. With complete diets, specific nutrient deficiencies are uncommon.

The major problem is the efficiency of utilization of the different feeds throughout the life cycle of the pig. The nutrient requirements of the pig at various phases of growth from birth to market weight and for breeding stock are well established. The remaining questions appear to concern the levels of feed that should be provided during the different phases of the growth of the pig in order to achieve optimum production and to yield the best carcass. Proper nutrition can greatly increase the efficiency of swine production, since feed represents such a large percentage of the cost involved. Following are some recommended practices for increasing efficiency of feed utilization with swine:

1. Feed well-balanced diets with adequate levels of crude proteins, amino acids, energy, vitamins, and minerals necessary to meet the particular demands. Protein is normally overfed to meet the needs of the most limiting essential amino acids. The finishing pig is normally fed 2.0 more percentage units of protein than required so that it will receive

adequate lysine. This results in a decrease of 10 to 15% in the efficiency of converting total diet protein to tissue protein. Lower levels of protein will eventually be used as amino acid supplementation becomes better understood and the economics of amino acid use justifies their addition to swine diets.

2. Use least-cost formulation to the extent that it is feasible.

3. Restrict the level of a properly balanced diet for sows during gestation to avoid over-feeding. Sows that have lost excessive body weight in the previous lactation need supplemental feed during the dry period to avoid the thin-sow syndrome.

4. Feed sows according to litter size during lactation and avoid overfeeding. The composition of the diet should not be changed between dry sows and lactating sows. Only the total amount of feed should be changed at the time of farrowing to avoid digestive upsets in early lactation.

5. Provide a creep-feed for nursing piglets beginning at about one week of age. An attempt is made to encourage piglets to be eating a significant amount of creep-feed at weaning time at three weeks of age so that digestive upsets are held to a minimum. Early weaning diets must be highly digestible (Fowler 1980).

6. Feed growing-finishing pigs for optimum, but not always maximum, gains to optimize feed energy costs per unit of pork produced. Marketing at 100 to 110 kg. live body weight is most economical (Sather et al. 1980).

7. Slaughter pigs as close to optimum slaughter weight as possible to minimize excess, trimmable fat.

8. Use antimicrobial agents and chemotherapeutics for short periods (two to three weeks) during stress rather than continuously.

9. Avoid feed wastage by using well-designed feeding systems.

10. Consider restricting feed intake if it will increase carcass quality and feed efficiency. In most cases, however, a premium for improved carcass quality will be needed to offset the increased time the pigs are handled.

11. Consider pellet feeding, which is most beneficial with the young pig. Pelleting is more helpful with bulky or high-fiber feeds with growing-finishing pigs. The economics of pelleting needs to be considered to ensure that the advantages are greater than the cost involved.

The veterinarian should examine the feeds and feeding systems at each visit. Changes in feed formulation and amounts of feed fed should be recorded.

The feed efficiency of the pigs from weaning to market should be monitored regularly. It is often difficult to obtain accurate data on this item for specific groups of pigs, because the amount fed to the groups may not be calculable because of a common feeding system. However, the total amount of feed used and the total weight of pigs marketed will give an estimate of feed efficiency.

Genetics and the Selection and Acquisition of Breeding Stock

Veterinarians have traditionally not provided advice on genetics and breeding programs in swine herds. However, veterinarians who become involved in providing a complete swine herd health and production program should be aware of the components of a breeding program, which include the basic concepts of swine genetics, heritability estimates of the economically important performance and carcass traits, the importance of records in selection, performance testing procedures, the value of cross-breeding, and the problems associated with the acquisition of breeding stock free of infectious agents. Performance and carcass traits in swine are affected by both heredity and environment. Heredity is the sum total of genes, and combinations of genes, the offspring received from its parents. These are fixed at the moment of conception and cannot be changed thereafter. Environment includes all nonhereditary factors such as feed, management, and disease. The environmental effects can be controlled to a certain extent by the swine producer. Both heredity and environment must be optimum in order to produce swine efficiently. For example, the best feeding and management system possible will be disappointing if the animals produced do not have the genetic ability to perform well and produce superior carcasses. On the other hand, a poor feeding and management system will also give disappointing results even if the swine produced are genetically superior.

The improvement of swine through breeding may be accomplished in two different ways. One way is to find the best animals for important traits when all are compared under similar conditions and then mate the best to the best. The second way is to cross unrelated strains or breeds to obtain heterosis, or hybrid vigor. The details of the different selection programs for purebred herds and commercial herds using cross-breeding systems are available in standard textbooks on genetics of livestock improvement (Lasley 1980). Annual reports of the Canadian Record of Performance (ROP) swine testing program provide no evidence of genetic trends in the purebred seed stock herds enrolled. Small herd size (<8 sows), short average life span of these herds (<5 years), and the geographically diffuse nature of the seed stock industry appear to have major impediments to the application of cohesive and sustained selection programs. The commercial industry, in contrast, has shown a marked improvement in average carcass merit between 1970 and 1980. This trend, stimulated and guided by the 1968 revision of carcass grading standards, has been accompanied by a 60% reduction in the number of commercial herds and a threefold increase in the average number of pigs marketed annually per unit. There has been a steady growth in the use of systematic cross-breeding programs, and producer demand for boars with performance credentials has greatly intensified. This has fostered a fivefold increase in ROP testing activity, given impetus to the evolution of swine AI programs, and encouraged the development of large closed herd seed stock operations with self-contained performance test facilities. The central objective of performance testing programs, both private and public, is the genetic improvement of traits directly relevant to efficient lean meat production. Future production requirements are unlikely to alter this basic objective, but advances in the technology for live animal carcass evaluation and changing economic circumstances—specifically changes in rations to accommodate the increasing competition for cereal grain supplies—will necessitate continuous review and revision of testing procedures (Fredeen 1980).

Efficiency of production varies greatly among production units. It is not uncommon to find the amount of feed required to produce a unit of market weight to be as low as 3.3 to 3.7 for farms with excellent management and as high as 4.5 to 5.0 for farms with somewhat poorer management schemes. Differences of this magnitude in production efficiency are not totally due to genetic differences; however, one should always be aware that performance never exceeds the genetic potential of the breeding stock used in a herd. Therefore, the genetic potential should not be the weak link in preventing a production unit from attaining the efficiency of 3.3 units of feed per unit of live hog marketed.

Basic Concepts

Most traits of economic importance in swine may be classified as quantitative traits, that is, traits that exhibit some measurable or observable quantity, such as litter weight, growth rate, or backfat thickness. It is true that many qualitative traits such as coat color do exist, but the economic significance of these traits is usually much less than for the quantitative traits. The exception may be some detrimental recessive traits such as lethals or blood disorders that result in either prenatal or postnatal death. These genetic defects should simply be selected against by selecting breeding stock that are free from defects and whose relatives and ancestors were as free as possible. Basically, qualitative traits are influenced or determined by only one or a very small number of pairs of genes, and the environment plays little or no role in determining phenotype. On the other hand, quantitative traits are influenced by many pairs of genes, maybe even many thousands of pairs of genes, and the environment may play a major role in determining the phenotypic (performance) value for these traits. The majority of the genes that influence quantitative traits act in an additive manner to influence phenotype. Consequently, selection to improve quantitative traits is aimed at selecting breeding stock with the greatest additive value for a given trait. The fact that the environment also influences phenotype prevents one from always being certain that the pig with the highest phenotypic value also has the highest sum of additive genes for the respective trait.

The concept of heritability confronts the problem of separating or partitioning the influence of genes and the environment upon phenotype. Heritability may be defined as the degree to which quantitative traits are transmitted from parent to offspring or the degree to which relatives are more alike than nonrelated individuals. Heritability may also be defined as the per cent of phenotypic variability among a population of animals that is due to the variability in additive gene action among the members of the population. In simpler terms, heritability refers to the proportion of the variability for a trait in a population that is due to additive genes. The remainder of the variability is the result of environmental influences and other types of gene action or interactions. Heritability estimates for several economically important traits in swine are presented in Table 11–4.

It should be quite clear that through selection, genetic progress will be more rapid for more highly heritable traits. By simply selecting the boars and gilts with the most desirable phenotypic values (production records) and following the practice of "mating the best to the best," one should be able to make rather rapid change for the more highly heritable traits. However, both generation interval and intensity of selection play a role in the rate of genetic progress.

Traits that relate to linear measurements, shape, or composition of pigs are generally high in heritability, and therefore genetic progress can be quite rapid within purebred swine herds for these traits. It is for this reason that breeders have been successful in reducing the fat composition and increasing the lean or muscle tissue in pork carcasses. Rate and efficiency of gain are also improved through selection but not as rapidly as traits relating to composition. The best method for improving feed efficiency is to select for increasing the rate of lean growth. This may be accomplished by selecting to increase the rate of growth and decrease backfat thickness.

It is unfortunate that the most important traits from an economic standpoint (fertility, prolificacy, liveability, libido, and longevity) are quite low in heritability. In fact, almost all traits that relate to physical fitness or environmental adaptability are low in heritability. This does not mean that purebred breeders should ignore them but rather that genetic progress will be quite slow in improving these traits by selective mating.

Cross-Breeding

Commercial producers for herds producing slaughter pigs should use selective breeding in a similar manner to purebred or nucleus herds for improving the highly heritable traits; however, the producer of slaughter pigs has available a major tool that is not available to the purebred breeder. That tool is cross-breeding, which results in hybrid vigor or heterosis. It is by taking full advantage of hybrid vigor that the slaughter pig producer may attain production levels for low to medium heritable traits that are much greater than production levels for purebred or nucleus herds.

Hybrid vigor or heterosis may be defined as the difference in performance between crossbred progeny and the average performance of their purebred parents. The formula for calculation would be:

$$\% \text{ Hybrid vigor} = \frac{\text{Average of offspring} - \text{Average of parents}}{\text{Average of parents}} \times 100$$

As an example, assume that the average production for Breed A is 100 for a hypothetical trait and the average production for Breed B is also 100. If an average boar from Breed A is mated to an average gilt from Breed B, the resulting cross-bred progeny, AB, has a performance of 120, so the

$$\% \text{ Hybrid vigor} = \frac{120 - 100}{100} = \frac{20}{100} = 20\%$$

Results of this nature are not uncommon for those traits that are low in heritability in swine. Traits that are highly heritable show little or no change due to hybrid vigor. Rate of growth shows an intermediate to high response due to hybrid vigor; however, efficiency of gain generally shows no response. This must mean that efficiency of gain is primarily a function of composition of gain. It is significant to note that whole-herd feed efficiency values will be improved by an increase in reproductive rate and an improvement in pig liveability. Since the hybrid vigor response for traits low in

Table 11–4. HERITABILITY ESTIMATES FOR TRAITS IN SWINE

Reproductive Traits	% Heritability
Number of pigs farrowed	0–15
Number of pigs weaned	5–15
Fertility	0–15
Age at puberty	0–15
Libido	0–15
Performance Traits	
Growth rate	25–45
Feed efficiency	25–35
Milking ability	20–30
Carcass Traits	
Length	40–60
Backfat depth	40–60
Longissimus dorsi area	40–60
Thickness of belly	40–60
Per cent muscle	40–60
Muscle quality	30–40
Other Traits	
Disposition	30–50
Udder quality	40–50
Skeletal shape	40–60

heritability is so great and since most of these traits are of significant economic importance in pork production, the breeding program or mating system for the slaughter hog producer should be planned to attain maximum or near maximum hybrid vigor in both the brood sow herd and slaughter pigs. In addition, the slaughter hog producer should combine breeds in a cross-breeding program to take advantage of the potentially desirable attributes of each breed.

Breeding Systems

As stated previously, the breeding system for producing slaughter pigs should be planned to attain maximum or near maximum hybrid vigor in both brood sows and slaughter pigs. The system should also be planned to take advantage of the inherent desirable attributes of the breeds selected for the cross-breeding system. Common practice in the U.S. from 1960 until about 1975 was to use a three-breed rotational cross-breeding program, but more specialized programs have been used recently. Attempts have been made to produce more pigs per sow per year and to produce pigs that grow fast, convert feed efficiently, and produce desirable carcasses.

Research results from the U.S. and other countries generally show the Landrace and Yorkshire breeds to excel other breeds for prolificacy, milking ability, and mothering ability. It has thus been logical to use these breeds for the "maternal line" and to seek other breeds to use as "terminal or meat line" sires. The breeds most popular as terminal sire breeds in the U.S. are the Duroc, Hampshire, and Spotted. The criteria for selecting a terminal sire breed should be growth rate and carcass cuttability. The breed combination preferred on a given farm is greatly influenced by the rearing environment.

Rotational cross-breeding systems may allow one to attain near maximum heterosis (two-breed = 67%, three-breed = 86%, four-breed = 93%); however, the major disadvantage of the rotational system is that both maternal and meat or growth breeds are used in the sow herd. A further complication is that of identifying the breed combinations in the cross-bred females. It becomes difficult from a management standpoint to get the females mated to the boar breed necessary to attain maximum hybrid vigor. Most producers never attain the degree of heterosis theoretically possible because of this difficulty.

The mating system of using F_1 Landrace ×

Yorkshire gilts mated to a Duroc boar will give maximum hybrid vigor in both sows and slaughter pigs. A cross-bred boar such as a Duroc × Hampshire, Duroc × Chester White, or Duroc × Spotted would also allow maximum hybrid vigor and give the advantage of using a hybrid terminal cross boar. This system requires a nucleus herd or purebred herd(s) to supply the F_1 gilts and/or the purebred or cross-bred terminal boars. With this system, all the genetic improvement through selection would be accomplished in the nucleus or purebred herds.

An alternative program is to use a two- or three-bred rotational cross-breeding program for the gilts and to use a static terminal program for the boars. The Landrace × Yorkshire (LY) sow seems quite popular in most areas; therefore, these two breeds may be used in a two-breed rotation for producing replacement gilts. This approach should give 67% of maximum hybrid vigor in the sows and 100% in the slaughter pigs if a terminal sire is used. If a third breed is used for the sow herd, it is possible to attain 86% of maximum hybrid vigor in the sows; however, the third breed to be utilized may be poorer for maternal traits than the Landrace and Yorkshire, and therefore the use of the third breed would result in a net loss in maternal performance. It is also more difficult to manage the three-breed rotational system than the two-breed rotational system. The LY sows may not be the most desirable for every herd. If there are problems with the LY sows maintaining condition and rebreeding or if the LY sows lack longevity, then a more rugged breed could be utilized in the sow herd.

The development of several useful tests for the prediction of genetic traits responsible for pale, soft, exudative pork (PSE) and the porcine stress syndrome (PSS) in the live pig now makes it possible to include these in selection programs (McGloughin 1980). The available predictors of meat quality in the live animal include the halothane test, serum enzyme analysis, muscle biopsy analysis, genetic markers, and the erythrocyte fragility test. The choice of testing procedure employed to improve meat quality in a population or breed will depend to a large extent on the frequency of meat quality problems and stress susceptibility in that population.

Sources of Breeding Stock

One of the major management decisions of commercial swine producers is to determine the source of breeding stock to be utilized in the breeding program. A major concern of both the producer and the veterinarian should be to introduce breeding stock with the greatest genetic potential for improving production efficiency.

However, a major concern is the introduction of breeding stock that are latent carriers of pathogens that may spread to the home stock. The swine producer has three basic alternatives for introducing breeding stock.

The first alternative is to maintain a closed herd except for the introduction of semen, embryos, or litters taken from their dams by cesarean section. This approach involves the least risk from the standpoint of disease introduction but often results in the lowest level of production efficiency of the three alternatives. The problem with the use of semen on a few selected cross-bred sows is that boars and gilts that will be produced are already cross-bred and are probably related to many animals in the herd. There is often a major loss in potential heterosis for herds in which this procedure is attempted. If the commercial producer attempts to maintain a few purebred sows to prevent the loss of hybrid vigor, often the genetic level of these sows will be questionable. If these sows are bred artificially to superior boars, frequently there is little or no selection pressure placed upon the progeny.

The second alternative is to purchase all breeding stock from a single supplier. This supplier should meet four basic criteria:

1. The health program of the supplier should satisfy the commercial producer and his veterinarian.

2. The selection and breeding program of the supplier should be planned to make near maximum genetic progress for the economically important traits.

3. The supplier must have available for sale the breeds or cross-bred combinations desired by the commercial producer so that maximum or near maximum hybrid vigor may be attained by the producer.

4. The supplier must have enough boars available for sale so that the commercial producer may "select" boars with superior performance records. This approach appears safe from the herd health standpoint. Most of the genetic improvement is left to the supplier, who should be devoting a major portion of his time and resources toward continued genetic progress. Selection of replacement gilts should continue in the commercial herd.

The third alternative is to use multiple suppliers of breeding stock. These suppliers would likely be two, three, or four purebred breeders of different breeds. If each of the breeders involved has a sound breeding and selection program, then this approach may allow the commercial producer to make optimum genetic progress. There are likely to be more problems with the introduction of disease by using this approach. Many commercial producers have been successful with this program by using careful introductory isolation and testing followed by a planned exposure program.

Consultation with Other Specialists

Other specialists such as nutritionists, geneticists, agricultural engineers, economists, and swine specialists should be consulted as necessary. *A single discipline specialist cannot provide reliable advice on every important aspect in the swine herd or facility.*

Veterinarians should not give advice in areas of the operation in which they are not competent. The veterinarian should accompany the specialist to the farm and indicate the animal health problem and how it may be related to genetics, nutrition, building design, or whatever. A report should be submitted by the specialist outlining the nature of the problem and the corrective action required.

Slaughterhouse Inspection

Meat inspection data have been used in many countries in the surveillance of farm animal populations for occurrence of specific diseases as well as in tracing of affected herds as part of national disease control programs. The Danish Swine Slaughter Data System provides surveillance of health disease among Danish bacon pigs (Willeberg 1980). The keystones of the system are a centralized, computer-based accounting system for cooperative abattoirs and a uniform code list of diagnosis from the meat inspection regulations to specify the lesions causing partial or total condemnation of affected carcasses. Pigs shipped to market are identified by herd or origin using a slap-tattoo. At slaughter, all lesions are examined and diagnosed by licensed veterinarians. The diagnostic data are stored and processed on a central computer from which owners receive payment for the pigs with specifications of any deductions for partial or total condemnations. The routine reporting of all slaughter inspection findings for a particular swine herd has been very useful for the individual manager. The information obtained on a country-wide basis is useful in identifying research priorities and extension service to the farmers about the prevalent diseases. The data may also be used to conduct epidemiologic investigations on farms with a high prevalence of diseases such as enzootic pneumonia and compare them with farms with a lower incidence.

Necropsy Examination

Necropsies should be done on as many pigs that die as possible and on selected sick pigs when the clinical diagnosis is not clear.

Records System and Preparation of Reports

It is the responsibility of the producer to keep adequate records as discussed in an earlier section (p. 293). The records must be analyzed and interpreted regularly by the veterinarian, and a report with recommendations for corrective action must be submitted to the owner.

Effect of Housing on Performance and Disease Incidence

Complete confinement of swine production has created many managerial and environmental problems that affect reproductive performance, growth performance, and the incidence of disease. Inadequate housing and ventilation, poor sanitation and hygiene, and overcrowding are predisposing causes of disease and poor performance. The most economically important health and production problems are multifactorial in origin. Thus, veterinarians providing a complete swine herd health service must acquire a sound knowledge of the optimum environmental requirements of all age groups of pigs raised indoors in total confinement. The various aspects of housing and ventilation must be examined at each visit to the farm. *An agricultural engineer knowledgeable about housing and ventilation should be consulted when problems are suspected.*

A checklist would include the following:

1. Sanitation and hygiene, cleaning and disinfection practices
2. Comfort of animals in their pens
3. Quality of air, adequacy of ventilation
4. Stocking density, overcrowding
5. Quality of floor material, evidence of traumatic injuries due to floor surfaces
6. Adequacy of temperature in each section of the pig house
7. Manure disposal

Some of the identifiable epidemiologic determinants that probably interact with each other to affect performance and disease include herd size, herd immunity, feeding systems, quality of flooring, pen cleaning systems, manure storage and disposal systems, ventilation systems, lighting, pen design, and abnormal animal behavior. The major problems appear to be stocking rates and pen sizes, quality of floor surfaces, sanitation of pens, ventilation, and offensive odors from manure storage pits.

As herd size has increased, there has been a corresponding increase in the incidence of disease and managerial problems that affect herd performance. The division of the herd into smaller units, each of which is operated as a single unit with the *all-in-all-out* system, is now recommended.

In large sow herds, a common practice is to divide the farrowing barn into smaller units with no more than 15 to 20 farrowing crates per unit. The dry sow units are usually much larger and may contain 100 to 150 or more sows per unit. Likewise, the nursery units for recently weaned piglets are operated as several small separate units with approximately 30 weaned pigs per unit.

Dry sows may be confined and fed in groups or in individual stalls. Confinement in individual stalls allows for controlled individual feeding, but heat detection may be a problem with large numbers of gilts and sows.

In most areas where pigs are raised in total confinement, a system of climate control using an effective ventilation system is necessary. The provision of an adequate ventilation system will optimize production, minimize the spread of aerosol infections, and provide a reasonable working environment for employees. Effective ventilation systems for swine barns are notoriously difficult for the engineer to design and for the producer to operate and maintain. Many systems are incorrectly planned or used and not maintained properly. Effective ventilation requires daily monitoring of the system, which often becomes too routine and consequently is ignored until the environment becomes obviously offensive.

Effective climate control involves maintaining the temperature at a desirable level with the aid of supplemental heat and adequate insulation of walls and ceilings, a relative humidity ranging from 50 to 75%, and satisfactory movement of air in and out of the building. There must be continuous removal of aerosol-contaminated inside air and a continuous supply of fresh outside air. Supplemental heat may be required to permit continuous ventilation while maintaining an ambient temperature for optimal animal health. The cost of energy for supplemental heat for swine barns in cold climates is now a major economic consideration.

The ventilation needs for confined swine can be calculated from a consideration of the size of the building, the number and ages of pigs, the building materials used, and the outside ambient temperature. Standard formulae are available, and the assistance of an agricultural engineer should be sought.

The major health problems that have been epidemiologically associated with inadequate ventilation include enzootic pneumonia, atrophic rhinitis, *Hemophilus* pleuropneumonia, tail-biting and other behavioral abnormalities, and manure gas poisoning.

The nature of floor surfaces used in swine barns has contributed to a wide variety of injuries to the feet and skin and possibly to the locomotor system (Cement and Concrete Assoc. 1978). The lack of bedding, such as straw, and rough concrete surfaces can result in skin abrasions of the teats and carpal joints of nursing piglets and abrasions and fissures of the soles and hooves of older pigs (Svendsen et al. 1979; Newton et al. 1980; Conrad and Mayrose 1979; Penny et al. 1971). A wide variety of concrete floor surface finishes, plastic-coated expanded metal floors, concrete and metal slatted floors, and asphalt-covered surfacing have been used with varying success. There is a need to scientifically determine the optimum floor surface for pigs of all ages in a swine herd.

Performance of growing-finishing pigs—rate of gain and gain per unit of feed consumed—have in general been comparable on partially and totally slatted floors. Where sizeable differences in performance have occurred, factors other than slatted floors alone are usually involved. Among these factors are environmental temperature, space per pig, number of pigs per pen, management practices, variable spacings between or careless installation of slats, improper ratio of slat width to space width, insecurely fastened slats, or rough surface or jagged edges of slats. Frequently, the effects of of these factors are difficult to assess.

The rapid intensification of the swine industry led to the use of many building materials that were attractive economically but undesirable for optimal swine production. The use of various floor materials and designs preceded research information, and the culling rates of breeding animals have been high. This has necessitated the remodeling of older facilities and the building of new facilities after careful consideration of animal comfort and economic reality.

The handling and disposal of swine manure is a major problem in total confinement production of swine. The daily accumulation of manure on solid floors may contribute to the spread of infectious diseases. Mechanical or hand scraping and cleaning in conjunction with total hauling and spreading on open fields has been the most widely used system. However, it is the situation that the progressive swine producer is trying to avoid. It is laborious and in general undesirable because the frequency of cleaning that will maintain relatively acceptable sanitary conditions is prohibitive from a labor and cost standpoint where large numbers of animals are confined. A combination of scraping and flushing the wastes into a holding pit or a lagoon has certain advantages. Less labor is required, and waste can be stored in an area other than the pen for hauling as a liquid or a solid at a more appropriate time.

With the introduction of partially or fully slatted floors a completely new series of alternatives and problems presented themselves. More than any other factor, the adoption of slatted floors for swine housing has accelerated the trend to total confinement. However, there has been much concern about the quality of the air inside confinement swine buildings with slatted floors, since the wastes may be held in the building long enough to produce gases and odors. Noxious gases and odors formed from stored wastes can be irritating to both the animal and the animal attendants and have been the cause of numerous complaints and litigations by neighbors. The most important gases generated in a swine confinement unit are carbon dioxide, ammonia, hydrogen sulfide, and methane, and a large group of trace organic compounds such as amines, mercaptans, and skatoles.

In geographic areas where the climate is favorable, the trend in manure handling and disposal in confinement rearing of swine is toward the use of flushing-lagoon systems. Animals will be reared in totally enclosed buildings on partially or fully slatted floors.

Wastes will be flushed from beneath the floors periodically but probably not more than once daily. These flushed wastes will be deposited in a nearby lagoon equipped with a floating aerator. Effluent taken from the upper surface of the lagoon will be recycled to the end of the swine building where it will be used to flush new wastes into the lagoon. Effluent containing both liquid and suspended fine solids from the lower part of the lagoon can be used in a nearby irrigation system (Conrad and Mayrose 1971).

Cleaning and Disinfection of Swine Barns. Experience in swine herds has shown that increased losses and lowered productivity may occur if rearing accommodation is not satisfactorily cleaned and disinfected between batches of pigs.

Cleaning and disinfection routines are designed to remove most of the microbial population from pig pens during washing and cleaning procedures, followed by the destruction of accessible residual infection by chemical disinfectants, the application of heat or steam, or fumigation. Farrowing, nursery, and follow-on accommodations must be meticulously treated and an all-in–all-out policy adopted where possible. Finishing pens need less attention, and breeding areas and dry sow accommodations need only be swept clean unless disease problems dictate otherwise. In fact, the spread of pathogens in the breeding area could be encouraged to ensure that breeding stock develop an immunity to the agents associated with reproductive failure and neonatal diarrhea.

Cleaning and disinfection routines should follow a final pattern as follows:

1. Remove bulk manure, litter, adherent dirt, and dust from floors, walls, and upper reaches, and dismantle equipment.
2. Soak and pre-wash pens and equipment with a suitable detergent or detergent-disinfectant solution liberally applied from a watering can or knapsack sprayer or, where conditions are suitable, a pressure sprayer. If necessary, complete the removal of organic material left after initial cleaning, then re-soak the area before rinsing and allowing to dry.
3. Apply the appropriate disinfectant to the floors, walls, equipment, and upper reaches, and allow to dry.
4. Leave the pens vacant for 7 days or more if possible.

Pathogens persist in residual dust, porous walls, and floors, and thorough cleaning and disinfection routines using the appropriate product are needed to achieve any significant reduction in their numbers. Buildings continuously populated with pigs need modified routines, and advice on the detergent-disinfectant combination that can safely be used under these circumstances is usually needed.

The characteristics and qualities of detergents and disinfectants that are suitable for cleaning and disinfection of swine barns are reviewed (Thomas 1982).

Housing the Sow from Weaning to Parturition. There is now almost universal adoption of individual confinement of pregnant sows and pubertal gilts in stalls or tether stalls. A major advantage of individual stalls is the ease with which individual feeding according to the conditions of the sow can be accomplished. However, because they are individually housed—usually on concrete with no bedding—and they cannot huddle, pregnant sows are particularly vulnerable to low house temperatures. It is therefore important that sows on restricted energy intakes and particularly those with energy reserves depleted by lactation should be housed in the correct thermal environment. At 12°C to 18°C the animals are in conditions considerably below their lower critical temperature and would require additional feed to achieve the projected live-weight increase. When straw bedding is provided, no extra feed may be required (Baxter and Robertson 1980).

A major problem with individual stalls for pubertal gilts and sows following weaning is the delay in the onset of estrus and a consequent increase in the average days from weaning-to-conception interval. This has a major impact on sow productivity, which is presented later under reproductive performance. The design of the dry sow barn and the proximity of the boar may be important contributing factors that should be kept under constant surveillance by the veterinarian. The use of small groups of uniform sizes of gilts and sows and controlled daily presence of the boar may be necessary to improve the onset and detection of estrus.

Housing the Sow During Lactation. Considerable effort has been expended by the swine and building industries to develop the most suitable farrowing crate. The incidence of crushing is still unacceptably high, but crates can be designed so that the sow is made to lower herself to her knees before flopping over to the fully recumbent position by narrowing the width between all but the bottom rails of the crate. However, the most significant improvements in sow productivity have come through better management of farrowing houses rather than through the buildings themselves. More attention is now being paid to sanitation and hygiene in the farrowing crates—leaving the crates vacant for at least a few days between sows, cross-fostering, the maintenance of small farrowing groups, and the planned induction of parturition of batches of sows using prostaglandins.

The ideal floor surface for the newborn piglet, as part of the farrowing crate, still remains elusive. Many different perforated floor surfaces have been developed that are non-slip and non-abrasive for the piglets and that are also easy to clean following weaning of the piglets.

Housing the Young Pig from Weaning to 30 Kg. Live Weight. Early weaning at three weeks or less has become commonplace. This trend has precipitated a demand for accommodations capable of housing piglets weighing less than 5 kg. with no maternal protection, often with low feed intakes, and in groups matched for size rather than in litter groups. Older pigs can be housed in single-tiered pens with mesh floors after weaning at 21 to 28 days. The lower critical temperature of pigs weaned at 5 kg. is about 27°C; consequently, weaner accommodations must be capable of maintaining temperatures of 30°C, especially in the immediate postweaning period when feed intake is low. All of the three-tier and first-stage flat-deck accommodations for young pigs will require some form of supplementary heating if the required house temperature is to be maintained when the temperature difference between outside and inside is greater than 12 to 15°C. Housing problems that occur in weaner pens include overcrowding, insufficient feeder and waterer spaces, postweaning check, and the spread of infections.

Housing the Growing Pig from 30 Kg. Live Weight to Market. Housing for pigs from 30 kg. live weight to market weight has not changed significantly compared with other classes of pigs. Pens with partially slatted floors with little or no bedding and holding 15 to 20 pigs are common. The urine and feces collect in the pit under the slatted floor and are removed as a slurry on a regular basis. Considerable field research in being directed to the handling of the slurry.

Flow of Pigs Through the Unit

The flow of pigs through a farrow-to-finish operation must occur with optimum efficiency. There must be adequate space in each section

of the operation, and a continuous breeding cycle must be established so that there is optimum utilization of space and a steady supply of pigs. The *all-in-all-out* system should be used to minimize infectious disease. In this system, each unit of the swine enterprise is fully occupied by pigs for the necessary time, which is then followed by a complete depopulation of the unit followed by cleaning, disinfection, and a period of vacancy for several days before being occupied by animals again.

Use of Antimicrobials as Growth Promotants and for Control of Infectious Disease

Antimicrobial feed supplements have been used extensively in swine rations since the introduction of antibiotics in the early 1950s. (Hays and Muir 1979; Hays et al. 1978). Antimicrobial agents commonly used in swine rations include bacitracin, bambermycins, chlortetracycline, erythromycin, neomycin, oxytetracycline, oleandomycin, penicillin, streptomycin, tylosin, virginiamycin, arsenicals, and nitrofurans. They are used to improve rate of gain and feed conversion in growing pigs and to control specific infectious diseases such as swine dysentery. Antimicrobials have been used in the rations of pigs extending from weaning until the end of the growing period. Maximum economic gains from improved rate of gain and feed conversion are obtained from the use of growth-promoting levels of the drugs during this period. Prophylactic or therapeutic levels of certain antimicrobials are commonly used when outbreaks of disease occur. Examples include swine dysentery, atrophic rhinitis, and *Hemophilus* pleuropneumonia. The use of antibiotics in the feed of sows has also improved reproductive performance.

Microorganisms resistant to antimicrobials emerge in the intestines of animals that are fed subtherapeutic amounts of antibacterials and there is a theoretical possibility that these resistant organisms may be transferred to man. Such problems do not appear to have developed to any appreciable extent during the 28 years of usage (National Academy of Science 1980).

Role of the Producer

The success of a health management and production program in a swine herd is dependent primarily on the willingness of the producer to strive to achieve the targets of performance, combined with his ability to keep the costs of production sufficiently below the returns received for market pigs or breeding stock so that a suitable profit is made.

The producer is with the herd on a continuous basis, and the level of health management and production applied on a daily basis will be reflected in the herd. A selection of the responsibilities of the producer includes the following:

1. Accurate daily record-keeping
2. Routine procedures and treatments such as iron injection in newborn piglets, the treatment of clinically affected pigs, the identification of animals, and vaccinations
3. Reproductive performance, which includes daily heat detection, mating gilts and sows, ensuring optimum use of boars, the selection of breeding stock, and following a predetermined breeding program
4. The purchase of feeds and the daily operation of the feeding system
5. The daily operation of the housing and environmental system to ensure an optimum environment. This includes adequate sanitation, hygiene, and ventilation
6. The submission of dead pigs for necropsy
7. Notification of the veterinarian of any significant changes in management, vaccinations, treatment, feed formulations, and outbreaks of disease. Too often the veterinarian is not notified of epidemics of infectious diseases like *Hemophilus* pleuropneumonia in finishing pigs or of abortions in sows for several days or weeks after the peak incidence
8. The education of animal attendants in the herd. This has become a major problem in large swine herds, which require several people to operate the entire enterprise
9. Flow of pigs through the herd. A well-operated farrow-to-finish operation is dependent on the establishment and maintenance of a continuous cycle of sows farrowing and uninterrupted movement of the pigs through the system. This requires constant surveillance of each aspect of the herd and adjustments in production where necessary. This is probably the most important facet of efficient swine production and one that is heavily dependent on the level of expertise of the people managing the herd
10. Financial management. The cash flow is traditionally the responsibility of the producer. The costs of production continue to spiral upward while the price of market pigs fluctuates. This requires sound financial management and adjustments when necessary. Traditionally, the veterinarian has not been involved in this aspect of production. However, as herds become larger, the annual cash flow becomes a major consideration, and veterinary advice on costs of production will assume major importance

In summary, the success of a health management and production program depends on the competence and skills of the veterinarian and the willingness and ability of the producer to produce pigs as efficiently as possible.

REPRODUCTIVE PERFORMANCE IN THE SWINE HERD

Reproductive performance has long been considered economically important to the swine producer. Present methods of intensified swine production, however, have created in the industry an increased awareness of the impact of reproductive rate in the sow herd on overall production efficiency.

Swine units have become larger and more specialized, and investment in buildings and equipment has increased greatly. Confinement production has placed increased demands on reproductive performance, created new problems to be solved in order to maximize reproductive efficiency, and made precise scheduling extremely important in the operation of an efficient swine production unit. Delays in breeding create major problems in efficient use of facilities and equipment.

As swine management systems have changed, the measurements of farrowing rate and litter size at birth have failed to provide a satisfactory evaluation of reproductive performance. Instead, a fertility index based on the average number of pigs weaned per year for each female in the breeding herd is often considered to be a more useful measure of reproduction. When presently accepted methods of swine reproduction are used, including three-week weaning, a sow can farrow 2.5 litters per year. Perhaps an immediate attainable goal for the industry would be 2.0 litters per female annually with an average of 8.0 pigs per litter at weaning, or a total of 16 pigs weaned per year for each female maintained in the breeding herd. Some herds exceed this level of reproductive performance at the present time, but the percentage of herds in this category is not known. In one survey of Illinois swine producers involving 21,536 farrowings, gilts and sows farrowed 1.25 and 1.71 times per female per year and weaned 8.3 and 13.3 pigs per year respectively (Leman et al. 1972). Therefore, weaning 16 pigs annually per female would represent considerable improvement in present levels of reproductive performance of the breeding herd.

The most obvious troublesome problem appears to be the failure or delay of gilts and sows to exhibit estrus. This results in both scheduling difficulties and reduced sow productivity (Day 1979).

A second major limiting factor is reduced fertility, as measured by farrowing rate and average number of live pigs per litter.

Monitoring Reproductive Performance

Some form of continuous monitoring of the breeding herd is necessary to detect reproductive failure. Often it is only by the close scrutiny of certain indices that disease problems underlying the poor performance of a herd are recognizable.

Wrathall (1977) has provided an excellent summary of appropriate reproductive performance indices in the pig herd, which appear in Table 11-7. If performance assessed by any of these indices falls below a *tolerance limit,* then investigation is required. The reference value given represents a normal standard of production as a general guide. The tolerance limit or the decision boundary is the level of production or disease incidence above or below which action is needed to correct the production problem or disease. Decision boundaries and reference values can be set out in graphical form as control charts for ease of examination and comparison of performance between different times of the year. The analysis of data in graphical form may also indicate possible diagnoses. For example, an epidemic of infectious infertility in sows at one point in time will be reflected in a reduced number of pigs born alive per litter at subsequent farrowing. Such analysis can suggest the most appropriate clinical and laboratory examination.

Once an appropriate recording system is in operation, it must be exploited by regular analysis of the data to produce herd performance statistics. One well-known and useful measurement of overall performance is the total number of piglets born alive (or, alternatively, weaned) per sow during the year, half-year, or other suitable period as cited in Table 11-5. This, when compared with a suitable standard or target figure, will show whether herd productivity has been satisfactory during the period in question. Because it is retrospective and general, however, the

Table 11-5. REPRODUCTIVE PERFORMANCE IN THE PIG HERD°

Output per Female per Year	Gilts	Sows	All Females
Litters per year	1.84	2.24	2.14
Live piglets born per litter	10.0	11.0	10.75
Live piglets born per year	18.40	24.64	23.01
Live piglets born per month	1.53	2.05	1.92

°Overall production to be expected from an efficient herd.

Note: Figures represent optimal output and refer to herds weaning piglets at 5 weeks of age and culling females after 4 litters (on average).

overall performance figure will not provide any early warning of problems or show where in the breeding cycle they are occurring.

The herd inventory is a vital component of any recording system and, when carried out regularly at a specific time in each week or month, identifies the exact number of males and females of breeding age (production units) and also the percentages in different categories (Table 11-6). This will show whether the herd is carrying its full complement and provide early warning of a bottleneck in the breeding cycle. Basic data for other calculations, such as average costs and performance of gilts and sows, are taken from the inventory as well. Inclusion of boars in the inventory will indicate whether there is adequate capacity on the male side, not only for insemination but also to provide "male influence" and social stimuli. Even when artificial insemination is used extensively, it is important to carry some boars and to locate them strategically in the herd; otherwise anestrus, subestrus, and other problems may occur.

For precise and up-to-date indicators of herd

Table 11-6. IDEAL INVENTORY OF BREEDING STOCK IN THE PIG HERD

	Gilts (%)	Sows (%)	All Females (%)
Unserved	23	6	9
Served—not yet farrowed	60	72	70
Farrowed—not yet weaned	17	21	20
Weaned—awaiting disposal	<0.2	1	<1
All classes	28	72	100

performance, it is necessary to identify and extract specific data from those records related most closely to sensitive stages and events in the breeding cycle (Table 11–7). Some of these stages, together with the kind of data expected from a normal herd, are shown in Table 11–8. The number of analyses and their frequency and detail will depend on such factors as size of unit, degree of personal involvement by management, and overall production figures. A large herd with a poor production record, for example, may benefit from frequent and detailed record analysis, at least until the problems have been resolved. Sometimes it may be necessary to carry out in-depth analysis of data pertaining to a specific problem area in order to characterize it fully and, if possible, to identify any causal relationships.

Factors Influencing Reproductive Performance (Sow Productivity)

The reproductive performance or sow productivity in a swine herd is dependent upon many identifiable factors. The number of piglets per sow per year is a direct result of the farrowing interval and the litter size. These two indices are in turn influenced by several other factors, which are shown in Figure 11–11 and described here.

The number of piglets per sow per year can be increased by reducing the interval between farrowing and conception and by reducing the lactation period. The length of gestation is almost constant (Table 11–9), but it can be decreased by two to four days by the induction of parturition. Litter size can be enlarged by increasing ovulation and conception rates or by reducing losses in the perinatal and postnatal periods.

The identifiable factors that affect reproductive performance in swine include the following:
1. Anestrus in pubertal gilts
2. Weaning-to-conception interval in sows
3. Infertility:
   Failure to conceive
   Embryonic mortality
   Fetal mummification
   Abortion
   Stillbirths
4. Neonatal mortality (birth to weaning):
   Low birth weight of piglets
   Small litters
   Low viability of piglets
5. Fertility and serving capacity of the boar
6. Effects of seasonal influences
7. Housing, nutrition, and management
8. Infectious diseases (parvovirus, leptospirosis)

Anestrus in Gilts

Pubertal estrus is expected in most gilts between six and eight months of age. The natural range in the attainment of puberty is from 135 to 250 days; this range is due to various stimulatory and inhibitory influences, including genotype, nutritional status, environment, and the presence or absence of the boar (Hughes and Varley 1980). With such a range it is hardly surprising that it is difficult to manage the introduction of gilts into a breeding program in a herd (Varley 1983). The failure or delay of gilts reared under total confinement to exhibit a detectable estrus is one of the most common causes of inferior reproductive performance in swine (Day 1979; Christenson and Ford 1979).

The need to plan, predict, and control estrus in groups of cycling gilts has emerged from structural changes in the pig industry. Swine herds are now very large and have large capital investments. Instead of a few gilts per year being reared haphazardly with a high wastage rate, it is now necessary to plan the rearing and systematic introduction of hundreds of gilts per year into a breeding herd. The more the operation is out of phase with the sow culling program, the greater the economic losses. If the breeding of gilts becomes erratic, overall production fluctuates four to six months later,

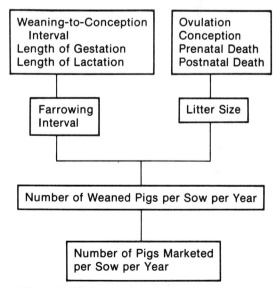

Figure 11–11. Factors influencing numbers of pigs per sow per year. (From Nielsen, H.E. and Danielsen, V. Sow productivity. Vet. Annual 19:102–107, 1979.)

Table 11-7. RECORDING REPRODUCTIVE PERFORMANCE IN THE PIG HERD†

Cycle	Breeding Cycle Events (Recorded as They Occur)	Performance Data (Calculated from Records)	Reference Figure (or Normal Standard)	Decision Boundary (Above/Below Which Action is Needed)
1. (Gilt)	Birth date			
	puberty			
	Service date	*Age at first service	225 ± 10 days	≥240 days
		Regular returns (21 ± 3 days)	10%	≥20%
	repeat service date(s)	*Conception rate to 1st service	90%	≤80%
		Irregular returns (24 days)	3%	≥6%
	abortion	Abortions	1%	≥2.5%
		Failures to farrow	1%	≥2%
		*Farrowing rate	85%	≤80%
	Farrowing date	*Piglets born alive per litter	9.5–10.0	≤9.0
	piglet losses	Piglets born dead	4%	≥6%
		Piglets born malformed	1.5%	≥3%
	Weaning date	*Piglets weaned per litter	9.0–9.5	≤8.5
2. (Sow)	Service date	*Weaning-to-service interval	6–9 days	≥10 days
		Regular returns (21 ± 3 days)	10%	≥20%
	repeat service date(s)	*Conception rate to 1st service	90%	≤80%
		Irregular returns (24 days)	3%	≥6%
	abortion	Abortions	1%	≥2.5%
		Failures to farrow	1%	≥2%
		*Farrowing rate	85%	≤80%
	Farrowing date	*Piglets born alive per litter	10.5–11.0	≤10.0
	piglet losses	Piglets born dead	5%	≥7.5%
		Piglets born malformed	1.5%	≥3%
	Weaning date	*Piglets weaned	9.5–10.0	≤9.0
		(Data for 3rd and subsequent cycles usually resemble those of 2nd cycle and may be lumped together with them)		
3. Other				
Final	Weaning date			
	Culling date	Age at culling	Varies, but usually after 3–5 litters	Depends on management policy

†Normal reference data and figures above/below which action may be needed.

NOTES: (1) Parameters indicated by stars (*) are those most suitable for regular monitoring; the others may be needed for analysis of specific problems.

(2) Frequency of data monitoring should be inversely proportional to the herd size, with at least 25 but not more than 100 female cycles being included on each occasion: e.g., herd size <50 females at 6-month intervals and >250 females at 1-month intervals.

(3) In large herds it is generally preferable to record and monitor gilt and sow data separately.

(4) Reference figures shown in the table are given as a general guide to performance of the more prolific "white" breeds, in herds practicing 5-week weaning.

From Wrathall, A.E. Reproductive failure in the pig: Diagnosis and control. Vet. Rec., 100:230–237, 1977. Reprinted with the permission of the Veterinary Record.

Table 11–8. REPRODUCTIVE FAILURE INVESTIGATION[*]

Pre-service	a. Gilts	Origin (purchased/home-reared), selection, age or cycle at which served, physical condition and health, feeding (flushing if any), housing, group size, boar proximity
	b. Sows	Physical condition, weaning procedure (± starvation) and feeding, housing, group size, boar proximity
Service	a. Boars	Origin (purchased/home-reared), selection, ages, physical condition and health, libido, frequency of use, housing, proximity to females
	b. Gilts and sows	Estrus detection, supervision of matings, number of matings per estrus, A.I. (source and technique), layout of mating area
Pregnancy	Gilts and sows	Methods for checking returns to estrus, pregnancy diagnosis, physical condition, timing of movement(s) (e.g., to the pregnancy accommodation), feeding (individual or group), housing, group size, bedding, comfort, exercise
Farrowing	Gilts and sows	Timing of movement into farrowing accommodations, construction of pens, crates, etc., proximity to other pigs, climatic control, comfort, supervision of farrowing (day/night), feeding
Lactation	a. Gilts and sows	Physical condition and health, comfort, feeding, usual lactation length
	b. Piglets	Physical condition and health, size and growth for age, creep environment and comfort, bedding, castrations and other procedures
Rearing		

[*]Checklist for clinical inspection of the pig herd.
From Wrathall, A.E. Reproductive failure in the pig: Diagnosis and control. Vet. Rec., 100:230–237, 1977.

with a major deleterious effect on cash flow.

The causes of anestrus include immaturity, the stress of confinement by tethering or individual stalls, the absence of a boar near the gilts, the breed of the gilt, and failure of management to detect estrous behavior in the gilt. Gilts raised in confinement have delayed puberty and either "quiet estrus" or "behavioral anestrus."

Total confinement can reduce the proportion of gilts that attain puberty by eight to nine months of age by up to 50%; time of year may also affect onset of puberty (Rampacek et al. 1981).

The incidence of gilts that do not show regular estrus cycles at nine months of age ranges from 10 to 40%, and breed of gilt is an important factor contributing to this percentage. The percentage of Landrace gilts that show regular estrus cycles at six months of age is much higher than that of Hampshire, Large White, Yorkshire or Duroc gilts (Christenson and Ford 1979). Of noncyclic gilts slaughtered at nine months of age, 55% were gilts with immature reproductive tracts (delayed puberty), and 45% were gilts with fully developed uteri and ovaries that had corpora lutea at different stages of development or preovulatory follicles and corpora albicans (behavioral anestrus). There is some indication that the percentage of gilts showing regular estrus activity would not increase significantly if gilts were checked for estrus for three more months (nine to 12 months of age). Maintaining noncyclic gilts beyond 8.5 to nine months of age for replacement cannot be recommended from an economic standpoint.

Various techniques have been employed to stimulate the onset of regular estrus cycles in the gilt. The more successful of these have been hormonal therapy, stress situations such as transportation, and boar contact (Hughes and Cole 1976).

The exposure of prepubertal gilts to a boar will advance the onset of first estrus. The timing of initial boar exposure has been shown to be of major importance, the gilt age at the start of boar exposure regulating to a large extent the response obtained (Kirkwood and Hughes 1982). Boar exposure at a very young age (three to four months) or at a later age (six months or older) is inefficient. However, exposure of the boar to the gilts at about 160 days results in the highest incidence of onset of regular estrus cycles. Continual boar contact with groups of gilts at this age will result in 80 to 88% ovulating within 17 days (Kirkwood and

Table 11–9. NUMBER OF FARROWINGS PER YEAR ACCORDING TO LENGTH OF LACTATION AND WEANING-TO-CONCEPTION INTERVAL

Weaning-to-Conception Interval (Days)	115 Days of Gestation Plus Lactation (Days) of		
	21	35	56
28	2.2	2.0	1.8
21	2.3	2.1	1.9
14	2.4	2.2	2.0
7	2.5	2.3	2.1

[*]From Fahmy, M.H. Factors influencing the weaning to estrus interval in swine: A review. World Review of Anim. Prod., (2):17:15–28, April–June 1981.

Hughes 1982). The first estrus will usually be followed by a second and third estrus at between 18- and 21-day intervals. The gilts may then be bred on the second or third estrus for optimum ovulation rate (Young and King 1981). It is now also known that olfaction plays an important role in porcine reproductive processes. Acceleration or delay of puberty can be effected by the presence or absence of mature boar odor. This knowledge should be utilized by farm building designers so that management objectives are not interfered with by inadequate pen layouts or inappropriate ventilation systems (Perry 1982). Embryonic loss, a low ovulatory rate, and small litter size are major factors against breeding at first heat (Paterson et al. 1978).

Techniques used to stimulate the onset of estrus in gilts include the induction of ovulation with either pregnant mares' serum gonadotropin (PMSG) or human chorionic gonadotropin (HCG), the imposition of a new estrus rhythm using HCG, the destruction of corpora lutea using either estrogens or progesterone, and the suppression of estrus and ovulation using either progesterone or analogues of progesterone. The most promising method appears to be that of suppression of estrus and ovulation. Groups of randomly cycling gilts are treated with an agent to maintain all of the animals in a state of mid-cycle quiescence. Withdrawal of the treatment is followed by a rapid follicular phase, and the gilts come into heat all at the same time. Methallibure, a nonsteroidal compound, will suppress estrus and ovulation when fed at 100 mg. daily for 18 to 20 days. Following withdrawal of this treatment, most gilts will exhibit estrus at between five and seven days. However, methallibure was found to be teratogenic and could not be licensed for sale. More recently, allyl-trenbolone, a progestogenic compound, has been tested as an effective heat-synchronizing agent in gilts (Varley 1983). A reliable synchronizing agent would provide considerable scope for planned mating of groups of gilts. The breeding of large numbers of gilts in a short period of time requires considerable planning of boar management to ensure that a sufficient number of highly fertile boars are available.

Anestrus due to inactive ovaries may be treated with a combination of 400 I.U. pregnant mares' serum gonadotropin (PMSG) and 200 I.U. human chorionic gonadotropin (HCG) (King et al. 1982; Meredith 1979). Approximately two thirds of the animals will exhibit estrus in seven to 10 days, but the fertility level and number of pigs born alive are less than desirable.

Weaning-to-Conception Interval in Sows

The mean weaning-to-conception interval is determined by three components: (1) the average interval from weaning to the appearance of heat; (2) the proportion of sows that return to heat three weeks later and are then mated successfully; and (3) the sows that take an extended period of time to return to effective service following weaning.

At the time of weaning, after a 42-day lactation, the reproductive tract of the sow resembles that of a prepubertal gilt or anestrous sow (Dyck 1983). From weaning to day 6 (estrus), the ovarian vesicular follicle population changes from predominantly small follicles (on the day of weaning) to large preovulatory follicles, a few medium-sized follicles, and a large number of small follicles (by day 6 postweaning) (Dyck 1983).

The factors that affect the weaning-to-conception interval in sows include endocrine activity, uterine changes, genotype, parity of the sow, season of the year, and level of nutrition during the preceding lactation.

Delayed Estrus in Sows

Under ideal conditions, the sow usually exhibits estrus within 10 days after her pigs have been weaned following a lactation period of at least three weeks. Postweaning anestrus in sows may be any or a combination of the following:
□ True anestrus due to failure of ovulation
□ Silent estrus with normal ovarian activity
□ Failure of the herdsman to detect estrus because of mismanagement

Slaughterhouse examinations of the ovaries of sows culled for anestrus reveal the presence of corpora lutea in about 50% of primiparous and 80% of pluriparous sows, which indicates that silent heat is a major cause of anestrus (Karlberg 1980). Progesterone profiles of postweaning sows reveal that 90% of pluriparous and 68% of primiparous sows resume ovarian activity within 10 days. Ovulation within 10 days with overt estrus occurs in 46% of primiparous and 54% of pluriparous sows. Ovulation without detectable heat (silent heat) may occur in 30% of all sows during the first 10 days after weaning (Benjaminsen and Karlberg 1981).

The season of the year also has a significant deleterious effect on return to regular estrus cycle, which is more severe in primiparous sows than in pluriparous sows. Postweaning anestrus is most common in the period from July to October, which may be associated with the change in length of daylight. These observations are recorded from the U.K. (Stork 1979), Australia (Paterson et al. 1978), and North America (Hurtgen and Leman 1980).

Underfeeding during lactation and following weaning, particularly of primiparous sows, is considered to be a significant cause of postweaning anestrus (Benjaminsen and Karlberg 1981).

Weaning the piglets before three weeks of age can be a major cause of postweaning anestrus in sows and cannot be recommended. Earlier weaning results in a reduced conception rate, increased cystic ovarian degeneration, and a net reduction in sow productivity (Elliot et al. 1980). The uterus requires 14 days to return to its normal size and weight after farrowing and a further 10 days before it is ready to accept further implantation. Zero-weaning of sows (within a few hours of birth) results in an increase in the interval from farrowing to conception, a concomitant increase in the farrowing interval, an increased incidence of cystic ovarian degeneration, and a reduced conception rate as compared with sows that have their pigs weaned at 30 days post partum (Elliot et al. 1980).

Practical Recommendations for Management of Anestrus

The minimization of the mean interval from weaning to conception is of paramount importance if maximization of sow productivity is to be achieved.

The most important management procedure to minimize the incidence of delayed estrus in sows following weaning is to move the sow to a breeding barn specifically designed for housing sows from weaning until successful breeding and conception. Following weaning, sows may be placed in individual stalls or in groups of four to six and observed carefully twice daily for the first 10 days following weaning. An intense surveillance system of heat detection in the recently weaned sow is necessary. Boar contact should begin within a few days after weaning to detect estrus in any of the sows. The presence of the boar during lactation (21 days post partum) stimulated sows to come into heat 2.28 days after weaning compared with 10 days for controls (Pitchey and English 1980). Sows in heat should be bred under supervision and a repeat service carried out in

12 to 24 hours. Bred sows should be identified and observed 18 to 21 days later for any returns to heat.

The level of nutrition during lactation should be adequate, particularly for first- and second-litter sows. A deprivation of feed and water for 24 hours following weaning is not considered necessary as was once advocated.

Hormonal therapy has been advocated for the treatment of sows with prolonged postweaning anestrus. Pregnant mares' serum gonadotropin (PMSG) at 400 I.U. combined with human chorionic gonadotropin (HCG) 200 I.U. may induce a fertile estrus in about 66% of animals within seven days after treatment (King et al. 1982). Prostaglandin analogues in combination with gonadotropin-releasing hormone are not as successful. A combination of estradiol benzoate and human chorionic gonadotropin is also ineffective (Friendship et al. 1982).

The induction of ovulation and conception in lactating sows has been examined as a possible method of reducing the overall mean farrowing interval. Treatment using pregnant mares' serum gonadotropin (PMSG) 1500 I.U., followed 96 hours later by human chorionic gonadotropin (HCG) 1000 I.U., followed by artificial insemination 24 and 36 hours later will induce ovulation and conception as early as 15 days after farrowing (Hausler et al. 1980). The conception rates, number of corpora lutea, and average number of embryos obtained were comparable to those obtained in a natural breeding program. The sow can be successfully inseminated without interruption of lactation or removal of piglets. Pregnancy is thus concurrent with lactation, eliminating the need for early weaning and reducing the interval between successive farrowings.

It is not possible to synchronize estrus in the pig with two doses of prostaglandins at a fixed interval as is possible in the cow (Jackson and Hutchinson 1980).

Infertility

Failure to Conceive. Failure to conceive is characterized by return to service less than 20 days after a normal mating or insemination and may be due to any of the following factors: (1) The spermatozoa fail to reach the ova. This may be due to an abnormal uterus or occlusion of the oviducts. (2) Death of ova post fertilization due to inherent defects of the gametes, incompatibility between them, or failure of the spermatozoa to penetrate the ova. Insemination too early or too late in the estrus cycle or the use of boars with temporary infertility may also be causative factors. (3) Death of the developing blastocysts within 12 days of fertilization is usually followed by the sow returning to estrus within the normal 21-day cycle. Causes of blastocyst death include overfeeding, environmental stresses, and systemic illness. In the Australian experience, there is a relationship between high summer temperatures, which exceed 32°C, and an increase in the incidence of sows that exhibit delayed, irregular returns to estrus (Paterson et al. 1978). In Britain, manifestations of seasonal reproductive inefficiency in large breeding units, mainly in animals bred during the summer months of July and August, include an increase in the returns to service, abortion, and sows remaining barren 95 days after service (Stork 1979).

Embryonic Mortality. Embryonic mortality is characterized by return to estrus more than 21 days after service. Embryonic loss between 14 and 40 days after fertilization is followed by fetal resorption of the uterine contents. Causes include infections of the uterus occurring at mating or by transmission in semen.

A calorie intake in excess of requirements during early gestation results in embryonic deaths, obese sows at farrowing, and breeding difficulties after weaning. Reproductive efficiency is at a maximum with a daily metabolizable energy intake of approximately 6000 kcal. (Michel et al. 1980).

Fetal Death. The common causes of fetal death in swine are leptospirosis and infection with parvovirus and pseudorabies.

Leptospirosis usually causes abortion without any significant illness of the sow. The diagnosis is made by serological examination of the sow and laboratory examination of the fetuses.

Parvovirus infection before 70 days of gestation in nonimmune gilts or sows will commonly cause mummified fetuses, which are carried to term with the net result of a small number of live piglets per litter (Mengeling et al. 1975; Mengeling and Paul 1981; Cutler et al. 1983). Parvovirus infection is widespread in the pig population, but the degree of reproductive failure will depend on the number of susceptible females introduced into the breeding herd from outside sources. Maternal immunity must be established before conception occurs. In some surveys, parvovirus infection may account for up to 45% of fetal deaths in swine herds (Sorensen and Askaa 1981a). Outbreaks of reproductive failure may occur fol-

lowing introduction of the infection into a susceptible herd (Donaldson-Wood et al. 1977). Severe fetal mummification can be expected in sows that become infected at between 45 and 65 days of gestation. Vaccination using a parvovirus vaccine before breeding will prevent experimental transplacental infection and fetal death (Sorensen and Askaa 1981b). A bivalent vaccine containing the parvovirus and the pseudorabies virus is also highly effective (Mengeling et al. 1981) and provides protection against the infection occurring in young pigs. Susceptible gilts and sows are vaccinated two weeks before breeding.

Pseudorabies infection during gestation in nonimmune sows may cause fetal resorption, fetal mummification, and abortion (Wohlgemuth et al. 1978). In some outbreaks, maternal illness occurs prior to the fetal deaths, whereas in others there may be no significant illness in the dams. Diagnosis is dependent on examination of the fetuses and serological examination of the dams. Control of the disease may be achieved using an eradication scheme of serological testing and the culling of positive animals or the use of vaccines in susceptible animals at least two weeks before breeding.

Other causes of fetal death that may occur sporadically include infections with enteroviruses, reoviruses, and adenoviruses, and miscellaneous bacterial and fungal infections (Kirkbride and McAdaragh 1978).

Stillbirths. Five to 7% of piglets are born dead, and approximately 10% of these die before the act of parturition begins. Most stillbirths occur during the process of parturition as a result of anoxia following the premature separation of the placenta or following intrauterine rupture of the umbilical cord, which may be shortened (Randall 1972a, 1972b). Prolonged parturition or uterine inertia in older sows may also be involved. The presence of meconium on the skin, in the mouth, and in the trachea of the piglet differentiates the Type II anoxic intrapartum stillbirth from Type I prepartum cases.

Perinatal Mortality

Low-Birthweight Piglets, Small Litters, and Low Viability. *Low-birthweight piglets* occur in most litters, especially in large litters and in those born to older sows. They are usually the piglets associated with small areas of placentation that are established at the implantation phase but particularly where uterine overcrowding has also occurred.

Small litters are usually the result of an above-average degree of embryonic loss. It has been shown that a pregnancy will not be maintained if four or less conceptuses are present in the uterus in the implantation phase or if one horn is devoid of developing blastocysts. Thus when two to five piglets are born, embryonic loss beyond the average has taken place. Reduced litter size may also occur in sows inseminated late or early in the estrus cycle, or following the use of subfertile boars or semen that has been delayed in transit.

Low viability can be expected in underweight or overweight piglets or where the number of stillbirths in a litter is higher than normal. If, however, it occurs in apparently normal piglets, other factors are involved. Prenatal virus infection and vitamin A deficiency can be responsible for congenital malformation with subsequent low viability. Pregnancies that are terminated two or three days early or those that end at day 117 or later also produce this effect. Inbreeding, estrogenic mycotoxins, or nutritional inadequacies such as manganese or vitamin B_{12} deficiency may also be responsible for some reduction in viability.

The inherent weaknesses of all newborn piglets, namely the absence of subcutaneous fat, an undeveloped thermoregulating mechanism, and low glucose reserves, all contribute to early perinatal loss, particularly if the environmental or nutritional conditions are also inadequate.

Fertility and Serving Capacity of the Boar

A sudden marked increase in the number of gilts and sows returning to service in 21 days after breeding suggests sterility of the boar. The semen of the boar should be examined and his serving capacity evaluated. Mating failure results from a variety of causes, including physical unsoundness, deficient sex drive, and inability to breed following mounting. Recommended boar management practices—particularly with young boars—that minimize problems include physical conditioning, acclimation, sexual training, and restricted use of the young boar. Decreased conception rates may also be due to excessive use of boars, particularly young boars.

Boars should be purchased at least six weeks prior to the beginning of breeding to allow for a two-week quarantine and a four-week preconditioning period. They should be at least eight months old before routine usage.

The number of boars required to achieve optimum fertility depends on the age of the boars, the size of the breeding pens, and the desired mating system. Ideally, young boars should not be used more than once daily. Because mating each female two or more times will increase conception rate and litter size, there should be enough breeding boars to mate each female twice. The number of boars needed is equal to the maximum number of females in heat per day $\times$ 2 (Leman and Rodeffer 1976).

Boars should be purchased from reputable herds that will delineate the exact guarantee and the condition under which the boar will be replaced. Only boars over eight months of age should be guaranteed, and breeders should void the guarantee if the new owner does not follow recommended boar management practices. Before delivery of a new boar, it should be tested serologically for diseases such as leptospirosis, brucellosis, pseudorabies, and other endemic diseases that can be detected serologically. Newly introduced boars should be kept in isolation for at least two weeks, then mixed with the other nonpregnant breeding females about one month before use in breeding in order to promote the spread of infectious agents such as parvovirus and porcine enteroviruses well before breeding to ensure that immunization occurs. During this preconditioning period, boars should be test-mated by exposure to females in heat.

Mating Systems. Double-mating can significantly increase conception rate and subsequent litter size. Maximum conception rates are obtained when females are mated approximately 12 hours before ovulation. Much of the benefit gained from double-mating may be the result of breeding nearer to the optimum time. Double-mating can be achieved by mating at 12- to 24-hour intervals with the same boar or mating at the same intervals with two different boars. In a hand-mating program, after the first mating, the female is served again, either later the same day or the following morning. In the commonly used pen-mating system, double-mating can be achieved by twice-daily boar rotation.

Boar Examination and Culling. Examination of boars for breeding soundness includes observation of prebreeding and breeding behavior with an estrous sow. The penis should be examined during copulation. Semen may be collected during copulation or by electro-ejaculation. Several common problems include aberrant sexual behavior, including insufficient libido; unsatisfactory conception rates due to inferior semen quality; diseases of the penis; and locomotor dysfunction due to diseases such as osteochondrosis, nutritional osteodystrophy, diseases of the feet, and infectious arthritis. Boars should be culled immediately if they are affected with any incurable abnormality that interferes with successful breeding and conception.

Seasonal Influences of Reproductive Performance in Swine

Seasonal infertility occurs in swine herds and is commonly associated with the hottest and most humid period of the year (Hurtgen and Leman 1980). The infertility is characterized by a decrease in farrowing rate and a delay in the return of sows to estrus after mating (Love 1978; Hurtgen et al. 1980). Litter size is not adversely affected, but gilts and first-parity sows are most frequently affected. It is thought that the infertility is caused by heat stress imposed more than seven days after mating, causing whole litter loss and the return of the sow to estrus. These observations are important in the management of swine breeding farms and in the diagnosis of reproductive problems. The provision of shade and the sprinkling of water on sows, gilts, and boars during the hottest periods of the year have been recommended but appear to be of questionable value. The effects of seasonal infertility may be minimized by intensifying postservice estrus detection from 17 to 35 days after breeding, especially during the heat stress periods. Early diagnosis of pregnancy should be made by 35 days after breeding so nonpregnant females can either be returned to the breeding area for surveillance or be culled.

Artificial Insemination

Artificial insemination has not been used in the swine industry as extensively as in the cattle industry. Artificial insemination can be applied to swine production, increasing the possibility of genetic improvement, disease control, and intensive management. The most critical problem when breeding sows artificially is determining the correct time to breed. Ovulation occurs approximately 40 hours after the beginning of standing heat, and the ova remain viable for only one to two hours. Thus maximum conception is achieved when fresh spermatozoa are waiting to fertilize the ova as soon as they leave the ovary. Ideally, a sow should be inseminated early on the second day

of standing heat to ensure that fresh, viable sperm are ready to fertilize the ova. However, with variation in sows and the fact that most producers only check for heat once daily, sows are usually bred on the first and second days of standing heat to ensure maximum conception rate.

Mating Management of Gilts and Sows

Maximum reproductive efficiency begins by breeding gilts at an early and predictable stage so that they farrow a good-sized litter at 10 to 11 months of age, nurse the pigs well, and maintain moderate body weight to ensure an early return to heat after weaning. They should proceed from there and produce good litters approximately every 150 to 160 days up to about the sixth litter, with a weaning program at four weeks of age. Factors that influence the age at which gilts reach puberty include genotype, nutrition during the growth period, contact with boars, and stresses associated with transportation and co-mingling with other gilts. Gilts are usually selected at approximately 170 days of age, mixed with other gilts, and given short periods of supervised daily contact with a boar. Following this stimulation, groups of gilts will usually exhibit their first standing heat in six to 10 days. The second and third heats will usually follow in a synchronized fashion and "flushing" (increasing the level of feeding 10 days prior to the breeding heat) can be done to increase the ovulation rate.

The factors that influence successful rebreeding of sows following weaning include the following.

Feeding. Sows should be fed a high level of feed following weaning to ensure that they come into heat as early as possible, preferably within five to seven days. The feed intake must be reduced immediately after mating, because high feed intakes after mating increase embryonic loss, especially in gilts.

Housing. Following weaning, sows are usually housed in individual stalls or groups. There are advantages and disadvantages of both systems. In individual stalls, estrus detection may be more difficult than when sows are in groups. However, when sows are grouped, fighting can be a major problem. Feed intake can be more effectively controlled in stalls, particularly for those that need an extra amount, than in groups. The housing system should allow for comfort; easy detection of heat; the sight, smell, and sounds of the boar;

easy movement of sows to the boar; and a good service area.

The Boar. The boar should be housed comfortably adjacent to newly-weaned sows. It should not be used excessively (four to six services per week) and should be evaluated for breeding soundness.

Age at Weaning. Under conventional conditions, weaning should occur when the piglets are three to four weeks of age. This will ensure that the sows will come into heat between five and seven days following weaning. Earlier weaning will result in an increase in the interval from weaning to heat and conception.

Litter Number. Sows are difficult to breed following their first lactation. This is usually associated with excessive weight loss of the gilt during her first pregnancy and lactation. As parity increases, the weaning-to-conception interval decreases. Excessive weight loss during the first lactation can be minimized by increasing feed intake during the lactation period.

Failure to conceive, embryonic mortality, and abortion also interfere with successful rebreeding of sows; these have been described earlier.

The influence of housing and management factors on reproductive efficiency in swine have been reviewed (Hurtgen 1981).

Selection of a Farrowing Cycle

The complete reproductive cycle of mature swine involves mating, gestation, farrowing, lactating, weaning, and the interval of remating; adequate facilities must be available to accommodate a number of animals at each of these stages. Farrowing time is relatively inflexible, and the parturition/nursing unit requires the greatest investment of capital. Thus, it is advisable to plan the entire reproductive program to optimize use of this facility (Table 11–10). Batch-farrowing allows better organization and more efficient use of facilities and labor, and reduces disease problems in newborn piglets. In a batch-farrowing system, a group of females bred at about the same time move into a farrowing unit just before the first sow is due, remain in the unit until the youngest litter reaches weaning age, and are then moved into the rebreeding area. The farrowing room is completely cleaned and sanitized before the next group moves in. The length of the farrowing cycle or time that the group occupies the farrowing room can be as short as four weeks with early weaning but is usually five to six weeks in most commercial practices.

Table 11–10. PRACTICAL WEANING-REBREEDING CYCLES FOR BATCH-FARROWINGS IN HERDS OF 100 TO 125 SOWS PRODUCING 250 LITTERS PER YEAR

Week	Three Farrowing Rooms (A, B, and C), 10 Crates/Room	Two Farrowing Rooms (A and B), 15 Crates/Room
1	Wean A	Wean A
2	Rebreed A	Rebreed A
3	Wean B	
4	Rebreed B	Wean B
5	Wean C	Rebreed B
6	Rebreed C	
7	Wean A	Wean A
8	Rebreed A	Rebreed A

In a herd that practices four- to five-week weaning, sows should be moved into the farrowing crates three to four days before they are due, and one or two days will be required for cleanup as the litters are weaned. Thus, the farrowing room will be tied up for six weeks with each batch. If 250 litters are expected, this requires $250 \times 6 = 1500$ crate-weeks or a total of 28.8 crates. This could be organized with two farrowing rooms of 15 crates each, operating with a farrowing every third week; or with three rooms of 10 crates each, operating on a two-week cycle. Both systems can spread the farrowing, weaning, cleanup, and rebreeding uniformly throughout the year.

In a three-week cycle, 15 sows will be weaned, and 12 of these should conceive the following week. The herdsman should attempt to mate four or five gilts at the same time to maintain his batch of 15 pregnant animals. With a two-week cycle, eight out of the 10 weaned animals should conceive the week after weaning, and about three additional gilts should be mated to maintain the batch number. Additional gilts must be mated if some of the group are culled prior to remating. The advantage of the three-week cycle is that females that fail to conceive at first mating usually return during the period when the next group is being mated. However, working replacement gilts into the system is easier with a breeding every second week. Larger units with populations in excess of 125 to 150 sows should consider batch-farrowing a group of sows every week.

Whatever system is adopted, it should be organized to produce a uniform flow of batches through the mating, gestating, and farrowing areas and then back to the mating area for rebreeding. To achieve efficient breeding performance with batches over prolonged periods necessitates adequate housing, sound nutrition, and a disease control program that maintains the entire herd in continual good health. In addition, the operator must plan and execute a management routine that ensures prompt initiation of estrus after weaning, detection of this estrus, high pregnancy rates, and large litters.

Pregnancy Diagnosis

The recurrence of estrus following service is a traditionally accepted method of diagnosing nonpregnancy in sows. In large herds where sows are penned individually, the detection of heat can be difficult and unreliable. The commercial gain through the routine use of pregnancy diagnosis is dependent on the accuracy of the results, the overall fertility of the herd, and the costs of the test. The most practical methods are vaginal biopsy, ultrasonic detection, and rectal examination (Meredith 1981). Rectal examination is possible in sows, not gilts, and has an accuracy rate of about 94% when done between 30 and 60 days of gestation (Cameron 1977). Where laboratory facilities are readily available, the vaginal biopsy technique is considered more efficient than the ultrasonic technique. Neither system allows routine detection of animals that have failed to conceive before the first anticipated return to service. False-positive results may occur due to embryonic or fetal death. The vaginal biopsy technique is highly accurate at between 18 and 22 days after mating (McCaughey and Rea 1979). The ultrasonic technique is most accurate between 27 and 35 days after breeding. A comparison of the rectal palpation and ultrasound techniques indicates that pregnancy can be accurately diagnosed in 98.8% of sows by rectal palpation and 96.6% by ultrasound (Balke and Elmore 1982).

Management During Gestation and at Farrowing

Nutrition

Following breeding, the amount of feed should be reduced to a maintenance level for pregnancy. High energy intakes during the first few weeks of pregnancy may result in increased embryonic mortality (Michel et al. 1980). Reducing the feeding level at the time of mating results in two separate and antagonistic effects on reproduction (Dyck and Strain 1983). Initially, there is an increase in embryonic survival. This is followed by a reduction in conception rate if the feed restriction is continued beyond a critical point in time. The accepted procedure of flush-feeding before mating for maximum ovulation rate, followed by a 10-day level of feeding near body weight maintenance, and a subsequent level of feeding to provide the desired growth rate during gestation, should result in increased litter size. Daily feed intake and body condition are easily controlled for sows fed and housed individually. However, body weight and condition may vary considerably in sows fed and housed in groups.

Immunization

Vaccination of pregnant sows against endemic infectious diseases may be indicated and should be done on a regular basis. Some vaccines must be given at least two weeks before breeding to avoid the effects of live vaccine antigens on the developing embryo. Sows may be vaccinated about one month before farrowing against diseases of the newborn piglet, such as transmissible gastroenteritis and colibacillosis, using commercially available vaccines. In cases where vaccines are not yet available, late pregnant sows may be deliberately exposed to the infected tissues of piglets affected with such diseases as vomiting and wasting disease.

Pregnancy Loss

The lesions of embryonic and fetal life are the sequelae of death of the conceptus at different stages of development (Wrathall 1977). These are summarized as follows:

1. Damage or disease in eggs and blastocysts (0 to 14 days) is usually fatal, and they are very quickly resorbed.

2. Damage or disease in embryos (14 to 35 days) often interferes with gastrulation, morphogenesis, or the formation of organ rudiments, thereby leading to structural malformations. If death occurs, it is followed by autolysis and gradual resorption so that little or no trace remains at term.

3. Damage or disease in fetuses (35 days to term) can produce various effects, including abnormality of tissue differentiation and function, distortion of body structure, and growth retardation. The onset of immune competence takes place at about 65 to 70 days, and after this, antibody production and inflammatory processes can take place. Fetal death is followed by autolysis and then mummification or maceration if sufficient time elapses before parturition or abortion. Bones of dead fetuses are not usually resorbed so that age of death, and sometimes even events that preceded

death, can be determined by x-ray examination.

4. Deaths that occur during the process of parturition (stillbirths) often result from fetal asphyxia. Sometimes, however, prior disease renders the fetus incapable of successful transition; thus careful postmortem study may be needed to ascertain the exact mechanisms of stillbirth. Distinction between late fetal death, intrapartum death (stillbirth), and early neonatal death is not always easy when parturitions are not actually observed. However, late fetal deaths, i.e., those occurring 24 to 48 hours prior to term, usually show signs of early autolytic degeneration (e.g., cloudy cornea, subcutaneous and intraabdominal hemolysis, friable liver, and kidneys), whereas evidence of lung expansion will be seen in cases of neonatal death. Piglets asphyxiated in utero often have meconium and mucus in their tracheas and bronchi.

In some abortions, all the embryos and fetuses are expelled without obvious abnormalities other than subcutaneous congestion, hemolysis, and early autolysis. On other occasions, however, some or all members of the litter may be diseased or long dead. Careful examination of aborted litters is therefore important not only because it enables distinction between maternal and embryonic failure but also because, in embryonic failure cases, it sheds light on what kinds of disease processes were involved. Radiography may once again be useful to ascertain the ages when fetuses died and to detect abnormalities preceding death. Furthermore, if all fetuses in the litter are x-rayed it may be possible to determine whether all were affected simultaneously on a particular date (as in cases of maternal illness or transplacental toxemia) or whether a sequential process was involved with spread from fetus to fetus in utero (as in cases of certain intrauterine infections).

When fresh fetuses are available, as, for example, when pregnant sows are slaughtered specifically for the purpose, or in instances where stillbirths or early neonatal deaths are identified as the major problem, there may be a need for postmortem dissection and perhaps other detailed studies. First, however, the conceptual age of the litter must be ascertained from the service date, and then other quantitative information can be recorded and compared with appropriate standards (i.e., means and tolerance limits) for normal fetuses or piglets of that particular age. Such standards can be of special value in assessing normality of fetal and newborn piglets.

Placentae should be examined when necessary, although recognition of pathological abnormalities presupposes familiarity with the normal.

Farrowing

Pregnant sows and gilts should be moved into the farrowing facility at least six days before the expected farrowing date. In a batch-farrowing system, a group will usually be brought into the farrowing crates at least one week before the mean expected due date. One week allows for individual variations in gestational length, which will vary up to four days, and for an adequate period of adjustment to the farrowing crate. The farrowing crates should have been cleaned, disinfected, and left vacant for at least three days before pregnant sows are moved into them. Also, all sows and gilts should be washed before entering the farrowing facilities. This removes gross fecal contamination of the skin and reduces the population of the bacterial flora of the skin, which aids in the control of bacterial diseases of the newborn piglet.

Farrowing may be induced in sows using a single injection of a prostaglandin or its analogues. A successful induction of parturition has practical application in commercial swine units operating a batch-farrowing system. Individual sows, within groups weaned on the same day, usually commence their postweaning estrus between four and eight days later. If these animals are served over a four- or five-day period with a gestation period lasting between 114 and 118 days, the farrowings would normally extend over about 10 days. With an induction treatment, initiated just after the first natural farrowings, it should be possible to reduce the farrowing range for an individual group to perhaps five or six days and maintain a better batch effect. This should increase the efficiency of utilization of the farrowing facility. A reduction of two to three days in the interval from first to last farrowing could allow more groups through the unit in a fixed time and give one or two extra days for cleaning and sanitation between groups. Concentrated farrowings would have other potential advantages: piglets could be readily transferred from the larger to smaller litters, routine activities like iron injections or castrations could be carried out on more piglets at the same time, and the age range at weaning would be reduced. Also, weekend and holidays farrowings could be avoided, which would minimize labor requirements during these periods.

Successful induced farrowings also allow a high percentage of farrowings to occur at predetermined times, when maximum surveillance and supervision can be provided to minimize the incidence of perinatal mortality (Hammond and Matty 1980; King et al. 1979; Dziuk 1979).

The prostaglandin products are usually given two to three days before the expected farrowing date (day 112, 113, or 114 of gestation). Farrowing usually occurs within 36 hours following the injection, with a mean time of about 26 hours. Induction of parturition on day 110 may be associated with a slight increase in perinatal piglet mortality compared with inductions on days 112 and 113 (Jainudeen and Brandenburg 1980). It is essential to have reliable breeding records in order to induce two to three days before the expected natural farrowing date. New prostaglandin analogues are being made available and are as effective as cloprostenol (Boland and Herlihey 1982).

Parturition in the pig is relatively simple, and dystocia and uterine inertia are uncommon. The duration of farrowing is approximately two hours, and a piglet is born approximately every 15 minutes. Posterior presentations are common, but most piglets are born in a dorsosacral position. The most common cause of perinatal mortality is intrapartum death of piglets born during the last third of the litter. Premature rupture of the umbilical cord is a major factor in the cause of intrapartum deaths that may be related to prolonged farrowing times (Randall 1972a, 1972b). In approximately 70% of intrapartum deaths, the piglets are alive at birth, although the clinical signs of viability are often limited only to the presence of a slow heart beat, which gradually fades and ceases within several minutes after delivery. These piglets are in a state of hypercapnia and acidosis, and resuscitation may be possible (Randall 1979).

Surveillance and supervision of farrowing to minimize perinatal mortality includes obstetrical assistance of sows with dystocia, resuscitation of piglets that are almost dead (intrapartum asphyxia), removal of placenta envelopes to prevent suffocation of piglets, placing piglets under the heat lamp immediately after birth to prevent hypothermia and crushing by the sow, assessment of the sow's milking potential and interfostering accordingly, identifying piglets that did not suck early enough, and clipping all piglets' teeth and treating navels with an antibacterial spray immediately after birth.

Control of Diseases of the Farrowing Sows. The most important disease complex of the sow at the time of farrowing is the mastitis-metritis-agalactia syndrome (Jones 1979; Einarsson et al. 1975, 1978). The etiology is not clear, but there is considerable clinical and laboratory evidence that toxemic mastitis, most commonly due to *E. coli*, is the predominant lesion and that metritis is usually not present (Nachreiner and Ginther 1971, 1972a, 1972b). Intramammary infections are common in sows at the time of farrowing (McDonald and McDonald 1975).

The prevention of the mastitis-metritis-agalactia syndrome in the sow is vital because of the effects of agalactia on the newborn piglets. It has been difficult to develop a rational approach to prevention because the disease has been considered as a complex syndrome caused by several different factors. However, the control of infectious mastitis would seem to be of major importance. Farrowing crates should be vacated, cleaned, disinfected, and left vacant for a few days before pregnant sows are transferred from the dry sow barn and placed in the crates. Pregnant sows should be washed with soap and water before being placed in the crates. Farrowing crates must be kept clean and hosed down if necessary, particularly a few days before and after farrowing, to minimize the level of intramammary infection. In problem herds, it may be necessary to wash and disinfect the skin over the mammary glands immediately after farrowing.

To minimize the stress on the sow of adjusting to the farrowing crate and the farrowing facilities, the sow should be placed in the crates at least one week before the expected date of farrowing. The nature and composition of the diet fed to the sow while in the farrowing crate should not be changed. The only change that is necessary is to increase the daily intake (compared with the intake during the dry period), beginning on the day after the sow has farrowed and thereafter as lactation proceeds. The inclusion of bran at the rate of one third to one half of the total diet for two days before and after farrowing has been recommended to prevent constipation. In some herds, the use of lucerne meal at the rate of 15% of the diet at all times has been recommended. However, under intensified conditions, it may be impractical to prepare and provide these special diets on a regular basis. Although field observations suggest that a bulky diet at the time of farrowing will minimize the incidence of toxic agalactia, there is little scientific evidence to support the practice.

Antimicrobial agents used prophylactically have apparently been successful in controlling some outbreaks. A sulfadimidine-trimethoprim-sulfathiazole combination fed for three to five days before the expected farrowing date may reduce the incidence of the disease in problem herds (Fiebiger et al. 1975).

The use of prostaglandins for the induction of parturition has not been associated with a consistent decrease in the incidence of the disease. Some field trials have shown a reduction, whereas others have had no effect.

Other diseases of the sow that may occur within a few days before or after farrowing include pyelonephritis, cystitis due to *Corynebacterium suis*, uterine prolapse, sow hysteria, and agalactia due to ergot-infested feed (Anderson and Werdin 1977).

Epidemics of infectious disease are uncommon in sows raised under confinement, presumably because of age-dependent immunity and lack of exposure to pathogens such as *Erysipelothrix insidiosa*, which may cause epidemics in nonvaccinated exposed animals. Cystitis and pyelonephritis due to *Corynebacterium suis* may occur in several animals over a period of several months.

An investigation of the causes of mortality and morbidity in sows in a commercial herd over the course of one year revealed a variety of sporadically occurring diseases (Jones 1967). The mortality rate was 10%, and 27% of the sows were culled. Reproductive failure and locomotor disturbances were the main reasons for culling. The sows lost from the herd had produced an average of 3.7 litters, but 44% had produced no more than two litters. In a one-year survey of 106 herds (2488 sows), there was a mortality rate of 4% (Jones 1968). The major causes of death were complications of parturition, cystitis, nephritis, endocarditis,

and acute hemorrhage. Bacterial infection was an important factor in 43% of the deaths.

Culling of Gilts and Sows

Sows are culled when, for a variety of reasons, they are considered to be unsuited for further breeding. The factors leading to culling may be complex and are a reflection of management, housing, genotype, disease status, and nutrition. The major reasons for culling sows, recorded by four different sources, are shown in Table 11–11.

Other important reasons for culling sows from commercial herds are as follows (Dagorn and Aumaitre 1979):

Reason	Per Cent
Failure to breed after one or several matings	31.0
Decrease in productivity due to old age	27.2
Lameness (leg weakness)	8.8
Low farrowing and weaning performances	8.4
Sow deaths	6.5
Anestrus	5.4
Farrowing difficulties	4.0
Abortion	2.8
Miscellaneous	5.9

Most sows are culled between three and five years of age, when litter size begins to decline.

Knowing when to cull a gilt or a sow that will be nonproductive is a major asset in ensuring continued high reproductive performance in the herd. Some criteria would include the following:

□ Persistent anestrus in gilts over nine months of age. In some studies up to 66% of gilts over nine months of age were culled for this reason (Ehnvall et al. 1981)
□ Persistent anestrus in sows lasting for more than 30 days after weaning
□ Failure to conceive after two successive matings
□ Chronic illness of any kind in which there is loss of appetite, loss of body weight, and failure to respond to treatment

Table 11–11. REASONS FOR CULLING SOWS

Reason	Percentage of Total Culled			
	POMEROY (1960)	P.I.D.A. (1964)[*]	DAGORN AND AUMAITRE (1979)	PATTISON ET AL. (1980)
Age	15.0	6.0	29.1	24.4
Failure to breed	21.4	21.8	41.8	37.5
Performance	32.5	28.2	9.0	13.8
Locomotor disturbance	N.A.	10.7	9.4	11.8
Milk failure or udder disease	6.1	10.9	2.5	0.6
Disease	7.5	5.2	1.4	3.3
Miscellaneous	17.5	17.2	6.8	8.6

[*]Pig Industry Development Authority, 1964, unpublished.

CONTROL OF DISEASES OF THE PIGLET FROM BIRTH TO WEANING

Preweaning Mortality Statistics

From surveys made in different countries on different breeds under various management and climatic conditions, it is known that preweaning losses average 20 to 25% of piglets born alive (Table 11–12) (Nielsen et al. 1974).

Approximately 75% of the preweaning losses occur within the first week after birth, 60% occurring from birth to three days of age. The mortality according to age groups is as follows:

Age Group	Per Cent of Total Preweaning Loses
0–3 days	60
4–7 days	12–15
1–3 weeks	12
3–4 weeks	18

More than 50% of the preweaning losses occur during the perinatal period from birth to three days of age (Bille et al. 1974). The perinatal mortality rate is particularly influenced by litter size, by the age of the sow, by the type of confinement of the pregnant sows, and by the degree to which the farrowing is attended.

In an Australian survey, diseases of the piglet associated with parturition accounted for about 25% of the preweaning losses, whereas the postparturient conditions accounted for 75% (Glastonbury 1977c). The pathologic findings in the piglets that died before, during, or immediately after parturition indicated that the antiparturient deaths accounted for 13% and were of undetermined etiology. The parturient deaths accounted for 75%, and intrapartum hypoxia was considered to be the major cause (Glastonbury 1977a).

The postparturient causes of preweaning mortality were as follows (Glastonbury 1977b):

Cause	Per Cent of Total Preweaning Losses
Physical factors (trauma and suffocation)	33.0
Starvation	12.8
Septicemia	10.9
Alimentary tract infectious diseases	5.2
Viral infections	2.6
Congenital abnormalities	0.8
Miscellaneous	2.4
Unknown	5.7

A survey over a two-year period of 54 Norwegian Landrace herds revealed an average litter size of 11.1 at farrowing and 8.6 at weaning, with an average preweaning mortality, including stillbirths, of 22.2%, with a range from 10.5 to 29.8% (Simensen and Karlberg 1980). Litter size at farrowing had the greatest influence on preweaning mortality, which was 12% in litters of eight or less piglets, rising steadily to 32.7% in litters of 15 or more. Litter size at farrowing and preweaning mortality were lowest in litters from gilts and highest in litters from sows with five or more farrowings. The higher mortality in the latter appeared to be related to a higher percentage of stillborn pigs. Among environmental factors, the most important was the standard of care. Mortality was lowest in herds with the farrowing and dry sow sections in the same room and highest in herds with the farrowing and slaughter pig sections in the same room.

Information on neonatal piglet mortality in the U.K. reveals that the majority of losses occur by the end of the second day after birth (English and Smith 1975). Mortality also increased as litter size and the age of the sow

Table 11-12. CAUSES OF PREWEANING MORTALITY[*]

Cause	Per Cent of Total Losses from Birth to Weaning	Per Cent of Total Pigs Born Alive	Herd Variations
Stillborn	26.1	5.9	2.6–8.7
Trauma	18.0	4.0	1.3–6.6
Starvation/undersize	11.8	2.6	0.7–4.6
Gastrointestinal disease	11.9	2.7	0.6–4.5
Pneumonia	4.5	1.1	0–2.0
Generalized bacterial infection	2.7	0.6	0.3–1.7
Congenital malformation	5.2	1.2	0.5–2.4
Polyarthritis and bacterial meningitis	6.2	1.4	0.4–3.5
Miscellaneous	10.8	2.4	
No etiology determined	2.8	0.6	

[*]According to Nielsen et al. 1974.

increased and as birth weight decreased. In one study, five groups of primary factors were found to contribute to 88% of the deaths of 236 liveborn piglets from one herd. The factors and their contribution to death are shown in Table 11-13.

Control of Preweaning Mortality

The newborn piglet requires an adequate intake of colostrum within a few hours after birth, a continued daily intake of milk, a warm environment of 30 to 34°C for at least the first three days of life, and protection from traumatic injuries such as crushing by the sow. Every economical effort must be made during the first three days to provide the optimum environment that will minimize crushing, chilling, starvation, and infectious disease.

Several epidemiologic determinants (contributory factors) have been associated with preweaning piglet mortality. Large litters (over 12) are associated with undersized piglets, which are weak and are more susceptible to crushing and starvation than heavier piglets (English and Smith 1975). Mortality is usually higher in piglets born from sows that have had eight or more litters. Mortality is also occasionally high in piglets born from gilts because of sow hysteria. There is also considerable variation in mortality rates between herds, which is probably a reflection of the level of management.

Because perinatal mortality (birth to three days of age) accounts for approximately 60% of preweaning piglet mortality, the level of management and supervision at farrowing time and the quality and the environment of the facilities assume major importance. The frequency of stillbirths can be reduced by allowing sows in late pregnancy some daily exercise and by attendance at the time of farrowing to assist pigs that are hypoxemic and may be covered by placenta. Farrowing may be induced and synchronized to occur at a time during the day or week when maximum supervision is available. Piglets from large litters can be cross-fostered most successfully when done as soon after birth as possible to ensure one functional teat per piglet, thus securing sufficient colostrum for each suckling pig in the litter.

The acquisition of an adequate level of colostral immunoglobulins is of vital importance. Some surveys indicate that piglets that fail to survive absorb only 10 to 50% as much immunoglobulin in the first 12 hours after birth as their age-matched surviving controls (Klobasa et al. 1981). Several factors may affect the levels of serum immunoglobulins achieved in the newborn piglet by 24 to 48 hours after birth. The concentration of immunoglobulins in the colostrum may vary from one sow to another by a factor of 10 (Inoue et al. 1981). The parity of the sow, the kind of feed used, the type of farming, the number of sows raised on the farm, and the level of management may affect the concentration of immunoglobulins in the colostrum of the sow.

Any factor that interferes with the movement of the piglet from its birthplace to the mammary gland will affect the time when the animal begins to suck colostrum and the amount it ingests. The feet of the piglet may

Table 11-13. SUMMARY OF CONTRIBUTION OF PRIMARY FACTORS TO DEATHS BEFORE WEANING OF 236 LIVEBORN PIGLETS

Primary Factors in Death	Average Birth Weight of Piglets (g.)*	Contribution to Death (%)	
Congenital and genetic abnormalities	1134	12.3	
Extreme weakness at birth	803	8.5	
Weakness at birth relative to littermates, associated with incomplete lung inflation	807	6.4	
Crushing and trampling of apparently normal and thriving piglets	1148		
1. Restlessness and/or awkwardness of sow predisposing to problem	1188	7.6	
2. No predisposing cause evident	1120	10.6	18.2
Clinically normal piglets at birth failing to achieve a regular and adequate suckle			
1. Adequate milk available on sow	871	31.4	
2. Sow suffering from agalactia	1039	11.4	42.8
Miscellaneous factors (e.g., born enveloped in afterbirth, savaging and primary infection)	1211		11.8
Total			100.0

*The average birth weight of all piglets born alive was 1243 g.
From English, P.R. and Smith, W.J. Some causes of death in neonatal pigs. Vet. Ann., *15*:95–104, 1975.

become stuck in perforated floors in which the holes are too large, or solid floors may be too slippery, and the piglet may become crushed by movements of the sow. The sow may refuse to allow the piglets to suck because of sow hysteria, agalactia, or any other illness. Generalized weakness of the piglet may not allow it to compete successfully for a nipple during sucking. Exposure to cold may affect the amount of colostrum ingested by newborn piglets (LeDividich and Noblet 1981). Piglets kept at an ambient temperature of 18 to 20°C consume about 37% less colostrum than piglets kept at 30 to 32°C. The effects of exposure to cold on the absorption of colostral immunoglobulins by the newborn piglet is not clear (Kelley et al. 1982).

The major immunoglobulin component of sow milk is secretory immunoglobulin SIgA, which is synthesized locally within the mammary gland and which forms a continuous defense, protecting the nursing piglet from disease caused by enteric pathogens (Husband and Bennell 1980). Most of the immunoglobulin in the milk of the sow is thought to originate from the immune system of the intestinal tract (Bourne and Newby 1981). Stimulation of the immune system of the gut of young pigs wll result in the production of intestinal SIgA, which can protect weaning pigs from infectious enteric disease. In the sow, stimulation of the intestinal tract by oral vaccination will result in the production of SIgA, which is transferred to the mammary gland and into the milk.

The reduction of traumatic injuries to newborn piglets can be accomplished by provision of farrowing crates that are designed to prevent the sow from lying down in one motion and by the surveillance of sows to ensure that any evidence of sow hysteria, sow aggressiveness, and other illnesses of the sow at farrowing time are recognized and treated accordingly (Bille et al. 1974).

The common infectious diseases of newborn piglets can be controlled by a combination of batch-farrowing; regular cleaning and disinfection of the farrowing crates between sows; a closed-herd policy, which minimizes the introduction of infectious agents through carrier breeding stock; and vaccination of pregnant sows to stimulate the production of specific antibodies to transfer to the newborn through colostrum (Nielsen et al. 1975; Svendsen et al. 1975). The early recognition and treatment of postparturient diseases of the sow are also indicated to prevent the spread of infectious diseases to the piglets and to minimize starvation and hypoglycemia due to agalactia.

An important environmental requirement of the piglet from birth to three days of age is supplemental heat to prevent chilling (Adams et al. 1980). This is usually done most effectively and economically with heat lamps. The lower critical temperature of the newborn piglet is estimated to be about 34°C, and the highest proportion of piglet death loss due to chilling occurs during the first 72 hours after birth. In draft-free farrowing units with an ambient temperature of at least 21°C, the provision of supplemental heat beyond three days of age is usually not necessary. Supplemental heat from three to 21 days of age will improve rate of gain compared with piglets with no supplemental heat, but it is not economically advantageous under ideal management conditions.

The causes of low birth weight in piglets are difficult to identify retrospectively. It is not unusual to find littermates differing by as much as 200% in body weight at birth. Possible influences on birth weight include maternal factors such as the size of placental development in early gestation and the effect of nutrition on the sow during pregnancy (Clauson 1978). However, it is not yet possible to achieve uniformity in birth weight through feeding or by selection. The most effective method to achieve uniformity in birth weight within litters is to batch-farrow and cross-foster piglets between simultaneously farrowed litters so that all the small piglets are allocated to one sow and the heavier ones to another sow. Cross-fostering should take place within six hours of farrowing for maximum benefit.

Procedures that are performed routinely in piglets from birth to weaning at three weeks of age include clipping needle teeth after birth, the injection of iron dextran at three days of age, the docking of tails at two to three days of age to prevent tail-biting, castration at two weeks of age, the provision of a creep-feed at seven to 10 days of age with increasing amounts up to weaning time, the provision of a water supply, and identification of the litter or individual pigs. Records should be kept of the birth date, the number of pigs born alive and dead, and the number of pigs treated and that died during the nursing period. If possible, necropsies should be done on each dead pig and the information recorded.

CONTROL OF DISEASES AND PRODUCTION OF THE WEANED PIG

Following weaning, at three to five weeks of age and weighing 5 to 7 kg., the piglets are reared in groups in weaning or nursery pens until they are about 10 to 12 weeks of age and weight 20 to 25 kg., when they are then moved into the growing and finishing pens. During the last 20 years, major advances in the science of nutrition of the weaned pig and the pathogenesis of enteric disease of pigs have made it possible to wean pigs successfully and to control diseases such as postweaning diarrhea.

The weaning process and postweaning performance are the most critical times of a pig's life next to the problems associated with survival in the first few days of life. Therefore, every economical effort must be made to make the transition from the dam to the weaning pen as carefully as possible. This requires attention to the management of nutrition, housing, sanitation, and hygiene, and measurement of actual performance, including weight gain and feed efficiency.

The common diseases or causes of suboptimal performance that may occur at high morbidity and cause significant economic loss within a few weeks following weaning are:

□ Postweaning decrease in body weight gain (postweaning check)
□ Coliform gastroenteritis (postweaning *E. coli* diarrhea)
□ Swine dysentery
□ Sarcoptic mange
□ Ascariasis

Less common diseases that usually occur sporadically are:

□ Epizootic viral diarrhea
□ Intestinal adenomatosis complex
□ Meningitis due to *Streptococcus suis* type 2
□ Pityriasis rosea

The factors and procedures that are important for optimum health and production of the weaned pig are:

□ Optimum age at weaning and postweaning growth performance
□ Method of weaning and mixing litters
□ Nutrition of the weaned pig
□ Maintenance of systemic and intestinal immunity
□ General and specific antibacterial prophylaxis
□ Housing and environment
□ Control of behavioral vices

Postweaning mortality rates from weaning to the beginning of the growing-finishing period range from 0.5 to 8.0% and higher. With good management, the mortality rate can be kept down to 1 to 3%.

Optimum Age at Weaning and Postweaning Growth Performance

Under commercial conditions, the optimum age for weaning is between three and four weeks of age. Weaning at this age results in optimum subsequent reproductive performance of the sow (Aumaitre 1978). Weaning at an earlier age would not increase the number of litters per sow per year because sows will not usually return to estrus until 30 days following farrowing. Early weaning at two to three weeks of age may also decrease cellular immunity compared with pigs weaned at five weeks (Blecha et al. 1983).

Over the last 20 years, the age at weaning of piglets has been steadily reduced from eight to three weeks of age. The theoretical annual productivity of pigs per sow based on age at weaning is presented in Table 11–14. Under practical conditions, weaning between three and four weeks of age has been most successful for the majority of producers. Weaning at an earlier age can be more profitable if the producer can cope with the critical factors involved, such as weaning-to-conception interval, an increased culling rate of the sows, and a decrease in number of pigs born per litter. All of these may be affected by decreasing the weaning age below three weeks of age (Gadd 1981).

Between three and 10 weeks of age, the average daily gain of weaned piglets fed an appropriate weaner ration under good management and adequate housing will reach 400 to 500 g./day (O'Grady 1978). Postweaning performance can be increased by using complex diets containing several different energy and protein sources, but these diets are also more expensive, and the increased gain may not always be economical (Okai et al. 1976).

The growth rate of the pigs during the postweaning period should be monitored weekly if possible. A practical method for weighing pigs on a weekly basis is not yet available, but performance must nevertheless be monitored if optimum performance is to be achieved.

Table 11–14. EFFECT OF AGE AT WEANING ON OUTPUT PER SOW PER YEAR

| | Theoretical Weaning Age (Days) | | | | |
	10	14	21	35	42
Gestation (days)	115	115	115	115	115
Lactation (days)	10	14	21	35	42
Weaning-to-conception interval (days)	10	10	10	10	10
Total cycle length (days)	135	139	146	160	167
Litters/sow/year	2.7	2.6	2.5	2.3	2.1
Weaners/sow/year at 9/litter	24.3	23.6	22.5	20.7	19.7
at 10/litter	27	26	25	23	21.2

Method of Weaning and Mixing Litters

The procedure of weaning should be done with the least stress possible. Under ideal conditions, the litters that are to be mixed and moved into a weaner pen should be allowed to mix together before they are weaned. This is done by removing the partitions between the farrowing crates and allowing the litters to mix for two to three days before weaning. At weaning, the sows are removed and the piglets left in the farrowing crates for an additional few days. This will encourage the piglets to eat the dry feed and to drink water in familiar surroundings. Two to four litters may then be placed together in a weaner pen that has been previously cleaned, left vacant for a few days, and equipped with a fresh supply of feed and water. The entire group should be weighed when placed in the pen and again when moved out, and the amount of feed used in each pen recorded for determination of feed efficiency.

Swine producers should be encouraged to weigh pigs in and out of the weaner pens on a regular basis. This will provide an excellent monitor of performance that can be evaluated; action can be taken when there is suboptimal performance. Producers are initially reluctant to weigh weaner pigs, but after seeing the results of a few batches, they will commonly recognize the benefits of such a practice.

Nutrition of the Weaned Pig

A major problem of early weaning at three weeks of age has been the nutrition of the weaner pig (Fowler 1980). At three weeks of age, the piglet is still heavily dependent on sow's milk, which is highly digestible, and the digestive enzyme capacity of the piglet at this age is just beginning to adapt to digestion of nonmilk proteins and carbohydrates (Kidder 1982). Thus, changing the diet of the nursing piglet at three weeks of age from sow's milk to a dry diet suddenly—without a period of

adjustment—is an additional stressor. The sudden change commonly results in an obvious depression in the rate of gain called the *post-weaning check*. The check lasts from seven to 14 days depending on managerial and environmental factors and is characterized by little or no weight gain and low feed intake accompanied frequently by diarrhea (Lecce et al. 1979). The poor weight gains are largely a reflection of low feed intake and not the result of inefficient feed conversion. They can be minimized by management schemes that keep the pig eating through the weaning period. Experimentally, frequent liquid feeding is one method that can be used to accomplish this goal (Lecce et al. 1979; Armstrong and Clauson 1980).

The inadequate ingestion of creep feed before weaning has a priming effect and a transient hypersensitivity to feed antigens in the immediate post-weaning period, which causes an enteropathy and predisposes to enteritis caused by *E. coli* (Miller et al. 1984). Total creep-feed intakes of 600 g. per piglet before weaning result in a mature intestine and minimize the incidence of post-weaning diarrhea.

The provision of high-energy, high-protein milk and milk by-products–based preweaner diets (creep-feed) to piglets, beginning when they are about 10 days of age, is used commonly to encourage piglets to eat dry feed early in life and through the weaning period. The concept is sound, and a large number of creep-feeds have been developed, all of which have as their primary purpose to make the pig eat, to become less dependent on sow's milk, and to wean onto a weaner diet with a minimum of nutritional stress. The major problem has been failure of the pig to eat a significant amount of dry diet before weaning. Therefore, after weaning, there is a period of from seven to 14 days before the pig adjusts to the diet. The presence of other stressors at weaning, such as the mixing of litters, crowding, uncomfortable weaner pens, and behavioral abnormalities such as fighting and tail-biting, may exacerbate the effects of the postweaning check due to inadequate feed intake.

A common practice among swine producers is to restrict feed intake during the early postweaning period to reduce the incidence of diarrhea in pigs. Some reports indicate a higher frequency of digestive disturbances in weaned pigs when fed ad libitum than when feed is restricted. However, restriction of feed intake will significantly reduce performance (Ball and Aherne 1982); diarrhea also reduces performance, but feed restriction reduces performance more than diarrhea. Restriction of feed intake by limiting weight of feed fed per day will reduce the incidence of and severity of postweaning diarrhea, but the overall performance of pigs to 90 kg. live weight may be unaffected by feed restriction or diarrhea (Ball and Aherne 1982).

The average daily gain of piglets weaned at three weeks of age will depend on the energy and protein concentration of the diet (Fowler 1980). Feeding trials indicate that the requirements of early-weaned pigs for protein and lysine in a diet with 3.6 MCal DE/kg. are approximately 19.0 and 1.0% for optimum growth performance but approximately 21.5 and 1.12% for the most efficient conversion of feed into lean carcass tissue. With a diet containing 19.0% protein, the average daily gain of piglets from 5 to 20 kg. live weight is approximately 445 g./day, and from 10 to 20 kg. live weight, 590 g./day (Campbell 1977).

Maintenance of Systemic and Intestinal Immunity

During the first month of life, the piglet is dependent on the sow's colostrum and milk for both systemic and intestinal immunity. The intestine of the newborn piglet absorbs intact immunoglobulin molecules from ingested colostrum for 24 to 48 hours after birth, which provides an umbrella of protection primarily against systemic infection for the first few weeks of life. Whereas colostrum provides the piglet with circulating immunoglobulins, the sow's milk provides secretory antibody (IgA), which becomes the predominant immunoglobulin in milk and which provides passive intestinal immunity from a few days after birth until weaning. At about the time of weaning, piglets develop their own intestinal antibody, which can be extra-stimulated by the use of oral vaccines administered through the feed (Bourne 1980). The endogenous production of

intestinal IgA begins to develop rapidly in the pig at about three weeks of age (Husband and Bennell 1980).

Vaccination of young pigs for diseases such as erysipelas is usually done at six to eight weeks of age when maternal immunity is waning.

General and Specific Antibacterial Prophylaxis

Antimicrobials as feed additives are used extensively in weaner starter diets to improve rate of gain and feed conversion (Hays and Muir 1979). Growth-promoting concentrations of antimicrobial agents modify the microflora of their products within the gastrointestinal lumen and probably within the host's immediate environment. Growth promotion has been greatest with unthrifty animals maintained under adverse managerial and environmental conditions. Agents that are widely distributed in the body and have a broad spectrum of antibacterial activity produce a greater growth response (Visek 1980).

Antimicrobials at therapeutic levels are also used in weaner pig starter diets over a short period of time—10 days to two weeks—if the pigs have been subjected to unusual stressors such as long transportation or an outbreak of infectious disease in the herd. Swine enterprises that purchase recently weaned pigs at four to six weeks of age from several different farms will often encounter outbreaks of coliform gastroenteritis and pneumonia, which may be controlled by the use of medicated feed containing broad-spectrum antimicrobials at therapeutic levels for 10 days to two weeks.

It is well recognized that the economic returns from the use of antimicrobials as feed additives are substantial. There is some evidence that the observed improvements in average daily gain and feed conversion resulting from the use of antimicrobials in the feed of pigs under commercial conditions are nearly double those observed in experimental station trials. This suggests that their real economic impact is underestimated if based only on experimental station trials.

A system of medicated early weaning to obtain pigs free from pathogens endemic in the herd of origin has been proposed (Alexander et al. 1980). Groups of sows are induced to farrow on the same day, and at five days of age the thriftiest piglets in the litter are weaned and reared in pens in groups of 12 per pen. The sows are treated with an antimicrobial before entry into the farrowing unit and until the piglets are weaned at five days of age. The piglets are dosed daily from birth to 10 days of age. The method is considered effective for obtaining pigs free of *Mycoplasma pneumoniae* and *Bordetella bronchiseptica*.

The use of subtherapeutic levels of antimicrobials in the diet of pigs and other food-producing animals has been questioned because of the development of drug-resistant bacteria that could be transferred to man. Drug-resistant enteric bacteria do emerge following the use of antibacterials in the diets of animals. But there is no evidence that the use of subtherapeutic levels of the antibiotics in animal feeds compromised subsequent treatment of clinical disease in animals (Solomons 1978). Also, after their use for over 30 years, there is no significant evidence of any adverse effects on human health (National Academy of Sciences 1980).

Housing and Environment

The environmental and housing factors that influence the performance of the early weaned pig include temperature, humidity, air velocity, light, animal space, and hygiene. Weaning houses (nurseries) have now been designed and adapted to provide sufficient space and volume and suitable environment for the weaned pig. In addition, reduction of labor requirements for piglet care has led to the design of weaner pens with wire mesh floors. However, wire mesh floored cages favor an increase of radiative and convective heat losses, and consequently the critical temperature of the piglet is probably increased (Le-Dividich and Aumaitre 1978). The optimum air temperature for piglets weaned from five weeks is about 25°C. At lower temperatures, growth rate and feed efficiency are reduced. Cold weather also increases pig mortality by affecting the immune system of the pig (Kelley 1982). The presence of bedding such as straw or wood shavings may help the piglets to create a microclimate that protects them from the adverse effects of climate and considerably reduces heat losses.

Experimentally, exposure of pigs weaned at three to four weeks of age to short-term chilling will increase the rate of passage of digesta, which could have an additive effect on the severity of nutritional diarrhea (Pouteaux et al. 1982). However, the role of chilling as a primary or contributing cause of diarrhea in recently weaned pigs is inconclusive.

There are no documented data on the optimum relative humidity for early weaned piglets.

Because of the considerable magnitude of convective heat losses from piglets reared in batteries, air velocity is an important factor to consider in addition to air temperature. Weaned piglets are more comfortable, grow faster, and consume less feed in a draft-free environment than draft-exposed pigs (Le-Dividich and Aumaitre 1978).

Rearing in complete darkness is considered to be favorable to a reduction in aggressiveness in mixed animals of different litters after early weaning.

The all-in–all-out management system is recommended for early weaned pigs. The weaner pens are depopulated, cleaned, disinfected, left vacant to dry for a few days, and then restocked with newly weaned pigs. Average daily gain and feed conversion are better in pigs reared in an all-in–all-out system compared with the continuous system. The improvement is probably due to the reduction of the microbiological flora in the environment due to the cleaning and disinfection. Continuous occupation of weaner pens by successive litters of weaned pigs without a clean-out and disinfection between litters results in a marked increase in the population of infectious agents, which increases the incidence of infectious diseases.

As swine producers continue to intensify to increase productivity, the need to increase the density of nurseries to reduce building and operating costs per pig is important. Increasing the density of groups of weaned pigs to a crowded level will decrease average daily gain, increase the feed:body weight gain ratio, and promote aggressiveness (Randolph et al. 1981; Lindvall 1981).

As floor space decreases from 0.25 to 0.17 to 0.13 m.^{2}/pig, average daily gain will decrease and continue to do so with each successive growth period (Lindvall 1981). A depression in growth rate during the weaner phase caused by overcrowding will affect subsequent growth rate throughout the growing period (Van Lunen 1983). In weaner pigs reared at densities of 0.37, 0.18, and 0.12 m.^{2}/pig on decks or on floors, there were marked differences in rate of gain, days to market, and backfat thickness in favor of the lower density of 0.37 m.^{2}/pig.

Decking is an effective way of increasing nursery density. Properly designed double- and triple-deck environmentally controlled nurseries can provide the means of meeting the environmental needs of the pig during the critical postweaning period. The building and operating costs per pig can be reduced without adversely affecting pig performance (Kornegay, 1980a, 1980b). There are no significant behavioral problems and the pigs usually remain clean because the feces pass through the expanded metal floors. Field trials suggest that 10 weaned pigs from 5 to 12 kg. body weight may be housed per 1.2×1.2 m. cage and that a maximum of eight pigs from 12 to 22 kg. may be housed. Factors influencing the space requirement include the starting weight, length of time that pigs will be kept in the nursery, environmental conditions and the degree of environmental control, type of floor, amount of feeder space per pig, type of feeder, and number of pigs per pen. Space recommendations for optimum performance of weaned pigs with an initial weight of 5 to 11 kg. range from a low of 0.09 m.^{2}/pig to a high of approximately 0.25 to 0.28 m.^{2}/pig.

Behavioral Adjustments and Stresses

Tail-biting, ear-biting, ear-chewing and -sucking, belly-rubbing, and fighting are all described as behavioral vices when observed in groups of pigs (Jeppesen 1981). When outbreaks of these vices occur, productivity may be markedly reduced. Tail-biting can result in systemic infection and in abscesses that are incurable. Poor ventilation, faulty nutrition, overcrowding, and boredom are among the suspected predisposing factors. However, there is no clear explanation of the etiology. Some observations suggest that behavioral vices could develop from the normal nosing behavior of pigs maintaining their hierarchy. Piglets still desiring oral stimulation may be rewarded by touching pig flesh. Presenting pigs with a textured, mobile surface providing stimulation to the sensitive nose and mouth region after weaning—but before behavioral vices occur—may prevent unsatisfied feeding behavior from being redirected toward other pigs. Attention to the environment, stocking rate, feed and water space, and the removal of particularly aggressive pigs will also help to control the problem.

Over the first six weeks after birth, the main behavioral changes consist of an increase in overall activity and in behavior associated with the ingestion of solid feed (feeding, drinking, rooting, and defecating) (Fraser 1978).

During the first few days following weaning, there is a sudden increase in general activity and aggression, coupled with restless behavior when the animals lie down together. Pawing the floor is also common and may be a form of nest-building for comfort. There is also a very rapid increase in feeding behavior during the first day after weaning with a much slower rise in the frequency of defecation (Fraser 1978). It has been suggested that perhaps the combination of the restless activity, the difficulty of lying together, and the stress of physiological adaptation to the new diet may lead to a state of fatigue and predispose to infectious diseases, which are common in the recently weaned pig. The importance of a consistently high ambient temperature for the early-weaned piglet is also recognized and may be a factor in postweaning behavior.

CONTROL OF DISEASES AND PRODUCTION OF THE GROWING AND FINISHING PIG

Following rearing in the weaning pens, the pigs are transferred to the growing and finishing pens at about 25 kg. body weight, where they are fed until they reach market weight at about 100 kg. body weight and are sold for pork, selected as breeding stock and kept as herd replacements, or sold as breeding stock to other farms.

The major objective during this feeding phase of pig production is to grow and finish the pig as rapidly as possible and still obtain a lean pig that will yield the highest carcass score possible in order to obtain maximum economic returns. Because feed represents approximately 70% of the cost of production, obtaining maximum feed efficiency during the growing-finishing periods is a major determinant of net profit.

The most important measures of performance in the growing-finishing period are:

▢ average daily gain
▢ feed conversion efficiency
▢ the cost per unit of live-weight gain
▢ the mortality rate from weaning to the end of the finishing period

The magnitude of the economic losses due to clinical disease, but more particularly subclinical disease, which causes suboptimal performance during the growing-finishing period, is potentially the largest of all the losses in a farrow-to-finish enterprise. Under good management, a feed conversion:daily live-weight gain ratio of 3.0:1 or lower is possible. A ratio of 4.0:1 represents a major economic loss in a herd of 100 sows marketing about 2000 pigs per year. It is generally not appreciated that these economic losses may be greater than those from preweaning mortality, which have traditionally been regarded as the source of the greatest economic loss in a herd.

The mortality rate in growing and finishing pigs has decreased in recent years. In a report in 1969, the mortality rate in pigs aged two to seven months in a commercial herd was 8.0%, and the major causes of death were pneumonia, enteritis, and intestinal hemorrhage (Jones 1969). The Pig Management Scheme Results for 1982 indicate mortality rates of 2.1% in the most profitable breeding and feeding herds. The suggested production standards indicate 3.5, 2.3, 1.0, and 0.0%, respectively, in poor, average, good, and best herds (Ridgeon 1982).

The major responsibilities of the veterinarian during these periods are to collect and analyze the data, make regular clinical inspections of the pigs and the facilities, do necropsies on dead and selected clinically affected pigs in order to obtain a rapid field diagnosis when epidemics are encountered, and consult with other specialists such as agricultural engineers and nutritionists when problems arise that may require examination by a specialist. All of this is then followed by the submission of a report by the veterinarian, which should include specific recommendations for any action deemed necessary.

Targets of Performance

The suggested targets of performance in interference levels (when action should be taken) during the growing-finishing period (feeding period) are as follows:

Index	Target of Performance	Interference Levels
Average number of days from birth to market	160	170
Average daily live-weight gain from weaning to market (kg.)	0.60	0.55
Feed conversion from weaning to:		
60 kg. B.W.	2.7	2.9
85 kg. B.W.	2.9	3.2
90 kg. B.W.	2.9	3.2
115 kg. B.W.	3.6	3.8
Per cent mortality from weaning to market	<2.0	3.5
Cost of production per kg. live-weight gain from weaning to market	Depends on local conditions	

Monitoring Health and Production During the Feeding Period. The information and data that must be collected on a regular basis, at least monthly and perhaps weekly in large units, include the following:

1. Average days from birth to market and average daily live-weight gain from weaning to market. This requires positive identification of pigs and accurate birth dates.

2. Feed conversion from weaning to market. This requires weighing groups of pigs in and out of their pens and the total amount of feed used. This is an extremely important production standard because subclinical respiratory and enteric diseases have a major deleterious effect on average days to market and feed efficiency. However, it is commonly difficult to obtain these data because pigs may not be identified, feed may not be weighed, considerable feed may be wasted depending on the feeding system, and not all pigs in a pen go to market at the same time.

3. The number of pigs affected with clinical disease each day, in which pen, the treatment given, the clinical diagnosis made, and the results of necropsies. A necropsy should be done on as many of the dead pigs as possible. When epidemics of clinical or subclinical disease occur and the diagnosis is not apparent, the submission of representative clinically affected, untreated animals will often provide valuable information. The incidence and nature of clinical disease will usually indicate the possible presence of subclinical disease. This information will indicate the route of spread of disease within the herd, accuracy of clinical diagnosis, and cause of death. A master file with the information for each pen should be centrally available.

4. Case fatality rates and population mortality rates. The case fatality rate will provide some indication of the efficacy of treatment. The population mortality should be consistently below 2%.

5. Performance indices in purebred herds. These include measurement of the thickness of backfat, number of days to maturity, and other selection criteria used in the selection of breeding stock and animals to be culled and sold as pork.

6. Pathological lesions in pigs at slaughter. If available and possible, every effort should be made to determine the nature and severity of lesions present in the pigs sent to slaughter. The incidence and nature of the lesions may reflect the disease status in the herd and assist in the diagnosis, treatment, and control of clinical and subclinical disease. The relationship be-

tween the prevalence of lesions at slaughter and environmental factors in the herd is complex and extremely variable (Flesja et al. 1982; Flesja and Solberg 1981; Flesja and Ulvesaeter 1980). Some environmental factors may be associated with certain diseases such as tail-biting, whereas on the other hand, there may be no relationship between certain infectious diseases and environmental factors that might be expected to be predisposing factors. This illustrates the complexity of relating managerial and environmental factors to disease.

The slaughter inspection system in Norway reveals that in bacon pigs the thoracic cavity is the most commonly affected part of the body because of the frequent occurrence of pleuritis, pericarditis, and pneumonia (Flesja and Ulvesaeter 1979a). Sarcoptic mange and ascariasis are also common. In culled sows sent to slaughter, there is a higher incidence of pyemia and abscesses than in bacon pigs (Flesja and Ulvesaeter 1979b). In bacon pigs, pyemia and abscesses occur, very often in combination with tail lesions, severe pneumonia, and anemia. Pyemia is also associated with polyarthritis and lesions of the claws. There is a strong relationship between the serositides and pleurisy, pericarditis, and peritonitis, which suggests that they may be caused by the same agent.

Other studies have revealed a positive correlation among the rates of respiratory disease in feeder pigs and the incidence of clinical disease, the mortality, and the prevalence at slaughter (Willeberg et al. 1978). It appears that meat inspection may be a more sensitive surveillance method for respiratory disease than clinical observation of the pigs. Evidence of subclinical respiratory disease can be discovered at slaughter, particularly among penmates of clinical cases rather than among pigs from respiratory disease pens. The monitoring of pigs at slaughter is an inexpensive method to obtain extensive information on clinical incidence, prevalence at slaughter, seasonal and age incidence, the efficacy of treatment, and possibly the effects of disease on live-weight performance and carcass evaluation. It is a powerful tool for the clinicoepidemiologic study of some of the common infectious diseases of growing and finishing pigs.

Diseases of Growing and Finishing Pigs

The most economically important diseases of pigs during the growing and finishing period are the infectious diseases of the respiratory and digestive tracts. Raising pigs in total confinement has successfully controlled several soil-borne infectious diseases, but the pneumonias and enteritides still occur clinically and subclinically and cause major economic losses. Pigs affected with acute pneumonia are relatively easy to detect. The major problem, however, is the presence of the subclinical pneumonias like enzootic pneumonia due to *Mycoplasma* spp. and pleuropneumonia due to *Hemophilus pleuropneumoniae*. Atrophic rhinitis (turbinate atrophy) occurs commonly, but the economic effect of the disease is probably minor under most circumstances.

The important diseases of the pig during the growing and finishing period are those that are endemic and cause subclinical disease and those that cause epidemics of clinical disease. A list of the diseases that occur is presented here with an indication of how commonly they occur and whether they are usually endemic or cause epidemics.

Respiratory Diseases
COMMON:
Enzootic pneumonia due to *Mycoplasma* spp.—commonly endemic
Hemophilus pleuropneumonia due to *Hemophilus pleuropneumoniae*—endemic and epidemic
Pneumonic pasteurellosis due to *Pasteurella* sp. and commonly secondary to enzootic pneumonia—sporadic
Atrophic rhinitis (turbinate atrophy) due to *Bordetella bronchiseptica*—endemic
LESS COMMON:
Swine influenza—sporadic
Glasser's disease—sporadic

Gastrointestinal Diseases
COMMON:
Swine dysentery due to *Treponema hyodysenteriae*—endemic and epidemic
Intestinal helminthiasis—endemic
LESS COMMON:
Adenomatosis complex—endemic and sporadic acute clinical illness
    Porcine intestinal adenomatosis
    Necrotic enteritis
    Regional ileitis
    Proliferative hemorrhagic enteropathy
Enteric salmonellosis—sporadic
Esophagogastric ulcers (gastric ulcers)—sporadic
Rectal strictures—sporadic
RARE:
Foot and mouth disease; swine vesicular disease; vesicular exanthema of swine
Septicemias (occur sporadically)
Salmonellosis

Erysipelas
Hog cholera
Pasteurellosis
Eperythrozoonosis
Diseases of Nervous System
Pseudorabies—rare
Nutritional Deficiencies
Mulberry heart disease, hepatosis dietetica, exudative diathesis due to vitamin E and/or selenium deficiency—sporadic

Osteodystrophy due to absolute deficiency or relative imbalance of calcium and phosphorus—uncommon
Genetic Defects
Porcine stress syndrome and pale soft exudative pork—occurs commonly in some herds
Behavioral Vices (common)
Tail-biting, ear-chewing, belly-rubbing
Skin Diseases (uncommon)
Parakeratosis (zinc deficiency)
Sarcoptic mange
Ringworm
Poisonings (rare)
Mycotoxicosis
Salt, arsenical, organophosphate
Diseases of the Feet and Musculoskeletal System
Leg weakness, osteochondrosis—common
Sore feet, cracked feet, foot rot—less common
Mycoplasma arthritis—sporadic

EPIDEMIOLOGY OF RESPIRATORY DISEASE IN GROWING AND FINISHING PIGS. The etiology and the factors that predispose to respiratory disease in pigs are complex. It is often difficult to interpret the significance of the presence of pathogens in the tissues of affected animals (Smith 1977). Respiratory disease in finishing pigs is probably the result of complex interaction between many environmental factors and mixed infections rather than simply the result of single infections (Little 1975).

Pneumonia is a major cause of decreased productivity in finishing pigs being fed for market. The economic losses are due to mortality, decreased rate of gain, and increased marketing of undersized or cull pigs (Straw et al. 1983a). In pigs located at a central performance test station, the presence of lung lesions at slaughter was associated with a decrease in mean daily weight gain. For every 10% increase in lung tissue affected with pneumonia, mean daily weight gain decreased by 5.3% (Straw et al. 1983a). Of the pigs examined at slaughter, 8.5% had no evidence of pneumonia, 52% had pneumonia in 1 to 5% of the lung, 22.5% in 6 to 10%, 8.5% in 11 to 15%, and 3.5%

of the pigs had pneumonia in 16 to 20% of the lung volume. There was involvement of more than 20% of the lung in 5% of the pigs. This illustrates the large percentage of pigs that may be affected with subclinical pneumonia and the potential for large economic losses due to suboptimal performance.

The effect of atrophic rhinitis on growth rate and feed efficiency is inconclusive. Some studies indicate that turbinate atrophy assessed at the abattoir was not related to growth rate; however, in a few herds, pigs with severe turbinate atrophy had slower growth rates (Straw et al. 1983b).

The relationship between turbinate atrophy and pneumonia is variable (Straw 1983a). In some studies, there was no difference in prevalence of pneumonic lesions at slaughter when comparing pigs with turbinate atrophy and those without turbinate atrophy. In another study, there was a greater frequency of pneumonia in pigs that had turbinate atrophy than in those that did not.

There may be a strong relationship between the incidences of pneumonia, pleurisy, and white spots in the liver of pigs examined at slaughter and environmental factors in the herd (Backstrom and Bremer 1978). The environmental factors associated with a high incidence of these lesions at slaughter include large herd size, poor hygiene and sanitation, overcrowding in pens, continuous occupation of pens instead of the all-in–all-out system, an inefficient manure storage-handling system, and an inefficient ventilation system.

Cohort epidemiologic analyses of the occurrence and treatment of pigs with respiratory disease and the effect of clinical disease on growth rate and the presence of lesions at slaughter indicate that the commonly applied treatments of clinical cases have limited effect (Willeberg et al. 1978). Also, in some situations, productivity is affected more by clinical epidemics than by subclinical occurrence, which may be due to a prolonged decrease in feed intake in clinically affected animals. The number of pigs culled for disease during the finishing period is often closely related to the prevalence of lesions at slaughter (Andersen 1981).

A well-designed epidemiologic analysis of the effect of environmental factors on the health of finishing pigs is recorded by Lindquist (1974). Clinical inspections were made in 99 finishing herds involving 209,815 pigs delivered for slaughter over a three-year period. The study attempted to answer several important questions about the role of housing and environment on the health and production of finishing pigs. Out of a possible 150 environmental variants, the following were studied:

□ Production strictly in batches. Units where the house is completely emptied of animals and cleaned between batches

□ Continuous production in batches. Units where a small number of animals from the previous batch still remained when the next batch arrived

□ Continuous production. Units where different age groups are present in the same house

□ Floor versus trough feeding

□ Number of pigs per section of the house (less than or more than 500)

□ Volume per pig (less than or more than 3 m.^{3})

□ Lying area per pig (less than or more than 0.5 m.^{2})

□ Total area per pig (lying area and area in dunging passage) (less than or more than 0.7 m.^{2})

□ Open dunging passage versus slatted floorings in the dunging passage

□ Free versus restricted access to drinking water

The effect of the different environmental factors on disease was assessed from the incidence of lesions recorded at slaughter and how the lesions affected the growth rate. Some of the conclusions were as follows:

□ Mortality was lower in houses with solid manure handling and an open dunging passage than in those with liquid manure handling and slatted flooring in the dunging passage

□ The incidence of pneumonia was lowest in pigs housed under the following conditions: Production strictly in batches Stocking density less than 500 pigs per section Space volume of more than 3 m.^{3} per pig Floor space of more than 0.7 m.^{2} per pig Solid manure handling system rather than liquid manure handling system

□ The average daily gain in pigs with severe pneumonia at slaughter was significantly lower than in pigs without lung lesions at slaughter. There were no differences in growth rate between pigs with mild pneumonia as the sole pathological lesion and those without lung lesions at slaughter

□ The incidence of pleurisy and pericarditis was also lowest in pigs housed in sections with less than 500 pigs per section, when production was strictly in batches, and when

the available floor space was more than 0.7 m.^{2} per pig. The incidence of pleurisy was highest during the warm period from May to October, and the average daily gain was lower in pigs with pleurisy than in those without pleural lesions at slaughter

In an overall assessment of the results, it is concluded that health status would generally appear to be better in houses with production strictly in batches, less than 500 pigs per section, a volume of at least 3 m.^{3} per pig, a total area (lying area + area in dunging passage) of at least 0.7 m.^{2} per pig, a solid manure handling system in the house, and free access to drinking water. It also is concluded that, of the studied environmental factors, the system of rearing has the greatest influence on animal health.

Lindqvist also indicates that 250 to 300 pigs would appear to be an optimum number per section and that trough feeding is preferable to floor feeding, the latter promoting the fecal-oral route of infection.

It was also evident that an assessment of the health status based entirely on observations made at slaughter must—for drawing definite conclusions—be complemented by a veterinary assessment of the animals in their environment during the period of production. If this is not done, essential information on the general clinical condition and behavior of the animals will be lacking, as will be data on diseases that are not recorded at slaughter.

The best evidence suggests that infection of the respiratory tract combined with environmental stressors such as inadequate ventilation and overcrowding results in clinical and subclinical pneumonia. The control of respiratory disease will depend on preventing the introduction of infected animals into the herd and on the provision of adequate housing and ventilation.

EPIDEMIOLOGY OF THE INFECTIOUS ENTERITIDES IN GROWING AND FINISHING PIGS. There is very little published information on the epidemiology of the infectious enteritides in growing and finishing pigs. Swine dysentery due to *Treponema hyodysenteriae* is the most common infectious enteritis of feeder pigs, and the intestinal adenomatosis complex and enteric salmonellosis occur sporadically. The factors that would be important in the epidemiology of an infectious enteritis that is transmitted by the fecal-oral cycle, such as swine dysentery, would logically include the feeding system and whether or not the pigs are fed on the floor or in feed troughs; the stocking density of the pen and the degree of over-crowding; the ease with which the pen can be cleaned; the adequacy of partitions between pens; the effectiveness of the dunging area in the pen; the effectiveness of regular complete depopulation of the pen when the pigs are marketed, followed by cleaning and disinfection and a period of vacancy before being occupied by the next group of pigs; and whether or not carrier pigs are introduced into the pens at the beginning of the feeding period.

In general, the housing and feeding systems must be designed and maintained so that transmission of disease by the fecal-oral route is minimized.

Management of Disease and Production During the Growing and Finishing Periods

The control of the economically important diseases and the management of production of pigs during these periods require a high level of animal production management and the adoption of disease control techniques designed for intensively reared animals. These will include the following:

1. Specific disease eradication policy
2. *All-in-all-out* production system
3. Adequate housing and ventilation (pen design, manure disposal, floor surfaces, ventilation system)
4. Feeds and feeding
5. Strategic medication of feed and water
6. Vaccination and use of anthelmintics and insecticides
7. Performance testing and selection of breeding stock
8. Continuous surveillance of animal health and production
9. Careful handling and transportation

A description of each of these requirements or techniques is presented here.

1. Specific Disease Eradication Policy. Certain diseases such as enzootic pneumonia and swine dysentery can be eradicated from the herd by the adoption of the Specific Pathogen-Free Herd or Minimal Disease Herd policy in which the breeding stock are cesarean- or hysterectomy-derived. The piglets are not in contact with the sows and are reared in isolation until they reach puberty, when they are transferred to the facilities. All breeding stock in the new herd are derived this way, and with strict security precautions, the herd remains free of the specific pathogens.

In self-contained, purebred, or commercial farrow-to-finish enterprises, the common infectious respiratory and enteric diseases can be controlled satisfactorily by the adoption of techniques designed to prevent entry of disease into the herd and by the provision of an adequate housing system.

2. All-in-All-out. Every effort should be made to ensure that a previously cleaned and disinfected pen in the finishing barn is filled with a group of pigs on one day, reared as a group throughout their growing and finishing periods, and if possible, the pen is completely depopulated at the end of the finishing period. However, not all pigs in the pen will be ready for market on the same day. If possible, pigs moved from the weaner pens (nursery) should be maintained as a group and placed in a pen by themselves in the finishing barn. This minimizes the stress associated with the change in feeding and environment.

3. Housing and Ventilation. Confined housing for growing-finishing swine may be provided in the form of completely enclosed, modified open-front, and open-front buildings. Most enclosed buildings are insulated and have mechanical ventilation, auxiliary heat, and partially or fully slatted floors or solid floors. Modified open-front buildings rely on natural ventilation, do not have auxiliary heat, and may be open on one side, whereas open-front structures are generally uninsulated, open on one side, and have feeders and waterers located in outside concrete lots.

The basic requirements for housing growing-finishing pigs include a warm, dry, and draft-free environment. Extremes of ambient temperature in the building, excessive air movement, and extremes of relative humidity can adversely affect rate of daily gain, feed consumption, and feed efficiency (Wahlstrom 1981).

Floor surfaces in swine barns can influence foot health (Cement and Concrete Assoc. 1978). Surveys indicate that 50 to 60% of pigs examined at slaughter may have foot lesions (Newton et al. 1980). Field trials to determine the effect of types of floor slats on performance and certain feet and leg characteristics of growing-finishing swine indicate the complex nature of the effect of floor surfaces (Newton et al. 1980). Lack of adequate exercise and hard flooring in confinement rearing systems are suggested as major contributing factors to leg weakness and osteochondrosis in growing-finishing swine, especially young boars in performance (Nakano et al. 1981). However, placing affected animals on pasture only slightly improves the gait. Shortening the length of the performance test period and increasing the opportunity for animal exercise may help to alleviate the problem (Fredeen and Sather 1978). The genetic aspects of feet and leg soundness in swine have been examined and the results are inconclusive (Bereskin 1979).

The design of the pens should provide for adequate floor drainage, easy cleaning, ease of daily inspection of pigs, adequate ventilation, and effective manure disposal. The walls between pens should be of solid construction and not wire-mesh fence, which allows the spread of infections between pens. The stocking rate should follow recommended guidelines. The location of the feeders, waterers, and dunging areas must reduce the fecal-oral route of infection.

It is assumed that an adequate ventilation system is necessary for the control and prevention of infectious respiratory disease.

4. Feeds and Feeding. The nutritional diseases of pigs during the growing and finishing phases of production are largely under control. The nutritional requirements of the growing and fattening pig are sufficiently well known that specific nutritional deficiency should not occur. The exception would be selenium and vitamin E deficiency diseases, which may occur in pigs receiving an adequate diet. Most of the activity in nutritional research of the growing and finishing pig deals with refinements of specific nutrient requirements and the source, digestibility, and utilization of specific nutrients. Major problems still exist in the systems of feeding the finishing pig in order to achieve the optimum carcass score within the genetic capability of the pig. A variety of feeding systems are available; each has advantages and disadvantages, which vary from farm to farm depending on the level of management, the type of housing, and the feeds used.

Veterinarians specializing in swine herd health and production are providing nutritional consultation to swine producers who mix and formulate their own rations on the farm. Home-grown or purchased grains are mixed with a purchased protein-mineral-vitamin concentrate mix. This requires a regular system of analyses of the feed grains used. A record of the total amount of feed used during the period is vital information for the assessment of feed efficiency from weaning to market.

5. Strategic Medication of Feed and Water. When epidemics of infectious diseases occur during the growing-finishing periods, antimicrobials may be added to the feed and water supplies, initially at therapeutic levels for up to several days, then followed by prophylactic levels for a few weeks. They should be used selectively and strategically to control or eradicate specific infectious diseases. Their routine indiscriminate use should be avoided because of cost, the possible development of drug-resistant pathogens, and the false sense of security that develops in the herdsman.

Swine dysentery can be eradicated from a herd by the judicious use of mass medication of the feed of the entire herd.

In swine feeder operations that purchase weaned pigs from a variety of sources, each with a different spectrum of diseases, the incidence of infectious disease of the respiratory and intestinal tracts is usually much higher than in self-contained herds, and there is no reliable method for control. The best that can be done is to provide the most comfortable environment that is economically possible, treat individual sick pigs as they are detected, submit dead pigs for necropsy, mass medicate at strategic times if appropriate, and practice the all-in–all-out method of filling and complete emptying of the pens, including the cleaning and disinfection of the pens between groups of pigs.

The diagnosis must be as accurate as possible if mass medication of the feed and water is used as a method of treatment of the herd. Mass medication of feed and water supplies of feeder pigs is not without problems. In addition to the costs, it is not always possible to medicate feed supplies that are already in place in storage on the farm, and the medication of water supplies is often difficult to do selectively unless there is a double waterline in each pen, one of which can be turned off. Medication of the entire watering system may not be necessary and is expensive. The withdrawal period for each feed additive must be followed to avoid drug residues in meat supplies.

6. Vaccination and Use of Anthelmintics and Insecticides. In herds that encounter epidemics of pneumonia due to *Hemophilus pleuropneumoniae*, vaccination with a bacterin of all pigs in the growing-finishing group may be indicated. Vaccinations for atrophic rhinitis and erysipelas are done at an earlier age.

Anthelmintics and insecticides should be used when indicated for the control of intestinal helminthiasis and skin diseases caused by arthropods. However, control of these diseases is most effectively accomplished by regular treatment of the adult stock, which minimizes spread to the weaned and growing pigs.

7. Performance Testing and Selection of Breeding Stock. In purebred herds, the selection of breeding stock as herd replacements or for sale to other herds will begin when the pigs are about four to five months of age. Selection will be based on conformation, number of functional teats in gilts, and backfat thickness determination in boars, combined with weight for age.

Those herds that sell breeding stock must ensure that their pigs are not subclinical carriers of infectious disease agents such as the virus of transmissible gastroenteritis, *Leptospira* spp., Aujeszky's disease virus, and *Treponema hyodysenteriae.*

Herds that import breeding stock from other herds should attempt to determine the infectious disease status of the herd of origin. Under ideal conditions, imported breeding stock would be quarantined in isolation facilities and subjected to several laboratory examinations for the presence of the common pathogens. However, these examinations are not yet sufficiently reliable to be recommended for general use.

In commercial herds producing hybrid pigs for market, positive identification of pigs and their dam and sire is necessary for an effective cross-breeding program.

The role of the veterinarian in assisting the producer in the selection of breeding stock and breeding programs has been minimal. However, swine veterinary specialists should be familiar with the general aspects of the breeding program and how breeding stock are selected and should ensure that genetic progress is being made.

Congenital defects in newborn piglets should be identified and action taken to cull carrier parents.

8. Continuous Surveillance of Animal Health and Production. Pigs in the growing and finishing pens must be visually inspected twice daily for evidence of clinical disease. Dead pigs must be removed from the pen and submitted for necropsy as soon as possible. A daily record of the number of pigs with clinical disease and the treatments given must be kept and reviewed by the veterinarian at each herd health visit. An annual report should be prepared, and recommendations for specific action should be submitted to the producer.

The average days to market and the amount of feed used for a group of pigs or the total number of pigs over the entire feeding period is vital information.

9. Careful Handling and Transportation at Time of Shipping to Abattoir. Finished pigs identified for shipment to the abattoir must be handled as carefully as possible during sorting and loading to prevent the porcine stress syndrome and pale soft exudative pork. Overcrowding in the transport vehicle must be avoided, and during hot weather, transportation should be done during the cooler parts of the day.

The handling facilities at the abattoir should be designed to minimize excitement and stress associated with the movement of animals during weighing, crowding, sorting, and killing (Grandin 1982).

THE WELFARE OF PIGS

The aims of modern pig rearing are directed toward a constant improvement of productivity. The resulting rearing conditions are more and more removed from the original way of life of the wild animal. The fundamental characteristic of wild boar and feral hog populations is their great adaptability to environmental conditions. This characteristic permits the use of a large range of rearing systems, extensive or intensive, to which the species can adapt (Mauget 1981).

There is now growing worldwide concern for the welfare of pigs raised intensively in total confinement. Some countries have enacted legislation that states the minimum housing and management requirements (Bogner 1981). These minimum requirements include the following:

1. The possibility of being able to stand up or lie down in a manner characteristic of the species and to adopt a relaxed position, e.g., pigs lying on their side with stretched limbs. This necessitates sufficient space.

2. During the rearing period, young animals should be given enough space to satisfy their instinct of play (running, play, and fighting). This requires a suitable floor.

3. The floors of stalls or pens should allow the animals to tread and stand safely and to lie down without suffering injury. Perforated floors do not always fulfill these demands. Therefore, at least the resting area should be bedded with a material like straw. Dry straw is an irresistible attraction to any pig, since it occupies and distracts them. Behavioral dis-

turbances such as ear-chewing or tail-biting may be reduced by the presence of straw. Bedded floors also decrease the need for high ambient temperature.

4. A restricted feeding system requires sufficient space for each animal at the trough. Care should be taken that the animals disturb each other as little as possible.

5. To avoid placing individual animals at disadvantage, they should be kept in groups of uniform sizes.

6. The environment (microclimate) of the animal must be appropriate for the particular age group.

The welfare of the intensively reared pig, its environment, and the incidence of disease are interrelated (Ekesbo 1981). Sows kept in confinement are exposed to more stress factors than sows kept free in pens. Backstrom (1973) found a definite relationship between herd size and increased frequency of toxemic agalactia, traumatic injuries in sows, piglet morbidity, and mortality. The health of litters in pens with straw as bedding was superior to that of litters in pens with other bedding materials. Litters in pens without bedding showed the poorest results. Herds in houses with liquid manure handling systems were associated with poorer pig health than those with solid manure handling systems. Postlactational anestrus as presented in an earlier section is a major problem in sows confined in individual stalls compared with being free in pens.

IMPORTATION OF BREEDING STOCK INTO BREEDING UNITS

A major problem in the establishment of new swine breeding units and introduction of replacement animals into existing herds is the source of the breeding stock. Clinically normal gilts and boars may be latent carriers of infectious agents, which may be shed and spread to resident animals in the herd, resulting in an epidemic. This is particularly important in large herds of 250 to 500 sows, in which an epidemic can cause major economic losses. The larger the unit, the greater the investment and the loss if disease occurs. Outbreaks of infectious disease tend to be more serious, to persist longer, and to be more difficult to control in larger units. Some notable examples of diseases that can be introduced by carrier animals include transmissible gastroenteritis, enzootic pneumonia, Aujeszky's disease, swine dysentery, leptospirosis, and turbinate atrophy. This creates a conflict between the desire to prevent the introduction of infectious diseases and the need to introduce new genes in order to make genetic progress.

Until about 1960, the purebred breeder was the source of pedigreed gilts and boars. The only assurance that the purchaser had of obtaining breeding stock free of the endemic diseases was the statement made by the seller that the herd was not recently affected with the diseases. This was not and is still not reliable. There is no effective method for determining that imported breeding stock are not carriers of the diseases previously mentioned.

Government-sponsored central performance-test stations were popular from 1960 to 1975, and they emphasized the identification of select breeding stock by testing animals for highly heritable traits such as growth rate, feed conversion, and carcass quality. Disease control in these centers was less than desirable because test animals came from many sources and were housed together at the stations, and following the test, the boars would be purchased as breeding stock and be introduced into herds.

The need for high-quality breeding stock free of several common diseases soon became obvious and led to the development of multiple-herd breeding networks known as a breeding pyramid (Fig. 11–12) (Heard 1978). In this network, nucleus herds supply breeding stock to multiplier herds, which in turn supply breeding stock to commercial farms. The nucleus herd is established from hysterectomy-derived piglets raised in isolation and known as Specific Pathogen-Free or Minimal Disease pigs. In the simple pyramid system, the nucleus herd is a closed unit, and all replacements are hysterectomy-derived pigs (Melrose 1977). The health standard and disease security system must be of a high standard. The multiplier herds supply breeding stock to the commercial herds, which in turn produce pigs for slaughter.

Theoretically, a 500-sow nucleus herd can provide replacements for 6000 grandparents in

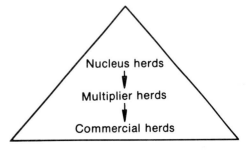

Figure 11–12. The pyramid system.

Table 11-15. CONSTRAINTS ASSOCIATED WITH POSSIBLE METHODS FOR CONTROL OF INFECTIOUS DISEASES IN SWINE BREEDING HERDS

Program Applicable In	I Minimal Disease (MD) or Specific Pathogen-Free (SPF)	II Eradication of Specific Diseases	III Health Control by Improved Husbandry, Preventive Medicine, and Medication
National herd	Very expensive, difficult to implement and maintain	Adopted in most countries for appropriate disease, i.e., hog cholera	Very expensive in terms of special advisers; usually available specialist manpower is inadequate
Cooperative herds	Herd breakdowns (approximately 6% per year) can be expected	Not commonly adopted for this alone; if disease suitable for eradication, national program is preferable	Can be applied and if discipline is good, groups will protect each other; some disciplinary control of groups necessary
Individual herds	Nucleus breeding herds have found this very beneficial when there is no lateral interchange of pigs	Can be applied to diseases that are not eradicable on a national basis, but there is a risk of herd breakdown unless strict isolation is practiced	A practical approach; can be cost-effective

multiplier herds. Multiplier herds can provide replacements for 90,000 parents in commercial herds, which in turn can produce 1.5 million slaughter pigs per year.

Pyramids are becoming popular in North America and Western Europe. In the U.K., they supply 75% of the replacement gilts and 50% of the boars.

Disease Control in Breeding Herds

Disease control is necessary at three levels—the national level, the cooperative herd level, and the individual herd level (Table 11-15).

Diseases such as foot and mouth disease, swine vesicular disease, vesicular exanthema, hog cholera, African swine fever, and other so-called exotic diseases are controlled at the national level. National disease eradication schemes, which economically benefit the whole swine industry, have been effective in controlling these diseases.

In the cooperative or multiple-herd breeding pyramid system, disease control is directed toward those common diseases that can cause epidemics and large economic losses. They include transmissible gastroenteritis, Aujeszky's disease, enzootic pneumonia, swine dysentery, atrophic rhinitis, parvovirus infection, vomiting and wasting disease, and sarcoptic mange. Successful control begins in the nucleus herds, which are hysterectomy-derived and remain closed to the introduction of live pigs. Animals move from the nucleus herds to the multiplier and commercial herds, never back to the nucleus. This is known as straight-line distribution (Alexander 1978). Some modification exists for the lateral exchange of breeding stock between nucleus herds and between multiplier herds.

Review Literature

Agriculture Canada. Confinement Swine Housing Publication 1451, 1981.

Bosc, M.J., Martinat-Botte, F. and Terqui, M. Practical uses of prostaglandins in pigs. Acta Vet. Scand. 77 (Suppl.): 209-226, 1981.

Bruce, J.M. Ventilation and temperature control criteria for pigs. In: Environmental Aspects of Housing for Animal Production. J.A. Clark (Ed.), Butterworths, London, 1981.

Christenson, R.K. and Ford, J.J. Puberty and estrus in confinement-reared gilts. J. Anim. Sci., 49:743-751, 1979.

Close, W.H. The climatic requirements of the pig. In: Environmental Aspects of Housing for Animal Production. J.A. Clark (Ed.), Butterworths, London, 1981.

Curtis, S.E. Environmental management in animal agriculture. Iowa State University Press, Ames, 1983, pp. 1-409.

Edwards, B.L. Causes of death in new-born pigs. Vet. Bull., 42:249-258, 1972.

Fredeen, H.T. and Marmon, B.G. The swine industry: Changes and challenges. J. Anim. Sci., 57(Suppl. 2): 100-118, 1983.

Heard, T.W. Methods of approach to the diagnosis and resolution of pig health problems. Br. Vet. J., 137:337-347, 1981.

Henry, D.P. Mating management in pigs. Aust. Vet. J., 48:258-262, 1972.

Hughes, P.E. Factors affecting the natural attainment of puberty in the gilt. In: Control of Pig Reproduction Proc. 33rd Easter School in Agric. Sci., Univ. of Nottingham, 1982, pp. 117-138. D.J.A. Cole and G.R. Foxcroft (Eds.).

Hughes, P.E. and Varley, M.A. Reproduction in the Pig. London, Butterworths, 1980.

Hurtgen, J.P. Influence of housing and management factors on reproductive efficiency of swine. J. Am. Vet. Med. Assoc., 179:74-78, 1981.

Kirkwood, R.N. and Hughes, P.E. Puberty in the gilt—the role of boar stimulation. Pig News and Info., 3:389-394, 1982.

LeDividich, J. and Aumaitre, A. Housing and climatic conditions for early weaned piglets. Livestock Prod. Sci., 5:71-80, 1978.

LeDividich, J. and Aumaitre, A. Housing and climatic conditions for early weaned piglets. Livestock Prod. Sci., 5:78-80, 1978.

Meredith, M.J. The treatment of anestrus in the pig: A review. Vet. Rec., 104:25-27, 1979.

Meredith, M.J. Anestrus in the pig: Diagnosis and etiology. Ir. Vet. J., 36:17-24, 1982.

Muirhead, M.R. The methods and problems of practicing preventive medicine in the pig industry. Vet. Ann., 19:108-114, 1979.

Muirhead, M.R. Pig housing and environment. Vet. Rec., 113:587-593, 1983.

Penny, R.H.C. Preventive medicine for pigs. Vet. Ann., 18:117-125, 1978.

Perry, G.C. The role of olfaction in the reproductive behavior of pigs. Pig News and Info., 3:11-15, 1982.

Sybesma, W. (Ed.). The Welfare of Pigs. Current Topics in Veterinary Medicine and Animal Science. Vol. II, pp. 1-334, 1981.

Wrathall, A.E. Prenatal survival in pigs. Part 1. Ovulation rate and its influence on prenatal survival and litter size in pigs. Review Series No. 9 of the Commonwealth Bureau of Animal Health, 1971, pp. 1-108.

References

Adams, K.L., Baker, T.H. and Jensen, A.H. Effect of supplemental heat for nursing piglets. J. Anim. Sci., 50:779-782, 1980.

Alexander, T.J.L. Pig movement: Health and control in a breeding pyramid. Pig Vet. Soc. Proc., 3:21-28, 1978.

Alexander, T.J.L., Thornton, K., Boon, G. et al. Medicated early weaning to obtain pigs free from pathogens endemic in the herd of origin. Vet. Rec., 106:114-119, 1980.

Andersen, H. Studies of the relationships between herd size, the percentage of pigs culled during the finishing period and the prevalence rate at slaughter of pigs with lesions. Nord. Vet. Med., 33:413-416, 1981.

Anderson, J.F. and Werdin, R.E. Ergotism manifested as agalactia and gangrene in sow. J. Am. Vet. Assoc., 170:1089–1091, 1977.

Animal Housing Injuries Due to Floor Surfaces. Proc. Symp. held at Cement and Concrete Assoc., Fulmer, Grange, Slough, Berks, England. Nov. 1978, pp. 1–177.

Armstrong, W.D. and Clauson, A.J. Nutrition and management of early weaned pigs: Effect of increased nutrient concentration and(or) supplemental liquid feeding. J. Anim. Sci., 50:377–384, 1980.

Aumaitre, A. Optimum age of weaning piglets. Livestock Prod. Sci., 5:1–2, 1978.

Backstrom, L. Environmental and animal health in piglet production: A field study of incidences and correlations. Acta Vet. Scand. Suppl. 41, 1973, pp. 1–240.

Backstrom, L. and Bremer, H. The relationship between disease incidence of fatteners registered at slaughter and environmental factors in herds. Nord. Vet. Med., 30:526–533, 1978.

Balke, J.M.E. and Elmore, R.G. Pregnancy diagnosis in swine: A comparison of the technique of rectal palpation and ultrasound. Theriogenology, 17:231–236, 1982.

Ball, R.O. and Aherne, X. Effect of diet complexity and feed restriction on the incidence and severity of diarrhea in early-weaned pigs. Can. J. Anim. Sci., 62:907–913, 1982.

Baxter, S.H. and Robertson, A.M. Pig housing—the last ten years. Pig News and Info., 1:21–24, 1980.

Benjaminsen, E. and Karlberg, K. Post-weaning estrus and luteal function in primiparous and pluriparous sows. Res. Vet. Sci., 30:318–322, 1981.

Bereskin, B. Genetic aspects of feet and leg soundness in swine. J. Anim Sci., 48:1322–1328, 1979.

Beynon, V.H. The economics of pig disease: The cost of disease in the pig industry. Pig Vet. Soc. Proc., 2:83–92, 1978.

Bille, N., Nielsen, N.C. and Svendsen, J. Preweaning mortality in pigs. 3. Traumatic injuries. Nord. Vet. Med., 26:617–625, 1974.

Bille, N., Nielsen, N.C., Larsen, J.L. et al. Preweaning mortality in pigs. 2. The perinatal period. Nord. Vet. Med., 26:294–313, 1974.

Blecha, F., Pollmann, D.S. and Nichols, D.A. Weaning pigs at an early age decreases cellular immunity. J. Anim. Sci., 56:396–400, 1983.

Bogner, H. Animal welfare in agriculture—a challenge for the etiology. In: The Welfare of Pigs. Current Topics in Veterinary Medicine and Animal Science. Vol. II, pp. 46–50, 1981.

Boland, M.P. and Herlihey, M.J. Induction of parturition in pig using a new prostaglandin analogue (K11941). Theriogenology, 17:193–197, 1982.

Bolitho, W.S. The economics of pig disease: The cost to the meat processor. Pig Vet. Soc. Proc., 2:93–99, 1978.

Bourne, F.J. Humoral immunity in the pig. Vet. Rec., 98:499–501, 1980.

Bourne, F.J. and Newby, T.J. Mucosal immunity in the pig. Pig News and Info., 2:141–144, 1981.

Cameron, R.D.A. Pregnancy diagnosis in the sow by rectal examination. Aust. Vet. J., 53:432–435, 1977.

Campbell, R.G. The response of early-weaned pigs to various protein levels in a high energy diet. Anim. Prod., 24:69–75, 1977.

Christenson, R.K. and Ford, J.J. Puberty and estrus in confinement-reared gilts. J. Anim. Sci., 49:743–751, 1979.

Clauson, A.J. Influences on the neonatal pig. Feedstuffs. Sept. 4, 1978, pp. 20–22.

Conrad, J.H. and V.B. Mayrose. Animal waste handling and disposal in confinement production of swine. J. Anim. Sci., 32:811–815, 1971.

Cutler, R.S., Molitor, T.W., Leman, A.D. et al. Farm studies of porcine parvovirus infection. J. Am. Vet. Med. Assoc., 182:592–594, 1983.

Dagorn, J. and Aumaitre, A. Sow culling: Reasons for and effect on productivity. Livestock Prod. Sci., 6:167–177, 1979.

Davies, G., Basinger, D., Farndale, J., et al. Pig Health and Production Recording. 1983. Booklet 2075. Ministry of Agriculture, Fisheries, and Food. Central Veterinary Laboratory, New Haw, Weybridge, Surrey, England KT153NB, pp. 1–59.

Day, B.N. Reproductive problems in swine. Beltsville Symp. in Agric. Res., Anim. Reprod., pp. 41–50, 1979.

Donaldson-Wood, C.R., Joo, H.S. and Johnson, R.H. The effect on reproductive performance of porcine parvovirus infection in a susceptible pig herd. Vet. Rec., 100:237–239, 1977.

Dyck, G. Postweaning changes in the reproductive tract of the sow. Can. J. Anim. Sci., 63:571–577, 1983.

Dyck, G.W. and Strain, J.H. Postmating feeding level effects on conception rate and embryonic survival in gilts. Can. J. Anim. Sci., 63:519–585, 1983.

Dziuk, P. Control and mechanics of parturition in the pig. Anim. Rep. Sci., 2:335–342, 1979.

Edwards, B.L. Causes of death in new-born pigs. Vet. Bull., 42:249–258, 1972.

Ehnvall, R., Blomquist, A., Einarsson, S. et al. Culling gilts with special reference to reproductive failure. Nord. Vet. Med., 33:161–171, 1981.

Einarsson, S., Larsson, K. and Backstrom, L. On agalactia post-partum in the sow. II. A hematological and blood chemical study in affected and healthy sows. Nord. Vet. Med., 30:474–481, 1978.

Einarsson, S., Larsson, K. and Backstrom, L. On agalactia post-partum in the sow. 1. A clinical study. Nord. Vet. Med., 30:465–473, 1975.

Ekesko, I. Some aspects of sow health and housing. In: The Welfare of Pigs. Current Topics in Veterinary Medicine and Animal Science. Vol. II, pp. 250–266, 1981.

Elliot, J.I., King, G.J. and Robertson, H.A. Reproductive performance of the sow subsequent to weaning piglets at birth. Can. J. Anim. Sci., 60:65–71, 1980.

English, P.R. and Smith, W.J. Some causes of death in neonatal pigs. Vet. Ann., 15:95–104, 1975.

Fahmy, M.H. Factors influencing the weaning to estrus interval in swine: A review. World Review of Anim. Prod., (2)17:15–28, April–June 1981.

Fiebiger, K., Kaiser, H. and Traeder, W. Preventive treatment of metritis-mastitis-agalactia syndrome in sows. Tier. Umbschau, 30:251–256, 1975.

Flesja, K.I. and Solberg, I. Pathological lesions in swine at slaughter. IV. Pathological lesions in relation to rearing system and herd size. Acta Vet. Scand., 22:272–282, 1981.

Flesja, K.I. and Ulvesaeter, H.O. Pathological lesions in swine at slaughter. I. Baconers. Acta Vet. Scand, 20:498–514, 1979a.

Flesja, K.I. and Ulvesaeter, H.O. Pathological lesions in swine at slaughter. II. Culled sows. Acta Vet. Scand., 20:515–524, 1979b.

Flesja, K.I. and Ulvesaeter, H.O. Pathological lesions in swine at slaughter. III. Inter-relationship between pathological lesions, and between pathological lesions and (1) carcass quality and (2) carcass weight. Acta Vet. Scand. 74(Suppl.):1–22, 1980.

Flesja, K.I., Forus, I.B. and Solberg, I. Pathological lesions in swine at slaughter. V. Pathological lesions in relation to some environmental factor in the herds. Acta Vet. Scand., 23:169–183, 1982.

Fowler, V.R. The nutrition of weaner pigs. Pig News and Info., 1:11–15, 1980.

Fraser, D. Observation on the behavioral development of suckling and early weaned piglets during the first six weeks after birth. Anim. Behav., 26:22–30, 1978.

Fredeen, H.T. Pig breeding: Current programs vs. future production requirements. Can. J. Anim. Sci., 60: 241–251, 1980.

Fredeen, H.T. and Harmon, B.G. The swine industry: Changes and challenges. J. Anim. Sci., 57(Suppl. 2): 100–118, 1983.

Fredeen, H.T. and Sather, A.P. Joint damage in pigs reared under confinement. Can. J. Anim. Sci., 58:759–773, 1978.

Friendship, R.M., Bosu, W.T.K. and King, G.J. Reproductive performance in sows treated with estradiol benzoate human chorionic gonadotrophin combination at weaning. Can. J. Comp. Med., 46:410–413, 1982.

Gadd, J. The economics of weaning pigs at different ages. Pig Vet. Soc. Proc., 7:1–11, 1981.

Gardner, J.A.A. and Stewart, M.C. Pig production in Australia. Pig News and Info., 3:283–287, 1982.

Glastonbury, J.R.W. Preweaning mortality in the pig. Pathological findings in piglets dying before and during parturition. Aust. Vet. J., 53:282–286, 1977a.

Glastonbury, J.R.W. Preweaning mortality in the pig. Pathological findings in piglets dying between birth and weaning. Aust. Vet. J., 53:310–314, 1977b.

Glastonbury, J.R.W. Preweaning mortality in the pig. The prevalence of various causes of preweaning mortality and the importance of some contributory factors. Aust. Vet. J., 53:315–318, 1977c.

Goodwin, R.F.W. A procedure for investigating the influence of disease status on productive efficiency in a pig herd. Vet. Rec., 88:387–392, 1971.

Govier, R.J. The economics of pig disease: A method of calculation of the on the farm cost. Pig Vet. Soc. Proc., 2:101–111, 1978.

Grandin, T. Pig behavior studies applied to slaughter-plant design. Appl. Anim. Ethol., 9:141–151, 1982.

Hammond, D. and Matty, G. A farrowing management system using cloprostenol to control the time of parturition. Vet. Rec., 106:72–75, 1980.

Hausler, C.L., Hodson, H.H., Kuo, D.C. et al. Induced ovulation and conception in lactating sows. J. Anim. Sci., 50:773–778, 1980.

Hays, V.W. and Muir, W.M. Efficacy and safety of feed additive use of antibacterial drugs in animal production. Can. J. Anim. Sci., 59:447–456, 1979.

Hays, V.W., Krug, J.L., Cromwell, G.L. et al. Effect on lactation length and dietary antibiotics on reproductive performance of sows. J. Anim. Sci., 46:884–891, 1978.

Heard, T.W. Pig movement: Health and control in a breeding pyramid. Pig Vet. Soc. Proc., 3:29–36, 1978.

Henry, D.P. Mating management in pigs. Aust. Vet. J., 48:258–262, 1972.

Hughes, P.E. and Cole, D.J.A. Reproduction in the gilt. 2. The influence of gilt age at boar introduction on the attainment of puberty. Anim. Prod., 23:89–94, 1976.

Hughes, P.E. and Varley, M.A. Reproduction in the Pig. London, Butterworths, 1980.

Hurtgen, J.P. Influence of housing and management factors on reproductive efficiency of swine. J. Am. Vet. Med. Assoc., 179:74–78, 1981.

Hurtgen, J.P. and Leman, A.D. Seasonal influence on the fertility of sows and gilts. J. Am. Vet. Med. Assoc., 177:631–635, 1980.

Hurtgen, J.P., Leman, A.D. and Crabo, Bo. Seasonal influence on estrus activity in sows and gilts. J. Am. Vet. Med. Assoc., 176:119–123, 1980.

Husband, A.J. and Bennell, M.A. Intestinal immunity in pigs. Pig News and Info., 1:211–213, 1980.

Inoue, T., Kitano, K. and Inoue, K. Possible factors influencing the Ig concentration in swine colostrum. Am. J. Vet. Res., 42:1429–1432, 1981.

Jackson, P.S. and Hutchinson, F.G. Slow release formulation of prostaglandin and luteolysis in the pig. Vet. Rec., 106:33–34, 1980.

Jainudeen, M.R. and Brandenburg, A.C. Induction of parturition in crossbred sows with cloprostenol. An analogue of prostaglandin F-2 alpha. Anim. Rep. Sci., 3:161–166, 1980.

Jeppesen, L.E. Behavioral vices in young pigs. Pig Vet. Soc. Proc., 7:43–53, 1981.

Jones, J.E.T. An investigation of the causes of mortality and morbidity in sows in a commercial herd. Br. Vet. J., 123:327–339, 1967.

Jones, J.E.T. The cause of death in sows. A one year survey of 106 herds in Essex. Br. Vet. J., 124:45–55, 1968.

Jones, J.E.T. The incidence and nature of diseases causing death in pigs aged 2 to 7 months in a commercial herd. Br. Vet. J., 125:492–505, 1969.

Jones, J.E.T. Acute coliform mastitis in the sow. Vet. Ann., 19:97–101, 1979.

Karlberg, K. Factors affecting post-weaning estrus in the sow. Nord. Vet. Med., 32:185–193, 1980.

Kelley, K.W. Environmental effects on the immune system of pigs. Pig News and Info., 3:395–399, 1982.

Kelley, K.W., Blecha, F. and Regnier, J.A. Cold exposure and absorption of colostral immunoglobulin by neonatal pigs. J. Anim. Sci., 55:363–368, 1982.

Kelly, G.R. Feasibility and design of a microcomputer swine unit information system. M.S. Thesis University of Saskatchewan, Saskatoon, Saskatchewan, 1983, pp. 1–222.

Kidder, D.E. Nutrition of the early weaned pig compared with the sow-reared pig. Pig News and Info., 3:25–28, 1982.

King, G.J., Robertson, H.A. and Elliot, J.I. Induced parturition in swine herds. Can. Vet. J., 20:157–160, 1979.

King, G.J., Walton, J.S. and Bosu, W.T.K. Potential treatment for anestrus in sows and gilts. Can. Vet. J., 23:288–290, 1982.

Kirkbride, C.A. and McAdaragh, J.P. Infectious agents associated with fetal and early neonatal death and abortion in swine. J. Am. Vet. Med. Assoc., 172: 480–483, 1978.

Kirkwood, R.N. and Hughes, P.E. Puberty in the gilt—the role of boar stimulation. Pig News and Info., 3:389–394, 1982.

Klobasa, F., Werhahn, E. and Butler, J.E. Regulation of humoral immunity in the piglet by immunoglobulins of maternal origin. Res. Vet. Sci., 31:195–206, 1981.

Kornegay, E.T., Ogunbameru, B.O., Collins, E.R. et al. Double and triple decking of pigs to increase nursing capacity. J. Anim. Sci., 49:39–43, 1980a.

Kornegay, E.T., Thomas, H.R., Arthur, S.R. et al. Pigs per cage, flooring materials and use of soybean hulls in starter diets for pigs housed in triple deck nurseries. J. Anim. Sci., 51:285–293, 1980b.

Lasley, J.F. Genetics of Livestock Improvement. Prentice-Hall, Englewood Cliffs, NJ, 1980.

Lecce, J.G., Armstrong, W.D., Crawford, P.C. et al. Nutrition and management of early weaned piglets: Liquid vs. dry feeding. J. Anim. Sci., 48:1007-1014, 1979.

LeDividich, J. and Aumaitre, A. Housing and climatic conditions for early weaned pigs. Livestock Prod. Sci., 5:71-80, 1978.

LeDividich, J. and Nicolet, J. Colostrum intake and thermoregulation in the neonatal pig in relation to environmental temperature. Biol. Neonate, 40:167-174, 1981.

Leman, A.D. and Rodeffer, H.E. Boar management. Vet. Rec., 98:457-459, 1976.

Leman, A.D., Knudson, C., Rodeffer, J.E. et al. Reproductive performance of swine on 76 Illinois farms. J. Am. Vet. Med. Assoc., 161:1248-1250, 1972.

Lindqvist, J-O. Animal health and environment in the production of fattening pigs. A study of disease incidence in relation to certain environmental factors, daily weight gain and carcass classification. Acta. Vet. Scand. 51(Suppl.):1-78, 1974.

Lindvall, R.N. Effect of flooring material and number of pigs per pen on nursery performance. J. Anim. Sci., 53:863-868, 1981.

Little, T.W.A. Respiratory disease in pigs: A study. Vet. Rec., 96:540-544, 1975.

Love, R.J. Definition of a seasonal infertility problem in pigs. Vet. Rec., 103:443-446, 1978.

Mauget, R. Behavioral and reproductive strategies in wild forms of Sus scroba (European wild boar and feral pigs). In: The Welfare of Pigs. Current Topics in Veterinary Medicine and Animal Science. Vol. II, pp. 3-13, 1981.

McCaughey, W.J. and Rea, C.C. Pregnancy diagnosis in sows: A comparison of the vaginal biopsy and Doppler ultrasound techniques. Vet. Rec., 104:255-258, 1979.

McDonald, T.J. and McDonald, J.S. Intramammary infection in the sow during the peripartum period. Cornell Vet., 65:73-83, 1975.

McGloughlin, P. Genetic aspects of pigmeat quality. Pig News and Info., 1:5-9, 1980.

Melrose, D.R. Health control in pig selection programmes. Vet. Ann., 17:80-88, 1977.

Mengeling, W.L. and Paul, P.S. Reproductive performance of gilts exposed to porcine parvovirus at 56 or 70 days of gestation. Am. J. Vet. Res., 42:2074-2076, 1981.

Mengeling, W.L., Cutlip, R.C., Wilson, R.A. et al. Fetal mummification associated with porcine parvovirus infection. J. Am. Vet. Med. Assoc., 166:993-995, 1975.

Mengeling, W.L., Gutekunst, D.E., Pirtle, E.C. et al. Immunogenicity of bivalent vaccine for reproductive failure of swine reduced by pseudorabies virus and porcine parvovirus. Am. J. Vet. Res., 42:600-603, 1981.

Meredith, J.J. The detection of pregnancy in pigs. Part 1. Tests for pregnancy (audiotape, slides and booklet). Part 2. Choosing a pregnancy test (booklets). Unit for Veterinary Continuing Education, Royal Veterinary College, London, 1981.

Meredith, M.J. The treatment of anestrus in the pig: A review. Vet. Rec., 104:25-27, 1979.

Michel, E.J., Easter, R.A., Norton, H.W. et al. Effect of feeding frequency during gestation on reproductive performance of gilts and sows. J. Anim. Sci., 50:93-98, 1980.

Miller, B.G., Newby, T.J., Stokes, C.R. et al. Influence of diet on postweaning malabsorption and diarrhea in the pig. Res. Vet. Sci., 36:187-193, 1984.

Muirhead, M.R. Veterinary problems of intensive pig husbandry. Vet. Rec., 99:288-292, 1976.

Muirhead, M.R. The economics of pig disease: The veterinary surgeon's angle. Pig Vet. Soc. Proc., 2:113-122, 1978a.

Muirhead, M.R. Veterinary services to intensive pig production in England. Pig Vet. Soc. Proc., 3:1-19, 1978b.

Muirhead, M.R. The pig advisory visit in preventive medicine. Vet. Rec., 106:170-173, 1980.

Muirhead, M.R. Constraints on productivity in the swine herd. Vet. Rec., 102:228-231, 1978.

Nachreiner, R.F. and Ginther, O.J. Porcine agalactia: Hematologic serum chemical and clinical changes during the preceding gestation. Am. J. Vet. Res., 33:799-809, 1972a.

Nachreiner, R.F. and Ginther, O.J. Gestational and periparturient periods of sows. I. Serum chemical and hematologic changes during gestation. II. Effects of altered environment, withholding of bran feeding and serum chemical, hematologic and clinical variables. III. Serum chemical, hematologic and clinical changes during the periparturient period. Am. J. Vet. Res., 33:2215-2219, 2221-2231, 2233-2238, 1972b.

Nachreiner, R.F., Ginther, O.J., Ribelin, W.E. et al. Pathologic and endocrinologic changes associated with porcine agalactia. Am. J. Vet. Res., 32:1065-1075, 1971.

Nakano, T., Aherne, F.X. and Thompson, J.R. Leg weakness and osteochondrosis in pigs. Pig News and Info., 2:29-34, 1981.

National Academy of Sciences. The effects on human health of subtherapeutic use of antimicrobials in animal feeds. Washington, D.C., 1980, pp. 1-376.

Newton, G.I., Booram, C.V., Hale, O.M. et al. Effect of four types of floor slats on certain feet characteristics and performance of swine. J. Anim. Sci., 50:5-20, 1980.

Nielsen, N.C., Christensen, K., Billie, N. et al. Preweaning mortality in pigs. 1. Herd investigations. Nord. Vet. Med., 26:137-150, 1974.

Nielsen, N.C., Riising, H.J., Larsen, J.L. et al. Preweaning mortality in pigs. 5. Acute septicemias. Nord. Vet. Med., 27:129-139, 1975.

O'Grady, J.F. The response of pigs weaned at 5 weeks of age to digestible energy and lysine concentration in the diet. Anim. Prod., 26:287-291, 1978.

Okai, D.B., Aherne, F.X. and Hardin, R.T. Effects of creep and starter composition on feed intake and performance of young pigs. Can. J. Anim. Sci., 56:573-586, 1976.

Paterson, A.M., Barker, I. and Lindsay, D.R. Summer infertility in pigs: Its incidence and characteristics in an Australian commercial piggery. Aust. J. Exp. Agric. Anim. Husb., 18:698-701, 1978.

Paterson, A.M., Barker, I. and Lindsay, D.R. Ovulation rate at first mating and reproductive performance of gilts. Aust. Vet. J., 56:442-443, 1980.

Pattison, H.D. Patterns of sow culling. Pig News and Info., 1:215-218, 1980.

Penny, R.H.C., Edwards, M.J. and Mulley, R. Clinical observations of necrosis of the skin of suckling piglets. Aust. Vet. J., 47:529-541, 1971.

Pepper, T.A., Boyd, H.W. and Rosenberg, P. Breeding record analysis in pig herds and its veterinary applications. 1. Development of a program to monitor reproductive efficiency and weaner production. Vet. Rec., 101:177-180, 1977.

Pepper, T.A. and Taylor, D.J. Breeding record analysis in pig herds and its veterinary applications. 2. Experience with a large commercial unit. Vet. Rec., *101*:196–199, 1977.

Perry, G.C. The role of olfaction in the reproductive behavior of pigs. Pig News and Info., *3*:11–15, 1982.

Pitchey, A.M. and English, P.R. A note on the effect of boar presence on the performance of sows and their litters where penned as groups in late lactation. Anim. Prod., *31*:107–109, 1980.

Pomeroy, R.W. Infertility and neonatal mortality in the sow. 1. Lifetime performance and reasons for disposal of sows. J. Agric. Sci., *54*:1–17, 1960.

Pouteaux, V.A., Christison, G.I. and Rhodes, C.S. The involvement of dietary protein source and chilling in the etiology of diarrhea in newly weaned pigs. Can. J. Anim. Sci., *62*:1199–1209, 1982.

Rampacek, G.B., Kraeling, R.R., Kiser, T.E. et al. Delayed puberty in gilts in total confinement. Theriogenology, *15*:491–499, 1981.

Randall, G.C.B. Observations on parturition in the sow. I. Factors associated with the delivery of the piglets and their subsequent behavior. Vet. Rec., *90*:178–182, 1972a.

Randall, G.C.B. Observations on parturition in the sow. II. Factors influencing stillbirth and perinatal mortality. Vet. Rec., *90*:183–186, 1972b.

Randall, G.C.B. Studies on the effect of acute asphyxia on the fetal pig in utero. Biol. Neonate, *36*:63–69, 1979.

Randolph, J.H., Cromwell, G.L., Stahly, T.S. et al. Effects of group size and space allowance on performance and behavior of swine. J. Anim. Sci., *53*:922–927, 1981.

Ridgeon, R.F. Pig management scheme results for 1982. Agricultural Enterprise Studies in England and Wales, Cambridge University Economic Report No. 86, 1982, 36 pp.

Sather, A.P., Martin, A.H., Jolly, R.W. et al. Alternative market weight for swine. 1. Feedlot performance. J. Anim. Sci., *51*:28–36, 1980.

Simensen, E. and Karlberg, K. A survey of preweaning mortality in pigs. Nord. Vet. Med., *32*:194–200, 1980.

Smith, J.E. Analysis of autopsy data on pig respiratory disease by multivariate methods. Br. Vet. J., *133*:281–291, 1977.

Solomons, I.A. Antibiotics in animal feeds—human and animal safety issues. J. Anim. Sci., *46*:1360–1368, 1978.

Sorensen, K.J. and Askaa, J. Fetal infection with porcine parvovirus in herds with reproductive failure. Acta Vet. Scand., *22*:162–170, 1981a.

Sorensen, K.J. and Askaa, J. Vaccination against porcine parvovirus infection. Acta Vet. Scand., *22*:171–179, 1981b.

Stork, M.G. Seasonal reproductive inefficiency in large pig breeding units in Britain. Vet. Rec., *104*:49–52, 1979.

Straw, B.E., Burgi, E.J., Hilley, H.D. et al. Pneumonia and atrophic rhinitis in pigs from a test station. J. Am. Vet. Med. Assoc., *182*:607–611, 1983a.

Straw, B.E., Neubauer, G.D. and Leman, A.D. Factors affecting mortality in finishing pigs. J. Am. Vet. Med. Assoc., *183*:452–455, 1983b.

Svendsen, J., Bille, N., Nielsen, N.C. et al. Preweaning mortality in pigs. 4. Diseases of the gastrointestinal tract in pigs. Nord. Vet. Med., *27*:85–101, 1975.

Svendsen, J., Olsson, O. and Nilsson, C. The occurrence of leg injuries on piglets with the various treatment of the floor surfaces of the farrowing pen. Nord. Vet. Med., *31*:49–61, 1979.

Thomas, P. Cleansing and disinfection of pig housing. Pig News and Info., *3*:157–160, 1982.

Thomas, W.J.K. Efficiency, inflation and pig production in the U.K. Pig News and Info., *1*:81–85, 1980.

Van Lunen, T.A. Effect of rearing weaner pigs at three stocking densities on raised decks or solid flooring. Can. J. Anim. Sci., *63*:731–734, 1983.

Varley, M.A. Synchronization of estrus in gilts. Pig News and Info., *4*:151–156, 1983.

Visek, W.J. The mode of growth promotion by antibiotics. J. Anim. Sci., *46*:1447–1469, 1980.

Wahlstrom, R.C. Effect of housing system on growing pigs. Pig News and Info., *2*:271–274, 1981.

Willeberg, P. Abattoir surveillance in Denmark. Pig Vet. Soc. Proc., *6*:43–56, 1980.

Willeberg, P., Gerbola, M.A., Madsen, A. et al. A retrospective study of respiratory disease in a cohort of bacon pigs. 1. Clinico-epidemiological analysis. Nord. Vet. Med., *30*:513–525, 1978.

Wohlgemuth, K., Leslie, P.F., Reed, D.E. et al. Pseudorabies virus associated with abortion in swine. J. Am. Vet. Med. Assoc., *172*:478–479, 1978.

Wrathall, A.E. Reproductive failure in the pig: Diagnosis and control. Vet. Rec., *100*:230–237, 1977.

Young, L.G. and King, G.J. Reproductive performance of gilts bred on first versus third estrus. J. Anim. Sci., *53*:19–25, 1981.

12 Health and Production Management for Sheep

INTRODUCTION

The Sheep Industry's Need for Health and Production Management

Although there is interest in providing planned health and management programs to sheep flocks, it is not possible to be very specific about them. At the beginning of the 1980s, the sheep industry appeared to have come safely through a severe testing period and had survived the contest between wool and synthetic fibers. In addition, the needs of the Moslem world for sheep meat had added another source of income to the sheep farmer's budget. The present era of confidence lends itself to the introduction of programs directed at preventing unnecessary wastage and increasing the profitability of sheep enterprises. The emphasis has changed from the need to survive to estimation of the possibilities of enhancing profitability.

A number of flock health programs have been described (Boundy 1979; Quinlivan 1981a; Hindson 1982). There have been none that mirror the successful dairy herd health programs. We have reported briefly on preliminary responses to a pilot scheme conducted by the University of Melbourne in Australia (Morley 1979), but it is still too soon to be really confident about encouraging others to follow our example. For this reason, what follows in this chapter is largely a notional program based on known strategies for the control of diseases and the minimization of wastage due to bad management. It has been assumed that the program will need to monitor performance, analyze its own efficiency, and be cost-effective in the same way as the dairy cattle programs do.

Sheep flock health and productivity programs are faced with several problems inherent in the sheep industry. For example, there is a common assumption of responsibility for veterinary services to sheep flocks by government agencies, especially when strong government veterinary services are available. There are two consequences. Because no fee is involved, there is little incentive to carry out a study of the cost-effectiveness of what is being done. Also, a government veterinarian's attitude is strongly shaped by government policy rather than the motive to enhance an individual farmer's profitability. The lack of participation by practicing veterinarians in the sheep industry has also led to a much greater involvement of agriculturally trained animal husbandry advisers than in the cattle industries. This trend is encouraged by the greater importance of production management compared with that of disease control in sheep than in the cattle industries. It is our view, however, that the properly trained veterinarian is well fitted to be the primary counselor to sheep farmers—the sheep species specialist in fact—provided he/she maintains good contact with animal nutritionists and geneticists.

Sheep farmers are traditionally slow to change their practices and techniques of management. These characteristics are probably appropriate to the species they tend, but they also represent something of an impediment to the introduction of new or different practices. A new concept of flock health and production maintenance represents a sociological change of greater dimensions than the average sheep farmer is likely to be able to absorb quickly, if at all. Thus, it becomes necessary in this context to plan the program very carefully, to introduce it gradually, and to be particularly careful to attack only those disease problems that are sure to yield easily and whose control can be seen to have obviously advantageous financial results.

Where to Begin with a Health and Production Management Program

What predictions there are for the future of the sheep industries (e.g., Gruen 1967; Cole 1971/72) pay little attention to planned flock health and production programs as essential factors in survival. However, it does seem probable that increasing intensification of sheep farming, coupled with increased capitalization of the farms and greatly increased value of individual sheep, will stimulate a need for a cost-effective program of health and production maintenance. In most sheep-raising areas, a preliminary survey will reveal incomplete adoption, sometimes badly so, of well-tried and cost-effective health and production techniques. This provides an invitation to offer an advisory and technical service and a challenge in that there are assessable shortfalls from realistic targets (Thomas and Pout 1975).

In pastoral agricultural systems, it is common to have sheep and beef enterprises on the same farm. The opportunities for making contributions to the farmer's welfare via health and production management programs are probably greater in beef cattle than in sheep, so that combined programs can be mutually supportive. However, although the need is greater in the beef cattle herd, the relative stability of the sheep industry is more conducive to the introduction of a long-term strategy. There is good evidence (Bennett et al. 1970) that there are substantial advantages to be derived from running cattle with sheep, although the advantages are mostly for the productivity of the sheep and are likely to be significant only when stocking rates are heavy, when the pastures are improved, and in cool to temperate climates. For these reasons, it is likely to be easier to convince farmers to begin with a maintenance program for their sheep flock and to let that expand to include—and possibly support financially—a program in the resident beef cattle herd.

The program set out in this chapter is based on an average commercial flock of about 2000 ewes producing either wool or fat lambs.

Specialty farms producing heavyweight, very tender lamb meat or dust-free superfine merino wool produced indoors will make much greater demands on their programs, but a description of them is not attempted here. Even stud flocks will have special needs compared with commercial flocks, and the justification of planned health and production programs is not likely to be so difficult. On the other hand, the very large flocks grazing at sparse stocking rates over extensive range and with relatively low financial returns per sheep find these programs less attractive. To a large extent, this is due to the relatively low incidence of disease or at least its importance compared with nutritional and climatic stress. But there is also the factor of labor intensification. The smaller farm, run as a family unit, is likely to have an incompletely used resource of labor, which can be utilized profitably in more or better disease control activities. The larger farms are usually beset with the opposite problem of trying to reduce labor intensity and avoid further activities of any sort.

An initial problem that often has to be resolved when a health maintenance program is to be instituted is who should provide it. It is not a problem with a single solution, because so much depends on local factors of education and experience, and the question of whether it should be an agriculturalist or a veterinarian who services the program can be resolved either way. However, whoever does provide the program must have strong support from the other. The more important question in the sheep industry is whether the service would be provided by government veterinarians or private practitioners. Because of the traditional involvement of the former in sheep matters generally, it seemed until recently that government service involvement would be the common development, and there is no reason why that should not be so. However, the situation in most countries is a tendency to withdraw from big government and free services to private industry, and the trend is now veering sharply to the private practitioner force. This means that the costs of the programs will be borne directly by the farmer, and if he and his adviser are to have mutual respect for each other's problems and the financial implications involved in the solutions to these problems, the program must be cost-effective and must include a means of demonstrating its own economic efficiency.

When it actually comes down to starting a

program and telling a sheep farmer that the program is available, there are difficulties compared with the situation in a dairy or beef herd, where the veterinarian is likely to have been a frequent visitor. In sheep work, that is less likely. The problem is to bridge the credibility gap and to convince the farmer that there is a gain to be made. The following steps are recommended:

1. As soon as experience in the area permits, establish the degree of profitability that could ensue. On a wool-producing farm in South Eastern Australia, this could be a 100% increase over the previous profitability, with half of the gain due to management changes and half to disease management (Watt et al. 1981).

2. Enlist the support of the local government veterinary service in promoting the program and nominating the veterinarians who are willing and able to provide the service. This will be a more attractive proposition to the government service if it appreciates that such a system will mean personal protective coverage for many more farms than they can possibly provide. It also means that the government service can fill its proper role of supervision of all veterinary services to farmers.

3. Commence with a program aimed at the most serious disease and production problems and especially those that are most susceptible to the techniques that are available. A survey, perhaps by questionnaire, is often most helpful in finding out what the problems are. A survey of the literature on disease prevalence is discussed in the next section.

4. The attractiveness of the program is greatly enhanced if it includes services that the farmer already uses or is inclined to adopt if they are available. The most obvious items are in the following list:

- Pregnancy diagnosis to permit early culling of dry ewes
- Serving capacity and fertility assessment of rams
- Carrying out the Mules operation for the prevention of blowfly strike
- Artificial insemination and embryo transplantation
- Estrus synchronization
- Foot care
- Drenching, jetting
- Selection of males and females to be used in the flock's breeding program
- Teeth grinding
- A nutritional advisory service, especially for housed sheep and during long drought periods

- A pickup and postmortem examination service, especially for deaths in newborn lambs

The economic facts of life in providing a sheep flock health and production management service are that it is necessary for the person providing it to have one or more reasons for visiting the farm on several occasions each year and for carrying out some physical manipulations for which he can charge a fee. Once this pattern is established, it is easier to provide advice and to charge a fee for it.

Common Causes of Wastage Due to Disease

The published literature is not bursting with documented evidence on disease prevalence in sheep flocks. There are surveys based on abattoir surveillance (Cuthbertson 1983), but these have little validity except as indicators of change in prevalence from year to year or season to season. They reflect prevalence in mostly market sheep and are biased toward the young part of the population. Similarly, surveys carried out on material passing through postmortem examination rooms are biased toward fatal diseases and give no indication of the real wastage caused by nonfatal diseases such as foot rot, many helminthiases, and nutritional deficiencies. Nor do they often provide that most basic of all epidemiologic data, the size of the population at risk and the number affected. Such surveys are common for particular sectors of the sheep population— especially lambs—and these are reviewed in the section on neonatal mortality.

Disease wastage in weaners and adult sheep varies from place to place, depending on climate and husbandry practices. An Australian report (Watt et al. 1981) estimated that 75% of ewes, 50% of weaner, and 85% of wether flocks were drenched for worms either wastefully, insufficiently, or at the wrong time of the year. There was also a significant neglect of preventive procedures against blowfly strike and clostridial diseases, with more than 50% of susceptible sheep populations left unprotected. Wastage was also predicted in flocks in which a supplementary diet was fed to ewes to avoid pregnancy toxemia, because only 6.8% of ewes bore twins. The degree of susceptibility seemed to be much too low to warrant an across-the-flock feeding program. A New Zealand survey (Davis 1980) reported 5% per annum deaths in 24,000 sheep. The most common diseases were pregnancy toxemia, pneumonia, dystocia, blood poisoning, chronic facial eczema, and salmonellosis. In a similar survey covering 3000 adult sheep in Norway, the average loss was 2.7% per annum, most deaths occurring at pasture (Lutnaes 1982). The most common causes were diseases of the nervous system, mastitis, trauma, metritis, and abortion.

Opportunities for Improved Profitability by Improved Management

As stated previously, sheep farmers are not noted for making the greatest use of technological aids in increasing productivity. In fat lamb production, the potential gain available in cross-breeding programs—especially with exotic breeds—is often underutilized (Terrill and Tidwell 1975). In wool sheep, a similar neglect of high-yielding genotypes may cause a potential gain of 40% in profitability to be lost (Watt et al. 1981). A similar oversight is of a potential increase in stocking rate of 25% without encountering problems or a need for additional labor and a corresponding failure to take advantage of a profitability rise.

The greatest opportunities for making gains in sheep farm management, in rough order of priority, seem likely to be:

1. Saving on worm drench by cutting out unnecessary drenching or by improved drench timing to get better results
2. Reduction of neonatal mortality
3. Improved reproductive efficiency
4. More intelligent use of pasture by pregnancy diagnosing and segregating ewes and by avoiding wasteful feeding to prevent pregnancy toxemia
5. Careful purchase of supplementary feed to obtain best cost/food unit value
6. Cross-breeding
7. Performing the Mules operation to protect against blowfly strike early and consistently

All of these are subjects on which a sheep species specialist veterinarian could be expected to advise a group of farmers in a practice area. It is this sort of close personal contact from a professional adviser who is likely to visit the farm often on other matters that is the most valued source of information to the farmer. In other words, it is the final common path down which extension advice can most readily pass.

OBJECTIVES

The principal objective of animal health and production management is to provide each individual sheep farmer with advice and accompanying services that will enable him to best achieve his objectives. For the purposes of this discussion, it is assumed that economic efficiency is the farmer's sole objective. There are many other possible objectives, including economic efficiency to reduce income tax indebtedness and increase capital gain, but they do not appear to require our advice.

It is necessary to point out a common error—the assumption that maximum physical production of wool or mutton is the final goal. This is often not so, and data on production per hectare should be accompanied by an estimate of cost per unit of product produced.

Because economic efficiency is the objective, every strategy and technique included in the program must be tested for cost-effectiveness. This is relatively easy to do if the assessment relates only to the technique under discussion. For example, the cost of extra feed can be compared with the potential value of preventing deaths from pregnancy toxemia in a flock. It is surprising how often this is not done, and when it is done, it is equally surprising how often a decision not to introduce the particular technique is the obvious tactic on financial grounds. Although a decision on the cost-effectiveness of a simple technique is easy to make, a major difficulty arises when it is necessary to consider the other implications of the technique. For example, a wrongly made decision to start supplementary feeding of late pregnant ewes may have a significant effect on the birth weight of lambs and the milk supply of ewes. Lamb survival is likely to be improved as a result. Conversely, the expenditure may compete with other tactics such as a prelambing drench. Accordingly, a whole-farm approach is needed to every decision made about health maintenance and, because health and production are inextricably related to each other, to virtually all the decisions made on the farm. The farmer is in the position of having to receive advice from a number of sources—from his feed merchant, his accountant, his veterinarian, and his agricultural adviser—and the advanced, highly educated, or naturally gifted farmer can coordinate the several streams. However, most farmers do not have this capacity, and the principal objective of the programs we are discussing must be to provide this coordinating service, obviously through one coordinating adviser—a sheep species specialist.

There is a significant gap in the services available for providing whole-farm advice. It is the technique for accurately, mathematically predicting the effect of simultaneous and continuing variation in a large number of factors that affect productivity and efficiency. Computer simulation models are most likely to effectively provide the necessary mechanism, but they are expensive and still in their experimental stages. Deterministic mathematical models and linear programs have provided assistance in decision-making during the past 20 years, but their limitations make it essential to push ahead with simulation models. When they are available, it will be possible to come much closer to the ultimate objective. The efficiency of the system will then be limited only by the accuracy and the variety of the information on which the computer simulation model is based. It should be obvious that the greater part of that data can and should come from the records of properly conducted flock health and production management programs.

Principal Causes of Reduced Productivity

The causes of wastage in sheep flocks, in order of decreasing importance, are:

1. inefficient management, including especially neonatal losses, reproductive inefficiency, and failure to properly utilize the productivity of pasture

2. disease, especially parasitoses

3. wasteful use of pharmaceutical and, to a lesser extent, biological medicines to prevent disease

Advice and physical service to sheep farmers that combines a whole-farm approach to problems in these three areas would provide a flock health and production program that could be highly profitable.

The basic health maintenance program that is discussed in subsequent pages is proposed for a commercial flock of wool or mutton or dual-purpose sheep running at pasture. It is based on the control of five major groups of diseases that are thought to be the principal causes of wastage in flocks of this type: these are listed as *mandatory diseases*. There is a list of other diseases—*optional diseases*—that are not as universal in occurrence as those in the first group, and they are added to the list as required. Some of these diseases are very real

causes of loss in the areas in which they occur. For some of them, the areas in which they occur are very restricted. Thus, it becomes necessary to develop one's own list of disease targets. The following is a sample list:

Mandatory Diseases

□ Reproductive inefficiency, especially neonatal mortality. Ram infertility requires special attention because it is more likely to be impaired than in the males of other species
□ Intestinal parasitoses
□ Blowfly strike
□ Clostridioses
□ Foot rot (and other diseases of the foot)

Common Optional Diseases

□ Weaner ill-thrift
□ Fascioliasis
□ Pregnancy toxemia
□ Hypocalcemia
□ Obstructive urolithiasis

Thus, it is common in pastured sheep to use a program based on improved reproductive activity, restraint of internal and external parasitoses, and the prevention of blowfly strike and clostridial diseases. These disease control measures depend on a more intelligent use of chemical agents; better management, especially of nutrition; more efficient use of the resources available. Genetic management can be involved in a similar way in improving feed utilization and at the same time reducing susceptibility to such diseases as blowfly strike. The proper combination of these disease control strategies with others that maximize pasture production and utilization is what converts a flock health program into a flock health and production program.

Factors Impeding the Establishment of Sheep Flock Health Programs

Lack of Contact with Sheep Flocks

In sheep farming on extensive range, the risks of poor productivity or heavy losses are so great—because of natural influences such as drought, flood, and poor feed supply—that high profitability is very variable in its occurrence. The price of wool has also been extremely volatile until recent years and did not encourage unnecessary financial investment in the wool enterprise. Small sheep farms with intensive management on fertile ground in high-rainfall or irrigated areas have been more susceptible to a high-input veterinary service, but because of the low value of animals, small farm size, and the availability of free government services, there has been little development of private practitioner services. Because of the limited resources available to government services, the input has, therefore been small.

A survey of the U.K. (Pout and Thomas 1973) showed an annual expenditure of 16 to 80 pence (30¢ to $1.50) per ewe, and of this, 84% was spent on anthelmintics, fasciolicides, dips, sprays, vaccines, and sera. The amount is very small, and there is an obvious emphasis on prevention. This results from the method of operation of veterinary services in the sheep industry. Because of the low individual value of the animals and the difficulty of making a clinical examination and diagnosis in a live sheep, the principal preoccupation has been with lethal diseases. The method of operation developed to deal with this has been to deliver several dead or badly affected sheep to a diagnostic laboratory and, armed with the resulting diagnosis, to undertake the relevant treatment of the rest of the flock. Field services have operated in the same way. In the absence of repeated visits to farms to treat sick animals or to participate in disease eradication programs such as the brucellosis and tuberculosis eradication programs, which provided opportunities to get on cattle farms, the development of flock health programs has had no starting point. The primary objective must therefore be to devise ways of getting onto sheep farms regularly so that the veterinarian can develop familiarity with, and gain the confidence of, the sheep farmer.

Once having gained entry to the farm, it is still necessary to get full farmer cooperation. However, compared with the situation in dairy herds, there is great difficulty in ensuring that the regular submission of data by farmers is maintained. This is largely because of the infrequency of visits to the farms called for in most programs. If these can be increased without jeopardizing the cost-effectiveness of the program, the problem could be largely resolved. Failing this, the maintenance of telephone or mail contact, with reminders of seasonal activities that should be carried out, will help to maintain enthusiasm.

Failure of Farmers to Intensify

Flock health programs, requiring frequent visits to farms and the provision of whole-farm advice, function much better in intensive farming conditions. Housed sheep represent the ultimate in intensification and offer the biggest opportunity, because the environment is controlled, diseases are more prevalent, and the capital investment per sheep is high.

There has been a great deal of intensification with pastured sheep in the past 30 years. New species of grass and clover and heavy stocking rates to maximize use of good seasonal growth, matched by conservation of standing fodder, made it possible to carry 17 dry sheep to the hectare compared with the previous level of four. The predicted increases in infectious disease such as foot rot and internal parasitoses have not been difficult to combat (Salisbury 1967).

Improved management of improved pasture has made it possible to achieve much greater output per hectare, but still only part of the potential gain has been achieved. What is required is a better understanding of the interactions in the pasture-sheep-pathogen system (Spedding 1962, 1963), and this is achievable only by the use of a simulation model.

Low Reproductive Efficiency

Poor ewe fertility and high neonatal mortality combine in sheep flocks to drastically reduce reproductive efficiency (Bishop 1964). In merinos, the rate of increase in flock numbers in good years is only 5 to 6%, but a single bad drought year may reduce flock sizes by 10 to 20%. Such losses require a high level of reproductive efficiency so that the losses of bad years can be made good quickly. In mutton sheep in the U.K., it is recognized that profitability depends on the number of lambs reared per ewe and how many ewes can be carried per hectare (Sainsbury 1972; Lees 1971). For profitable production, 1.5 lambs are needed to be reared per ewe, and stocking rates of 12 ewes per hectare are considered to be necessary. Both targets necessitate heavy supplementary feeding.

Slow Rate of Gain from Genetic Selection

Improvement in yield of wool within existing popular breeds—for example merinos—has proceeded, albeit slowly, because of the introduction of objective measurement as distinct from visual appraisal. Collective breeding units in which each farmer contributes sheep from his best-producing families have also encouraged measurement of wool yield rather than breed type characteristics.

The latter have been the stock-in-trade of traditional stud owners, and they are still a powerful reactionary force.

In the mutton breeds, genetic selection pressure for productivity has been high so that some traditional breeds have faded. Others have prospered. More recently, there has been an introduction of exotic breeds, which have a high rate of reproduction. Most of them have serious disadvantages as pure breeds, but there appears to be a great deal to be gained by cross-breeding between them and by crossing with indigenous breeds (Wiener et al. 1973). One of the dangers of exotic breeds in any species is that they bring disease with them—especially the slow viruses—and the losses from them—for example, maedi-visna—may exceed the genetic gain (Turner 1971).

If the profitability of sheep farming is to be increased, or even maintained, to the level at which the average commercial sheep farm can afford a planned sheep flock health and production program, it will be necessary to improve nutrition, improve the multiplication rate to enhance culling pressure and rebuild flock numbers quickly, and enhance genetic selection pressure based on more vigorous culling.

Competition with Agricultural Scientists

In the sheep industry, especially in extensively grazed conditions, the inefficiency of production caused by disease is relatively small compared with the wastage, which has managerial and environmental causes. The bulk of the wastage caused by disease is due to dietary deficiencies and parasitic disease, both of which are controllable without immediate veterinary supervision. Even in the remaining diseases, there is a large component of managerial error. If all of these indications of the importance of management are taken into account, it is apparent that the veterinarian is likely to meet competition from the non-veterinary agricultural adviser.

There is no single solution to this problem. In some areas, the solution to providing a flock health and production service may be as an accessory to an existing, active farm management advisory service. The reverse arrangement might also be effective if the veterinarian had a strong interest and good expertise in the sheep industry. Because some veterinarians have developed this interest, and because of this interdependence of disease and management, it is important to decide whether a specialist sheep veterinarian can adequately provide sheep production and animal advice to the commercial sheep farmer. All of our experience indicates that the animal husbandry specialist does not have the basic training to enable him to develop significant expertise in dealing with animal disease but that the veterinarian does have enough animal science to enable him to develop the necessary skills in animal husbandry.

The Need for Integration with Traditional Veterinary Services

The only sizable commercial sheep meat and wool industries in the English-speaking world are in Australia, New Zealand, and South Africa, and they are still dependent on public or semi-public veterinary services. This appears to have derived from the historical origin of the sheep industry as a marginally profitable one capable of existing in the least hospitable environment. The fact is that both meat and wool sections of the industry have become financially stable and profitable. An early reaction to this improved financial status was the development of a corps of privately employed farm management advisers. This group fared badly when the boom economy to which it was geared collapsed in the early 1970s. The resurgence of the industry in the 1980s seems to provide an opportunity for flock health and production programs, tailored to fit the demands of the individual farm, to develop. The difficulty that bars the way is the existing competition between government and private services for the control of this kind of work. A combination of the two services in which government officers promote preventive programs and provide field and laboratory back-up services to private veterinarians who carry out the field visits and give the necessary management advice would seem to be an obvious and advantageous arrangement. It would embrace the present trend in most countries, to have the industries accept more financial responsibility for the services that they receive.

Education of the Species Specialist Veterinarian

If the veterinarian is to provide highly qualified advice on matters of nutrition, genetics, and pasture management, the education provided at present in most veterinary schools will need to be supplemented in those subjects.

Because the field of work is narrow and vocationally oriented, this additional teaching would be most logically provided in postgraduate courses. The types of additional subjects that would need to be included in such a course are:

- genetic management, including objective measurement methods; the handling of large numbers of sheep in a series of echelons of differing excellence
- grazing management; the economy of subdivision, selecting a level of grazing pressure, and selection of pasture species
- nutrition; other special nutritional supplies in drought feeding, wet ewe maintenance, and weaner management
- reproduction management; times of joining, duration of joining period, concentration of lambing, and selection of rams
- cost-effective control of the serious diseases in the particular area
- familiarity with the physical techniques of shearing, foot care, artificial insemination, ovum transplantation, wet and dry ewe selection, lamb postmortems, Mules operation, drenching, teeth grinding, fleece appraisal, and many others

TARGETS

The form taken by a flock health and production management program depends largely on what the targets are. For that reason, the basic target areas are outlined at this point:

1. Determination of the principal causes of wastage in the area or on the particular farm is an essential first step. Most often this is done based on information provided by farmers in an unstructured way. A properly structured and conducted survey offers much more chance of an accurate result. A permanent data collection service, covering a much wider area and coordinating returns from the health and production areas, would be better still. Assessment of the wastage in dollars and cents must be accompanied by estimated costs of control. The final decision on which forms of loss should be initial targets can then begin.

2. The method used to assess efficiency of production can also determine the structure of the monitoring program. For example, in sheep it is difficult to accurately measure lambing percentages, and it is more common to use marking or weaning percentages as the index of reproductive efficiency. This could direct a concentration of effort to those activities rather than to the lambing process.

3. A farm is often a combination of enterprises, and whole-farm advice may mean including the beef or other enterprise in the advisory system. This would then create a need for the development of appropriate targets and programs to measure whether specific targets are being achieved. In practical terms, it will also be highly desirable to have all of the management programs for the several enterprises on the farm coordinated in such a way as to effect economies of data collection. Thus, a sheep farm carrying a beef herd might reasonably expect to have both enterprises dealt with in terms of examinations and data collection at the same visit.

Indices of Productivity in Sheep Flocks

To measure health and production performance on the basis of the number of positive identifications of a worm, a bacterium, or a disease is of limited value. What is more important is to monitor productivity overall and in a number of indices. If overall productivity is below the target, it should be possible to determine which of the indices is indicating the source, and, if that is determined, to then decide which of the contributory worms or bacteria is the major cause of loss. There may, of course, be more than one such cause.

Thus, it is necessary to set out the relevant indices and the targets thought to be achievable in each one of them. Which of the commonly used indices is relevant varies with the particular circumstances. In extensively run flocks under ranch conditions, it is usually the survival rate—that is, the longevity—of the sheep that determines whether or not the enterprise is successful. In intensively managed flocks, survival is a prerequisite, and the final decision depends on the rate of gain in body weight of growing sheep or the weight of wool (related to micron measurement of the fiber) produced. An exhaustive index of techniques used in performance recording in sheep has been prepared (Owen 1971).

The indices set out below are relevant to southern Australian conditions in terms of work published and local experience. But they are still very theoretical even in our own case, and no actual targets are quoted because they have not been tested against a large bank of data to determine that they are, in fact, reliable in a practical way. Some levels of performance quoted in the literature follow.

$Reproductive\ index = \dfrac{\text{lambs born}}{\text{ewes joined}}$. This is the most informative index, but is often not measurable because of lack of surveillance at lambing. Additional indexes are:

Cycling index	= % ewes mated in first 14 days	=	65-70%°
Mating index	= % ewes mated in complete joining,	=	>95%
	i.e., % ewes that do not mate	=	<5%
Conception rate	= % ewes mated that lamb	=	>95%
Abortion rate	= % pregnant ewes that abort	=	<2%
Ewe death rate	= % ewes dead per annum	=	<5%
Twin rate	= % ewes with twins: merinos	=	10-20%°
	Romneys	=	80%

Lamb survival index

Marking percentage	= % lambs marked to ewes joined: merinos	=	80-100%°
	Romneys	=	110-120%
	% ewes that lose all lambs	=	10-20%°

Miscellaneous—mating management efficiency

Average age of ewes at first joining		18 months
Percentage of rams to ewes in mating groups	=	2%
Length of joining period (6 weeks in autumn, 9 weeks in spring)	=	6-9 wks.

Meat production in mutton flocks as measured by:
Average body weight at weaning (related to age at weaning) or —
Number of lambs (body condition score or weight and age)
   plus number of surplus adult sheep sold per hectare or —
Actual weight of lamb or mutton sold per hectare

Wool productivity indicated by:
Wool yield by weight (quality and price quoted) per hectare —

Longevity expressed as:
Percentage of deaths and culls per year in age groups or —
Percentage increase in flock size less reproductive index or —
Percentage of sheep sold as surplus to static requirements less reproductive index —

°The worse figure is for maiden ewes. Unless otherwise specified, the indices are for merinos in Australia (Plant 1981) and are for illustration only.

Management Efficiency. An assessment of the percentage application of recommended techniques is worthwhile. This can be further subdivided into the intensity of application of the adopted techniques as indicated, for example, by the number of lambs submitted to the Mules operation by six months of age. The assessment can also be made by measuring the rate of occurrence of specific diseases.

Specific targets are not supplied for most of the indices set out above because there is such great variation in them between countries and between breeds. Actual targets need to be developed for each locality and be based on known performance in pilot herds and on general local knowledge. The local knowledge will, for the most part, be hard data from field research, much of which is regionally based nowadays. Absence of such information will make target development more hazardous.

Some Notes on Special Productivity Targets

Meat Production

In terms of lamb—the common denominator in most countries—there should be an annual turn-off of 150% of lambs related to the ewe flock, and lambs should average 65 lb. (30 kg.) body weight at 14 to 20 weeks of age off pasture. But, as with wool, the range of normal values is very wide and is influenced by many factors, especially, in optimum feed situations, by the inheritance of the ram and the ewe. Thus, Southdown rams on Romney ewes produce a 34.5-1b. (16-kg.) lamb carcass, whereas a Dorset Horn ram will sire lambs weighing 38 lb. (17 kg.). On the other hand, the value of the Southdown carcass is likely to be higher because of its better grading and higher value per pound weight. The period taken to reach the desired weight is also critical, but insufficient data are available to give any worthwhile figure. The target in lamb feedlots in the U.S. is an entry weight of 70 to 80 lb. (33 to 36 kg.), a daily gain of 250 g. for 60 days, and an outweight of 105 lb. (47 kg.). The targets in intensive lamb feeding units are not so well defined, but a daily gain on milk replacer of 250 to 300 g. to reach 80 lb. (36 kg.) at 16 weeks at slaughter time is a reasonably satisfactory guide.

Wool Production

There is a large variation between breeds of sheep and in merinos, between strains of merinos, in the weight of fleece and the quality of wool produced. These differences are further magnified by the quality and quantity of food available and by geographical location. Thus, it becomes almost meaningless to quote any targets. However, the alternative is to derive an optimum figure based on the mean of a large mass of data collected in a specific area. One is then faced with the possibility that the entire area might be deficient in a specific nutrient, for example, selenium, and that might be the piece of information one wanted. It then becomes reasonable to state that under optimum conditions, classes of merino sheep are capable of producing the following weight of clean wool each year:

Fine wool merinos—19 microns diameter wool; 70's spinning quality; 6.5 lb. (3 kg.)

Medium wool merinos (Peppin strain)—21 microns; 60's spinning quality; 9 lb. (4 kg.)

Strong wool merinos (South Australian)—22-24 microns; 58-60's spinning quality; 20.5 lb. (9.5 kg.)

Longevity

Those sheep that survive disease, accident, culling for poor productivity, or sale because of high productivity achieve the ultimate goal of "cast for age." In practice, this means culling for dental wear—the sheep is broken-mouthed and unable to graze efficiently, and is rejected because of inability to maintain weight or produce wool. The age at which the teeth fade varies, depending on diet—especially the calcium, phosphorus, and fluorine intakes—and the degree of contamination of feed with soil debris. On moderately rough pasture, composed of native plants, the age at which ewes are culled is somewhere around six to seven years. Fertility is at a maximum about this time, and if tooth wear could be postponed for

another two or even three years there could be a distinct financial gain. With an average culling age of 6.5 years, an annual death rate of 2.5%, and an annual culling rate for disease of 2.5%, the average age of all sheep on the farm at any one time would be about 3.3 years. If the flock size is not stable because the management objective is to increase or decrease the size of the flock, these targets will vary.

Culling Rate

In meat flocks, the usual objective is to sell as many fat lambs as possible. Culling for age plus death losses and culling for disease usually amount to about 25%, leaving 75% of lambs born available for sale.

REPRODUCTIVE INEFFICIENCY
Criteria

The low rate of reproduction in commercial sheep flocks points to this as one of the prime targets for a flock health program. The rate of loss is high and has not changed much for many years. There are two parts to the problem:
- Failure to produce one or more live lambs by every ewe bred, which is presented as reproductive inefficiency in this section
- Loss of a full-term lamb in the perinatal period, which is presented in the next section as neonatal mortality

Because the subject is a complex one and because there is a great deal of information about it, it is necessary to discuss the problem in a structured way, related to the way in which the problem is encountered in the field. Therefore, we deal with it from the point of view of a reproductive inefficiency problem brought to us by a farmer in the ordinary course of practice. The same technique is used for handling a problem that begins to develop in a flock that is under a flock health management program. The final aspect of this discussion is the flock health program that should be instituted to avoid wastage due to disease but at a cost less than the benefit derived. Such programs will vary widely from place to place, and even from time to time, depending on the profitability of the sheep enterprise.

It is assumed that, as with other herd health management programs described in other sections of this book, the program must automatically assess itself so that the benefits of its operation are continually under surveillance.

There are two criteria used to measure reproductive efficiency in a sheep flock:
- *The lamb-marking percentage*—the per cent

of ewes joined that rear a lamb up to marking/docking

□ *The compactness of the lambing*—a compact lambing is desirable in order to concentrate the labor involved in, and the disruptive effects of, lambing. The desirability of getting all lambs at the same age at marketing has meant that a synchronized estrus has been a long-term quest in the sheep industry

The acceptable lamb-marking percentage varies so much with the circumstances that it is not possible to quote a figure that makes much sense. For example, in Australia's extensive merino flocks, which are exposed to inclement climate, predators, and indifferent nutrition, a lamb-marking percentage of 75% may represent efficiency. In meat sheep in the northern hemisphere, a lambing percentage of 120% may be the benchmark; and in Finnish Landrace, 200% may be the target. The objective in each environment must be the lambing percentage that contributes the greatest profitability per hectare. In intensively managed flocks, the number of lambings achieved and the number of lambs born per year is of vital importance (Lees 1971). In the U.K., the judgment to fit local circumstances is two lambs per ewe, but even this decision is not uncomplicated. So much depends on the effects of the additional lamb. If it is carried on the ewe and finished on summer grass, there is no great difficulty other than the need to balance ecological conservation against economic productivity. However, if it is to be provided for in winter housing and with artificial feeding, the advantages are not so obvious. At present, the advantage disappears if the lamb has to be weaned from the ewe and raised artificially.

Compactness of Lambing. To ensure that most ewes come on heat and become pregnant during a brief, e.g., 30-day, period, it is necessary to use either hormonal means or special management techniques as set down in the section on maximizing fertility. In well-managed flocks of Romney sheep in New Zealand for example, it is possible to get 95% of ewes bred during a 34-day joining period.

Financial Profitability. Because the final criterion is to ensure the greatest economic return in the circumstances that prevail on a particular farm at a particular time, there are no uncomplicated issues with respect to decisions on sheep breeding programs. At every joining period, it is necessary to make compromises in management to meet fluctuations in the variables of feed supply, climate, demand for replacement sheep, market de-

mand for sheep products, and especially the restrictions imposed by the physiology of the sheep. This is not a characteristic of the sheep industry alone, but the industry is more susceptible to the changes in these uncontrollable variables because it is so intensely pastoral and therefore exploitative.

Because of its traditional "poor man" image and its exploitative nomadic nature, heavy losses of sheep or inefficiency at reproducing them tends to be accepted much more readily than in other industries. However, when the consequences of such productive inefficiency are contemplated in the light of today's values, it is obvious that there is often room for investment in preventive medicine in sheep flocks.

One of the difficulties in any comparison of the relative importance of various forms of loss is the difficulty of defining rates of loss and the value of the productivity lost. There is also the extraordinary fluctuation that can occur in the price of wool. Almost for argument's sake then, and using 1969 values (Moule 1969), the effects of varying the lambing rate in merino flocks have been illustrated. Increasing it from 100 to 120% increased the profitability per ewe by $2.20; increasing it from 76 to 112% increased the profitability per ewe by $4. Examined in the light of Australia's prevailing 50% lambing percentages in Queensland, compared with 100% in Tasmania and a national average of about 70%, the potential gain to the national economy is obvious, especially because the lambing percentage is so easily improved by improvements in management. The manipulation of reproductive physiology by such techniques as hormonal control of estrus, termination of pregnancy, and embryo transplantation are unlikely to be extensively used except in very high-cost systems of production. Their use in the stud system is understandable. Their high rate of use in Europe to produce feeder lambs at unseasonable times to suit consumer demands is a surprising development in light of the extra cost of the product.

Modes of Reproductive Failure

The fact that reproductive inefficiency exists will have been established by comparing the lamb-marking rate (or other similar index) or the compactness of the lambing with the targets established by reference to performance of peer flocks. If the failed target is the marking rate, it is then necessary to decide whether the shortfall is due to (1) failure to produce a live lamb, (2) death of a live lamb after birth, or (3) a combination of the two. If the farm has accurate data on the pick-up of dead lambs, the answer is usually fairly obvious. Failing retrospective data being available, the first task becomes the one of accumulating prospective data so that the decision as to which mode of loss is critical can be made. However, there is no need to delay starting work on the problem because there are so often problems in both modes.

If the shortfall is one of failure to produce a live lamb, it is then necessary to decide which one of the following is the source of the error:
□ Failure to mate—ewe or ram
□ Failure of conception—ewe or ram
□ Early embryonic death—ewe problem
□ Abortion
□ Combinations of any of the above
In flocks where complete records are kept and good field observations have been made, it is usually possible to make an accurate diagnosis quickly. What follows is a discussion of techniques of assessment, a description of the individual errors encountered and how to counter them, and then a description of a sample flock health program to optimize fertility.

Techniques for Appraisal of Reproductive Efficiency

The diagnostic procedure for deciding in which mode the specific error lies in any problem of flock reproductive inefficiency has been described frequently. It is displayed diagrammatically in Figure 12-1. A more detailed account, suitable for field research, is also available (Moule 1965). The special techniques that will enable the appropriate decisions to be made include the following.

Farm Profile

This includes construction of a history of the problem plus a description of the managerial and physical resources that may be important in causing the problem. On a well-managed farm, good data will be available that can be analyzed as discussed below. In others, it may be necessary to use approximations from limited records. If neither of these is available, it may be necessary to create a data file prospectively by collecting data for one or more years. Suitable categories for analysis of the data are:

Geographical analysis—lamb-marking percentages on different farms, parts of farms, or even paddocks

Ewe flock performance as displayed in:
□ different age groups, e.g., maidens versus mature
□ indigenous versus introduced (brought-in) ewes
□ nutritional status
□ culling policy, e.g., culling on age, lamb production, wool production
□ shearing, dipping, drenching program
Ram management—the same sort of information is required about rams as about the ewes:
□ purchasing policy—age, origin, time of introduction to flock
□ shearing, dipping, drenching program
□ joining policy, including number of rams per 100 ewes, switching rams half way, length of joining period, time of year, prejoining teasing, joining as singles or as groups
□ culling policy, e.g., culling for age, fertility, serving capacity.

Examination of the Flock

Some of the information in the following items may be gained by personal inspection, some by advice from the owner.

Physical Examination of the Rams. Information about the rams that is critical to a good reproductive performance, and that should be included in a prejoining examination, is discussed here. In commercial flocks, rams are usually put into ewe flocks in groups equivalent to 2% of the population. The prevalence of individual infertile rams is so low that ram-induced infertility is unlikely. Such is not the case with stud flocks, where single-ram mating is the norm.

Examination of rams should include:
□ Physical examination, paying particular attention to teeth, feet, gait, body condition score, and testes for size and springiness
□ Serological examination for *Brucella ovis* if there is a suggestion of epididymal abnormality
□ Semen evaluation and serving capacity tests if there is any suggestion of ram infertility. A practice of examining a sample of normal rams is hazardous because a chance occurrence of one or more sterile rams in the unexamined group will result in a serious decline in credibility of the program as a whole
□ If the rams are isolated in a group separated from the ewes, it is likely that the ewes are not cycling. If the rams are moving around and obviously working, the ewes are cycling normally; if the activity continues at a high

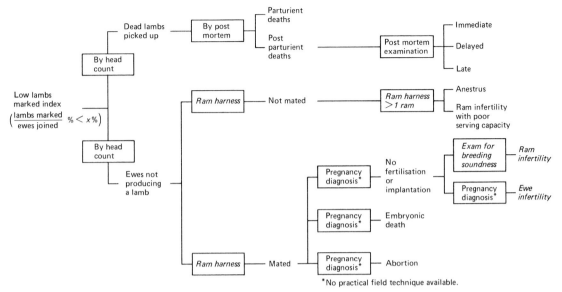

Figure 12-1. Determination of cause of low lambs marked index.

level, it is probable that the ewes are cycling normally but have a conception problem either because of an abnormality in the ewes or a fertility deficit in the rams

□ Serving capacity tests are used for rams as they are for paddock-mating beef bulls, but there is very little published about them. Rams are observed for their sexual activity in a group of ewes and in the company of other rams. Rams that complete the most services during a specified time interval are given the highest rating. It is thought that these rams produce the most pregnancies in limited joining periods and make it possible to use a lower percentage of rams

Physical Examination of Ewes. The ewes' body condition should be estimated about two months before joining so that there is time to supplement their diet if this is desirable. Special attention should be paid to the presence of a group of thin ewes among a flock of better conditioned ones; the presence of a "tail" to a flock indicates a heavy parasite infestation, old ewes, bad mouths, or inadequate feed supply.

Accurate Head Counts of Ewes and Lambs. These are basic and absolutely essential, especially at lambing. If they are carried out whenever the sheep are worked, irrespective of the reason, they provide a repeat monitoring of the size and composition of each flock. Because the data recording and analysis on sheep farms must be based on flocks or subflocks, their accurate identification at all times is essential. The means of identifying the

group may be by colored ear tag or by fleece brand.

Ram Mating Harnesses. These are available so that ewes that are mated can be identified. By the use of different colored crayons in the harness, the identity of the mating ram can be determined. If identification of those ewes that are showing estrus but that are not to be bred is the objective, vasectomized rams may be used. Failure to mate may result from anestrus in the ewe or failure of the ram to perform. The technique is not likely to be applicable in the field unless plenty of labor is available, because the flock needs to be examined at least once each week to record raddling and to allow adjustment of the harness. Changing of the colors avoids confusion about which marking is latest. Changing of colors every two weeks is a little easier on the color range if a six-week joining period is contemplated. The harnesses can be used during the mating period to determine whether a particular ram is working; if all the rams are idle, the probability is ewe anestrus or early embryonic death with a prolonged interestral interval. If the supply labor is short, the use of ram mating harnesses for, e.g., the last three weeks of the mating period will provide most of the information needed for half the outlay. For the first three weeks, the rams work unmarked.

If possible, the ewes that are marked as being served during a particular period should be kept as a group so that at pregnancy diagnosis they should all be at approximately the same duration of pregnancy. It is absolutely essential that the ewes retain their identification and that an accurate record of the events for each ewe be kept.

Pregnancy Diagnosis. Knowing whether or not a ewe is pregnant has three principal advantages:

1. Cost-effectiveness in today's sheep industry depends on the type of management in which pregnant ewes are provided with a particular level of nutrition and form of management, whereas dry sheep are provided with less. To do this effectively requires early and accurate pregnancy diagnosis.

2. Attention at lambing can be focused on the pregnant ewes and, if management is reasonable, on groups of ewes arranged in order of impending parturition.

3. In any investigation of a suspected reproductive problem, this is the most important piece of information.

There are a number of methods available:

1. Enlargement of the udder together with firmness and warmth. If in doubt, some fluid is expressed. It should be clear and sticky, like honey. Only ewes in the last four weeks of pregnancy can be detected this way. Doubtful ewes should be rechecked in another week.

2. A rectal probe technique, the probe being advanced with one hand to touch the fetus, while the other hand manipulates the abdomen. The technique is fast, safe, and reliable after 70 days of pregnancy, provided the operator is experienced. At 100 days it is 99% reliable (Plant 1980). The technique requires care and palpatory sensitivity; otherwise losses from peritonitis or abortion may occur (Turner and Hindson 1975).

3. Ultrasonic detection by Doppler instruments, operating on the basis of detecting fluid movement as through fetal heart or vessels. Confusion can occur with the effects created by maternal vessels. The technique is time-consuming but accurate.

4. Ultrasonic technique based on the detection of fluid-filled organs—the amplitude depth principle. Fluid-filled organs other than the uterus can give false-positive readings. Pyometra may also show positive. The instrument is accurate (Bondurant 1980) (83% during the period 61 to 151 days after mating commences) (Meredith and Madani 1980) but expensive, and only a high level of expertise makes it possible to test sheep economically. Facilities for holding and examining sheep need to be good for ultrasonic methods.

5. Miscellaneous methods, including a serological technique that has an unacceptable error in a high rate of false-negatives in early pregnancy (Cerini et al. 1976; Robertson et al. 1980); radiographic diagnosis, which is slow and expensive; and running vasectomized rams with the ewes after the rams are taken out (Knight et al. 1975). Information gained from pregnancy diagnosis should include the proportion of ewes pregnant out of the number of ewes joined, the proportion of ewes in early and late pregnancy, and the body condition score of the ewe and the condition of her udder at the time of the examination.

Surveillance for Abortion. Careful surveillance for evidence of abortion is recommended but is not really a rewarding technique in ewe flocks. It is virtually impossible to encounter an early fetus, and unless placenta is seen hanging from a ewe, many abortions go unnoticed.

Identification of Wet and Dry Ewes. Classification of ewes as soon as lambing is complete into groups indicating whether or not they have had a lamb is known as a wet/dry classification. It is best done by a veterinarian and is the basis for one of the regular farm visits. If the classification can also include the year of birth of the ewe, which is easily achieved by a colored ear tag, the fate of the ewe can be decided on the spot. The recommended classifications are as follows:

1. Wet-wet ewes, which have lambed and are now lactating, i.e., their lamb(s) is alive. They will have a lambing stain down the back of the udder. The udder is full and the teats are clean and large, giving a bespectacled clean appearance when viewed from below.

2. Wet-dry ewes, which have lambed but have lost their lambs. A lambing stain is evident. The udder is at first large and full, but within a day the teats are dirty. Within a few days, the cleavage between the two halves of the udder is very evident, but from then on the size decreases. Milk will still be present in the udder for periods sometimes exceeding two months, the secretion gradually becoming clearer and more sticky. Neither of these groups is in good condition.

3. Dry-dry ewes, which have not had a lamb this season, have no lambing stain, are in good condition, and have small udders with no milk in them.

Necropsy Examination. The ultimate examination technique in the quest for answers to infertility problems is the postmortem examination. This is obviously of greatest value in determining the cause of death in newborn lambs. Such examination of clinically infertile ewes is usually unrewarding.

Decisions About Reproductive Inefficiency

When sheep are housed or under close surveillance, it is possible to collect good data about demonstration of estrus; successful mating, as indicated by ram harness marking; failure to return to estrus; successful or unsuccessful parturition; and marking and weaning.

When sheep are at extensive pasture, the only opportunity for collecting information may be when they are gathered together and put through yards or a shearing shed. Thus, the first effective count may be at marking (tail docking and castration), when the only information still available is likely to be the identification of wet and dry ewes. If pastured ewes are lambed through a yard or shed system, as discussed under neonatal mortality, the same information can be collected more accurately.

Diagnosis of Mode of Reproductive Efficiency

This is shown diagrammatically in Figure 12-1. The scheme includes the use of techniques that may not always be available on commercial sheep farms. Without them, the questions cannot be answered. Since the questions also cannot be answered retrospectively, the investigation must be a prospective one. The modes of inefficiency—and thus their methods of detection—stated very briefly are:

□ failure of ewe to mate—no raddle marks present from ram harness
□ failure of ram to mate—only some of rams in group mate some of the ewes; both are identified by raddle marks from the harness. Note: If all rams have low fertility, it is impossible to differentiate a and b
□ failure of ewe to ovulate—peritoneoscopy or exploratory laparotomy
□ failure of rams to inseminate—mark of color unique to particular ram not seen, or reduced number, or single ram mating groups using harness, with succeeding ram successful
□ failure of conception—normal interestral periods as indicated by ram harness marks with different colors every two weeks
□ early embryonic death—long interestral periods as indicated by ram harness marks with different colors every two weeks. When

rams cease marking, conception may be assumed and rams are withdrawn. To determine that ewes do not return to estrus, run vasectomized rams with ewes
□ abortion—pick-up of aborted fetus, viewing of retained placenta
□ neonatal mortality—see next section

Failure of ewes to mate is not a common problem in adult merino ewes (Edey 1969; Mullaney 1966; Cannon and Bath 1971), although it can occur (Restall et al. 1976a). However, it is a significant occurrence in maiden ewes. The more common problem is a failure of fertilization or to maintain the pregnancy.

Diagnosis of Failure to Mate

The decision to be made is between anestrus in the ewe or inability to mate by a ram.

Ewe Anestrus. The most important single factor affecting estrus occurrence in ewes is nutrition. A dietary deficiency of total energy is manifested by a depression of ovulation rate or of fertilization and implantation. The result can be a decrease of the rate of mating to 70% for the first two weeks of the joining season. The management response is to "flush" the ewe with supplementary feeding before the joining period (Tassell 1967a).

Determination of the nutritional status of sheep can probably best be done by weighing a sample of them, but condition scoring, as described later under the heading of nutrition, is a highly satisfactory substitute. The difficulty with weighing is the lack of a standard weight scale on which to base the judgments. In merino flocks, the fertility level—in terms of lambs born—plateaus at about 85 to 90 lb. body weight at joining. A common figure quoted in Corriedale flocks is that the percentage of lambs born increases 1% for every one pound increase in body weight at joining. There is a special need to ensure adequate feeding of maiden ewes. The higher the live weights—within reason—at the first mating at 18 months of age, the higher the fertility index is likely to be.

The above are principles and examples of them. There is so much variation in body weight/fertility relationships between breeds and in different locations that any attempt to establish fixed standards would be futile.

The occurrence of estrus also varies with the season independently of nutritional status (Moule 1960). This is most marked in merinos and merino cross-breeds, which come in heat regularly in autumn, although they will breed in any season of the year in various geographical locations. There is also a seasonal influence on the number of ovulations occurring at one time, so that a higher proportion of twins is likely to occur in merino ewes bred in the autumn than if they were bred in spring. The differences are significant, the respective fertility indexes being 95% in autumn and 78% in spring. Fasting and shearing depress estrus display without affecting ovulation, but the field significance of the relationship is unconvincing (Mackenzie et al. 1975).

The presence of a teaser or ram, and in fact the population density and composition of the flock, all influence the occurrence of estrus and are used—especially the former—to improve reproductive efficiency in an economic way. Failure to mate because of poor serving capacity of rams is referred to under the heading of ram infertility. Other factors that affect the onset of estrus are:

□ access to clovers containing estrogenic substances
□ heat stress, cold stress
□ shearing ewes in the joining period
□ breed—some are less active and slower to start

Ram Impotence. Painful conditions of the feet and joints that prevent proper mounting and interfere with successful breeding activity by the ram are the commonest cause. Poor nutritional status and insufficient ram population may also reduce ram activity. The more important causes of ram infertility are listed under failure to establish pregnancy.

Diagnosis of Cause of Failure to Establish Pregnancy

This includes failure of fertilization and implantation, and early embryonic death.

Ewe—Failure to Conceive. Except for the infectious diseases, which cause abortion and embryonic death and which are discussed elsewhere, there are few known specific causes of failure to establish pregnancy. Very high ambient temperatures and genetic influences are listed as such causes (Moule 1960). Nutrition/fertility relationships are unclear. However, embryo survival is greatest in ewes fed a full maintenance diet. Poisoning by estrogenic substances in subterranean clover and other plants is the best-known cause. It may result in a failure to establish pregnancy in 70% of ewes and causes further losses of lambs at parturition (Tassell 1967b). Selenium deficiency in the diet

is suspected of causing early embryonic death; that is, the early embryonic mortality is prevented by the administration of selenium. It is suspected that fertilization by a ram affected with seminal degeneration may also be followed by a high level of embryonic deaths. The subject has been elegantly reviewed (Edey 1969). Season also has an effect on conception, the least efficiency being apparent in merino ewes bred in the spring months.

Ram—Failure to Impregnate. Rams contribute very significantly to infertility in sheep flocks, largely because of infectious diseases that affect the reproductive tract. In addition, there are environmental influences. Rams show most libido in autumn, and they may be relatively infertile in hot summers, especially if they are not acclimatized. Libido also tends to be low in late winter and spring, especially in British breeds of sheep. High environmental temperatures can also cause seminal degeneration. Because of the relative frequency of fertility breakdown in rams—5 to 10% is not remarkable in year-old rams and 35% may be impaired at 7 years—an examination of the rams before each mating period is well worthwhile (Ott and Memon 1968). Young rams should be examined first at nine to 12 months of age. A physical examination of the penis and scrotal contents is conducted first. Particular attention is paid to the epididymis because of the common occurrence of infection with *Brucella ovis*. Evidence of epididymitis, varicocele, orchitis, hypoplasia or atrophy of the testicles, or tunical adhesions is sufficient reason for culling the ram. Testicular size and tone are good indicators of fertility in mature rams, the size in particular being a good indicator of potential semen output. Impaired semen production occurs relatively commonly, usually as a result of high environmental temperatures, access to estrogens, overfatness, fever, dipping in arsenical dips during a mating season, and vitamin A deficiency.

Further examination is necessary if a diagnosis or a more accurate evaluation is required. Collection of semen by electroejaculation is a standard procedure, and examination of the semen makes possible a judgment on semen quality and the probable state of fertility. Bacteriological examination of semen has considerable merit, and serological examination for *Br. ovis* is a standard procedure. The specific diseases associated with ram infertility are presented in other textbooks, but a point that should be made here is that vaccination against brucellosis can cause a severe systemic reaction and should not be done during the three months immediately preceding joining.

There are many other diseases that can, by their local or systemic effects, cause a temporary or permanent infertility in rams. The length of the list precludes citing them, but fly strike, parasitism, foot rot, and arsenic poisoning are important diseases in this context. During any physical examination of a ram, the presence of a local dermatitis, for example due to mycotic dermatitis, arsenic "burn," or mange, would be noted as a possible cause of infertility and its prevention recommended. The scrotum is obviously important, but so are the feet, and a badly undershot jaw, preventing good prehension, can also cancel out the reproductive efficiency bestowed by a perfect set of genitalia.

Diagnosis of the Cause of Abortion

Watson (1973) suggests that 1 to 2% of abortions are acceptable in the average flock as being nonspecific in etiology, but that an occurrence rate higher than this should be investigated because of probability of intervention by an infectious or toxic agent. U.K. figures suggest that the national abortion and stillbirth rate is 4 to 5%. Australian data are sparse but suggest that infection is widespread but of low incidence (Gorrie 1962; Dennis 1972b). The principal problem in sheep is that so many abortions and stillbirths go undiagnosed. Australian data indicate that 42% of ovine abortions are not diagnosable by ordinary laboratory means (Munday et al. 1966). Information from the U.K. suggests that the undiagnosed figure is 58% (Linklater 1979) (Fig. 12-2).

The common infectious causes of abortion in ewes are *Vibrio foetus (Campylobacter foetus* var. *intestinalis)*, *Salmonella* spp., *Chlamydia* (causing enzootic abortion of ewes), and *Toxoplasma* spp. Other less common infections are *Listeria monocytogenes* and *Corynebacterium pyogenes*. The respective frequency of occurrence of these infections is not very well defined in Australia, but vibriosis and listeriosis are the ones most commonly recorded (Dennis 1975; Broadbent 1975). *Brucella ovis* has a variable reputation as a cause of abortion. It is thought to be a cause in New Zealand but not in Australia, where infection of rams with this organism is common. Enzootic abortion of ewes, caused by *Chlamydia* sp., is a less common cause, although the infection is relatively common. Although a heavy abortion

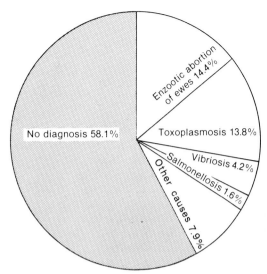

Figure 12–2. Causes of ovine fetopathy. (From Linklater, K.A. Abortion in sheep. Vet. Rec. (In Practice), 1:30–33, 1979.)

rate is not usually associated with border disease, there may be significant embryonic loss in this disease as well as the more widely recognized congenital defects. Other sporadic causes of infectious abortion are the rickettsiae, *Ehrlichia phagocytophila* (tickborne fever), and *Coxiella burnettii* (Q fever). Noninfectious causes include stress related to transport and handling, and pregnancy toxemia. Toxins are not well identified as abortifacients, but the evidence against fungi growing on *Romulea bulbocodium* (onion weed), or the plant itself, is very convincing. Other fungal toxins, e.g., from *Claviceps purpurea* and *Aspergillus fumigatus*, are commonly quoted as causes of abortion. Abortion caused by infection with fungi, as in cattle, is not recorded in sheep.

The difficulty in obtaining reliable data is due to the absence of suitable surveys; information based on material presented to laboratories is likely to be heavily biased. This is often due to the unsuitability of specimens for a complete laboratory examination or to lack of laboratory facilities to conduct these examinations.

Management Programs to Optimize Fertility in Sheep Flocks

It is not possible to devise a program to fit all circumstances of sheep husbandry. However, some general guidelines are possible, and the following points at least need to be taken into consideration in such programs. Unfortunately, reproductive efficiency in sheep is susceptible to inefficiency at many points, and combinations of factors often occur in nature so that it is seldom easy to diagnose a specific cause. Part of the difficulty also arises because of the vagueness of our understanding of how specific factors actually exert their influence on the reproductive process. It would help, too, if it were possible to be more definite about exactly which point in the reproductive process is the one at which the inefficiency arises. Two broad generalizations are:

1. When lamb marking percentages are consistently below acceptable levels, the fault probably lies in management, including climatic, nutritional, and genetic aspects of the environment.

2. When lamb marking percentages fluctuate temporarily, the fault is usually due to an infectious disease or exposure to a toxic agent, or to seasonally abnormal inclement weather or overall deficiency of feed (Moule 1969).

Joining (Breeding) Program

Time of Year for Joining. A joining period should be selected at which the serving capacity and fertility of rams, and the occurrence of estrus and pregnability of ewes, are at their best. This means avoiding very hot summers (because high environmental temperatures reduce ram libido and semen quality and ewe fertility) and very cold winters. There is a distinct preference for autumn over spring because of the greater fertility. For example, in fat lamb flocks, the variation may be as great as 130% lambing percentage for spring joining and 170% for autumn (Lees 1971). However, the joining period must also be compatible with good nutrition of the ewe in late pregnancy and with lambing occurring at a time when lamb survival is maximal. This means not only a time of clement weather but also that the stressful situation of lambing should occur at a time that is nutritionally appropriate for a good start in life. The optimum joining period will also need to be one of a high plane of nutrition. The time of shearing, because of the temporary loss of insulation, is an additional potential cause of stress that must be taken into account in arranging a sheep management year. Shearing causes a drain on metabolism, and if sheep are shorn immediately before the joining period, both ewes and rams are likely to be temporarily reduced in fertility. Another fertility-reducing operation, dipping, is also likely to be carried out soon after shearing. It is advisable to allow at least six weeks after shearing before joining.

The time of year of joining determines the lambing period and, to a large extent, the neonatal mortality rate. Besides the number of lambs found dead during a bad-weather, late spring, there is a more subtle form of loss. Ewe lambs that are born in spring show their first estrus in the next autumn at 120 to 200 days of age. Those born in late autumn are likely not to show estrus until the next autumn at 360 to 440 days of age. This greatly increases the difficulties already encountered in getting maiden merino ewes joined at an early age.

Length of Joining Period. In autumn, six weeks is a sufficient joining period in a reproductively efficient flock. In spring joining, eight to nine weeks is recommended.

Joining Paddocks. It is an advantage to have good paddocks with good shelter, water supply, and feed for joining.

Management of Ewe Flocks

Management of ewe flocks with an eye to their reproductive performance must emphasize a strong culling program, good nutrition, and avoidance of systemic or debilitating disease. The culling program should be directed toward performance, age, and inherited defects.

Genetic Selection for Fertility

Genetic methods of improving fertility are well recognized by merino breeders. Techniques include selection for twinning by selecting as many ewes and rams as possible from among twins. Twinning is highly inherited, provided the ewe's maiden performance is deleted. The remaining selection pressure is for fleece weight, also highly inheritable. Selection pressure is directed against "wrinkly" rams with heavy skin folding because they are more susceptible to heat stress and less fertile than plain-bodied rams. Similarly, wrinkly ewes have a high incidence of dystocia because of heavy birthweight lambs and have lower survivability than plain ewes. Universal support is lacking for the view that ewes with open faces are more fertile than ewes with heavy wool cover, i.e., "muffle-faced." However, there is enough evidence to suggest that selection against the character is desirable. This means that selection of merinos for high wool production as exemplified by wool covering the face and wrinkled skins is counterproductive because these sheep are less fertile. All reproductive indices are likely to be decreased, including proportion of ewes that lamb, proportion of multiple births, and survival rate. The degree of loss is estimated to be a 5% reduction in fertility due to excessive wrinkledness and a reduction of up to 15% associated with severe face-muffling. A total of 40% more lambs weaned from plain sheep compared with very wrinkly sheep is recorded.

Selection for Multiple Births. Provided the net effect on lambs weaned is beneficial, this practice is to be recommended. Twinning is a heritable characteristic, and some remarkable gains have been made using this knowledge.

Selection pressure should be directed against defects as follows:

◻ Young ewes for undershot or overshot jaw; wrinkledness, muffled face; faulty udders
◻ Mature ewes for faulty udders; no lamb in second or later breeding season

An alternative to selection within a breed is to cross-breed with a breed of known high prolificacy, like the Finnish Landrace. However, the gain of lambs born is often reduced by an increased rate of lamb loss in the immediate postpartum period (Maund et al. 1980).

Prejoining Examination—Ewes

A breeding soundness examination is not possible in ewes, but assessment of nutritional status is, and an examination of the udders and culling of ewes with faulty teats or udder is recommended. In ewes carrying a heavy fleece and with severe breech contamination it may be advisable to crutch or even shear before joining. Maiden ewes present problems, and timidity may be one of them. This can be overcome to an extent by putting them into a small paddock at night and using mature, vigorous rams. The identification of individual ewes is desirable but unlikely to be practicable except in stud herds. Some special method of identification of twins is desirable.

Ewe body weight, condition score, and nutritional status are not synonymous terms, but they are closely related. A high body weight enhances the occurrence of estrus and the conception rate of ewes (Hedges and Reardon 1975), and ewes in poor body condition and with low body weight have low estral activity and conception rates (Grant et al. 1981). There is also reliable evidence that a good nutritional status coincides with good ovulation and conception rates (Tsakalof et al. 1977). In merino ewes between 60 and 110 lb. body weight, each increment of 10 lb. is thought to increase the lambing percentage by

6% (Miller 1981). Although the above views are widely held, there is some dissent (Speedy and Clark 1981), but it is possible that the difference could be accounted for by differences between breeds. In flocks where worm infestations are a problem, prejoining and prelambing drenching with an effective anthelmintic may effect improvement in ewe fertility by 4 to 7% of lambs weaned (Mackay 1980).

The good nutritional status of ewes at the beginning of the joining season must be maintained for the six to nine weeks of joining; the ewes should be on a stable or rising plane of nutrition.

Feeding Program

The ewes need to be on a rising plane of nutrition for three weeks before joining and for three weeks afterwards. This is necessary to "flush" the ewes, to maximize ovulation and implantation. Maximum fertility depends on the ewes being in good condition without being fat. It is best to avoid pasture dominated by subterranean or red clover because of their potential estrogenicity. Unfortunately, the joining period often coincides with a domination of the pasture by these plants. Maiden ewes should receive special nutritional consideration at their first joining to ensure that they have optimum body weight.

Any operations such as shearing, drenching, or dipping, which are likely to interfere with normal food intake, should be avoided.

Benzimidazole anthelmintics and onion grass, *Romulea bulbocodium*, or a fungus growing on it, are known to cause embryological defects or serious losses in conception rate and should be avoided during the joining period and the first half of pregnancy.

Age of Ewes

The objective for age at first joining for ewes is 18 to 19 months, and the fertility at first joining declines 5% every six months from this age (Moule 1960). Up to six years of age, the fertility index increases so that there is a point in keeping ewes until at least this age. The exact optimum age will vary with the nutrition available and the amount of attention that can be given to maiden ewes at joining time. Other limiting factors are the increasing frequency with age of serious udder damage and, on hard grazing, dental attrition. Ewes are usually culled for age at six to seven years, and this is probably before they have reached maximum reproductive efficiency. Certainly in merinos the fertility index and lamb survival index reach their peak at about seven years and the twinning index at about eight years.

Systemic Diseases

Outbreaks of diseases that have general systemic effects can be disastrous for a breeding program. If blowfly strike is likely, the sheep could be jetted before and during the breeding season. In a bad worm season, drench three weeks before putting the rams in. Not much can be done to prevent outbreaks of foot rot or pinkeye, but it might be necessary to prolong the joining period. Poor body condition due to nutritional deficiencies of selenium, iodine, copper, or cobalt need correction. Where ewes are affected by debilitating diseases such as caseous lymphadenitis and chronic progressive pneumonia, their fertility is likely to be greatly reduced (Gates et al. 1977). The control of those other diseases that secondarily affect the fertility of sheep—and this includes most diseases—is presented in other books.

Stimulation of Estrus

Besides nutritional means of stimulating estrus, there are several other techniques available. One is to use the teasing effect of a ram. Ewe fertility is enhanced by a male presence, and the inclusion of a teaser ram with a ewe flock for one to two weeks before mating has the effect of condensing the mating and shortening the lambing period. Rotating the rams between ewe flocks overcomes to some extent the damaging effect that a sterile ram will have.

A number of hormonal methods of stimulating ovulation are also available (Boland et al. 1978, 1979). They can be used for synchronizing estrus but are also useful in overcoming acyclicity. A particular use is when it is desired to wean lambs early (e.g., at eight weeks) and remate the ewes because the last lambing percentage has been very low. The hormonal treatments available are:

- progesterone-impregnated vaginal sponges plus injected pregnant mare serum gonadotropin (Rawlings et al. 1983). These have some disadvantages. They require careful scheduling and the dose rate of PMSG must be calibrated carefully to suit the ewe's ovarian status, more being required when the ewe is suckling a lamb
- gonadotropin-releasing hormone. Because this hormone needs to be available over a long period, it may be administered via a subcutaneously implanted mini-pump. Instead of administering gonadotropin, its presence is stimulated by the drug
- prostaglandin $F_{2\alpha}$, two injections of 100 μg. 11 days apart, is effective and can be followed by paddock mating or artificial insemination of all ewes without estrus detection 64 hours after the second injection. Pregnancy rates are good
- immunization against androstenedione. This technique is in the developmental stage, but excellent results are recorded in increasing the ovulation rate (Smith et al. 1981; Grant et al. 1983). Its principal use appears to be directed at increasing the twinning rate rather than initiating estrus

All of these measures work best if the ewes are in good condition (body condition score of 2½ to 3½ out of 5) and have been exposed to virile male company during the previous three or four weeks. The response of the flock to whatever treatment is used should be monitored, either by pregnancy testing or by running rams wearing marking harnesses.

Artificial Insemination

Where it is desired to spread the influence of a sire or group of sires over a large population quickly, for example, the introduction of "polledness," artificial insemination has a significant part to play. Good techniques are available, and results with fresh semen are good (Miller 1981). Ewes are detected in estrus by teaser rams, usually vasectomized ones. Semen is usually collected by artificial vagina or, in some circumstances, by electrical stimulation. The semen is checked for quality by physical methods, diluted, and used immediately. Short-term storage for 24 hours at 2° to 5°C is used but is not universally favored. Results are conflicting. Deep-frozen semen has a conception rate of about 50%; thus it is unlikely to be used in ordinary circumstances. Insemination is into the cervical canal, using a lighted speculum, with the ewe's hindquarters elevated and the forequarters being downward to give maximum viewability and to restrict movement. The same problems that limit fertility of ewe flocks in paddock mating also operate in inseminated flocks.

Pregnancy Diagnosis and Surveillance

This technique has been described in an earlier section, but it has not been generally adopted in sheep preventive medicine because of the cost. It is used in the examination of flocks that have a problem in reproductive efficiency.

It is hard to justify the expenditure if the conception rate is high. The chief return for the examination is in terms of the supplementary feed saved if 20 to 30% of the ewes in a supposed lambing flock can be taken out and put onto dry sheep rations because they are not pregnant. It also enables the farmer to sell off those nonpregnant ewes over a longer time frame or to remate them quickly if that suits his annual pattern. Also, the closer surveillance needed for pregnant ewes can now be concentrated on a smaller group.

If the pregnant ewe flock is large enough, it is advantageous to divide it into groups with similar projected lambing dates. Vaccinations provided to pregnant ewes and directed at passive immunization of their lambs can also be given at a more exactly appropriate time.

Pregnant ewes are especially subject to a number of diseases for which special surveillance should be maintained. They are:

□ Failure to conceive. If the rams are taken out of the flock before pregnancy is in fact established in many ewes, failure to observe that would result in a serious drop in reproductive efficiency. Continuing to run vasectomized rams with the ewes will detect the error. The accuracy of the observation will be greatly increased if the rams are provided with sheep marking harnesses.

□ Abortion due to any cause. Because many abortions in ewes can go unobserved, a single occurrence should stimulate a very close surveillance. This is of particular importance if *Campylobacter fetus* var. *intestinalis* is the cause. Vaccination against this disease is usually not carried out routinely because of the sporadic abortions that occur. However, vaccination is recommended at the beginning of the outbreak (Gilmour et al. 1975).

□ Pregnancy toxemia is common during the last third of pregnancy, especially when the ewe is carrying twin lambs and the feed supply is declining.

□ Hypocalcemia may cause deaths in late pregnant ewes that are suddenly deprived of all feed during late pregnancy. It is more commonly a disease of lactating ewes.

During the last six to seven weeks of pregnancy, the plane of nutrition of the ewes needs to be rising, or at least maintained, in order to avoid pregnancy toxemia and also to promote lamb survival. As a general rule, ewes should gain 15 to 20 pounds (7 to 9 kg.) body weight during this period. One of the serious deficiencies of knowledge in sheep nutrition is the optimum curve of body weight for ewes over a year's cycle. What is needed is a knowledge of the nutritional, and therefore body weight, requirements to fit the needs of the lambs and ewes so that they can be fitted to the natural fluctuations in the pasture that is available. In general, spring lambing fits the pasture availability best.

Termination of Pregnancy

Surveillance over lambing ewes is a key factor in reducing neonatal lamb mortality and is dealt with in the next section. Hormonal intervention to terminate pregnancy is a valuable tool in sheep management.

Termination of unwanted early pregnancy in ewe lambs going into feedlots or in cases of misalliance is sometimes required. The injection of 125 or 250 μg. of cloprostenol (a prostaglandin analog) is reported to cause rapid luteolysis in 92% of ewes pregnant for 20 to 60 days, 83% showing estrus within seven days (Tyrrell et al. 1981).

Induction of parturition in late pregnant ewes can be effected by the injection of a corticosteroid, e.g., 8 to 10 mg. betamethasone (Lucas and Notman 1974) or 2 mg. flumethasone (Harmon and Slyter 1980). Parturition occurs about 45 hours after the injection. There are no lamb losses or retained placentae. The effect is much reduced in ewes less than 130 days pregnant, and treatment after pregnancy day 138 is recommended for best results (Emady et al. 1974). Estradiol benzoate (10, 20, or 40 mg. IM as a single dose) is also reported to be an effective inducer of parturition in ewes pregnant 140 days or more (Restall et al. 1976b).

Ram Management

The stud side of the sheep industry is engaged in producing rams to be used as sires in other studs and commercial flocks. The following program can be used as a protocol to follow when checking a ram for purchase as well as for maintaining ram fertility in a flock with a flock health program in operation.

Selection for Fertility

The known and suspected inherited defects of sheep are listed elsewhere. Those that are of particular importance to ram fertility are cryptorchidism, excessive skin wrinkling, "muffle-faced" strains, and inguinal hernias. Of indirect importance in fertility is the positive inheritance of twinning, a susceptibility to dystocia, and dental malapposition. It is probably wisest to select against testicular and scrotal abnormalities that are of unknown origin. For rapid genetic improvement, the average age of the ram flock should be kept low. This also encourages high fertility. Commonly quoted figures are that 10% of rams are infertile at four years and 35% at seven years.

Prejoining Examination

Six to eight weeks before the joining season begins, a physical examination should be made of all rams, followed by physical and bacteriological examinations of semen in rams with abnormal palpatory findings. During the physical examination, the presence of other diseases that may effect ram fertility can be identified. These include local abscesses caused by *Corynebacterium pseudotuberculosis*, chorioptic mange and mycotic dermatitis of the scrotum, blowfly strike, and lice and ked infestation.

The rams need to be in good body condition at the start of the mating season if they are to stand up to the intensive hard work of breeding 50 ewes in a six-week period. In one report of 160 rams examined, only 37% were in ideal condition, 50% were in acceptable condition, and 12% were in poor reproductive condition (Galloway et al. 1981). Bad feet, poor body condition, and poor teeth are commonly found, with testicular degeneration, epididymitis, spermiostasis, and preputial injury the commonest findings in the genitalia.

At the time of examination, the feet should be trimmed, the rams should be drenched for worms and blood samples taken for brucellosis testing, and they should be shorn if necessary. The ration should be adjusted if the ram is in too light condition for safety and the worm drench repeated at monthly intervals until the joining period.

The ram needs to be in good body condition before joining to a small band of active ewes. Rams are usually cared for well enough nutritionally that a deficiency of energy is unlikely to be an important cause of infertility, but a rising plane of nutrition in the immediate prejoining period is recommended with the objective of having the rams in good condition without being fat. A dietary deficiency of vitamin A of sufficient severity to affect fertility is not likely under normal pastoral conditions, but if there is a completely dry period of two months in the prejoining period, supplementation with vitamin A or lucerne hay should be provided.

The mating season is usually chosen to provide the best nutritional status at joining time for the ewes, and for the lambs at lambing time. However, the mating season also needs to be related to climate to ensure maximum fertility. Additional measures include shearing the rams twice a year with the aim of having about 3 cm. wool at joining. Insufficient wool leads to lack of insulation. Unnecessary driving during joining is to be avoided and, if possible, well-shaded paddocks should be provided. Fat, heavily wrinkled, and shorn rams are the most susceptible to infertility caused by heat stress.

Per Cent and Age of Rams

In commercial flocks, rams are usually used for a relatively short period, and rarely beyond seven years of age; culling at that age is largely for genetic reasons, although total fertility tends to decrease from four years of age onward. In stud flocks, rams give good service for much longer. For optimum results, mature rams are used at a concentration of 2 to 2.5% of the total ewe population. Young rams in their first season breed fewer ewes, and a concentration of 4% is recommended. A similar concentration may be needed on very sparsely populated farms to ensure that the rams can locate the ewes in estrus.

A commonly adopted measure to avoid poor reproductive efficiency because of ram infertility is to run ewes in groups of sufficient size so that more than one ram is needed for each group and then to rotate the rams between groups every two weeks. In the nonbreeding season, it is good practice to keep the rams divided into age groups. If numbers are small, the untried rams should be kept separate from the experienced rams. The recommendation is based on preventing transmission of *Brucella ovis* between rams and may have little other justification.

In a spring joining period, which is usually longer than an autumn mating, i.e., nine instead of six weeks, it is recommended that two drafts of 1% of rams be used one after the other. In autumn joinings, all the rams are put in together.

Monitoring Ram Performance

The efficiency of the rams can be gauged by the use of a mating detection harness. A number of rams can be observed in the one ewe flock by the use of different colored crayons in the harness. The same device can be used to indicate time periods. In the first three weeks of joining, the rams should be marking many ewes, but in the second three weeks, the numbers being bred should be much less. A harness ensures identification of those rams that are working, the percentage of the off-spring, and the identity of those ewes that are mated on the same day. It is of very great practical value in flocks where anestrus is likely. During a busy joining season, an active ram will lose a good deal of body weight, and this may also be used as a rough guide to the ram's breeding prowess.

The Special Targets of Flock Health Programs

NEONATAL LAMB MORTALITY

The Size of the Problem

In sheep flocks that are housed at lambing time, and in which surveillance of ewes and the provision of timely assistance in cases of dystocia are possible, neonatal mortality of lambs can be minimal—that is, provided the lambs are born at full term and that iodine deficiency, hypothyroidism, and colibacillosis are avoided. But when lambing is a pastoral exercise, the picture can be very different. The percentage of lambs surviving until weaning in southern Australia under average conditions can be as low as 70 to 80% compared with the number of lambs born, which can be 100% of the merino ewes joined.

Dennis (1972a) quotes an estimated loss of 20% of all lambs born in most countries before weaning. In Australia, 80% of these deaths occur during the first few days of life; the immediate and delayed parturient deaths are discussed below. A survey of the range flocks in the U.S. showed that there was a mortality rate of 23.5% between birth and weaning and that 73% of these deaths occurred during the first five days of life (Safford and Hoversland 1960). In Zimbabwe, 15% of lambs are recorded as dying before 16 weeks of age, with 70% of the losses being due to managerial errors (McKenzie and Grant 1976). In southern Australia, the average estimated neonatal lamb loss in a predominantly merino population is 15 to 20% (Dennis 1974), but losses as high as 70% of ewes losing all their lambs are recorded (Plant et al. 1976). English estimates of loss are 12% (Boundy 1979), and Scottish estimates vary from 5 to 15% (Houston and Maddox 1974) in milder climates but up to 20 to 25% in hill sheep, due mostly to starvation and exposure (Watt 1980). New Zealand figures (Gumbrell 1980) show that an average mortality of 8 to 10% of newborn lambs was composed of death due to starvation in 39% and exposure in 28%; 76% of lambs had lesions caused by dystocia. Of these deaths, 6% occurred before parturition, 33% during parturition, and 61% after parturition. A Norwegian summary showed an overall death rate of 9.7% from birth to five months of age, with 46% of these deaths occurring in the perinatal period of day 1 to 28. The ewes were housed and vaccinated against clostridial disease (Lutnaes and Paus 1981). The practical acceptable level of mortality in neonates is 7 to 8%.

Relative Importance of the Individual Causes of Neonatal Mortality in Lambs. The principal causes of neonatal mortality are those causing hypothermia in the lamb—excessive heat loss due to a high chilling factor in the environment, low heat production caused by prolonged birth, immaturity, and starvation (Eales 1982). However, it is not possible to give general figures because individual agents have varying importance in different environments. Especially important is whether or not the sheep are housed, and if not, whether they are farmed intensively with close surveillance or whether they are run under extensive pastoral conditions where such surveillance is not possible.

The most exhaustive survey of causes of neonatal loss is an Australian one (Dennis 1974, 1975). As might be expected in their extensive circumstances, starvation, dystocia, predation, and exposure accounted for most deaths. Pathological and microbiological causes were relatively minor. Even in housed ewes in the U.K., which were pastured after lambing, the losses were about 12%, most of them at birth and in the first day of life, with starvation and stillbirth representing almost half the deaths and neonatal infection the next biggest group

(Purvis et al. 1979). In northern Scotland, where the sheep run at pasture all year, the overall death rate has been recorded as 14.2%, again with stillbirths, starvation, and exposure as the commonest causes, accounting for over 50% of deaths (Johnston et al. 1980). In New Zealand, the most common cause of death in singles was dystocia due to high birth weights; in multiples, the commonest cause was starvation and exposure due to lower birth weight. Lambs of birth weight of 3.5 to 5.5 kg. and from four- to five-year-old ewes survived best (Dalton et al. 1980). In Queensland (Australia), exposure to high environmental temperature was a common cause, with small lambs (about 2.5 kg.) being most susceptible (Stephenson et al. 1980).

Similar losses occur in housed and feedlotted flocks in the western U.S., death losses varying from 8 to 12% of the lambs born, with the lower figure related to better management (Kirk and Anderson 1982). In housed and feedlotted ewes, starvation is still a significant cause of death, but exposure is less so.

There is a sequence in the occurrence of diseases of lambs that has been accurately identified for feedlot lambs but not for field lambs, although the sequence is likely to be very similar. The list of common causes of death in feedlot lambs (Kirk and Anderson 1982) is:

☐ death before birth—abortion, stillbirths
☐ birth to two days—exposure, starvation, dystocia (trauma)
☐ two to six days—trauma, starvation, pneumonia, diarrhea, enterotoxemia
☐ seven to 21 days—pneumonia, diarrhea, enterotoxemia, white muscle disease
☐ 22 days and on—pneumonia, enterotoxemia, coccidiosis

Classification of Causes of Perinatal Mortality

On any sheep farm there are losses of lambs in utero, during birth, and in the neonatal period. When recommending a preventive veterinary program to limit these losses, it is necessary to know the important modes of loss on the particular farm. In sheep flocks, it is common to find that more than one cause— and often a number of causes—contribute significantly to the total loss. This is shown pictorially in Figure 12–3.

Determination of the exact cause or causes of loss is usually difficult, because the principal requirements—to observe closely, record care-

fully, and classify accurately—are not easy tasks in the sheep-farming environment. A system of classification is shown pictorially in Figure 12–4. It is based on an overall group of perinatal mortality (Dennis 1972a) that includes all deaths from late pregnancy to 28 days after parturition. Failure to establish pregnancy, early embryonic death, and abortion have been presented in the previous section. Our concern at this stage begins at the point of diagnosis of stillbirth.

Diagnosis of Causes of Perinatal Losses

Diagnosis of Specific Cause of Lamb Death. On the basis of the history of the mortality and the gross changes at necropsy examination, it should be possible to categorize the cause as being environmental or as deriving from the characteristics of either the lamb or the ewe, as discussed here.

ENVIRONMENTAL CAUSES
Climate—inclement hot or cold weather
Nutritional error
    General inanition
    Iodine—goiter
    Copper—enzootic ataxia
    Selenium/vitamin E—white muscle disease
Predators

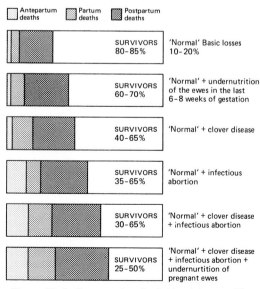

Figure 12–3. Causes of perinatal lamb losses. (From Dennis, S.M. Perinatal lamb mortality. Cornell Vet., *62*:253–262, 1972.)

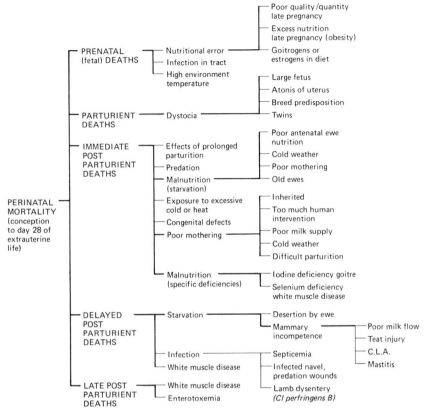

Figure 12-4. Classification of perinatal deaths of lambs.

Infections
Congenital ⎫ with or without
Extrauterine ⎭ immune deficiency
CAUSED BY EWE CHARACTERISTICS
Breed
Age
Mothering capability
Dystocia
CAUSED BY LAMB CHARACTERISTICS
Size of lamb—dystocia
—undersized and weak
Twinning
Congenital defects
Physical events, e.g., marking
Lack of vigor—many causes

Techniques

A high perinatal death loss may be obvious, with a large number of dead lambs. In other circumstances, it may only become apparent as a high level of positive pregnancy diagnoses followed by a low lamb-marking percentage. Perinatal lamb losses are therefore often much greater than farmers realize, and the first objective is to determine the extent of the problem. This section on techniques is recommended as a guide to examining a problem in a flock (Plant 1977) or to developing a monitoring system to include in a continuing flock health program.

As a general rule, it is recommended that losses of less than 15% of all lambs, or less than 10% of ewes losing all their lambs, are within the bounds of normality and are uneconomic to investigate in detail. It is unlikely that a cost-effective program could be mounted against the causes in these flocks.

1. Analysis of Retrospective Data. Careful examination of past lambing records should be combined with a description of the management of the farm and its physical resources. This analysis can pay excellent dividends if there are good records. It will give an assessment of the size of the problem plus an indication of which phase of the lambing sequence is the location of the error. Suitable areas for analysis are:

◻ time, season, prevailing weather at lambing, reasons for timing
◻ geographical location of lambing paddocks, shelter available

□ size of ewe flocks, degree of supervision, reason for group, e.g., similar joining or projected lambing dates

□ supplementary feeding during late pregnancy

□ number of ewes requiring assistance at lambing

□ quality of predator control

□ tranquility of ewe flock under supervision

□ length of the lambing season

□ lambing percentage; method of estimation should be $\dfrac{\text{lambs born}}{\text{ewes joined}} \times 100$. Ensure nonpregnant ewes have not already been taken out

□ losses at marking

□ losses at weaning

□ weaning policy, age, weight, amount of feed available

2. Special Examination of Flock to Decide Reproductive Efficiency at Lambing. The two recommended examinations are the ones for pregnancy diagnosis and the wet/dry ewe classification, both of which were discussed in earlier sections.

3. Observation of Flocks at Lambing. Differentiation between mismothering by ewes and lack of vigor in lambs as causes of death by starvation of lambs is important and is possible only by daily observation of the flock by the farmer. Starvation due to death or absence of the ewe or because of failure of lactation is usually clear-cut. The lambs, although still alive, are dejected, hunched-up, gaunt, and hungry. Eventually, they are comatose and hypothermic. Postmortem lesions are confined to dehydration, complete utilization of white fat, and replacement of it with red gelatinous tissue.

When the cause of the starvation is lack of vigor of the lamb, the signs and lesions of starvation are complicated by those of the primary cause, which may be infection, exposure to cold or heat, congenital defects, and so on. They are, accordingly, more difficult to identify, and the only really satisfactory way of identifying specific causes in lambs dying of starvation is the observation of the flock's behavior. When the cause of lack of vigor in lambs is undernutrition while in utero, it is necessary to identify this on the basis of low body weight at birth and an absence of placental lesions. The history of availability of feed and evidence of low body weight in the ewes is confirmatory evidence.

An accurate count of dead lambs is the only way to determine how many lambs have been lost. Ewes with twins may lose one and not come to notice easily.

When a large number of lambs are dying over a short period, it requires some thought to devise a system of carrying out necropsy examinations so as to get a significant result without an impossible cost. First, it is necessary to conduct examinations that answer the question, "Did this lamb die of dystocia, or starvation, or predation, or infection, or is it in a new category that requires investigation?" In other words, did the lamb die of a specific cause related to a proposed or existing control measure? Having categorized the death, it may be necessary to pursue a "new category" series of deaths to a more definite end-point. But it will be more necessary to examine a predetermined number of dead lambs to get a statistically significant result. This is not only a matter of numbers; it is also a matter of selecting the postmortem specimens in a quite random manner. It is easy to get a biased sample if it is left to the farmer to pick up the lambs selected for postmortem examination. If possible, the placenta should also be collected because it is a better source of any infectious agent. When the farmer is bringing the lambs in, it is usually possible to have him put all of one day's pick-up in a wet-proof bag and bring the dated bags every third day. The bags must carry the date of pick-up, information on weather, and so on.

A technique for a standardized postmortem examination has been described by McFarlane (1961, 1965, 1966) and is in general use. Its purpose is to establish whether or not the death was preparturient, parturient, or postparturient, and whether the postparturient ones were early or late after birth.

The system depends on a number of critical "lesions" that suggest that particular lambs should be classified into one of 21 time slots relative to parturition. Thus, lambs that have died intrauterine or intravaginal, i.e., preparturient deaths, show rapid autolysis of subcapsular renal cortex. Postmortem discoloration and mummification occur at further time intervals. Parturient deaths are indicated by local edema of parts of the body jammed in the pelvis and in which circulation has been obstructed; the lungs are aerated and there is often hemorrhage from the liver. Postparturient deaths are divided into immediate, delayed, and late time categories, and classification is made on the basis of aeration of lungs, the state of the umbilical artery, the degree of mobilization of body fat, the soles of the feet as an indication of whether or not the lamb has walked, and the presence of ingesta along the length of the gut. These findings are shown in Table 12-1. Severe cases of goiter are readily recognized at necropsy, but weighing of the thyroids may be necessary to make a diagnosis in flocks where hypothyroidism is suspected of being a contributory rather than a principal cause (Setchell et al. 1960).

4. Head Count of Ewes and Lambs at Marking (Docking). This provides an opportunity to segregate the lactating ewes from the ones that have not lambed. Ewes that have lambed, but have lost all their lambs, will have enlarged udders containing secretions of various kinds depending on when the lambs ceased to suck. Ewes that have not lambed will have small, empty udders and no staining of the perineal wool. Detection of these ewes will be greatly helped by a previous pregnancy diagnosis.

The valuable information that should be gained from a marking count includes:
□ marking percentage, i.e., of ewes joined
□ percentage of lambs to ewes present—the twinning index
□ wet ewes that have no lamb; loss of lambs due to various causes

Specific Environmental Causes of Lamb Deaths

Inclement Weather. The heaviest losses in Australian sheep flocks occur in the form of outbreaks when the weather is very bad. Deaths are the result of excessive body cooling due to low temperature, driving winds, and starvation. Wetness may or may not be involved. The starvation results indirectly from poor mothering by the ewe either because she is a poor mother, because the weather interferes with mothering, or because the lamb is weak owing to poor antepartum nutrition. These lambs often walk after birth, but at postmortem examination there is little to see. They may have sucked, but there is little digestion, and the intestine on the recumbent side is flaccid.

The relative importance of environmental and maternal factors is not easy to determine. The preponderance of evidence supports the view that inclement weather kills many lambs, probably more than would otherwise die, but principally those that are predisposed to be susceptible either because of their own reduced vigor—dependent upon poor preceding nutrition—or because of poor mothering—itself as dependent on poor nutrition of the ewe

as on her inherited lack of mothering ability (Alexander and Peterson 1961; Alexander 1962, 1964; Alexander et al. 1979). The vigor of the lamb, principally manifested as "sucking drive," is reduced by lack of reward, so that a vicious cycle is created if the ewe will not stand. Vigor is also greatly reduced by cold discomfort, giving inclement weather two points at which it influences lamb survival rates (Alexander and Williams 1966). The lamb dies of hypothermia and inanition.

Consistent, very hot weather during pregnancy results in lightweight lambs and sometimes in abortion. Environmental temperatures need to be of the order of 100°F (37.8°C). At this sort of temperature, newborn lambs soon die, e.g., neonatal lambs up to seven days old survive only two hours at temperatures over 100°F. Lambs with short coats are usually the first to die, apparently because of their poorer insulation. Some lamb deaths occur in these circumstances because of the need of the ewes to make frequent trips to water. The lambs may get lost or fall exhausted.

Lambs that have died of exposure have no specific postmortem lesions. If they are found while they are still alive, they are prostrate, comatose, and hypothermic. In either case, they are likely to be confused with lambs dead of other causes. In a series of postmortem examinations, it is the absence of clear-cut indications that helps to identify this cause; they may or may not show evidence of having walked, of having fed, of having absorbed fat, and of having utilized body fat.

Nutritional Errors. GENERAL INANITION. Lack of total food supply is the principal cause of death in most lambs in bad outbreaks. It can be caused by bad weather, by *too* much human intervention at lambing time in flighty ewes, by poor nutrition of the ewe, or by lack of vigor on the part of the lamb. Normal lambs are born with sufficient nutritional reserves to last them for one to four days, so that deaths due to starvation occur during this period. The starvation may be primary or secondary. Primary starvation is due to absence of the milk supply. Secondary starvation occurs when the lamb lacks sucking vigor due to another primary cause, which includes mismothering by the ewe, damage to teats or udder (Hayman et al. 1955), and poor nutrition of the ewe (Bareham 1976).

The nutrition of the ewe, inasmuch as it determines her body condition and milk flow, has a considerable effect on her mothering tendency and the energy supply to the lamb.

Table 12-1. GUIDE TO DETERMINATION OF TIME OF LAMB DEATH BASED ON POSTMORTEM EXAMINATION

	Blood-stained Subcutaneous Edema	Breakdown of Fetal Tissues	Renal Autolysis	Thrombosis of Umbilical Artery[1]	Aeration of Lungs[2]	Soles of Feet Worn[3]	Ingesta in Gut[4]	Body Fat State[5]
Acute parturient	Generalized extensive	Mummification or autolysis	Marked	−	−	−	−	Autolyzed
Parturient	Local to presented parts	−	Slight or nil	−	±	−	−	Stable
Immediate postparturient	−	−	−	±	+	±	−	Stable
Delayed postparturient	−	−	−	±	+	+	±	Stable or
Late postparturient	−	−	−	+	+	+	+	Marked catabolism

[1]Thrombosis of umbilical artery indicates that lamb has survived birth process.
[2]Aerated state of lungs indicates that lamb has breathed.
[3]Wear on soft sole of foot will indicate that lamb has walked.
[4]Milk in the intestine and milk fat in the lymphatics of the gut indicate that the lamb has sucked.
[5]Catabolism of the body fat (not white as normal, but yellow-brown gelatinous material) indicates lamb has mobilized fat to convert to energy and suggests that nutritional stress has occurred.

For example, the difference between survival rates on native and improved pasture can be 74% for the former as compared with 82% for the latter (Lax and Turner 1965).

Another way in which nutrition of the ewe exerts its influence on lamb survival is via the improved nutrition of the fetal lamb and its greater size and strength at birth. Overfeeding can also be harmful in that the lambs are overweight and may develop dystocia. As a general guide, it is recommended that ewes should maintain their own body condition in late pregnancy and at the same time gain 15 to 20 pounds in the six weeks before lambing.

Later on in the lamb's life, nutrition of the ewe exerts still another effect. High-plane nutrition of the ewe leads to a high milk yield and the maintenance of a strong ewe/lamb bond. Ewes on a low plane of nutrition tend to reach the threshold milk yield, which leads to voluntary weaning much earlier. The growth rate of lambs and even their survival may be affected at this point (Arnold et al. 1978).

SPECIFIC NUTRITIONAL DEFICIENCIES. The commonly occurring ones are iodine-deficient goiter, neonatal white muscle disease due to selenium deficiency, and congenital enzootic ataxia or swayback due to copper deficiency.

Orally Ingested Poisons. Plant poisons include *Veratrum californicum*, which causes brain defects and prolonged gestation and *Astragalus* and *Oxytropis* spp., which cause limb contractures. The anthelmintics albendazole and parbendazole are known teratogens. Apholate, a chemical sterilant used on insects, is suspected to be teratogenic. Experimental hyperthermia has been shown to cause limb deformities.

Infectious Diseases Causing Neonatal Lamb Mortality. The list includes:
- septicemias—*Escherichia coli, Listeria monocytogenes, Salmonella* sp.
- bacteremias with localization in joints, endocardium, eyes—*Toxoplasma gondii*
- streptococci, staphylococci, *Erysipelothrix insidiosa*
- diarrhea with dehydration—colibacillosis, rotavirus infection
- toxemias—gas gangrene of the navel; crowpicked eye (Smith 1965b) caused by *Clostridium septicum* or *Cl. edematiens;* lamb dysentery caused by *Cl. perfringens* type B

In sheep, much more so than in cattle, the infections that cause abortion also cause fetal and neonatal deaths. They are more accurately identified as fetal-neonatal syndromes (Dennis, 1972a; Hartley 1968). There is a long list of miscellaneous infections that occur in lambs, but they are not cited here.

The prevalence of neonatal infections varies. In New Zealand, up to 30% of total deaths and in Scotland (Watt 1980), 18% of total deaths are attributed to infectious disease. In Australia, a similar level of such infections, up to 30% of total lamb deaths, is reported (Hartley and Boyes 1964; Hughes et al. 1964; Haughey et al. 1967), and the viruses of bovine mucosal diseases and parainfluenza type 3 have also been isolated from perinatal mortalities in lambs (Hore et al. 1973). In general, the tendency is to make little of the role of neonatal infections in causing lamb mortalities because the mortality rate in flocks due to these infections is often as low as 1%. This happens often, especially in merino flocks, and more obvious reasons for lamb mortalities, such as deleterious climate and nutrition, are usually readily available.

Culture of every fetus in an investigation is not possible. The recommended alternative is to culture from those carcasses that show lesions suggestive of congenital infection. These include subcutaneous, usually bloodtinged, excess fluid and fibrin in body cavities, hepatomegaly, focal hepatic lesions, intestinal hyperemia, enlarged mesenteric lymph nodes, and bright yellow meconium. Although culture of the lamb and the placenta is preferred, the placenta is more important for diagnosis than the lamb.

Extrauterine Infections. Attention has also been given to infections in dead newborn lambs in which the infection is assumed to be picked up after birth because death occurred in the late postparturient period (Hughes et al. 1971). The incidence of such infection is very low, being 1.6% of all dead lambs. In terms of late postparturient deaths, the infections represented only 3.3%. A much higher incidence is frequently reported, and the result will depend a great deal on local conditions and the size of the sample. The infections recorded include the common pathogens of *Chlamydia, Pasteurella hemolytica, Fusobacterium necrophorum,* and *Clostridium* spp. but without emphasis on any particular agent. *Brucella ovis* has been identified as causing abortion in some sheep flocks and is suspected as a cause of perinatal lamb deaths via congenital infections in others (Haughey et al. 1968). Tetanus is one of the more common infections, but it is much less common nowadays. In lambs at pasture, especially under intensive management systems on lush pasture, enterotoxemia due to *Cl. perfringens* type D is a common enough occurrence to warrant routine prevention by vaccination of ewes before lambing and of lambs at tail-docking time. When the disease occurs in lambs that have not yet had their tails docked, it is a common recommendation to check their growth by docking them immediately. Ecthyma is always likely to be a problem in unweaned lambs, especially when they are artificially reared. Vaccination provides complete protection.

Postmortem lesions that suggest extrauterine postnatal infection are omphaloperitonitis, focal suppurative lesions in any solid viscera or skeleton, and pneumonia, arthritis, and enteritis. The specific infection with *Cl. perfringens* type B (lamb dysentery) is uncommon nowadays but is accompanied by a hemorrhagic enteritis. Clostridial infections of navels, predator-inflicted wounds, and marking wounds are also uncommon because of the awareness by farmers of the need for hygiene or prophylactic treatment at these times.

The clinical picture associated with neonatal infections, whether prenatal or postnatal, is likely to include a range of septicemia with sudden death or navel-ill accompanied by one or all of the following: meningitis, arthritis, endocarditis, and panophthalmitis. By far the most common occurrence is arthritis, either suppurative and caused by streptococcal or staphylococcal infections or nonsuppurative and caused by *Erysipelothrix insidiosa*. These diseases are amenable to early treatment. Hygiene at lambing to avoid umbilical infection and sterilization of instruments at tail docking and castration are appropriate preventive measures.

As in other species, there is a relationship between poor husbandry, low immune globulin intake, and a high level of neonatal infection (Ducker and Fraser 1973). Poor mothering by the ewe or interference with mothering by too much human intervention can thus predispose to neonatal infection. As in other species, some short-term reduction in losses that arise in this way can usually be effected by the injection of a suitable antibiotic, or a mixture of them, into the ewe before lambing and into the lamb for the first week of life. Some spectacular results are claimed (Hamdy et al. 1967), but the technique is scarcely practical for large-scale commercial flocks. Fortunately, these problems are not common in these circumstances.

Blowfly strike of navels or castration wounds can occur but are uncommon because it is not usual to perform these operations in a dangerous period. It is a more common practice to carry out the Mules operation when docking and castrating, and the usual recommendations about hygiene to prevent infection via these wounds should be instituted.

Predation. Predatory birds and animals are responsible for much postmortem mutilation of carcasses and some deaths of lambs weakened by other influences. In developed countries, they are unlikely to be a major factor in pulling down a significant number of live lambs (Dennis 1974). Under extensive conditions, a wide range of animals and birds, including eagles, ravens, foxes, and feral pigs, are considered to cause significant losses (Smith 1965a). In Australia, crows are a significant cause of loss, but their significance is much less than that of foxes, and feral pigs are the worst of all, being capable of killing 80% of the lambs born (Plant et al. 1978). In the U.S. (Dennis 1980), more than 8% of all lambs born may die because of predation. Most deaths are caused by coyotes, which are credited with 93% of the losses. One point to be noted is that overall lamb losses in hardy wool-type sheep are often less than 10%.

Determination that predatory injuries have occurred antemortem depends on the presence of massive hemorrhage in the region of the injury. Tissue disruption and broken bones may occur ante or post mortem. There may be mutilation, but extensive hemorrhage will not be present when the damage occurs after death. Deaths in this group should be classified as predation killing of a healthy animal or as mutilation by a scavenger when the subject is ill or dead when first attacked.

Some information about the identity of the predator may be deduced from an inspection of the cadaver. Foxes and coyotes bite the neck, head, and face of lambs, causing extensive hemorrhage in the area and often crushing or tearing open the larynx. Death occurs as a result of suffocation or hemorrhage. Fang marks through the skin are accompanied by teeth marks, often more visible on the inside of the skin. Coyotes may eat part of the carcass, a hind leg of an older lamb or the internal organs, heart, liver, and abomasum full of milk of newborn lambs. Foxes favor the tongue, lower jaw, tail, and thigh. Dogs, which usually hunt in pairs, do not kill for food, and many lambs or sheep may be killed in one attack. There are usually many bites anywhere on the body. Older sheep are torn about the flanks and thighs. Lambs are often crushed and the limbs stripped of flesh. Crows are poorly equipped to predate and are restricted to gaining access to the interior through a natural opening of an animal already attacked by another predator or already ill from another disease. Common targets are the tongue, eyes, anus, and umbilicus. Eagles and other avian predators and scavengers have the same predilections for tongues and eyes. Eagles usually leave talon marks along the back of a predated lamb.

Specific Ewe Causes

Breed of Sheep. Breed of sheep does have an effect on survival rate (Wiener et al. 1973). There are also apparent differences between families. But the differences between strains of sheep within a breed have not been shown to be significant (Lax and Turner 1965; Arnold and Morgan 1975). Among breeds, merinos are notoriously poor mothers, especially young ewes. Desertion of a lamb at birth is common, and the lambs die of starvation. There is a great deal of difference in mothering traits among ewes, and ewes that are poor mothers often respond poorly to intensive lambing techniques. They also often have prolonged labor and lose most weight before lambing. Selection of the breed of sheep also determines the rate of twinning and, because twins are much more sensitive to environmental insults in early life than singles, they are likely to have a much higher mortality rate. Selection for twinning, especially in merinos, should not be attempted unless intensive lambing facilities are available. The lower average birth rate of twins probably contributes to this higher mortality rate. Certainly, high- and low-weight singles have less chance of survival than those in the median zone (Purser and Young 1964).

Age of Ewe. There is a significantly higher survival rate in lambs from middle-aged merino ewes than those from two-year-old or seven-year-old merino ewes. In part, this is due to the better milk supply and mothering instincts of the middle-aged ewe, but there are other factors, such as the higher birth weights of the lambs, which favor the lamb of the middle-aged ewe. The preponderance of deaths in lambs from young ewes is likely to be due to dystocia. In old ewes, it is more likely to be due to starvation (McDonald 1966). Similar findings are recorded for Norwegian sheep (Lutnaes 1982).

Dystocia. Most cases of dystocia in ewes are due to fetal-pelvic disproportion, with emphasis on the large fetus. This may be encouraged by heavy nutrition, but it is also genetically disposed by the presence of large heads, as in Dorset Horns, Southdowns (Dennis 1970), and Romneys (Hartley and Kater 1964). The proportion of dystocias can be 70% in Southdowns, 28% in Romney Marshes, and as low as 4% in fine-wooled merinos (George 1975). Correspondingly, the percentage of neonatal deaths that result from dystocia is lower (10% of all neonatal mortality) in merinos than for cross-breds (10 to 34%) and for Dorset Horns (36%) (George 1976).

Most dystocias are caused by high birth weights or twinning, with very few cases resulting from malpositioning. When malposition is the error, it usually affects the front legs, with or without deviation of the head.

In the long term, the positive approach to reducing the losses caused by dystocia depends on genetic selection against small pelvic diameters and large lambs or lamb heads. These criteria have been used effectively in a culling program to greatly reduce the occurrence of dystocia in Romney Marsh sheep (McSporran et al. 1977). In Dorset Horns (Fogarty and Thompson 1974), a close relationship between pelvic size and dystocia has been observed; and in Australia, a relationship between fetal size (Whitelaw and Watchorn 1975; Smith 1977) and dystocia has been observed in fine wool merinos and Cheviots. It is also generally agreed that ewes with twins or triplets encounter dystocia more commonly than ewes with single lambs, so that selection for multiple births is likely to lead to more losses at birth. If the pelvis is measured as an aid to selection, it is the internal measurement that is of importance; the external measurement is not a reliable guide (McSporran et al. 1979). Death is usually due to asphyxia, and this may also occur in births of long duration without obvious obstructions. Occasionally, death is due to rupture of the liver. Lambs dead of dystocia are characterized by localized edema of head, tongue, and forelimbs in anterior presentations and of the perineum and tail in posterior or breech presentations (Hartley and Kater 1964). It is important to determine whether there has been fetal-pelvic disproportion or uterine inertia such as occurs with hyperestrogenism in poisoning by subterranean clover. Lambs that survive a difficult birth may subsequently die of starvation because of poor mothering by the ewe. Others may die of injury incurred during parturition, including intracranial hemorrhages (Haughey 1973) or stretching of the meninges (Haughey 1980). The injury to the CNS appears to be the critical factor rather than an indirect effect on food intake (Duff et al. 1982).

Mothering Capability. The mothering ability of the ewe is dealt with in a number of places, especially under breed of sheep. There are some other management points. Lambs are not discriminatory and will suck any ewe. However, ewes are discriminatory, and they vary in their selectivity. Some ewes, before lambing, are receptive and actually search out and steal lambs from other ewes. Others are antagonistic to their lambs and desert them readily. This mothering trait may be innate and inherited. It may be interfered with by managerial factors such as too much human interference; prolonged parturition, including dystocia; poor milk supply; and poor vigor of the lamb. The teat-seeking activities of lambs are subject to the same sorts of influences and may be absent or weak at birth. In normal lambs, there is a high level of teat-seeking activity at birth, but it declines rapidly to about 10% at 12 hours of age. It declines when the lamb is starved and when the weather is cold and the lamb is hypothermic, especially in the first few hours of life. Maternal behavior is likely to be interfered with by flocking behavior, in which the ewe tends to move to the rest of the flock rather than to its lamb. This tendency is likely to increase as the lamb gets older.

Mammary Adequacy. At some suitable time during the ewe's lactation, an examination should be conducted to ensure that both halves are functional and the teat canals are patent. Significant losses can occur in ewes with teats damaged during shearing and halves destroyed by *Corynebacterium pseudotuberculosis* (Hayman 1955), and in ewes with fibrosed udders (Kirk et al. 1980). The prevalence of defective udders may be as high as 12% in abattoir surveys (Madel 1981).

Specific Lamb Causes

The characteristics of lambs that lead to their becoming diseased are as follows.

Congenital Defects. The frequency of defects in newborn lambs appear to be much less than in cattle, and they are not usually recognized as a cause of significant mortality, e.g., an American survey recorded nine out of 36 listed inherited defects in 21,000 Rambouillet lambs born over a 15-year period (Ercanbrack and Price 1971). Another estimate is of 2%

congenital defects for lambs compared with 0.5 to 3% for calves (Hughes 1972). However, higher figures are also quoted (Priester et al. 1970). The nature, cause, and diagnosis of congenital defects in lambs has been reviewed (Dennis and Leipold 1979).

Inherited Defects. The known or strongly suspected inherited defects are:

□ corticocerebellar atrophy (Stamp 1967)
□ a clinically similar disease in Border Leicesters characterized by lesions in neck muscles
□ inherited goiter in merinos and possibly Polled Dorsets
□ ceroid lipofuscinosis in South Hampshires
□ generalized glycogenolysis of Corriedales
□ globoid cell leucodystrophy of Polled Dorsets
□ multiple tendon contracture in merinos
□ osteogenesis imperfecta
□ mandibular underdevelopment of merinos and Rambouillets
□ epidermolysis bullosa in Suffolks and South Dorset Downs
□ dermatosparaxia in merinos
□ bilateral lip cleavage in Texels
□ redfoot in Scottish Blackface
□ inherited photosensitization in Corriedales and Southdowns
□ atresia of gut segments
□ entropion in several British breeds of fat sheep
□ prolonged gestation and fetal giantism in Karakuls (also caused by poisoning with *Veratrum californicum* or *Salsola tuberculata*)
□ hairy birthcoat*
□ cryptorchidism (Claxton and Yeates 1972)
□ scrotal anomalies*
□ crooked legs*
□ ventricular septal defect in Southdowns (Dennis 1970)

The diseases against which control programs have been mounted are corticocerebellar atrophy, photosensitization, and entropion. Selection against the defect can be practiced, but the selection pressure for profitable traits is likely to be high. Accordingly, there is great difficulty in conducting a genetic control program in a single flock. On the other hand, participation in a group breeding scheme (see under genetic management) may make the program feasible (Hight and Rae 1970; Jackson and Turner 1972).

---

*Genetic controllability reported.

Sporadic and Environmental Congenital Defects. The defects known to result from the effects of noxious items in the environment include:

◻ hairy shakers or border disease caused by a virus

◻ brain deformity (porencephaly) caused by attenuated bluetongue virus

◻ arthrogryposis and hydranencephaly caused by Akabane virus infection

◻ white muscle disease due to vitamin E/selenium deficiency in the diet

◻ poisoning by weeds in pasture, e.g., *Veratrum californicum, Astragalus,* and *Oxytropis* spp., *Lupinus sericeus*

◻ poisoning by farm chemicals, especially parbendazole and cambendazole

◻ experimentally by high environmental temperatures

◻ enzootic ataxia (swayback) caused by copper deficiency in the diet

◻ goiter caused by a deficiency of iodine in the water supply

There is a very long list of sporadic defects in sheep. Lists are available for New Zealand (Hartley and Kater 1964) and Australian merinos (Dennis 1965).

Twinning. Although the mortality rate among twins is higher than among singles, the difference may be obvious only under extensive conditions where the general mortality rate is already high. Some of the deaths are the result of unobserved dystocias, which are more likely with twins than with singles. There is also a behavior problem, especially with merino ewes, which are inclined to walk away from one of a pair of twins, especially if it lacks vigor for some reason. However, many of the separations and subsequent deaths from starvation are in robust lambs (Stevens et al. 1982).

Surgical Procedures. Given the absence of the rare disaster at castration, this operation does not significantly alter the survival rate. Excessive blood loss is very rare in young animals, even with knife castration and tail-docking. Internal bleeding, when the spermatic cords are removed by traction rather than being severed with a knife, occurs and makes a dramatic postmortem picture, but the overall importance of these losses is very small. Strong rubber rings (elastrators) are commonly used for docking and castration, and avoid blood loss. An early suggestion that their use might be followed by a higher incidence of tetanus has been disproved.

Lack of Vigor. This is a clinical sign that develops secondarily to a primary disease. There is no intrinsic disease by this name, and it should not be used as a diagnosis.

Control Programs to Optimize Perinatal Survival

Principles of Preventing Neonatal Lambing Losses

An overall control program to suit all circumstances is difficult to propose because the relative importance of the etiological factors varies so much from place to place, from farm to farm, and even within one farm from year to year. In general terms, a program should at least give consideration to each of the following techniques:

1. Close supervision of lambing to detect ewes with dystocia early and provide assistance with the birth. This principle can be practiced by close examination on horseback of ewes at pasture three times a day, by continuous supervision of individual ewes in single pens indoors, or by any variation between these two extremes. The farmer must be instructed in the technique of providing aseptic assistance with parturition.

2. Close supervision of ewe and lamb immediately after birth to ensure proper mothering. The amount of activity required varies with the mothering tendency of the ewe, merinos being the worst as a breed. The objective is to ensure that the lamb receives adequate colostrum—and thus antibodies—in the first few hours after birth and then receives sufficient energy to maintain it through the sensitive first few days when it is very susceptible to hypoglycemia. It is very important to avoid excessive, officious interference, especially with merino ewes and particularly with maiden ewes. A heavy-handed bustling attentiveness may cause more disturbance of mothering than it prevents.

3. Provide protection for the lamb from inclement weather either by lambing in clement weather or by shedding or other protective wind baffles. These include leaving rows of hay bales arranged to give shelter from prevailing winds and cutting of swathes through a standing cereal crop or overgrown pasture (Watson et al. 1968; Egan et al. 1976). The provision of windbreaks around the edges of large paddocks has very little value; the ewes and lambs are too far away to be protected. In effect, they need to get in among the protective material. In very hot climates,

the two critical needs are proximity to water and overhead shelter from the sun. Shedding may be done in the shearing shed or in a shelter constructed especially for the purpose. The latter has obvious advantages, especially if the shed can be put to other uses in the lambing off-season.

4. Adequate nutrition may necessitate supplementary feeding either by hand-feeding of the ewes in late pregnancy or by moving them faster through a paddock rotation system or even by advancing or delaying lambing by four or more weeks. Autumn and spring may be times of feed shortage in some years.

5. Providing surveillance for dystocia and providing shelter and mothering assistance require significant concentration of effort during the lambing period. Ewes getting close to lambing must be brought into an intensive care group, and the ewes and lambs are passed out of this group as soon as possible but only when the dangers of starvation and exposure are past. In shed lambing, this is an obvious maneuver, but it can also be utilized in pasture lambing by a technique of "drifting" lambs and ewes away from the lambing group and into new rearing groups, which are watched less intensively.

6. Measures to ensure an adequate supply of milk for the lambs when they come as single or twins include the prelambing inspection of the ewes' udders. If shearing methods are rough, many ewes can have damaged teats, which reduce the availability of one or both sides of the udder. The lesion needs only to be a small one to block the teat canal. A high incidence of caseous lymphadenitis, with lesions occurring in the supramammary lymph nodes, or of mastitis can also have disastrous effects on lamb survival. Udders surrounded by excessive wool, very pendulous udders, or grossly distended teats also reduce the availability of the milk supply. Ewes with any of these defects should be culled at the earliest opportunity.

7. The choice of the lambing method to be used on a particular farm is largely dependent on the financial gains to be achieved. Managerial expertise is also important. For example, some farmers are excellent in their ability to pick ewes coming up to lambing. Unless there is reasonable expertise at this, the number of ewes that need to be under intensive surveillance at one time becomes so great that the shed required becomes too big to be financially practicable. Many of the problems of intensive lambing could be eliminated by an efficient system of estrus synchronization or

batch-lambing. The farmer must also be able to grasp the concept of asepsis. An outdoor penning or indoor shedding system requires disinfection of pens between ewes to avoid cross-infection of neonatal infections. Manual assistance to a ewe with dystocia requires hygienic precautions. Intensive lambing practices without the farmer appreciating the need for great care with these activities could lead to serious losses.

8. Ability as a shepherd is a large factor in preventing lambing losses, but in present times a more important restricting factor is the relative absence of people to work in this and other agricultural activities. It may be that an excellent intensive system has to be scrapped and the flock reverted to "sink-or-swim" pasture lambing with minimum supervision.

9. The financial gain achieved is the final criterion, but some factors need to be included in it. For example, if a particular farmer is very anxious to increase his flock size without purchasing sheep, the value of twins is raised, and the value of individual animals saved also rises. Because of the need to "capitalize earning power" when it is possible, the opportunity of increasing stocking rate must be kept constantly in mind, but the return to the new management technique must be set against its cost. The price of additional lambs has to be managed so that the cost of additional labor and the interest on the capital invested in a lambing shed are not greater than the value of the lambs provided. Thus, the whole project becomes much more important when the prices of wool and mutton are high and all farmers are seeking to enlarge their flocks.

10. The availability of capital may be as important as the availability of labor. Unless capital is available for shed construction or another similar device, it may be impossible to proceed. One of the functions of a "flock health program" is to assist farmers in getting financial assistance by providing expert advice to money-lending organizations.

11. Other factors that affect the time of lambing may have managerial and financial implications that outweigh inclemency of weather problems. For example, autumn joining and spring lambing has the advantage of high fertility but the disadvantage of higher neonatal losses. The net effect of switching to spring joining and autumn lambing may be nil in terms of lambs on the ground, but a seasonal poor supply of feed in early summer may mean that a high lambing percentage may be offset by a poorer growth rate in early lamb life.

12. The overriding consideration in any flock health program is the need to know the forms of neonatal loss and their important causes. On most farms, it is not possible to do this because the necessary records are not available. In most cases, a count is kept of lambs marked and lambs weaned, but it is usually necessary to run a surveillance year to accumulate data on which to base a decision that the reproductive loss is due to poor fertility or high neonatal mortality. The records needed include:

□ careful, accurate pick-up at least once a day of all dead lambs
□ careful, accurate postmortem examination of a large random sample of dead lambs
□ accurate head count of ewes that lamb and the number of lambs born

This form of examination should be accompanied, as discussed earlier in the section on reproductive inefficiency, by a program including the use of a ram harness to mark ewes in estrus and pregnancy diagnosis. A complete examination is the only way of avoiding an error when both ends of the reproductive cycle have errors.

A completely successful program to cover all eventualities, without regard to cost-effectiveness, is not likely to be a desirable objective. Following are programs of increasing sophistication and cost. The program likely to be chosen will be the one most suited to the economic status and managerial system of the property (Beggs and Campion 1966).

Extensive Lambing

Leaving the ewes to their own devices and examining them once daily at most is a time-honored and satisfactory method where sheep grazing systems are extensive. To do anything more than this would be financially impracticable in most cases, because the usual mortality rate under this system of management is very low. Predators are one of the main causes of loss, and shepherding during the day and corraling at night are about the only practicable preventive measures. Changing the lambing date to avoid the inclement weather of late winter and early spring offers some attractions but has the serious disadvantage of missing the heightened fertility obtained by mating in early autumn (Watson and Elder 1961). The net effect is likely to be no gain. Selection for more motherly ewes would be a worthwhile objective in a very timid ewe flock, but care would be needed to avoid losing some of the fine wool

characteristics. The use of the sheltered paddocks and pastures with the best available feed are routine recommendations for lambing ewes and may be applicable here. The system has the advantage of avoiding excessive interference with the ewes.

Intensive Lambing at Pasture

In this system, the ewes are run at pasture but at a high stocking rate, with surveillance at least twice and preferably three times daily. This provides an opportunity for early correction of dystocia and mismothering, and allows a more accurate identification of lambs and their dams. The system is improved by having a series of small fields available as close as possible to the house to permit almost continuous observation. Maiden ewes should have the closest surveillance, and if feed can be saved in the paddocks before lambing commences, this is an advantage. Shelter provided by putting out hay bales in rows or by cutting swathes in long pasture, especially phalaris or an oat crop, is much used by the sheep and is a great help (Watson 1968; Egan et al. 1972). It is essential that lanes be cut in the long grass or cereal crop. This enables the sheep to move about freely. Failure to do this can result in ewes and lambs being fatally separated. One of the advantages of the system is the number of lambs that can be salvaged that would otherwise die of starvation and exposure. But these solutions require a vehicle for use as an ambulance, a makeshift nursery in a shearing shed, heat lamps and infrared lamps, hot water bottles, cartons, bottle feeding equipment, and a store of antibiotics. Lambs that are likely not to have had colostrum need a prophylactic injection of antibiotics daily for three days after birth.

This system is the one most used and most recommended in southern Australia for average circumstances. It is possible to detect and correct dystocias and mismothering problems but with difficulty in catching the subjects, so that it is sometimes necessary to drive the particular group all the way to the nearest sheep yards. There is also the disadvantage that all the ewes must be inspected. There is no opportunity to separate the flock into ewes that are about to lamb within the next few days and those that are still distant from lambing. This is wasteful of time, and if the lambing percentage is good anyway, there is a tendency to dispense with the inspection, especially when other matters are pressing or when the weather is bad; these tend to be the times when the need is greatest. On the other hand, doubling the amount of time taken in the inspection may give very little improvement in the lambing percentage.

Drift Lambing

This technique is used to overcome the disadvantage of having to examine all the lambing ewes at every inspection. About six small paddocks are needed; the ewes that are reasonably close to lambing are put into the system each day and the nonpregnant ones moved on, leaving the ewes with recent lambs behind. Those left behind are watched to make sure that a firm ewe/lamb bond is established and that both the lambs and ewes are well. After three or four days, they are moved out to other larger groups. The ewes are fairly easy to move in autumn, when feed is inclined to be short and some supplementation by feeding out is occurring. In spring, when there is ample pasture available, the ewes are not easy to move. Drift lambing can be combined with shed lambing as an emergency program to be adopted when weather is bad and losses are likely to be very high. There is one thing that is lacking in the drift system—protection from bad weather. The smallness of the paddocks makes feeding, surveillance, and identification much easier.

Outdoor Pen Lambing

In this technique, the ewes at the point of lambing are moved out of a set of drifting paddocks and into a set of individual pens. It may be that all ewes go into a pen, or perhaps only the problem ones that present mismothering or dystocia difficulties. If all ewes go through, it may be that they are put in individual pens before they have lambed or after they have lambed. The former requires a very sharp midwife-type eye; some farmers have it, some do not. A technique used to improve accuracy of selection is to use a ram marking harness during the mating period and separate the ewes into groups of one week's matings. These groups can then be moved up to the shed in rotation as their anticipated lambing date arrives. Persons who are good at selecting ewes that are close to their time are very valuable—almost essential—for the efficient running of an intensive lambing operation (Watson 1967). Experience is also valuable.

Some of the points on which selection of ewes is based are:
- relaxation of pelvic ligaments as indicated by "falling in" of the tail and pin bones
- slackness of the vulva and surrounding skin, giving the vulval lips a boxing-glove shape
- bright red to purple color of vulva and posterior vagina
- firmness and swelling of the udder with division of the udder into two halves very evident; the presence of colostrum

For both outdoor and indoor pen lambing, it is usually safest to have a group pen into which the ewes go first—about 20 to the pen. From here, the individual ewes are selected for the lambing cubicles.

The number of cubicles required varies with the efficiency of the operator in detecting impending parturition. An average operator can manage one cubicle per 20 ewes to lamb. A highly skilled person can manage one cubicle per 35 ewes. A common practice is to limit shed lambing to the maiden ewes where the greatest losses occur and the most gains are to be made. As efficiency increases and more ewes can be handled through the shed, additional age groups are added.

Again, there is the disadvantage that inclement weather could still cause many deaths, but if the pens are carefully located or protection is provided against strong winds by natural or temporary artificial windbreaks, these losses will be reduced. The result will not be as good as that obtained by providing a shed, but the capital cost of the latter is avoided. The costs and returns have been identified (Clarke 1977), and the profitability of shed lambing was good at that time because of the high value of sheep.

Shed Lambing

Like outdoor pen lambing, this system provides an individual pen or crate for each ewe as she lambs. The ewe and lamb stay in the pen sufficiently long to ensure that the mothering bond is established and that the lamb has its quota of colostrum. The lamb lacking in vigor can receive special attention. They are then moved out to the flock, the pen is cleaned and possibly disinfected if there is any indication of need for it, and the next patient is admitted. The provision of a shed is a considerable economic investment and is not recommended unless the sheep are stud sheep and individually valuable or unless cold, wet, windy weather is common at lambing time. One of its principal advantages is that it gives shelter to the workers when they are providing assistance to the animals. It is a great advantage if the shed can be used for several purposes; at least it should be of the simplest and cheapest construction.

As soon as the lamb is born, it is kept under observation to make sure it stands and sucks. Those that are lacking in vigor profit from warmth provided by an infrared lamp and from an injection of glucose solution injected intraperitoneally or subcutaneously. These lambs should be checked for progress about every six hours. Continuous surveillance is not justified. Ewes that are disinclined to stand for the lamb to suck can be tied up short or restrained in some similar way. If there is a limit to the number of ewes that can be handled through a shed, preference should be given to maiden ewes because they need more assistance than older ewes. The logical extension of a shed lambing program is the harvesting of the lambs at early weaning, e.g., three weeks, and artificially rearing them. The way is then clear for two crops of lambs each year and two uses of the shed.

General Provisions in All Lambing Systems

The systems just described are directed at the principal causes of loss at lambing—inclement weather, poor mothering, insufficient food supply, lack of assistance for ewes that are in trouble, and deaths caused by predators. All of these programs need to have specific provisions for the control of specific causes of loss if and when they occur. These include:

- specific nutritional deficiencies of iodine, copper, selenium, and vitamin E
- congenital defects conditioned by inheritance
- specific bacteriological, chlamydial, and viral causes of abortion and neonatal death due to intrauterine infection
- similar infections occurring postnatally
- estrogenic pasture causing uterine atony
- ewes with defective udders
- a high incidence of dystocia due to inherited characteristic of large head or whole lamb
- other causes of ewe-induced lamb losses, particularly "ring-womb," uterine prolapse, and vaginal prolapse
- trauma and blood loss resulting from dystocia, tail docking, and castration
- protection against predators

PRODUCTION MANAGEMENT

Nutrition on Pasture

Good sheep management depends more than anything else on the judicious use of pasture. Pasture management is a science in itself, and it is not proposed to attempt a presentation of it here. However, it is important to give some indication of the types of factors that have to be considered in a pasture management program. They include:

The Pasture as Feed
    Composition of the pasture
    Use of fertilizers
    Availability of irrigation
    Subdivision
    Pasture resting, pasture saving
    Fodder conservation from pasture—hay and ensilage
    Fodder cropping
    Supplementary feeding

Animal Management—Utilizing the Feed
    Stocking rates
    Composition of the grazing flock
        Breeding sheep vs. dry sheep
        Date of joining
        Date of weaning
        Date of marketing
    Disease control—restraints on animal movement

There are many interactions between all of these factors, and between them and the uncontrollable variables of climate; environmental disasters, including fires and floods; and the site factors of geographical location. It is not possible to do much more than generalize about the subject unless one has access to a computer simulation model, which enables one to test the effect of variations in each of these variables. For a good summary of the subject, the reader is referred to a series of papers (White and Morley 1982).

In general terms, pasture management for sheep requires that heavy spring and autumn growths be heavily stocked, saved as standing feed, or hayed. In the poor growth periods, the standing fodder and hay are used to subsist the sheep through the period of undernutrition. Special attention is required in breeding sheep to provide optimum nutrition at the critical periods of joining, late pregnancy, and lactation, especially the first few weeks. For lambs, the critical period is from weaning until time of sale. These are the periods when supplementary feeding with grain or concentrates is most likely to be needed. On farms with mixed enterprises, grain growing is an advantage because of the stubble that becomes available, and beef cattle are also helpful in that they permit better management of the pasture, especially if it is overgrown.

Live Weight vs. Body Condition. It is not possible to set down feed requirements for sheep at pasture in terms of megajoules or kg. of dry matter. For practical sheep farming, the need is to be able to measure the sheep's biomass and feed so as to maintain, lower, or raise it as the occasion demands. Body weight has always been a poor guide because it takes no account of breed, height and age, and these things are important if weight is to be interpreted. Of much more value is the now commonly used technique of estimating body condition score. The system is the same as that used in dairy cattle, but there are 5 gradings instead of 8. The system developed by the U.K.'s Meat and Livestock Commission is shown in Table 12-2 (Speedy and Clark 1981).

The ewes to be mated should have a body condition score of greater than 2.5 if good lamb production is to be achieved. During pregnancy, it is the last six weeks that are most important, because most fetal growth occurs then. It is important that ewes get the highest possible allowance of protein at this time. It is not energy that the fetus requires, but protein. A good supply increases the chance of producing a good-quality strong lamb.

Early and mid-pregnancy are unimportant nutritionally except that they provide an opportunity to put weight on ewes that have come into the pregnancy in too light a condition. It may be desirable to divide the flock into two groups or else risk overfattening the residual ewes.

A high-protein, high-energy diet in early lactation ensures a good supply of milk and a robust lamb. In practice, the characteristic that is most likely to determine success or failure is the farmer's ability to decide when to change feeds or paddocks in order to fit the needs of the animals. It is also an advantage if he can predict what response there will be to the strategic application of nitrogen fertilizers.

It is quite critical that the dry sheep on a farm be kept separate from the late pregnant and lactating ewes and lambs because of their different feed requirements. During the periods of least feed requirement, some paddocks are cropped for hay or closed up for later feeding as conserved fodder. It is for this reason that pregnancy diagnosis has come to be such an important management tool—it makes segregation of the flock possible.

The health problems that occur in sheep, especially on pasture, are too numerous to even list here. Some of the groups of diseases follow.

Poisonings. Poisoning may be caused by fungi on grasses, e.g., facial eczema, possibly rye grass staggers. Toxic agents in pasture grass, e.g., phalaris poisoning, fescue, and *Panicum* sp. poisoning, may occur. In special circumstances, any lush grass may contain toxic amounts of nitrate (converted in the rumen into nitrite).

The list of poisonous weeds is very long indeed. Two important groups are the *Astragalus* sp., because of their palatability and extensive occurrence in North America, and the plants containing pyrollizidine alkaloids and other hepatotoxic agents in Australasia and South Africa.

Cyanide poisoning is no longer common because the common plant causes, especially sorghum and Johnson grass, are not grown much. Large areas of sheep country can be rendered unfarmable by the presence of subterranean clover containing estrogens, or by a variety of plants containing high levels of oxalate.

Nutritional Deficiencies. Phosphorus, copper (primary or secondary due to a high molybdenum intake), cobalt, iodine, and selenium/vitamin E deficiencies are causes of naturally occurring diseases. Zinc deficiency has been produced experimentally. Vitamin D could be deficient in housed sheep, but this is unlikely in grazing animals. Animals on pasture during very long droughts may become

Table 12-2. BODY CONDITION SCORING

Score	Description	Farmer Term
1	Spine sharp Back muscle shallow No fat	Lean
2	Spine sharp Back muscle full No fat	
3	Spine can be felt Back muscle full Some fat cover	Good condition
4	Spine barely felt Muscle very full Thick fat cover	
5	Spine impossible to feel Very thick fat cover Fat deposits over tail and rump	Fat

vitamin A–deficient, but this is unlikely given the long hepatic storage of the vitamin.

Miscellaneous Dietary Diseases. Bloat is much less common in pastured sheep than in cattle. Urolithiasis is a more common occurrence, especially in some areas where silica uroliths prevail, and calculi containing benzocoumarins occur on diets high in subterranean clover. Periodontitis and premature wear of sheep teeth achieve a high prevalence in some areas, especially New Zealand, and cause premature culling. Pregnancy toxemia commonly occurs because of inability to maintain nutritional status in late pregnancy in a bad season. Hypocalcemia is also an important disease for the same reason but mostly in lactating ewes. It is often accompanied by hypomagnesemia.

Nutrition in Housed Sheep and Sheep in Feedlots

The only significant intensive system for fattening sheep is the standard lamb feedlot used in the western states of the U.S. The system is not very popular because of the small price margin and the large fluctuations in the price of lamb—both feeder and fat lambs. The objective is to have lambs gain weight at the rate of 0.25 kg./day at a cost of 10¢/day, with a gross margin of $1.00/head.

The lambs enter the feedlot at 70 to 80 lb. (30 to 35 kg.) B.W. If they are smaller, some come in at 55 lb. (25 kg.) and must go onto high-quality pasture until they make the entrance weight. Specially grown alfalfa pasture is commonly used, although there is also a preference for stubble from cereal crops or crop residues, e.g., sugar beet tops. The objective on this feed is to gain about 125 g./day at a cost of about 1¢/head/day. When they enter the feedlot, they are introduced to the heavy grain ration slowly and usually with a good supply of ensilage. The target is to have the lambs gain 250 g./day and be ready to market at 105 lb. (47 kg.) after 60 days in the lot.

Because most lambs in the area are weaned in autumn, feed-lotting is seasonal and largely restricted to winter months. This has a sizable effect on the kinds of disease that occur. There is little information available about the types of diseases that frequent lamb feedlots, but a mortality rate of 5% is not unusual. A target of 2.5% is a fairly readily attainable figure. Although death losses are important, they tend to exert an exaggerated influence over preventive veterinary thinking in feedlots. A much greater form of loss is the reduced rate of gain caused by chronic or subclinical disease.

Pierson (1970) has described a flock health program in a lamb feedlot that reduced death losses from 4 to 1.5% in the first year. The greatest loss was associated with management and poorly designed corrals. A weekly visit of two to four hours was made during the feeding season of August to July. An accurate record of all health data was kept and updated at each visit. All newly arrived batches of lambs were examined closely for evidence of disease, a close watch kept on lambs in the hospital area, and autopsies done on dead lambs whenever possible.

The program for the owner to follow included the following steps:

- vaccination of all lambs with *Clostridium perfringens* type D toxoid on arrival
- identification of each group by a paint brand
- sorting for size, only lambs of 35 kg. or more going into pens, lighter lambs going onto pasture
- a period of five to six days in starting pens under very close surveillance and on fattening ration, with added antibiotics (100 mg. oxytetracycline and 100 mg. neomycin daily), for three days

The lambs were then combined into suitable sized groups with others and put into the feeder pens with grain supplied in self feeders, alfalfa and corn silage being provided in troughs. After three weeks in the feedlot, all lambs are given a broad-spectrum anthelmintic, and sick or unthrifty lambs are removed to a hospital pen for diagnosis and treatment.

It is necessary in such a program to keep very accurate records of losses and expenditures related to health maintenance. Where possible, body weights at entrance and sale, and the gain related to weeks required to gain it, should be used in addition to deaths, to indicate to the owner how well the health program is succeeding. Because the profitability of a feedlot depends on the efficiency with which the capital investment and the heavy recurring costs of labor are used, one of the two critical indices is the speed with which lambs go through the lot. Thus, inadequate feeding, climatic stress, and chronic disease become greatly important.

Among the important sources of loss are those that occur during transit to the lot. The lambs may become exhausted and go down to be trampled by the others so that they die of multiple injuries, exhaustion, or asphyxia. In hot weather, heat stroke may be an important cause of death. Most such problems can be prevented by avoiding overcrowding and by careful, easy-going transportation.

Hard data on disease prevalence in sheep feedlots are not readily available. What data exist are based on very small numbers, with mixed lots of age groups and no data on the numbers at risk (Moteane et al. 1979).

Of the death losses, those caused by enterotoxemia are usually the greatest. Vaccination with *Cl. perfringens* type D toxoid as they go into the feedlot is almost mandatory (Pierson 1967). Although this removes the bulk of the losses, some deaths can still occur during the first 10 days, and there would be an economic advantage in having the lambs vaccinated before they leave the home farm. The management technique of keeping the lambs on a low level of feed intake for the first two weeks in the feedlot may be necessary in a very high-risk situation, but the effects are so unrewarding financially that a more positive approach is usually necessary. During their sojourn in the feedlot, the provision of a ration containing adequate roughage is an added protection against the disease occurring even in vaccinated lambs. Focal symmetrical encephalomalacia is also a cause of significant loss, and a more intensive campaign against enterotoxemia should also reduce the occurrence of this disease. Serious losses are sometimes caused by outbreaks of polioencephalomalacia. They present a problem, not only because of the ease with which they can be confused with outbreaks of enterotoxemia but also because of uncertainty about the cause and prevention. A routine preventive program would not appear to be necessary, but the administration of thiamine prophylactically is necessary if cases occur. To avoid the possibility of salt poisoning contributing cases of a similar disease, it is essential that water be available at all times, especially when freezing prevents drinking. Salt, if it is provided, must be available at all times. An intermittent supply, combined with an intermittent water supply, can cause salt poisoning.

Once in the feedlot, and with enterotoxemia under control, the other important causes of loss include pneumonia and septicemia caused by *Pasteurella hemolytica*. This disease appears to be readily promoted by stress of transport or by inclement weather. There is no effective prevention, although a vaccine appears to have some merit if administered twice. In countries where psoroptic and other manges occur, dipping or spraying sheep as they enter the lot is almost obligatory.

During their stay in the lot, lambs are commonly affected by coccidiosis, which usually commences from two to three weeks after they enter. Prevention depends on hygienic arrangement of feeding and watering troughs to avoid their fecal contamination and early isolation and/or treatment of infected animals to prevent unnecessary contamination of the environment. Internal parasitism is always a very real threat, and a routine dosing with a broad-spectrum anthelmintic as the lambs enter the lot is recommended on the basis that it must be beneficial in almost every case. One of the problems arising when lambs do have diarrhea is their predisposition to blowfly strike of the soiled area.

Because of the almost universal occurrence of wetness underfoot in outdoor feedlots and the high incidence of foot rot in outside flocks, this disease is a major problem. Good drainage, the provision of roofing shelter, sandy soil, and mounds in the middle of the corrals all help, but severe outbreaks are inevitable. Although paring the feet and foot bathing are effective as a control program, they are hardly economical when 10,000 lambs are affected. The injection of large doses of penicillin and streptomycin is expensive and much less effective when it is wet underfoot. The vaccines against foot rot, which are currently being developed, represent a much more significant potential weapon.

Obstructive urolithiasis occurs as a large problem in feedlots on many occasions. Affected groups of lambs usually come from well-defined geographical areas. The only generally applicable prophylaxis is the incorporation of 4% sodium chloride in the ration. Salt above this concentration will depress food intake unnecessarily. Other ailments likely to reduce effective weight gains are entropion and pinkeye, but the former should have been dealt with before the lambs enter the lot, and pinkeye is a summer disease; it may occur in an extended feeding season. There is no prevention other than early diagnosis and fast, effective treatment of early cases to prevent wider spread.

As well as traditional sheep feedlots, there are now those conditioning units in which sheep are held before being shipped overseas as live sheep, principally to Arab countries. They are, for the most part, adult male castrates with an emphasis on lean meat. Four-to five-year-old merino wethers are a common type of sheep for this trade in Australia (McAuliffe et al. 1978). The feeding program usually consists of hay, 0.4 to 1.0 kg./day, and pellets at the rate of 1.2 kg./day at the end of the period. The sheep are started on hay only, and the pellets are introduced and increased gradually to the full quota just before shipment. The death rate is very low (0.034%), and the principal causes of death are likely to be polioencephalomalacia and salmonellosis. A miscellaneous category includes clostridial infections and intoxications, trauma, transit tetany, toxemic jaundice, and obstructive urolithiasis.

Special Feeding Circumstances

Survival Feeding in Drought Times. For maximum economy and ease of handling, only grain is fed. Concentrate pellets may be used but add to the expense. Roughage is hard to handle economically and in drought times is usually prohibitively priced. The sheep being fed grain are usually left in their paddocks and fed on the ground. In sandy country, where sand eating can cause heavy losses, troughs in the paddocks are necessary, or the sheep are yarded and fed in a feedlot system. Recommended amounts of feeds to be fed are shown in Table 12–3. They are the amounts needed to completely support the sheep. They can be reduced if some natural feed is available.

Lactic acid indigestion is always a threat, especially if sheep are put onto grain suddenly. All feeding changes should be made gradually; the grain should not be in amounts greater than those cited below, and it must be spread out in such a way that all sheep can eat at the same time. Otherwise, the aggressive ones may get much more than their share. Molasses is also capable of causing lactic acid indigestion. During prolonged feeding, 1 to 1.5% finely ground limestone added to the ration compensates for calcium loss and reduces the

osteoporosis that is likely to occur. In the initial stages, it is important to feed every day to avoid lactic acid indigestion, but once the sheep are trained, better survival is obtained by intermittent feeding. A recommended regime for dry sheep is to commence with 50 g./day, increasing to 350 g./day by day 14. The feeding is then changed to every second day, and by day 24 the sheep can be getting 1050 g. (preferably 1400 g.) every third day. Pregnant and lactating ewes get proportionally more, as shown in Table 12–3. Lactating ewes need some roughage, and 500 g./day would be a good investment. The economic advantage of knowing whether or not ewes are pregnant is most obvious during drought feeding.

Miscellaneous Problems During Drought Feeding

1. The feed is usually simply spilled in a long tortuous trail on the ground. Some dirt will be eaten, but cocciodiosis can be avoided by moving the trail slightly from time to time. Long-term feeding of the smaller grains on the ground leads to digestive upsets from the ingestion of surface soil. Troughing is much to be preferred—one foot of double-sided trough for each three to four sheep.

2. Drought feeding of parasitized sheep is poor economics, and all sheep should be dosed with a broad-spectrum anthelmintic before drought feeding commences.

3. Lambs are a problem, especially if it is necessary to wean them early to save the ewe's life. They should not be weaned until they are at least 15 lb. (merino) or 20 lb. (cross-breeds) body weight. At this weight, they should be about six weeks old. They should be fed roughage at all times; at the beginning there should be at least 50% of the feed as chaffed roughage mixed with the grain. Vitamin A is probably best provided from the beginning— give 250,000 I.U. vitamin A at marking. A straight grain ration or poor hay will also be low in protein, and the addition of 5 lb. linseed meal or 2 lb. meat meal per 100 lb. grain is

Table 12–3. DROUGHT FEEDING TABLE°

Class of Sheep	Wheat, Sorghum Barley Grain	Oat Grain	Proprietary Sheet "Nuts"	Hay
Adult dry sheep including rams	350	400	450	750
Ewes in last six weeks of pregnancy	450	550	600	900
Lactating ewes	650	750	800	1250
Lambs and weaners	250	300	350	500
NB: The amounts quoted are just adequate; a 33% increase would be safer.				

°Amounts in g/d/sheep.

recommended. At this age, lambs need ample water, some good shelter from wind, and not too much space. A stocking rate of 600 to 800 lambs per acre is recommended. A hospital will be needed for the weak ones.

4. Lambing ewes should not have to compete too hard for their feed, and if possible some roughage should always be available. Intermittent grain feeding then does not cause too much mismothering and desertion of lambs.

5. Weaners and chronic "shy feeders" may not eat the grain and may die of starvation if they are not drafted off and driven up to the feed and held on it. In any group on subsistence rations, there will be some sheep that do not fare well. If losing them is to be avoided, they should be moved to a hospital group that is given special treatment.

6. Sheep and cattle should not be fed together. The sheep are too exposed to traumatic injury.

7. If urea is used, poisoning can occur if maximum amounts are fed and sheep are put onto these amounts suddenly. Preferably, it should be fed with a carbohydrate-rich concentrate such as grain or molasses and only when roughage is also fed. Feed no more than 10 g. urea/head/day and ensure that it is thoroughly mixed with the feed.

8. If the period of feeding is prolonged, the young sheep up to 1½ years of age will need supplementation with vitamin A. Weaners at three months of age, if they have not had access to green feed, should receive 500,000 I.U. vitamin A, which should protect them for six months.

9. Other specific nutritional deficiencies that may be encountered are vitamin E, leading to cardiac and skeletal muscular dystrophy, and osteoporosis resulting from a high-phosphorus, low-calcium diet. Agalactia in ewes is also noted on purely grain diets. This can be corrected by inclusion of some roughage in the diet.

Grazing on Lush Pasture or on Green Cereal Crop. These practices are subject to two potential errors. On this kind of feed, late pregnant and lactating ewes are likely to suffer a high prevalence of hypocalcemia, with or without hypomagnesemia. In some bad outbreaks, even dry sheep can be affected, especially on cereal crops. There is little that can be done to prevent the disease unless the sheep can be moved to a less lush feed, an unlikely prospect in a good spring. Most situations in which hypocalcemia is a likely

hazard are dealt with by maintaining close surveillance and treating cases early.

Inadequate Diet in Late Pregnancy. This occurs commonly enough because ewes are often mated to catch a spring or autumn flush when they are at the point of lambing. Failure of the appropriate rain to appear may result in an outbreak of lethal pregnancy toxemia.

Breeding Plans—Quality Control

Quality control in sheep breeding is still largely a matter of visual appraisal by show judges, with the high prices at sales going to the progeny of animals that fill the eye of a recognized authority. Objective measurement of wool and meat has been available as a technique for many years, but the rate of adoption of the policy has been slow. This has been largely due to the slowness of the commodity dealers to switch to a more equitable system of payment. Purchase of lamb and mutton meat on the scale at abattoirs and payment for wool on the basis of the quality of a sample are gaining popularity, and this will encourage performance testing. Genetic selection pressure can then be applied to these marketable qualities. Much less importance will be ascribed to "wool-classing" in the shearing shed, although that will still be necessary in order to cull out damaged and discolored fleeces.

Production is not the only criterion for selection. Longevity and reproduction are also important, especially because high wool production may be inversely related to fertility. Other characteristics in wool sheep that need to be kept in mind are freedom from wrinkles on the breech and low susceptibility to fleece rot, both of which predispose to blowfly strike. An exhaustive discussion of breeding plans for wool-producing flocks has been provided by Miller (1981).

Because of the conservative attitude and reluctance to use objective measurement by the traditional stud breeders, there has been a development of cooperative ram breeding societies (Hight and Rae 1970; Jackson and Turner 1972). These assume that the major influence on inheritance is the ram and that selection of ewes is unlikely to have any significant effect on succeeding generations. They also assume that there are a sufficient number of good genes in the total population to make it worthwhile to find them, test them for performance—preferably in a central, controlled location, mate them to selected ewes, and harvest their ram progeny. The ewes are selected by the cooperating farmers from their own flocks because of their superior performance. The ram offspring are sent to the seed farms. This has the same effect as selecting for good characteristics in a flock but at the same time increasing the size of the flock many times.

Cooperative ram breeding has been highly successful in merinos in Australia and is also well developed in meat and long wool sheep in New Zealand (Quinlivan 1981b). The selection priorities recommended are:
□ reproductive efficiency
□ fleece weight
□ structural soundness
□ growth rate
□ weaning weight
□ easy care
□ appearance (breed type)
□ wool quality

Because of the slow rate of gain by genetic selection in standard sheep breeds, there has been a turn toward cross-breeding or to new breeds. Cross-breeding has been in vogue for many years in the fat-lamb–producing section of the industry. This has been given a new fillip by the introduction of exotics. The Border Leicester × merino mother may now be mated to a fat-tailed Persian sire instead of a Polled Dorset, but the impact of the exotics is still too small to be properly evaluated. New breeds (Perendale ≡ Romney × Cheviot, Coopworth ≡ Romney × Border Leicester) were also produced in New Zealand and continue to thrive.

A point of some importance with respect to the introduction of exotic breeds is the opportunity that this provides for further spread of exotic diseases, especially slow viruses. Scrapie and maedi-visna are prime examples, the former in Suffolks, the latter in Texels.

THE BASIC FLOCK HEALTH AND PRODUCTIVITY PROGRAM

A basic sample health program for the commercial breeding flock is discussed here. It is based on the effective control of internal parasitoses, blowfly strike, clostridioses, and foot rot, and on the maintenance of an efficient reproduction program. To do this and still maintain maximum cost-effectiveness requires special care in avoiding overcapitalization and excessive use of labor in an effort to provide for all emergencies. This would be contrary to one of the principal needs of the sheep industry, which is to reduce the intensity of the permanent labor force employed and to cater to the peak needs for shearing, drenching, lambing, and so on by the use of contract labor. It should be possible to provide for a health service by utilizing such contract labor and even organizing it and providing it as part of the service. This consideration is of most importance to large flocks. In smaller flocks, the profitable utilization of what is in effect a potential oversupply of labor may include the development of additional health maintenance techniques (Morley 1979).

It would be foolhardy to commence a flock health program without experience and expertise in the control of the diseases that are the principal targets of the program and without the back-up services of labor and laboratory to support these activities. It is a job for experienced professionals and must pay the professional standard rates of pay. To do this, it must be financially self-supporting (Quinlivan 1981a).

General Outline of the Program

The basis of these programs is the frequent and repeated stimulation of the farmer to carry out the recommended procedures that are essential to the maintenance of health and production. It is common experience that farmers left to carry out these procedures themselves often fail to do so or, if they do carry them out, do so in a way that reduces or destroys their effectiveness. This problem is greatest with sheep and beef cattle farmers because they see their animals infrequently and make decisions and carry out procedures only a few times a year. This makes them reluctant to make additional decisions or carry out additional tasks. These problems are most easily countered by a specific series of contacts with the farmer. These contacts are all essential to the overall strategy of the program and include:

1. An initial *farm profile* to ensure that the farmer's objective is understood. The objective is usually maximum profitability, but it may include a factor for gracious living. Additional information must be obtained on the resources of the land, water, animals, labor, and money available to the enterprise. Discussion of the major problems and the probable plan of attack should be combined with preliminary arrangements made for the data collection system. An analysis of the data of the previous

one or two years is a great help in defining productivity and problems.

2. A system of *timely checks and reminders*, adapted to the needs of each farm and sent by mail at times appropriate to the expected occurrence of the problem. For example, the farmer is advised to vaccinate *now* against enterotoxemia or to drench *now* for liver fluke.

3. Periodic *solicitation from the farmer of data* on performance in production and health maintenance tasks. This information is used to determine whether production targets are being achieved and whether recommended disease control procedures are being carried out. Failure to perform elicits a specific reminder of the need to do so.

4. A *system of regular visits* by the veterinarian, usually three each year, to carry out physical work and to discuss past performance and future behavior. This personal contact is vital to provide for discussion and argument about the value of the program.

5. An *annual discussion* by a small group of farmers (15 to 20 is a good number) on additions, deletions, and modifications of the program or its recommended techniques and targets, and to provide an opportunity for community discussion on difficulties encountered in achieving objectives.

6. The program must concentrate on the key issues, the ones that cause a lot of wastage, those that can be controlled with little expenditure, and those that are highly profitable. In most sheep-raising areas, the same problems have the top priorities:

□ reproductive inefficiency
□ neonatal deaths
□ the need for intensive cross-breeding
□ greater culling rate based on objective measurement of body weight gains and fleece quality and yield
□ better mangement of pastures and their best utilization, including selective supplementary feeding
□ getting maiden ewes to optimal mating weight at first joining
□ optimal body weights of adult ewes
□ flushing feed levels at mating and at end of pregnancy and early lactation
□ restraining prevalence of infectious and other diseases to a level consonant with optimal profitability

7. Professional scientific advisers in other disciplines should be retained only as consultants. This means avoiding referring a client to, e.g., a specialist agronomist.

Programed Visits

It is desirable to arrange two or three visits to each farm each year (Quinlivan 1981a; Boundy 1981). This is not as simple as in cattle work unless there is the opportunity to do practical things such as pregnancy diagnosis, but if the major disease problems are identifiable, it is possible to arrange the visits at critical times in the proposed disease control programs. Many of these do not require the participation of a veterinarian. Vaccination against the clostridioses, foot paring and foot bathing, the Mules operation, jetting for blowfly, lamb marking (docking and castration), and dipping for lice and ked are usually farmer or contract layoperator techniques. That is not to say that the veterinarian should not or would not carry out these tasks. In the development of sheep flock health programs, some veterinarians begin by involving themselves in these techniques, but to be financially attractive to the farmer, the method would require speed and ingenuity. A recommended program of visits is shown in Table 12–4. It includes:

1. A *ram check visit*. The most important visit is the one before joining, specifically to examine the rams for breeding soundness and preferably the ewes for body condition. These activities require a veterinarian.

2. A *prelambing visit*. This provides an opportunity to ensure that all the necessary preparations for lambing and attempts to minimize losses in the newborn have been taken.

3. A *postlambing visit*. This visit is primarily to review the performance at lambing and make plans for the next mating season. It also provides an opportunity to class ewes into wet and dry groups, a classification best done by veterinarians. Ewes with defective mammary glands can also be identified and marked for culling. Ewes to be culled for age or bad teeth can also be identified at this visit.

Optional Visits During Lambing. These are not usually undertaken unless there is a specific problem to solve. However, it is a most critical period, and if lambs can be preserved for some days, a visit at this time to conduct necropsies might produce the answers to the local problems in neonatal mortality. Although reliable necropsies are best done in a regional laboratory, it is often difficult to do a large number in a central place. A visit to the farm to view the physical circumstances in which lambing occurs, performance of some nec-

Table 12–4. ANNUAL SCHEDULE FOR HEALTH MANAGEMENT VISITS TO SHEEP AND BEEF CATTLE COMBINED ENTERPRISES

Visit No.	Sheep Activities (Spring Lambing)	Cattle Activities (Autumn Calving)
1 Spring (Sept.–Oct.)	Review results of spring lambing. Arrange joining for next autumn lambing. Check on efficiency of blowfly control procedures. Arrange drenching program in light of recent drenching. Assess wool yield.	Pregnancy diagnosis; if applicable, strain 19 vaccination; check that calf growth rate is satisfactory.
2 Late Summer (Feb.–Mar.)	Examine rams for breeding soundness, arrange joining for next spring lambing. Check fluke and worm control programs for efficiency of execution. Finalize culling of ewes. Arrange further drenching program.	Final pregnancy check. Inspect yearling growth rate. Assess efficiency of worm control and arrange future drench program.
3 Late Autumn, Early Winter (May–June)	Check parasite status by egg count. Review of year's performance for sheep and cattle.	Examine bulls for breeding soundness. Advise on cow culling.

A more detailed program, suitable for use in an intensive sheep farming environment, is set out in Figure 12–5. Many similar charts are available, e.g., one for merinos in Western Queensland (Fig. 12–6) (Miller 1979) and one for all sheep in Scotland (Fig. 12–7) (Hindson 1982). These are reproduced by courtesy of the authors.

ropsies, and the return of selected specimens to the laboratory is often a more practical answer. The visit may extend over a period of a few days. If there is a major problem and no effort is to be spared, it is recommended that the investigator carry out a series of visits, the first just before lambing commences to assess the body condition of the ewes, the state of the lambing paddocks, and arrangements for surveillance of the lambing. Subsequently, one or more visits should be made to assess the functioning of the system as a whole. At these visits, the necropsies would be done on the lambs that had died during the preceding 48 to 72 hours.

Timing of Visits. Periodic visits by the supervising veterinarian to sheep farms using flock health programs need careful timing. The schedule needs to take into account other managerial activities on the farm, so that visits do not conflict with them unnecessarily but take place at a time when sheep would ordinarily be handled for other purposes. Whenever possible, the visits should avoid being simply for the purpose of looking and advising. There is also an advantage in having the visits synchronize with a relevant farm activity, such as drenching or marking, which could be profitable to observe.

Conjoint Beef-Sheep Enterprises

It is common practice, especially in Australia, for sheep and beef cattle enterprises to be conducted on one farm. These circumstances require a sheep flock health program and a beef herd health program with the planned visits to both arranged to be simultaneous. A program (courtesy of Dr. F.H.W. Morley) for a flock lambing in spring and beef cows calving in autumn is as follows (Table 12–4) (see also Figs. 12–5 to 12–7):

Data Collection and Storage

Management Data. It is necessary to have some method of recording management details in such a way as to provide information on the quality of animal management and the intensity with which the program's recommendations are applied. It is therefore necessary to record details of sheep groups and their numbers, age, and genetic composition without necessarily identifying each sheep; also, management details such as supplementary feeding, shearing body weights, fleece weights, numbers and dates of sales of sheep, and prices received for products all need to be recorded.

The best arrangement is to set up groups of sheep on an age basis and to retain them in these groups for as long as possible. The group is identified by ear marks or ear tag, and this is usually sufficient for the maintenance of adequate records. The difficulty arises when sheep from a number of groups are co-mingled. It is then necessary to identify a new group composed of the residues of a number of groups, each of which may have a different history.

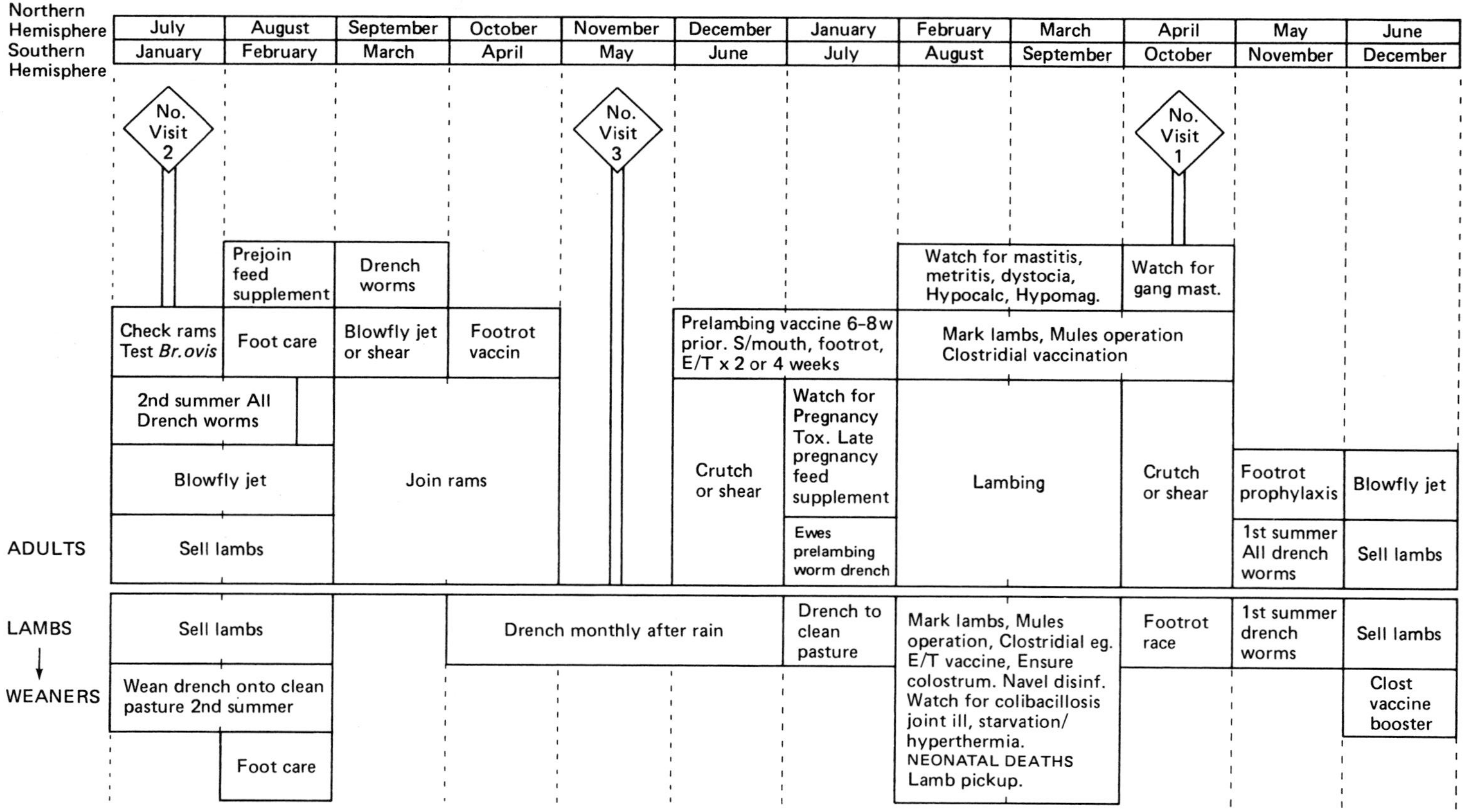

Northern Hemisphere	July	August	September	October	November	December	January	February	March	April	May	June
Southern Hemisphere	January	February	March	April	May	June	July	August	September	October	November	December

No. Visit 2 (January/July) · No. Visit 3 (May/November) · No. Visit 1 (October/April)

General / Rams:
- Check rams, Test *Br. ovis* (January/July)
- Prejoin feed supplement (February/August)
- Drench worms (March/September)
- Foot care (February–March)
- Blowfly jet or shear (March/September)
- Footrot vaccin (April/October)
- Join rams (March–May)
- Prelambing vaccine 6–8w prior. S/mouth, footrot, E/T x 2 or 4 weeks (June/December–July/January)
- Watch for Pregnancy Tox. Late pregnancy feed supplement (July/January)
- Crutch or shear (December/June)
- Ewes prelambing worm drench (July/January)
- Watch for mastitis, metritis, dystocia, Hypocalc, Hypomag. (August/September)
- Mark lambs, Mules operation Clostridial vaccination (September/March)
- Lambing (August–September)
- Watch for gang mast. (April/October)
- Crutch or shear (April/October)
- Footrot prophylaxis (May/November)
- Blowfly jet (June/December)

ADULTS:
- 2nd summer All Drench worms (January–February)
- Blowfly jet (February/August)
- Sell lambs (January–February)
- Drench monthly after rain (May–July)
- Drench to clean pasture (July/January)
- 1st summer All drench worms (November/May)
- Sell lambs (June/December)

LAMBS:
- Sell lambs (January/July)
- Wean drench onto clean pasture 2nd summer (January/July)
- Mark lambs, Mules operation, Clostridial eg. E/T vaccine, Ensure colostrum. Navel disinf. Watch for colibacillosis joint ill, starvation/hyperthermia. NEONATAL DEATHS Lamb pickup. (September/March)
- Footrot race (April/October)
- 1st summer drench worms (May/November)
- Sell lambs (June/December)

WEANERS:
- Foot care (February–March)
- Clost vaccine booster (June/December)

Figure 12–5. Sample sheep calendar—Southwest Australia.

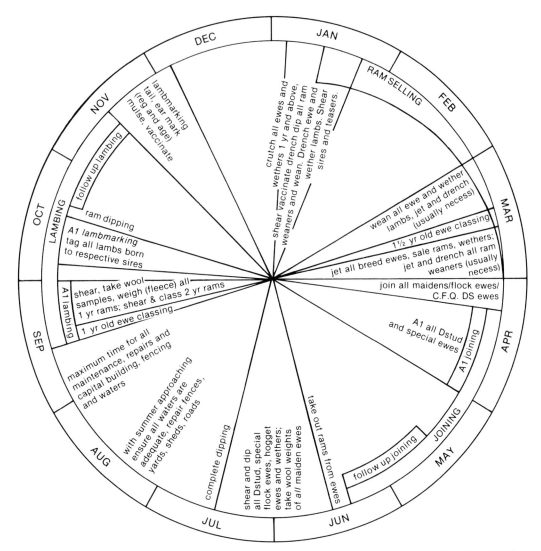

Figure 12-6. A sheep management calendar for merinos in Western Queensland. (From Miller, S.J. 1979.)

An alternative or supplementary method is to group ewes on the basis of their joining dates, so that they are all likely to be lambing at about the same time. As the ewes lamb, they are drifted off until the group is sufficiently large; then a new group is commenced. The alternative method of doing this is to identify the ewes joined by using a mating indicator harness on the ram and removing the ewes from the original group as they are marked. Both techniques are inclined to confuse the original groups and their histories. A code for each group should indicate that it contains ewes or wethers, year of birth, and breed.

The basic requirement for collecting all information, managerial and disease-related, is a structured diary with tear-off sheets that are filled in and sent into the data processing bureau each month. This permits the record keeping to be constantly monitored and the data to be stored at a constant rate during the year. Each monthly report should include a statement on:

□ the climate, feed supply, comfort index, and rainfall
□ management procedures, including sales, births, data on rams in and rams out, supplementary feeding, shearing, crutching, marking of lambs
□ preventive veterinary procedures, e.g., drenching for worms or flukes, jetting, dipping, Mules operation, vaccinations, examination of rams for breeding soundness, and so on
□ deaths and illnesses, postmortem examinations conducted

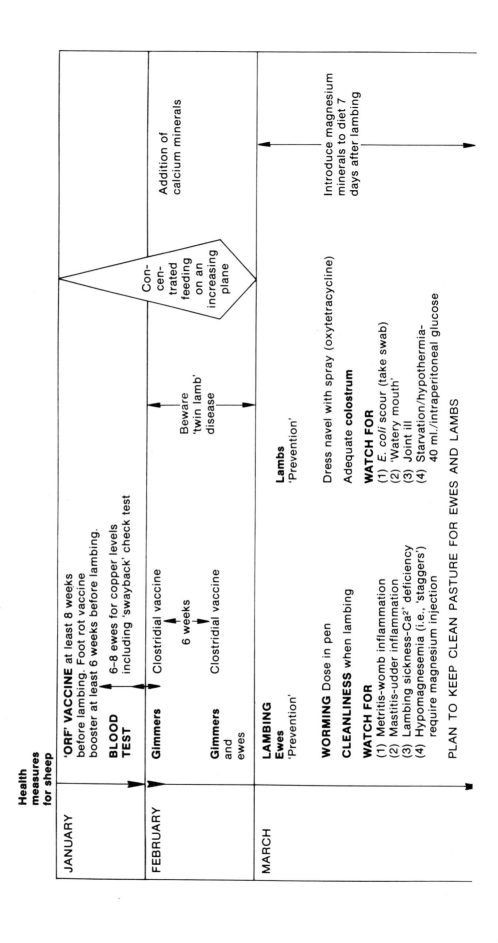

Health measures for sheep

JANUARY

'ORF' VACCINE at least 8 weeks before lambing. Foot rot vaccine booster at least 6 weeks before lambing.

BLOOD TEST 6–8 ewes for copper levels including 'swayback' check test

FEBRUARY

Con-cen-trated feeding on an increasing plane

Beware 'twin lamb' disease

Gimmers Clostridial vaccine

6 weeks

Gimmers and ewes Clostridial vaccine

Addition of calcium minerals

MARCH

LAMBING Ewes 'Prevention'

WORMING Dose in pen

CLEANLINESS when lambing

WATCH FOR
(1) Metritis–womb inflammation
(2) Mastitis–udder inflammation
(3) Lambing sickness–Ca^2 deficiency
(4) Hypomagnesemia (i.e., 'staggers') require magnesium injection

Lambs 'Prevention'

Dress navel with spray (oxytetracycline)

Adequate **colostrum**

WATCH FOR
(1) *E. coli* scour (take swab)
(2) 'Watery mouth'
(3) Joint ill
(4) Starvation/hypothermia– 40 ml./intraperitoneal glucose

Introduce magnesium minerals to diet 7 days after lambing

PLAN TO KEEP CLEAN PASTURE FOR EWES AND LAMBS

APRIL

Foot rot vaccine 2 ml. for **lambs** aged 2 weeks +

LAMBS-Diarrhea **WATCH COCCIDIOSIS** take **feces** samples to laboratory

MAY

EWES-Watch for **GANGRENOUS MASTITIS** from now on

Worm lambs every 4–6 weeks if clean pasture not available

JUNE

LAMBS-Clostridial vaccine 'booster' at 12–16 weeks of age

Magnesium should be available to ewes at least until end of June

JULY

Drench and wean onto clean pasture

AUGUST

Ewes, tups and gimmers

Foot care
(1) Severe trimming affected feet
(2) Spray antibiotic
(3) Foot bath 5% formalin

Ovine abortion vaccine-**GIMMERS**

Feed small amount concentrate or equivalent 2 weeks before and 6 weeks after tupping to increase lamb numbers. Any 'unusual' foods, e.g., brussels sprouts, *must have minerals balanced.*

SEPTEMBER

'**Tupping**'   Tups may be blood tested for *Toxoplasmosis* on entry

OCTOBER

Foot rot vaccine

NOVEMBER

DECEMBER

Figure 12–7. Disease control program for a United Kingdom sheep flock. (From Hindson, J. Sheep health schemes. Vet. Rec. (In Practice), 435–458, 1982. With contributions by Dr. Plenderleith, Glasgow University.)

405

A second document considered to be essential to this exercise is the annual management profile, which records in detail the resources, management, and objectives for the farm. By this means, significant changes in these activities or aspirations are recorded.

If a cash-flow report is to be provided, there will need to be additional information on prices obtained for wool and stock and prices paid for feed and other supplies.

No details of the types of forms used in these programs are provided here but are available on request to the authors. They are inclined to be very specific to the particular areas, methods of husbandry, and economic status of the animal industry in question.

Because the amount of data is relatively small, there usually being only a few groups of sheep on each farm, the data is susceptible to being handled manually. Manual handling would already be necessary for much of the data because it is qualitative rather than quantitative in character, for example, the state of the pastures. Comparisons of results between farms and before-and-after on individual farms, including partial budget estimations of financial status, will require a combination of descriptive and numerical/ financial data.

Health Data. Information on health matters, including deaths, necropsy results, illnesses, treatments, and prophylactic techniques, are recorded in the diary provided and copies forwarded periodically to the data laboratory. More detailed reports of work done by veterinarians or the diagnostic laboratory are supplied to the data laboratory, and the information is coded and stored. It is usually desirable to construct a disease identification code that is relevant to the particular area.

A complete necropsy examination should be carried out on each sheep, but in a pastoral economy that is run on extensive lines, it is impossible to do this. The best that can be hoped for is that if more than one or two cases occur, sufficient interest will be aroused to stimulate the farmer to present one or two cadavers for necropsy examination.

Analysis of Data— Reporting to Farmers

The number of reports provided to the farmer each year will depend on the amount of stimulation required by the farmer and the additional costs raised by each additional report. It is usual to supply a report after each visit, that is, two or three per year. One of these is an annual report containing a review of the entire performance of the flock for the past year. The others are interim reports covering the period since the previous report.

Annual Report. This should include a report on all the indices that have been monitored, including those relating to health and those dealing with production. It would also be simple to predict sheep numbers for each of the succeeding months, based on numbers of ewes mated, joining date, and anticipated fertility index. This would permit forward planning of feed supplies. Also included should be a listing of the activities carried out in each group, together with its record of production. This is comparable to an individual cow's record of a lactation performance in a dairy herd.

Eventually, it will be found to be practicable to analyze and report annually on the quality of performance of individual paddocks, or families or crosses of sheep. This may assist management to decide which paddocks need pasture improvement or other agronomic interference. Cross-breeding of sheep may be able to be rationalized in terms of what actually happens on the particular farm. This sort of analysis will probably require that the records be computerized and that interfarm comparison be available.

In terms of timing, the logical occasion for an annual report is when lambing is completed and the analysis of reproductive performance is completed; thus, July or January 1 is suitable, depending on whether the lambing is in the spring or the autumn.

Interim Reports. One of these would be best supplied after the ram evaluation visit, the other as appropriate. These are supplemented by error messages when examination of the records indicates that a recommended procedure has not been carried out, and reminders are sent out to advise farmers of specific tasks that should be carried out at specific times.

Interfarm Comparison. If an annual meeting of a study group of farmers is arranged, it is common practice to discuss a comparison between farms so that each knows how his performance rates with others. Identities are masked by a code number, and performance in each of the indices is listed. There may be good reasons for a farmer to not achieve, or even to attempt to achieve, one or more targets, and these often serve as good points around which to arrange a discussion.

Manual or Computer Analysis of Data. Provided the expense of the computer program can be borne, it is preferable because it is so error-free, so consistent, and so successful at carrying out boring, repetitive bookkeeping and examining of records. In comparison with dairy cattle, there are relatively few incidents to record, and a manual data processing system is adequate if there are only a few flocks. But if there are a large number of sheep or if many additional procedures such as individual identification, weighings, use of a crayon marking breeding harness, and so on are used, the manipulation of record cards becomes very tiresome.

The Special Targets of Flock Health and Production Programs

Accurate information on the relative economic significance of the various forms of wastage in sheep flocks is not generally available and would, in any case, be of little significance in areas other than where they originated. The available surveys quote only losses by death, that is, measurement is by head count, and almost no attempt has been made to measure loss by reduction in productive efficiency by surviving sheep. For example, in extensively run flocks in semi-arid climates, the total losses of lambs and ewes may reach 10% of the flock per year (Nass 1977), and for adult sheep alone the losses may be 3% (Moteane et al. 1979). In these environments, of the total sheep and lamb losses, 25% may be due to predators (Tigner and Larson 1977), and climatic and nutritional stresses account for a large proportion of the remainder.

English estimates of loss in a more intensive, less nutritionally stressful environment are 16% total losses per year, including 4% for ewes and 12% for lambs (Boundy 1979). Scottish figures for lamb losses are 15 to 20% (Houston and Maddox 1974) and 14.2% (Johnston et al. 1980).

Because of the absence of detailed wastage figures, it is not possible to accurately identify the major diseases. However, the losses of lambs are sufficiently large to suggest that reproductive inefficiency is preeminent as a cause. For pastured sheep, internal parasitism, blowfly strike, foot rot and allied diseases, and clostridioses are universal causes of productive inefficiency and are included in the section on special targets of flock health and productivity programs.

Costs and Income

Costs. The cost-effectiveness of these programs in the hands of experienced veterinarians who are advising average sheep farmers is excellent. There will always be a few farmers whose management and disease control is so good that the program offers them little financial gain, but they will be recognizable early if a retrospective analysis of data is done at the time of the original farm profile. Some of these farmers will decide not to continue but most will, in order to have insurance against error.

Charges for advice and visits are difficult to decide. It is best to charge by the hour for time spent on the farm but to charge much more than one would for doing purely mechanical things like TB testing. What is involved, in addition to physical presence on the farm, is:
□ arranging for laboratory tests
□ answering telephone calls for advice
□ analysis of data, often by computer
□ discussions with and arranging visits by other consultants
□ preparation of reports

A factor of 2 is suggested as a reasonable way of multiplying the standard fee. A reasonable total fee would be $50/hour. The time spent on the farm would vary with the numbers of animals and problems to be dealt with, but four visits of three hours each would cost a farmer with 2000 breeding ewes a total of $600/year or about 30¢/ewe/year. This does not include mileage, which may be expensive for farms in an extensive farming area. Nor does it include other than minimal computer charges because the program is not computerized. The sheep are dealt with in groups of about 300, and the volume of data to be handled is small. For stud herds in which the sheep must be recorded individually, there would be additional computer charges, probably of the order of $1/head/year.

If it desirable to reduce costs, this can be done by retaining only two visits, the ram examination visit and the postlambing visit.

In feedlot practice, much of the work is by necropsy. Charging at the rate of $50/hour, the financial return to the investment is high (Kirk and Anderson 1982).

Income. If the cost-effectiveness of the program is to be assessed, the actual income needs to be known. Failing this, the income can be estimated on the basis of yield multiplied by value. For wool, the total wool sold comes from bale weights, and the yield per sheep from the bale weight divided by the number of sheep shorn. This figure is available from the shearing shed cut-out figures. Quality of wool can be determined by access to the objective measurements if they are used as a basis for the sale of the wool.

Body weights are harder to come by, unless

the lambs, hoggets, and wethers are sold to abattoirs on a weight basis or are weighed by the abattoir for its own purposes. Scales to be used on the farm have limitations because of the variations in gut-fill that occur from time to time during the day, making the assessment of carcass weight from live weight a haphazard arrangement.

OTHER MAJOR DISEASE PROBLEMS

The following diseases were chosen to be listed, out of the large number that afflict sheep, because they are universally present, cause significant wastage, and must be included in a basic program. The diseases are:
□ gastrointestinal helminthiasis—worms
□ blowfly strike
□ clostridial diseases
□ foot rot
They will be dealt with briefly here because they are included with details in most textbooks of food animal medicine.

Gastrointestinal Helminthiasis— Worm Control

In general, internal parasitoses in sheep are controllable by an intelligent use of anthelmintic programs and management of sheep and pastures. Uninformed and excessive use of anthelmintics has contributed to the development of anthelmintic resistance in some parasites. Control of these diseases by immunological means at one time appeared to offer an alternative or supplementary strategy for parasite control. However, their use has not prospered and seems unlikely to do so.

Details of the control programs used against individual parasitisms are not presented here. Attention is directed particularly to trichostrongylosis, ostertagiasis, esophagostomiasis, and hemonchosis, with some attention to nematodiriasis and cooperiasis. Control programs against these worms will differ markedly from place to place depending on the climate, the big variable being *Hemonchus contortus*. In its absence, e.g., in a winter rainfall area, it is necessary to drench adult dry sheep only twice each year, breeding ewes three times, and lambs twice. This is because the hot, dry summer is very damaging to larvae, and the larval pickup is very small. The same applies to countries with very cold winter climates.

Adult dry sheep should be drenched at least once in summer to empty out the sheep at a time when the pasture conditions are hard on larvae and thus clean the pasture of infection for the dangerous period ahead—a warm, moist autumn. The general recommendation is for two summer drenches, the first as soon as the pasture has dried off and the second in midsummer. A spring drenching can also be included with advantage. This disposes of any existing worm load so that the sheep can make best use of the spring flush of feed.

Breeding ewes get an additional drench either just before or within three weeks of lambing. The purpose is to avoid heavy contamination of the environment for the lambs and to enhance the ewe's milk flow.

Rams will receive a prejoining drench along with the other adult sheep in the summer drench program.

Lambs should get a drench at weaning to avoid their succumbing to the stress of weaning plus the burden of a parasite infestation. In lambs born in autumn into bad situations or if there is any evidence of worm infestation, another drench may be given in mid-winter while the lambs are still on the ewes. Lambs still on ewes should not need drenching while they are not yet grazing much.

The above is a sample program that would be applicable in certain circumstances. It is not possible to specify beyond this. It presupposes that a broad-spectrum anthelmintic is used and that there is no problem of anthelmintic resistance in the resident worm population.

Summer Rainfall Areas. In this kind of climate, the conditions on the pasture during the summer months are very favorable for larval survival, and pick-up may be very heavy indeed. This is especially so for heavy egg-layers such as *Hemonchus contortus*. One or two summer drenches cannot therefore restrain pasture contamination. For flocks that lamb in the spring, two drenches are given to the ewes at lambing, one before and one after. Lambs are drenched at weaning and then monthly for six months. This intensity may be reduced if clean pasture is available after each drenching. Conversely, a heavier drenching program still may be necessary on heavily contaminated farms during seasons of hot, humid weather.

Monitoring Results of a Worm Control Program. The biggest problem with any worm control program is to monitor its efficacy. In completely standard climatic conditions, the recommended programs are guaranteed to be effective, but only if there is no resistance and if the drenching program and use of rested pasture are carried out conscientiously. The only methods available to monitor the parasitic status are total worm counts on cadavers—a not very practicable method in a commercial flock health environment—and fecal egg counts. Egg counts are notoriously unreliable, but because of their ease of performance it is worthwhile to attempt a very cautious interpretation of what the counts mean. The problem is created by senior sheep, which have developed a resistance to parasitic infestation so that there may be heavy infestations with immature larvae, which are not laying any eggs at all. The resistance may be of a varying degree and may vary widely between sheep in the same flock. A simple way of overcoming this problem is to use only susceptible sheep as monitors. Weaners less than nine months old and ewes in early lactation are the obvious subjects. These should have been drenched with an efficient anthelmintic about one month previously. If they have then been grazed on a particular pasture for the ensuing month, their fecal egg burden should be an accurate indication of the infection status of that particular pasture. Individual sheep counts are not necessary; bulked specimens containing samples from 10 sheep each and two counts per flock are considered to be an adequate sample. The exercise might be carried out as the condition of the sheep dictates or at regular intervals, for example during veterinary visits plus other occasions, with the farmer collecting the samples.

It is possible, therefore, to assess the status of particular pastures, but the more common problem is to determine the parasitologic status of a particular group of sheep. If the sheep are a susceptible group, they can be tested, preferably at a time when larval pickup is at a high level, for example after autumn rain. If the sheep are likely to be partly immune, the testing will be much less reliable. Some of the sheep may be passing significant egg loads, but many of them will harbor only immature larvae and will be passing very few eggs.

Safe Grazing. The concept of a "clean" pasture, carrying no infective nematode larvae, is difficult to translate into reality. Nowadays, it is customary to think of "safe" grazing on which sheep will increase their worm load only slowly after going onto it, having had a prior effective drench. Reinfection is a very real threat and one to which relatively few farmers pay even lip service. Unfortunately, any

significant reduction of helminth larval burdens on pasture can only be relied upon in hot summer weather, in which it will take two to six months of high, subtropical temperatures. Paddocks that have been closed to sheep for some time, such as grain or forage crop stubbles and hay paddocks, are the best suited as "quarantine" areas, but they are obviously limited in their availability. It is therefore usually necessary to limit their use to the susceptible groups—the young sheep up to 18 months of age and the ewes with lambs.

An alternative and moderately effective procedure to spelling pasture is alternate grazing of paddocks by sheep and by cattle. Almost all helminths are species-specific, so that cross-transmission between sheep and cattle does not occur. The use of alternate grazing with resistant sheep is much less reliable because these sheep, although they are resistant to the growth of helminths, can produce significant levels of contamination of pasture. Whichever decision is made about how to achieve the least parasitic risk to young sheep, it is often the quality of the feed in a paddock that determines whether it is used for grazing.

Blowfly Strike

Blowflies and wet sheep's wool can create a dramatic and disastrous disease situation within a very short time. Blowfly strike is a preventable disease and continues to be a major disease whenever susceptible sheep are pastured in large groups, only because farmers fail to use available control techniques (Morley 1979). The only satisfactory way of dealing with the problem is to maintain a long-term strategy of reducing the susceptibility of the sheep and to combine this with a stand-by short-term emergency tactic that will deal with an infestation urgently and effectively.

The epidemiology of the disease is basically that it requires a particular environment to flourish, and when that environment is achieved, the growth of the infestation is very rapid.

The Mules Operation (or breeding for a plain breech). Correct mulesing and tail docking (Yeo 1981) are the long-term strategies that will effectively eliminate the greater part of the sheep's susceptibility. The operation is carried out with sharp shears on the skin wrinkles of the breech and tail, which are presented to the operator rump-down with the area exposed and accessible. The folds are removed by cutting with the shears, using a scissors action and making sure to start with sharp V cuts rather than blunt starts. The widest part of the denuded area should be just above the vulva. Docking of the tail is critical. It must be removed between the second and third vertebrae. Too long means fouling and strike susceptibility. Too short means a high prevalence of skin carcinoma of the vulva. The operation must be done in clean surroundings with disinfected instruments and the lambs left undisturbed for three to four weeks to give the wounds time to heal.

Properly done and performed over a period so that the flock is wrinkle-free on the breech, this operation reduces the size of the fly population and reduces the chances of infections occurring in the less common sites of the back and the pizzle.

Because of the possible importance of the pizzle as a site of carryover infection in winter, two methods have been devised to reduce the susceptibility of this area. A chemical ringing method creates a bare area of scar tissue around the pizzle and reduces the chances of wetting. The other technique—pizzle dropping—consists of severing the anterior attachment of the pizzle to the abdominal wall. This has a similar effect of reducing urine staining of wool.

The problem of convincing farmers to apply the Mules operation and pizzle-dropping to sheep can only be resolved by convincing them of the cost-effectiveness of the procedures. A careful study of costs and benefits does not appear to have been done. The principal disadvantage of the techniques is that they look painful and perhaps unnecessarily multilatory. Although considerations of animal welfare must direct increasing attention to the long-term project of breeding less susceptible sheep with plain breeches, this does not appear to have a high priority with farmers.

Timing Shearing Correctly. The less wool a sheep is carrying at the time of high risk, the less the chance of infection. If the time of major fly infestation can be coincided with a prior shearing, much of the risk to heavy-wooled sheep can be avoided.

Avoiding Fleece Rot. This disease has become very prevalent and is very conducive to blowfly body strike. Breeding to reduce susceptibility to it and development of a vaccine against it are strategies of potential prophylactic importance. Body strike is relatively uncommon, and outbreaks of it last for relatively short periods; but the disease is severe,

and heavy losses result (Watts and Merritt 1981).

Control of Gastrointestinal Helminthiasis. Prevention of the diarrhea that usually accompanies trichostrongylosis in sheep helps to keep the perineum clean and less attractive to blowfly strike.

Fast Application of Insecticide. When the first sheep are struck, the rest must be jetted (or some other effective means of application used) immediately. This means within 24 to 48 hours. The machinery needs to be adequate to the task. The sheep handling facilities need to be able to handle the numbers quickly, and the insecticide needs to be formulated so that it can be administered rapidly in the available equipment.

Use of an Effective Insecticide. The objective is to use a chemical to which the local blowfly larvae are least resistant. A very careful watch must be kept on this. Most areas with a local problem monitor the sensitivity of maggots continuously. *Lucilia cuprina* is the most prevalent fly in Australia (90% of strikes are by this fly) and the only one to be resistant. Resistance has developed to all modern insecticides, including aldrin and dieldrin, carbamates, and organophosphates, but the triazine compound Vetrazin is still effective (Hart 1981).

Foot Rot

Bacteroides nodosus, the causative agent of foot rot in sheep, is an obligate parasite and the disease is, therefore, eradicable. The carrier sheep—the only significant source of infection—can be identified and eliminated either by treatment or by sale for slaughter. However, there are many circumstances in which the degree of attention that has to be applied to each sheep is just not available. It is then necessary to retire to a continuous defensive position. The commonest defense is weekly dipping in a 5% formalin foot bath when climatic conditions of high temperature and moisture encourage rapid spread of the disease.

The long-sought solution of an immunization against *Bacteroides nodosus* is not yet a reality. Several vaccines are available, both oil adjuvant and alum-precipitated. However, the efficiency of the vaccine varies. The vaccination is sufficiently expensive and the sheep of such little value that the vaccine is expected to be a complete control program in itself and without any need for supplementary procedures. Because the antigenicity of different

Table 12-5. SUMMARY OF CONTROL PROCEDURES USED IN SOME DISEASES OF SHEEP

Disease or Production Procedure	Monitoring Technique(s)	Management	Prophylactic Techniques		
			Vaccination	Medication	Other
Anthrax	Sudden death is the only manifestation	Hygienic disposal of carcasses and other infected material	Excellent results. Annual in enzootic areas	—	—
Black disease	Sudden death is the only manifestation	Fluke control prevents	Excellent results with two vaccinations	—	—
Bluetongue	Clinical evidence of oral and coronet erosion lesions. Seroconversions indicate presence of one or more serotypes	Prevent introduction of virus into country	Many vaccines available	—	—
Botulism	Clinical cases of flaccid paralysis in groups of sheep on contaminated food or water	Avoid use of feed or water containing carcasses	Excellent results with type-specific toxoid for enzootic area	—	—
Brucellosis	Serological testing—complement fixation test. Plus physical palpation epididymitis	Run some groups separately. Vaccine and test and slaughter positive reactors	Vaccination effective	—	—
Caseous lymphadenitis	Observe enlarged lymph nodes at shearing	Cull affected sheep. Disinfect shearing and marking tools after each sheep	Vaccine available and reduces severity but does not prevent disease	—	—
Contagious ecthyma	Observe lesions on mouth, udder, coronets	Isolate affected sheep. Avoid abrasive material in environment	Very effective live virus vaccine	—	Bad outbreaks in lambs or ewes
Enterotoxemia	Sudden death of lambs usually	High feed and good body condition of sheep predispose—reduce them	Effective	—	A production disease due to over-stretching lamb's potential
Fluke infestation	Report from abattoirs. Fluke egg counts in feces	Control of snails in pasture water	—	Strategic dosing with effective flukicide	—
Hypocalcemia	Serum calcium and magnesium values may predict but not a practical exercise. Observe cases of recumbency and death	Avoid sudden changes of environment or feed in late pregnant or lactating ewes	—	—	—
Jaagsiekte	Chronic fatal pneumonia sporadic cases	Slaughter of clinical cases or slaughter all sheep in country	—	—	—
Johne's disease	Emaciation, soft feces, wool shedding. Serological tests, necropsy lesions best	Slaughter of positive reactors with eradication as aim	Vaccination possible and effective but not practiced unless prevalence high	—	—

Table continued on following page

411

Table 12-5. SUMMARY OF CONTROL PROCEDURES USED IN SOME DISEASES OF SHEEP (continued)

Disease or Production Procedure	Monitoring Technique(s)	Management	Prophylactic Techniques		
			Vaccination	Medication	Other
Listeriosis	Clinical cases of abortion, septicemia in lambs, circling in adults	Reduce access to ensilage. Very cold weather predisposes	No reliable vaccine available	Therapy not prophylactic	—
Louping ill	Clinical cases of incoordination, tremor, paralysis. Serological detection possible	Control of vector ticks by dipping program	Excellent vaccine available	—	—
Lumpy wool	Clinical cases very evident with lumpy discolored wool	Isolate affected animals and avoid grooming and other gear spread of infection	—	Antibacterial dip after shearing	Disease disappears in dry weather
Maedi-visna	Observe chronic pneumonia or encephalitis cases. Serological identification possible	Slaughter of serologically positive sheep. Isolate lambs at birth with no colostrum. Avoid shed lambing	—	—	Complete slaughter of whole flock advised
Malignant edema	Found dead	Hygiene at lambing, castrating, docking, shearing. Disinfect wounds	Highly effective	—	—
Mastitis	Clinical cases gangrenous mastitis	Cull affected ewes. Change pastures and bedding grounds	None available	Therapy not prophylactic	—
Nasal bots	Clinical rhinitis and sneezing	—	—	Strategic organophosphate treatment effective	—
Nutritional deficiency of:					
Calcium	Bendability and ease of fracture of bones	Improved general nutrition and provision of specific nutritional deficiency			
Cobalt	Poor weight gain. Urine concentration MMA or FIGLU			Reticular "bullet"	
Copper	Poor weight gain. Blood copper or ceruloplasmin			Depot injection	
Iodine	Birth of goitrous lambs			Depot injection iodine	
Selenium	Blood levels of glutathione peroxidase			Reticular "bullet"	
Pasteurellosis	Clinical cases of septicemia and pneumonia	Avoid environmental and feed stress	Vaccines used but efficiency not proven	Feeding tetracyclines common in feedlots	—

Pediculosis	Frequent inspection of fleece of live sheep	Avoid spread by inert objects. Maintain good body condition (body score)	—	Strategic dip or spray application	—
Pinkeye	Observe signs of blindness, eyelid spasm, conjunctivitis	Avoid close confinement, long grass, flies	—	Suitable collyrium medicine	—
Pizzle rot	Scabs at preputial orifice. Swollen prepuce	Reduce diet. Ring shear around prepuce	—	Implant of testosterone in wethers	—
Poisoning Pasture plants	Many clinical syndromes represented, especially uncoordination	Careful surveillance of pasture area for poisonous plants and elimination of them	—	—	—
Weeds					
Trees					
Arsenic	Clinical cases of abdominal pain, diarrhea, high mortality	Access to dipping fluids must be prevented	—	—	Use insecticides other than arsenicals
Polioencephalomalacia	Clinical cases of blindness, opisthotonus, nystagmus, tonic convulsions	Ensure adequate roughage in diet, also adequate continuous water supply	—	Dietary supplement with thiamin	—
Pregnancy toxemia	Observe late pregnant ewes with blindness, convulsions, recumbency, ketonuria	Ensure high caloric intake in last third of pregnancy—plane of nutrition needs to rise	—	Propylene glycol supplementation of diet effective but impractical	—
Scrapie	Pruritus, incoordination, paralysis. Very long incubation period	Slaughter clinical cases. Also slaughter contact sheep or goats in free area	—	—	Inheritance a significant factor in cause. Selection aids control
Squamous cell carcinoma	Tumors on vulva, ear at high level of prevalence	Leave tail docked at correct length. Suggested that susceptibility may be inherited	—	—	Correct length of tail left at docking
Tetanus	Clinical cases of fatal tetanic convulsions	Hygiene at birth, docking, castration, mulesing, shearing	Excellent results. Vaccinate ewes annually before lambing	—	—
Toxemic jaundice	High liver coppers. Obvious jaundice	Encouragement of grass growth. Compared with clover. Prevention of undernutrition	—	Administration of molybdenum daily	—
Weaner ill-thrift	Failure to make adequate weight gains in presence of adequate feed	Gentle handling of young sheep at weaning	—	Copper, cobalt, selenium, vitamin D supplementation	—

isolates of the organism varies, perhaps accounting in part for some of the breakdowns, vaccines containing a range of serotypes of the causative organism are now being used (Egerton 1981).

Clostridioses

Enterotoxemia, botulism, tetanus, blackleg, black disease, malignant edema, and focal symmetrical encephalomalacia can be significant causes of loss in sheep flocks, usually as massive outbreaks. Perhaps because they are easily controlled by vaccination and don't specifically require changes in management, they are generally kept under control. It is usually because vaccination programs are allowed to lapse or because the diseases occur out of season or in normally free areas that outbreaks happen.

A summary of the control procedures used in the management of other common disease entities in sheep is shown in Table 12-5.

Review Literature

Coop, I.E. Sheep and goat production. World Animal Science Series C1, Elsevier Scientific Publishing Co., Amsterdam, 1982.

Donald, A.D. Control of internal parasites of sheep. Univ. of Sydney Post. Grad. Cttee. Vet. Sci., Refresher Course for Veterinarians, No. 58, Sheep, pp. 441-451, 1981.

Moule, G.R. Field investigations with sheep. A manual of techniques. Commonwealth Scientific and Industrial Organisation, Melbourne, Australia, 1965.

New Zealand Veterinary Association Sheep Society (1975). Proc. N.Z. Vet. Assoc. Sheep Soc., 5th Seminar, Fac. Vet. Sci., Massey University, Palmerston North, June 13-14, 1975: Lamb Survival.

Plant, J.W. Field investigations into reproductive wastage in sheep. Univ. of Sydney Post Grad. Cttee. Vet. Sci., Refresher Course for Veterinarians, No. 58, Sheep, pp. 411-438, 1981.

Plant, J.W. Infertility in the ewe. Univ. of Sydney Post. Grad. Cttee. Vet. Sci., Refresher Course for Veterinarians, No. 58, Sheep, pp. 675-705, 1981.

Prichard, R.K., Hall, C.A., Kelly, J.D. et al. The problem of anthelminthic resistance in nematodes. Aust. Vet. J., 56:239-257, 1980.

Thurnley, D.C. Proc. N.Z. Vet. Ass. Sheep Soc., 2nd Seminar, Fac. Vet. Sci., Massey University, Palmerston North, June 9-11, 1972. Some factors predisposing to perinatal lamb mortality.

References

Alexander, G. Energy metabolism in the starved newborn lamb. Aust. J. Agric. Res., 13:144-164, 1962.

Alexander, G. Lamb survival. Physiological considerations. Proc. Aust. Soc. Anim. Prod., 5:113-122, 1964.

Alexander, G. and Peterson, J.E. Neonatal mortality in lambs: Intensive observations during lambing in a flock of maiden Merino ewes. Aust. Vet. J., 37:371-381, 1961.

Alexander, G. and Williams, D. Teat sucking activity in lambs. Effects of cold. J. Agric. Sci., 67:181-189, 1966.

Alexander, G., Lynch, J.J. and Mottershead, B.E. Use of shelter and selection of lambing sites by ewes in paddocks with closely or widely separated shelters. Appl. Anim. Ethol. 5:51-69, 1979.

Arnold, G.W. and Morgan, P.D. Behavior of the ewe and lamb at lambing—relationship to lamb mortality. Appl. Anim. Ethol. 2:25-27, 1975.

Arnold, G.W., Wallace, S.R. and Maller, R.A. Some factors involved in natural weaning of sheep. Appl. Anim. Ethol. 5:43-50, 1978.

Bareham, J.R. Behaviour of the lamb on the first day after birth. Br. Vet. J., 132:152-161, 1976.

Beggs, A.R. and Campion, E.J. Field techniques to increase lamb survival. Proc. Aust. Soc. Anim. Prod., 6:169-176, 1966.

Bennett, D., Morley, F.H.W., Clark, K.W. et al. The effect of grazing cattle and sheep together. Aust. J. Exp. Agric. and Anim. Husb., 10:694-709, 1970.

Bishop, A.H. Wool production in the high rainfall zone. A review of the industry's response to the pasture revolution. J. Aust. Inst. Vet. Agric. Sci., 30:219-231, 1964.

Boland, M.P., Kelleher, D. and Gordon, I. Comparison of control of estrus and ovulation in sheep by an ear implant (SC-21009) or by intravaginal sponge. Anim. Reprod. Sci., 1:275-281, 1979.

Boland, M.P., Lemainque, F. and Gordon, I. Comparison of lambing outcome in ewes after synchronization by progestagen of prostaglandin. J. Agric. Sci., 91:765-766, 1978.

Bondurant, R.H. Pregnancy diagnosis in sheep and goats. Field tests with an ultrasound unit. Calif. Vet., 34:26-28, 1980.

Boundy, T. Programming for preventive medicine and improved productivity in sheep. Vet. Ann., 19:79-82, 1979.

Boundy, T. Programming for preventive disease and improved production in sheep. Can. Vet. J., 22:221-225, 1981.

Broadbent, D.W. Infections associated with ovine perinatal mortality. Aust. Vet. J., 51:71-74, 1975.

Cannon, D.J. and Bath, J.G. Prenatal losses in Border-Leicester-Merino cross ewes in Victoria. Aust. Vet. J., 47:323-324, 1971.

Cerini, M., Findlay, J.K. and Lawson, R.A.S. Pregnancy-specific antigens in the sheep: Application to the diagnosis of pregnancy. J. Reprod. Fertil., 46:65-69, 1976.

Clarke, J. Intensive lambing will be profitable now. J. Agric., 75:251-253, 1977.

Claxton, J.H. and Yeates, N.T.M. The inheritance of cryptorchidism in a small crossbred flock of sheep. J. Hered., 63:141-144, 1972.

Cole, V.G. The future of the sheep industry. Implications for the veterinarian. Victorian Vet. Proc., 30:17-22, 1971/72.

Cuthbertson, J.C. Sheep disease surveillance based on condemnation at three Scottish abattoirs. Vet. Rec., 112:219-221, 1983.

Dalton, D.C., Knight, T.W. and Johnson, D.L. Lamb survival in sheep breeds on New Zealand hill country. N.Z. J. Agric. Res., 23:167-173, 1980.

Davis, G.B. A sheep mortality survey. Proc. 2nd Intern. Symp., Vet. Epidemiol. Econ., 1979, pp. 106-110.

Dennis, S.M. Congenital abnormalities in sheep in Western Australia. J. Dept. Agr. West. Aust., 6:691-693, 1965.

Dennis, S.M. Perinatal lamb mortality in a purebred Southdown flock. J. Anim. Sci., 31:76-79, 1970.

Dennis, S.M. Perinatal lamb mortality. Cornell Vet., 62:253–262, 1972a.

Dennis, S.M. Infectious ovine abortion in Australia. Vet. Bull., 42:415–419, 1972b.

Dennis, S.M. Perinatal lamb mortality in Western Australia. Aust. Vet. J., 50:443, 450, 507, 511, 1974.

Dennis, S.M. Perinatal lamb mortality in Western Australia. Aust. Vet. J., 51:11, 75, 80, 83, 1975.

Dennis, S.M. and Leipold, H.W. Ovine congenital defects. Vet. Bull., 49:233–239, 1979.

Dennis, S.M. Predation of lambs. Vet. Med. S.A.C., 75: 845–852, 1980.

Ducker, M.J. and Fraser, J. A note on the effect of level of husbandry at lambing on lamb viability and subsequent performance. Anim. Prod., 16:91–94, 1973.

Duff, X.J., McCutcheon, S.N. and McDonald, M.F. Central nervous system injuries as a determinant of lamb mortality. Proc. N.Z. Soc. Anim. Prod., 42:15–17, 1982.

Eales, F.A., Gilmour, J.S., Barlow, R.M. et al. Causes of hypothermia in lambs. Vet. Rec., 110:118–120, 1982.

Edey, T.N. Prenatal mortality in sheep. A review. Anim. Breed. Abstr., 37:173–190, 1969.

Egan, J.K., McLaughlin, J.W., Thompson, R.L. et al. The importance of shelter in reducing neonatal lamb deaths. Aust. J. Exp. Agric., 12:470–472, 1972.

Egan, J.K., Thompson, R.L. and McIntyre, J.S. Overgrown Phalaris tuberosa as shelter for newborn lambs. Proc. Aust. Soc. Anim. Prod., 11:157–160, 1976.

Egerton, J. Footrot. Univ. Sydney Post. Grad. Cttee. Vet. Sci. Refresher Course for Veterinarians, No. 58, Sheep, pp. 647–651, 1981.

Emady, M., Noakes, J.C. and Arthur, G.H. Corticosteroid induced lambing in the ewe. Vet. Rec., 95:281–285, 1974.

Ercanbrack, S.K. and Price, D.A. Frequencies of various birth defects of Rambouillet sheep. J. Hered., 62: 223–227, 1971.

Fogarty, N.M. and Thompson, J.M. Relationship between pelvic measurements and dystocia in Dorset Horn ewes. Aust. Vet. J., 50:502–506, 1974.

Galloway, D.B., Morley, F.H.W., Watt, B.R. et al. Current trends in sheep flock health. Vict. Vet. Proc., 39: 19–20, 1981.

Gates, N.L., Everson, D.O. and Huler, C.V. Effects of thin ewe syndrome on reproductive efficiency. J. Am. Vet. Med. Assoc., 171:1266–1267, 1977.

George, J.M. The incidence of dystocia in fine-wool Merino ewes. Aust. Vet. J., 51:262–265, 1975.

George, J.M. The incidence of dystocia in Dorset Horn ewes. Aust. Vet. J., 52:519–523, 1976.

Gilmour, N.J.L., Thompson, D.A. and Fraser, J. Vaccination against vibriosis in sheep in late pregnancy. Vet. Rec., 96:129–131, 1975.

Gorrie, C.J.R. Ovine abortion in Victoria. Aust. Vet. J., 38:138–142, 1962.

Grant I.M., Galloway, D.B. and Morley, F.H.W. Effect of condition and liveweight at mating on the percentage of ewes marked by raddled rams during a 10 week joining period. Victoria Vet. Proc., 39:20–23, 1981.

Grant, I.M., Galloway, D.B., Geldard, H. et al. Effects of active immunisation against androstenedione and/or grazing a lupine stubbles at joining on the reproductive performance of Corriedale ewes. Proc. 20th World Vet. Cong., Perth, 1983.

Gruen, F.H. Long term projections of agricultural supply and demand Australia 1965 to 1980. Dept. of Economics, Monash Univ., Clayton, Victoria, 1967.

Grumbrell, R.C. Preliminary report on the results of the first year of a five year survey on lamb perinatal mortality. Proc. 10th Seminar Sheep and Beef Cattle Soc., N.Z. Vet. Assoc., pp. 94–99, 1980.

Hamdy, A.H., Redman, D.R., Bell, D.S. et al. Influence of a penicillin streptomycin preparation on lamb mortality. J. Am. Vet. Med. Assoc., 150:196–199, 1967.

Harmon, E.L. and Slyter, A.L. Induction of parturition in the ewe. J. Anim. Sci., 50:391–393, 1980.

Hart, R.J. Blowfly control, resistance. Univ. Sydney Post. Grad. Ctte. Vet. Sci. Refresher Course for Veterinarians, No. 58, Sheep, pp. 51–65, 1981.

Hartley, W.J. Congenital infections associated with perinatal lamb losses. Post. Grad. Foundation in Vet. Sci., Univ. of Sydney. Vet. Review, March, 1968, pp. 1–10,

Hartley, W.J. and Boyes, B.W. Incidence of ovine perinatal mortality in New Zealand with particular reference to intrauterine infections. N.Z. Vet. J., 12:33–36, 1964.

Hartley, W.J. and Kater, J.C. Perinatal disease conditions of sheep in New Zealand. N.Z. Vet. J., 12:49–57, 1964.

Haughey, K.G. Vascular abnormalities in the central nervous system associated with perinatal lamb mortality. Aust., Vet. J., 49:1–15, 1973.

Haughey, K.G. The role of birth in the pathogenesis of meningeal hemorrhage and congestion in newborn lambs. Aust. Vet. J., 56:49–56, 1980.

Haughey, K.G., Hughes, K.L. and Hartley, W.J. The occurrence of congenital infections associated with perinatal lamb mortality. Aust. Vet. J., 43:413–420, 1967.

Haughey, K.G., Hughes, K.L. and Hartley, W.J. Brucella ovis infection. Aust. Vet. J., 44:531–535, 1968.

Hayman, R.H., Turner, H.N., and Turton, E. Observations on survival and growth to weaning of lambs from ewes with defective udders. Aust. J. Agric. Res., 6:446–455, 1955.

Hight, G.K. and Rae, A.L. Large-scale sheep breeding: Its development and possibilities. Sheep Farming Annual (New Zealand), pp. 73–85, 1970.

Hindson, J. Sheep health schemes. Vet. Rec. (In Practice), 4:53–58, 1982.

Hore, D.E., Smith, H.V., Snowdon, W.A. et al. An investigation of viral and bacterial agents associated with ovine perinatal mortality. Aust. Vet. J., 49:190–195, 1973.

Houston, D.C. and Maddox, J.G. Causes of mortality in young Scottish Blackface lambs. Vet. Rec., 95:575, 1974 (corresp.).

Hughes, K.L. Spontaneous congenital abnormalities observed at necropsy in a large survey of newly born, dead lambs. Teratology, 5:5–10, 1972.

Hughes, K.L., Hartley, W.J., Haughey, K.G. et al. A study of perinatal mortality of lambs from the Oberon, Orange, and Monaro districts of New South Wales. Proc. Aust. Soc. Anim. Prod., 5:92–99, 1964.

Hughes, K.L., Haughey, K.G. and Hartley, W.J. Perinatal lamb mortality: Infections occurring amongst lambs dying after parturition. Aust. Vet. J., 47:472–476, 1971.

Jackson, N. and Turner, H.N. Optimal structure for a cooperative nucleus breeding system. Proc. Aust. Soc. Anim. Prod., 9:55–64, 1972.

Johnston, W.S., McLachlan, G.K. and Murray, I.S. Sheep losses and their causes on commercial farms in northern Scotland. Vet. Rec., 106:238–240, 1980.

Kirk, J.H. and Anderson, B.C. Reducing lamb mortality: A two-year study. Vet. Med. S.A.C., 77:1247–1252, 1982.

Kirk, J.H., Huffman, E.M. and Anderson, B.C. Mastitis and udder abnormalities as related to neonatal lamb mortality in shed-lambed ewes. J. Anim. Sci., 50: 610–616, 1980.

Knight, T.W., Oldham, C.M., Smith, J.F. et al. Analysis of reproductive wastage in sheep in Western Australia. Aust. J. Exp. Agric. Anim. Husb., 15:183–188, 1975.

Lax, J. and Turner, H.N. The influence of various factors on the survival rate to weaning of Merino lambs. 1. Sex, strain, location and age of ewe for single-born lambs. Aust. J. Agric. Res., 16:981–995, 1965.

Lees, J.L. Some aspects of reproductive efficiency in sheep. Vet. Rec., 88:86–95, 1971.

Linklater, K.A. Abortion in sheep. Vet. Rec. (In Practice), 1:30–33, 1979.

Lucas, J.M.S. and Notman, A. Corticosteroids to synchronise parturition in sheep. Br. Vet. J., 130:i, 1974.

Lutnaes, B. Field investigations of illness and death among adult ewes. Norsk Veterinaertidsskrift, 94: 469–478, 1982.

Lutnaes, B. and Paus, H. A field study of diseases and mortality in lambs. Extent and time of episodes. Norsk Veterinaertidsskrift, 93:167–174, 1981.

Lutnaes, B. Field study of illness and death among lambs. II. Flock variation in losses, and mortality among single, twin and triplet lambs from ewes of various ages. Norsk Veterinaertidsskrift, 94:245–249, 1982.

Mackay, R.R. The effect of strategic anthelminthic treatment on the breeding performance of hill ewes. Vet. Parasit., 7:319–331, 1980.

Mackenzie, A. J., Thwaites, D.J. and Edey, T.N. Oestrus, ovarian and adrenal response of the ewe to fasting and cold stress. Aust. J. Agric. Res., 26:545–541, 1975.

McKenzie, R.L. and Grant, J.L. A survey of lamb mortality in commercial flocks of sheep. Rhodesian Vet. J., 6:69, 1976.

Madel, A.J. Observations on the mammary glands of culled ewes at the time of slaughter. Vet. Res., 109: 362–363, 1981.

Maund, B.A., Duffell, S.J. and Winkler, C.E. Lamb mortality in relation to prolificacy. Exp. Anim. Husb., 36:99–111, 1980.

McAuliffe, P.R., Hardefeldt, K.W. and Hucker, D.A. Health problems associated with the export of live sheep. Aust. Vet. J., 54:594–595, 1978.

McDonald, J.W. Variation in perinatal mortality of lambs with age and parity of ewes. Proc. Aust. Soc. Anim. Prod., 6:60–62, 1966.

McFarlane, D. Perinatal lamb losses. Aust. Vet. J., 37: 105–109, 1961.

McFarlane, D. Perinatal lamb losses. Part 1. N.Z. Vet. J., 13:116–135, 1965.

McFarlane, D. Perinatal lamb losses. Part 2. N.Z. Vet. J., 14:137–144, 1966.

McSporran, K.D., Buchanan, R. and Fielden, E.D. Dystocia in a Romney flock. N.Z. Vet. J., 25:247–257, 1977.

McSporran, K.D., Wyburn, R.S. and Fielden, E.D. Studies in dystocia in sheep. N.Z. Vet. J., 27:64–66, 75–78, 1979.

Meredith, M.J. and Madani, M.O.K. The detection of pregnancy in sheep by A-mode ultrasound. Br. Vet. J., 136:325–330, 1980.

Miller, S.J. A sheep management calendar for Merinos in Western Queensland. Aust. Adv. Vet. Sci., p. 52, 1979.

Miller, S.J. Artificial breeding techniques of sheep. Univ. of Sydney Post. Grad. Cttee. Vet. Sci., Refresher Course for Veterinarians, No. 58, Sheep, pp. 71–86, 1981.

Morley, F.H.W. Applications of research to flock health. Vict. Vet. Proc., 37:29–30, 1979.

Moteane, M., Middleton, D.M. and Polley, L.R. Survey of disease conditions in adult and feeder sheep in Saskatchewan. Can. Vet. J., 20:2–7, 1979.

Moule, G.E. The major causes of low lamb marking percentages in Australia. Aust. Vet. J., 36:154–159, 1960.

Moule, G.E. Field investigations with sheep. A manual of techniques. Commonwealth Scientific and Industrial Research Organisation, Melbourne, Australia, 1965.

Moule, G.E. The management of breeding sheep in Australia. Univ. of Sydney, Post. Grad. Foundation in Vet. Sci., Vet. Rev., 6:50, 1969.

Mullaney, P.D. Prenatal losses in sheep in Western Victoria. Proc. Aust. Soc. Anim. Prod., 6:56–59, 1966.

Munday, B-L, Ryan, F.B., King, S.J. et al. Preparturient infections and other causes of fetal loss in sheep and cattle in Tasmania. Aust. Vet. J., 42:189–193, 1966.

Nass, R.O. Mortality associated with sheep operations in Idaho. J. Range Mgt., 30:253–258, 1977.

Ott, R.S. and Memon, M.A. Breeding soundness examination of rams and bucks. Theriogenology, 13:155–164, 1968.

Owen, J.B. Performance recording in sheep. Commonwealth Agric. Bureau Technical Communication, No. 20, CAB, Farnham Royal, England, 1971.

Pierson, R.E. A survey of lamb health in feedlots. J. Am. Vet. Med. Assoc., 150:298–302, 1967.

Pierson, R.E. Herd health program for a large feedlot lamb operation. J. Am. Vet. Med. Assoc., 157:1054–1506, 1970.

Plant, J.W. Field investigation of perinatal lamb mortalities. Aust. Vet. Assoc., 54th Ann. Conf. Program, p. 157, 1977.

Plant, J.W. Pregnancy diagnosis in sheep by rectal probe. Vet. Rec., 106:305–306, 1980.

Plant, J.W. Field investigations into reproductive wastage in sheep. Univ. of Sydney Post. Grad. Cttee. Vet. Sci., Refresher Course for Veterinarians, No. 58, Sheep, pp. 411–438, 1981.

Plant, J.W., Ferguson, B., O'Halloran, W. et al. Causes of infertility in individual sheep flocks in New South Wales. Aust. Vet. Assoc., 53rd Ann. Conf. Program, p. 189, 1976.

Plant, J.W., Marchant, R., Mitchell, T.D. et al. Neonatal lamb losses due to feral pig predation. Aust. Vet. J., 54:426–429, 1978.

Pout, D.D. and Thomas, W.J.K. Veterinary and medicine costs and practices in lowland sheep. Agricultural Economics Unit, Univ. of Exeter, U.K., p. 34, 1973.

Priester, W.A., Glass, A.G. and Waggoner, N.S. Congenital defects in domesticated animals. General considerations. Amer. J. Vet. Res., 31:1871–1879, 1970.

Purser, A.F. and Young, G.B. Mortality amongst twins and single lambs. Anim. Prod., 6:321–329, 1964.

Purvis, G.M., Ostler, D.C., Starr, J. et al. Lamb mortality in a commercial flock. Vet. Rec., 104:241–242, 1979.

Quinlivan, T.D. Is there a role for practitioners in flock health programs? Univ. of Sydney Post. Grad. Cttee, Vet. Sci., Refresher Course for Veterinarians, No. 58, Sheep, pp. 269–290, 1981a.

Quinlivan, T.D. Cooperative ram breeding. Univ. of Sydney Post. Grad. Cttee. Vet. Sci., Refresher Course for Veterinarians, No. 58, Sheep, pp. 280–290, 1981b.

Rawlings, N.C., Savage, N.C., Scheer, H.D. et al. Estrus synchronisation in commercial sheep flocks in Alberta and Saskatchewan. Can. Vet. J., 24:236–237, 1983.

Restall, B.J., Brown, G.H., Blockey, M. deB. et al. Assessment of reproductive wastage in sheep. Aust. J. Exp. Agric. Anim. Husb., 16:329–352, 1976a.

Restall, B.J., Herdegan, J. and Carberry, P. Induction of parturition in sheep using estradiol benzoate. Aust. J. Exp. Agric. Anim. Husb., 16:462–466, 1976b.

Robertson, H.A., Chan, J.S.D., Hackett, R.J. et al. Diagnosis of pregnancy in the ewe at mid-pregnancy. Anim. Reprod. Sci., 3:69–72, 1980.

Safford, J.W. and Hoversland, A.S. A study of lamb mortality in a western range flock. 1. Autopsy findings on 1051 lambs. J. Anim. Sci., 19:265–273, 1960.

Sainsbury, D.W.B. Economics feature. Buildings and sheep. Br. Vet. J., 128:529–530, 1972.

Salisbury, J.R. Special disease risks associated with heavy stocking rates. Victorian Vet. Proc., 25:53–56, 1967.

Setchell, B.P., Dickinson, D.A. Lascelles, A.K. et al. Neonatal mortality in lambs associated with goitre. Aust. Vet. J., 36:159–164, 1960.

Smith, G.M. Factors affecting birth weight, dystocia and preweaning survival in sheep. J. Anim. Sci., 44: 745–753, 1977.

Smith, I.D. Some observations on ovine perinatal mortality in Western Queensland. Aust. J. Exp. Agric. Anim. Husb., 5:110–114, 1965a.

Smith, I.D. Role of avian predators in lamb mortality in Queensland. Aust. Vet. J., 47:333–335, 1965b.

Smith, J.F., Cox, R.I., McGowan, L.T. et al. Increasing the ovulation rate in ewes by immunization. Proc. N.Z. Soc. Anim. Prod., 41:193–197, 1981.

Spedding, C.R.W. The agricultural ecology of sheep grazing. Br. Vet. J., 118:461–481, 1962.

Spedding, C.R.W. The feeding of sheep at pasture. Vet. Rec., 75:1153–1156, 1963.

Speedy, A.W. and Clark, C.F.S. Lowland sheep: The nutrition and management cycle. Vet. Rec., 108:493–496, 1981.

Stamp, J.T. Perinatal losses in lambs with particular reference to diagnosis. Vet. Rec., 81:530–537, 1967.

Stephenson, R.G.A., Edwards, J.C. and Pratt, M.S. Causes of lamb deaths and some practical ways of reducing them. Queensland Agric. J., 106:411–418, 1980.

Stevens, D., Alexander G. and Lynch, J.J. Lamb mortality due to inadequate care of twins by merino ewes. Appl. Anim. Ethol., 8:243–252, 1982.

Tassell, R. The effects of diet on reproduction in pigs, sheep and cattle. Plane nutrition in sheep. Br. Vet. J., 123:257–264, 1967a.

Tassell, R. The effects of diet on reproduction in pigs, sheep and cattle. Part 4. Sheep—protein, vitamins, minerals. Br. Vet. J., 123:364–371, 1967b.

Terrill, C.E. and Tidwell, G.M. Crossbreeding of sheep. Proc. 3rd World Conf. Anim. Prod., Melbourne, pp. 620–625, 1975.

Thomas, W.J.K. and Pout, D.D. Veterinary costings in lowland sheep. Vet. Ann., 15:72–74, 1975.

Tigner J.R. and Larson, G.E. Sheep losses on selected ranches in southern Wyoming. J. Range Mgt., 30:244–248, 1977.

Tsakalof, T.S., Vlachos, N. and Latousakis, D. Observations on the reproductive performance of ewe lambs syncronised for estrus. Vet. Rec., 100: 380–382, 1977.

Turner, C.B. and Hindson, J.C. Manual pregnancy diagnosis in the ewe. Vet. Rec., 96:56–58, 1975.

Turner, H.N. Exotic sheep breeds of possible value in north Australia. Wool Technol. and Sheep Breed. 18:42–49, 1971.

Tyrrell, R.N., Lane, J.G., Nancarrow, C.D., et al. Termination of early pregnancy in ewes by use of a prostaglandin analogue, and subsequent fertility. Aust. Vet. J., 57:76–78, 1981.

Watson, R.H. Intensive lambing. J. Agric. Victoria, Oct., pp. 420–428, 1967.

Watson, R.H. Reduction of perinatal loss of lambs by shelter. Proc. Aust. Soc. Anim. Prod., 7:243–249, 1968.

Watson, R.H. and Elder, E.M. Neonatal mortality in lambs. Aust. Vet. J., 37:283–290, 1961.

Watson, W.A. The prevention and control of ovine abortion. Br. Vet. J., 129:309–314, 1973.

Watt, A. Neonatal losses in lambs. Vet. Rec. (In Practice), 2:5–9, 1980.

Watt, B.R., Morley, F.H.W. and Galloway, D.B. Causes of wastage in Western District sheep flocks. Victorian Vet. Proc., 39:17–19, 1981.

Watts, J.E. and Merritt, G.C. Body strike in sheep. Univ. of Sydney Post. Grad. Cttee, Vet. Sci., Refresher Course for Veterinarians, No. 58, Sheep, pp. 177–191, 1981.

White, D.H. and Morley, F.H.W. Analysis and management of sheep production systems—a series of 4 papers. Proc. Aust. Soc. Anim. Prod., 14:35–46, 1982.

Whitelaw, A. and Watchorn, P. Dystocia in a South Country Cheviot flock. Vet. Rec., 97:489–492, 1975.

Wiener, G., Deeple, F.K., Broadbent, J.S. et al. Breed variation in lambing performance. Anim. Prod., 17: 229–243, 1973.

Wilkinson, F.C. Footrot. Western Australian experience. Eradication, differentiating strains and role of cattle. Univ. of Sydney Post. Grad. Cttee. Vet. Sci., Refresher Course for Veterinarians, No. 58, Sheep, pp. 21–23, 1981.

Yeo, D. Mulesing. Univ. of Sydney Post. Grad. Cttee. Vet. Sci., Refresher Course for Veterinarians, No. 58, Sheep, pp. 653–656, 1981.

13 Computers in Animal Health Management

INTRODUCTION

Good animal management includes good animal sensitivity, good husbandry, and good records.

Good animal sensitivity is necessary so that the farmer knows instinctively which is the best of any two choices for the welfare and long-term productivity of his animals. Good husbandry, including animal health, animal nutrition, and genetics, requires also that the farmer have a capacity to integrate all of the activities on a farm into a coordinated, smooth-running, whole-farm system. This is the characteristic usually identified as general management. Good records are those that can be retrieved, analyzed, and used as measures of performance and for comparison of these performances with pre-set targets, with previous years, and for interfarm comparisons. All of this revolves around the objective of ensuring that a high level of performance efficiency is maintained. The data base created by these efforts can also be used to predict future productivity, future needs for feed and animal replacements, and cash flow.

An animal farmer may be lucky enough to be born with sensitivity for animals, but if not, it can be developed, provided there is sympathy and perceptivity. Nutrition, genetics, and health can also be learned, but more importantly, advice can be sought from experts who will set down details of a feeding, breeding, or health program. The biggest gap in the farmer's assembly of techniques has been that of recording,ʼ not accountancy, because that has been available. Big ranches and enterprises

418

have had the advantage of being able to employ bookkeepers who maintained inventories of livestock and farm supplies and could, hopefully, lay out plans for future financial investment on the cattle ranch or the sheep station. However, the bulk of animal farmers—those on the family farm—have had to depend on family help. All that is a thing of the past. Nowadays, the smallest farmer can hire an internationally renowned record keeper and data analyzer—the computer programer—who devises the computer program, i.e., the software, which indicates what data is to be collected and then does the rest itself. The quality of this data processing, and accordingly, the information that is provided by the analyses, depends almost entirely on the quality of that program. The computer and its attachments, i.e., the hardware, make some contribution albeit very little, and there is little difference in the performance of modern computers. The golden rule in this farm recording system is to choose the software that does the tasks best and *then*, and only then, find the computer that will run the program. This constraint arises because there are a number of computer languages, any one of which may be utilizable on only a few computers. To translate the desired program into another language is prohibitively expensive, and to buy a computer because it is marginally superior to another in size of memory or speed of handling is poor policy.

ADVANTAGES OF COMPUTERIZATION

Any veterinary practice deals in a vast amount of recorded data because it has many clients who buy from the practice a large number of individual services for which relatively small amounts of money are paid. For example, there are seven species of animals with which most veterinarians come in contact. Each species has its own diseases and their remedies. Another variable is the number of drugs and the variety and size of materials, which are multiplied many times over by the differences in size of the patients all the way from a Chihuahua bitch to a Hereford bull. In the modern-day food animal practice, there is added to this already formidable mass of data the need to provide a planned animal health and production service that monitors production and disease incidence; predicts performance, feed needs, and cash flow; and produces lists of animals to be examined or treated

or culled. All of this is quadrupled because these programs are now available for dairy cattle, beef cattle, sheep, and pigs.

If these data are to be stored, sorted, retrieved, and analyzed in many different ways so that their accumulation is not wasted by being used only for its original purpose, it can only be done in a realistic way by the use of a computer. No other system can possibly handle the mass of figures accurately and economically.

A large part of the demand for figures and analyses of them has arisen in recent times because of our newfound enthusiasm for cost-effectiveness. We not only need to know that there is more money in the bank at the end of the year than at the beginning, but we also need to know what our performance is compared with our peers. Within our own practices, we need to know which part of it is profitable and which is not, and what increase in fees is necessary to prop up a losing unit. It can all be done manually but no longer at the rates of pay that humans demand.

The rules of cost-effectiveness must also apply to a computerization proposal. Accordingly, the first rule of computerization is: ALL COMPUTERIZATION IS EXPENSIVE. IT SHOULD NOT BE CONTEMPLATED UNLESS IT CAN BE SHOWN THAT THE BENEFITS OUTWEIGH THE COSTS.

There are the usual difficulties in assessing any cost/benefit relationship, but they are compounded in a study of computers because of the variety of systems available. In simple terms, they are:

1. Microcomputers—in a stand-alone state
2. Microcomputers used as intelligent terminals to a large, central main-frame computer.
3. A central main-frame computer connected to many stations by "dumb" terminals, which can receive and dispatch data but cannot process any by themselves
4. A special adaptation of the main-frame-dumb terminal system aimed at a large data base—the VIEWDATA system

One of the pieces of information that would be most valuable when choosing between computers is the number of patients or annual accessions, or for preventive medicine purposes, the number of animals that must be under the practice's control before it is economically viable to establish a computer in the practice. Suggested thresholds are:

□ standard "fire-engine" practice—5000 accessions per year

□ herd health practice—5000 adult cattle under control

In a survey of veterinary practices in the U.S. in 1982, it was found that 4.5% of them used a computer or computer service. Most of this use was for the business management part of the practice (Wise 1972).

In the case of microcomputers, the initial costs of the machine plus the program are large, but maintenance costs are low. For terminals connected to main-frame computers, the initial costs are low, but rental is high. Every computer salesman will tell you that the computer will save you office time and improve cost-effectiveness by the reduction of labor required. The theoretical argument is true, but the actual result is often not what was predicted. To do the exact same tasks that were done previously, the computer saves time by about a third to a half, but the saved time may not be used economically by staff. The circumstance in which installation is most profitable is when office staff is stretched to the limit, or beyond it, and either an additional staff member or a computer must be added to the office work force.

Once the computer is installed, it is found to provide many more attractive services than were available beforehand. These are utilized, and the saved office time is suddenly taken up again. As a result, the administration of the practice is much more efficient, but it costs more. It would then be necessary to estimate whether the financial advantage conferred by the better administration had offset the computer charges. Conservative thinkers are not impressed, innovators are, and only time will really tell. To a large extent, the decision depends on whether you prefer money or efficiency—that is, if you have to make a choice.

A summary of the administrative advantages of a computer includes:

□ the production of useful analyses of income, expenditure, and so on, instantly, and at no extra cost
□ a 30 to 40% increase in the speed of processing data
□ long-term storage (archives) created cheaply, quickly, and at minimum requirement for storage space
□ replacement records (back-up) created quickly and cheaply, confirming complete safety on data storage, which cannot realistically be provided by any other data processing system. The usual practice is to store the back-up discs at some distant location

□ the provision of a very large range of administrative services to the practice and a large range of advisory services to clients. The latter are discussed in detail in later pages.

If a tentative decision is made to move into computer technology as a practice tool, it is wise to review all of the things that a computer can do for a food animal practice and, indirectly, for farmer clients. If the list is unimpressive, if really suitable software is unavailable, if the volume of data is not great, and particularly if office staff are not under pressure to expand, it may be premature to computerize. It may be wiser to stay away from the decision because the machines and the programs are in a phase of rapid development, and are decreasing (or not increasing) in price but are improving greatly in efficiency. More importantly for professional people who will want to use the systems but may not want to delve deeply into their electronics and engineering, they are increasing in "friendliness." Computer friendliness means the ease with which the operator can communicate with the data in the machine. It is a characteristic dependent to some extent on the thoughtfulness of the person writing the program, who appreciates that the bulk of users do not want to be computer buffs, and partly on the increased storage capacity of the machine. When the amount of storage is greatly restricted, the data to be stored is coded with the smallest possible numbers of characters. These codes are not particularly easy to remember. When space is not at such a premium because of improved storage technology, it is possible to use more characters. A four-character alphanumeric code is not unusual, so that REP5 can mean the fifth disease on the reproductive system list, and no great feat of memory is required to remember the code. Data transmission becomes easier and more accurate as a result. Friendliness also includes easier writing of programs and simpler, more easily remembered, commands.

The receptivity of the machine also depends largely on the language built into it. To a large extent, this depends on the manufacturers appreciating the needs of the operator.

CHOICE OF COMPUTER RESOURCES

If a decision is made to computerize a practice's record system, it is not desirable to rush out and buy a microcomputer. There are a number of ways of acquiring access to a computing service, and the pros and cons of these are discussed in the following paragraphs.

The criteria on which to base a choice between the various access routes to a computer vary from group to group of users, but in general the same basic list applies, especially to a selected closed group of users such as food animal veterinarians.

Main-Frame Computers

These are large computers usually operated by institutions or commercial firms that rent time to outside persons. It is possible to send data in by conventional mail or by electronic mail, i.e., by a remote terminal over telephone lines.

"Mail-Ins." The least satisfactory method is the "mail-in," when data or requests for results are mailed into a central computer service to be entered into a computer by an independent operator. The delays likely to result in the passage through mail services and within the data bureau make the system very susceptible to a long turnaround time and to error due to loss of material or unfamiliarity of the operator with the material, which is likely to be highly specialized.

Contact with a Main-Frame Computer Via a Distant Terminal and Telephone Link. This system has the advantage that a massive program, such as a computer simulation model of a dairy herd, can be accessed for information, and data from a large number of units can be stored centrally and can provide a large data base quickly. Its principal disadvantages are cost for computer time and inability to gain access at all times. At busy times, it may be necessary to wait for long periods, but there is usually a facility that allows the information to be put on standby until space is available, at which time the data is automatically loaded. All computers have "down-time," when they are not available because of electrical or similar problems, or more commonly because adjustments are being made to basic programs. Although optional down-time is usually scheduled at weekends, there will be periods when the computer is simply not available. On the credit side of the large computer are enormous storage, very large machine memory, and ability to carry out very complicated analyses in very fast time. For example, in a mastitis model used by us on a Cyber, the computer examines 1200×1 month of lactations for mastitis events in 0.5 seconds. The large number of terminals that are available on the one computer makes expansion of a system within an institution easy, and there is almost no limit to the expansion that can take place.

Microcomputers

Microcomputers are developing so rapidly that criticisms of them are often not valid within a short time. Their virtue is that they are totally at the command of the owner. There is no waiting, and delay is minimal. The programs used are exactly what the owner wants, not what a computer center decides you need. These advantages are sometimes theoretical. Within one's own organization or practice, there are conflicting demands for access, especially between the administrative services such as billing and client data and the needs of a herd health service. Also, the programs are usually purchased as a package and may have features that are not completely suitable for one's own needs. They have a fairly large capital cost (for a practice large enough to make good use of one, e.g., a five-person practice, the price for a hardware and software package capable of handling 20,000 clients and a fee income of $500,000, with three terminals and storage for 10 years of records, a price in 1985 would be $30,000 to $40,000), but after purchase, the only cost is a mechanical and program maintenance contract, which may cost 15% of the capital cost per year.

Disadvantages of microcomputers are slow speed (10 to 20 times longer for average data searching and analysis), small machine memory, which is a big reason for the slow speed, and limited capacity for extension by the addition of terminals. Data storage is usually smaller but can be added to, so that for all practical purposes it is sufficient for a practice.

Microcomputers Linked to Main Frames

A microcomputer can stand alone—it is, in fact, called that—a Stand Alone Micro, or it can be linked to a main-frame computer. The latter system has the advantage that when not in use as a terminal for the main frame, it can be used for stand-alone purposes. This provides the opportunity to keep some data or analyses on the farm or at the veterinary practice and to send other material, perhaps the analyses, to the central unit. This is important if an institutional service desires epidemiologic data without having to store all the raw data, for example, on production. The FAHRMX program at the

University of Michigan is an example of this system (Gibson et al. 1982).

In summary, in choosing which system to use, there are so many factors that influence the decision that the choice must be an individual one. For an institution that conducts research and needs a great deal of mathematical/statistical analysis of data done quickly, a link to a main-frame computer is an enormous advantage. The amount of data to be stored and the number of terminals using the computer also influence the decision. For example, a system with more than 10 terminals will overstress a microcomputer, and for comfort, a system with more than seven terminals will be better off with a connection to a main-frame computer. In terms of data to be handled, a microcomputer can probably deal with the recording and analyses of data for 10,000 cows without significant delays in processing. Microcomputers are already handling a sophisticated herd health and production program for 50 large dairy herds (Stephens et al. 1982). The only other factor likely to affect the decision in this circumstance is the distance from the terminal to the computer. The coupling to the terminal of the telephone can be a very fast (expressed in baudes) transmitter and reduce the telephone connect time greatly. However, the other charge—for rental of the landline—which is essential if there is to be avoidance of inaccessible telephone lines, is determined by distance from the computer. At distances of 200 to 300 km., the rental charges are prohibitive.

For a city practice, a microcomputer or a terminal connected to a commercially operated main-frame computer is a satisfactory solution. For a country practice, a microcomputer seems easily the best solution. The principal foreseeable development for veterinarians is a company producing and maintaining software especially produced or adapted for veterinarians in practice.

VIEWDATA—The Main-Frame Variant

These are programs that provide telephone access to telex or television displays of a data bank. There are several systems. The U.K. version of the television program is Prestel; the Canadian version is Telidon; and New Zealand has a VIEWDATA version of Prestel with a veterinary data bank.

The telex version is extensively used for getting access to library data. The best-known veterinary service is the Commonwealth Agri-cultural Bureau program, "DIALOG." The medical programs in most use, although there are many others, are MEDLINE and MED-LARS. There are other systems in other disciplines (Brodhauf et al. 1977). These systems do not have much to offer rural practitioners. However, we should know that the service is available from most scientific libraries. For a small fee, the veterinary literature can be searched for references to a particular subject, which must be very accurately defined, and authors, titles, and abstracts provided. Of more immediate importance are the following.

Telephone Access—
Television Display Programs

The computer programs offer the greatest opportunity for a major change in communication since the intervention of the printing press. The equivalent of a textbook can be written and stored so that it can be accessed by computer. The principal types of service are simple factual data, including dose rate, specific clinical signs, or postmortem lesions; the transmission of standard messages between participants; and problem-solving, especially in providing guides to diagnoses. By a decision tree–type program, it is possible for the computer to thread its way through the categories of disease until it reaches a diagnosis.

The system can be open to general access, but for the veterinary profession the best system is the closed group option in which only accredited users can access the system. Their fees provide the income for the program. In such systems, it is possible to arrange for contributors to add to the data base, an enormous opportunity for collection of such data as disease incidence (Robson and Richmond 1982).

The mechanics of the system are simple. A personal television set is fitted with a keyboard, an adaptor, and an acoustic coupler. The user dials a telephone number and places the telephone in the coupler. The television set is now connected to the computer at the other end of the telephone line. By dialing in the correct code on the keyboard, the available programs are called up on the television screen. The operator may simply view the data or, if the suitable arrangement has been made, can use the computer to which he is connected exactly as if the computer was in his own office. The system is described pictorially in Figure 13–1.

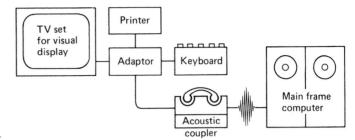

Figure 13-1. The view data system.

A summary of possible uses of VIEWDATA includes:

The *viewing of data* as in:
□ commercial advertising material
□ textbook standard information on drugs, dose rates, toxicity, on diseases and diagnosis
□ weather forecasting
□ telephone numbers
□ library data
Interaction with:
□ personal computer for billing and other administrative matters
□ cooperative computer, e.g., disease incidence recording
□ transmission of messages between participants—electronic mail
□ purchase of drugs and supplies
□ diagnosis by decision tree programs

CHOOSING A COMPUTER PACKAGE

If an appropriate program is available commercially, it is then necessary to find the best computer on which to run it. With present-day sophistication, it is possible to find business administrative programs that are written in a language that is acceptable to a number of microcomputers. Veterinary programs, especially those for food animal preventive medicine, are not yet generally developed to that stage. Exceptions are the dairy herd health programs, which have been adapted to run on a variety of microcomputers. Although there is this existing deficiency, it is our view that the microcomputer will be the machine for the practicing veterinarian, and what follows is a description of that class of machine.

Characteristics of the Hardware

The physical microcomputer machine consists of a number of parts that may all be within the body of the computer or may be separate and detachable, so that there is opportunity to include units of varying levels of cost, complexity, and capability. The parts are as follows.

Input Devices
From an operator by:
□ keyboard, directly or via a telephone system (by a modem or by an acoustic coupler)
□ voice recognition is available, but not for practical purposes
□ an optical reader of printed/typed material
From a data storage service:
□ magnetic discs (floppies or hard discs) or tapes
□ cards or paper tapes
Output Devices
□ Visual output via VDU (visual display unit)
□ Written output via a printer

The visual display is transient and displays input (messages typed in) and output (answers given by the central processing unit). It is customary to view the data or commands or results on the VDU and, if they are correct, have them printed. The visual display can operate at a very fast speed, far exceeding our capacity to read it. The printer is much slower.

Central Processing Unit (CPU). The heart of the computer, in fact, *is* the computer, and it does all the work of processing and sorting data. It must be told very precisely what to do. This is done by having an *operating system* or systems in the machine, which provide the advice the CPU needs. This advice refers to the control and sequencing of the input and output devices and to the commands provided by the application program. The *application* (or user) program is the one written for a specific task or application. A good operating system can take application programs written in different languages and use them via input/output devices not originally designed for the computer being used.

The application program carries specific commands, and these can now be directed to the proper places and organized correctly.

They are converted to binary code and then to electronic signals, the language that the CPU understands and to which it responds. The conversion takes place by reason of instructions received from the *Read Only Memory* (ROM), which is built into the CPU when it is constructed. The reaction to the electronic signals generated in this way passes back through the same circuits. The ROM is incorporated in the basic silicon chip and wiring configuration, which are the basis of each microcomputer. The silicon chips come in several families, only four of which are in common use, some but not all of which can run on the most advanced and versatile operating system—the CP/M. The other well-known operating system is MS-DOS. The important feature of the CP/M system is that it can convert most microcomputers to impersonate others so that they can operate other hardware and utilize other programs.

The CPU does all the mathematical work, directs all the searching and sorting of data, analyzes it when this is called for, and stores it all in the accompanying machine memory. This is the *Random Access Memory* (RAM), which is accessible at any point and is the portal through which all input enters and output leaves the CPU. It is the buffer to which data has to be brought if it is to be used in any way. Most of the data will be stored at a distance on discs or tapes, where it is not accessible. It cannot be viewed nor can it be manipulated. To do either, a segment of the data must be brought into accessibility in the RAM, the machine's memory.

Bulk Storage Discs and Magnetic Tapes.
The bulk of data storage in a computer system will be on one of these units. Hard discs and floppy discs of various degrees of density and diameter carry varying amounts of data, depending on their size and cost. Tape cassettes have been the basic bulk storage for small computers, but they are much too slow for work in a practice. This superficial description is shown pictorially in Figure 13–2.

The Computer's Memory

The efficiency with which a computer can operate, in terms of speed and in terms of the complexity of the problem it can resolve, depends to a large extent on the size and complexity of its memory. This includes the *Read Only Memory* (ROM), which comes with the machinery and is unalterable, and the *Random Access Memory* (RAM), which is accessible and alterable at any point. These

memories are like the nervous system in an animal. It is born with neurons and basic instinctive functions, like the ROM of the computer. These are added to by experience and practice, to perform additional functions, and are being added to and modified all the time, like the RAM of the computer. By way of analogy with human functions, there is a further step in handling information. In man, it is the capacity to bring some faintly remembered but little-used data from the subconscious mind or from further away still, for example to consult a textbook or other source of information not carried in the organism itself. In the computer system, the calling in of data stored in files is from discs—the small inexpensive floppies or the expensive hard metal discs—or from magnetic tape.

The Read Only Memory (ROM) is built into the machine and is its basic, instinctive functions. Its size and complexity is important when choosing a computer because it determines the size and complexity of the functions it can perform.

The Random Access Memory (RAM) is more important because it is the part that the operator can manipulate and is therefore the entry port into the computer when it is proposed to examine a problem. Its size is very important because it determines the amount of data that can be dealt with at one time. For example, the standard operation is to call in data from storage on a disc into the RAM and use it, either for computation, for printing it out, or for altering or deleting it. The more data that one can get into the RAM, the faster and easier it is to carry out these actions. Just as a person with a prodigious conscious memory can relate pieces of information together quickly and accurately, without the need to refer to textbooks, so a computer with a large RAM is very much faster in its calculations. For example, a small microcomputer for personal use will have 24K of RAM, a modest business computer will have 64K, and a monster mainframe instrument will have 2 million K. 64K is the common denominator in computers used in large veterinary practices.

Although the convenience and the efficiency of the peripheral instruments—the video screen, the printer, the disc drives, and so on—differ between computers, the differences are minor compared with the systems that are central to the computer—the CPU, the ROM, and the RAM. As in humans, these systems determine the kind of person who lives inside the case, the speed and accuracy of its

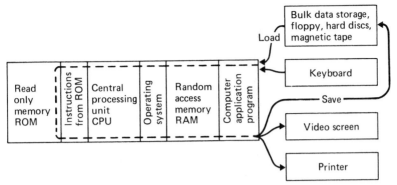

Figure 13-2. The basics of a computer.

reactions, its willingness and ease of communication, and its friendliness. Thus, the value of the computer depends on the size of its machine memory and the resourcefulness of its techniques—the basic wiring configuration and its ROM.

Loss of Memory. A characteristic of the random access memory is that it is not only accessible in terms of being able to alter it, but it is also capable of loss. Data that is called up from disc or tape into the machine will be lost if there is a power failure or if the machine is switched off. This will be of no importance in most cases because it will still be in the memory on the disc, but any alterations or additions that have been made will be lost. The rule to avoid such loss is to convert new material in the machine's memory to disc or tape whenever there is a pause in operations, or at least at the end of every day. To complete the insurance, the disc-stored data should also be copied onto backup discs at regular intervals.

Additions to Memory and to Video Displays and Printers. One of the principal characteristics of microcomputers is their capacity to grow. This would be an obvious attraction to persons wishing to start off in a small way and add on as a practice grew or when familiarity with the machine encouraged its use in additional spheres of work. It is possible to add to ROM and to RAM by purchasing additional packages of memory. This is how a basic microcomputer can be adapted to become a terminal for a main-frame computer or for a word processor.

It is also possible to add to a microcomputer or a main frame by converting it to more and more peripheral output and input units, usually a combination of a video display unit and a printer. The bigger the central processing unit in general terms, the more peripherals can be added. Because of the probability that, in a veterinary hospital, more peripherals will need to be added from time to time, it is essential when making a purchase to ensure that future needs for expansion can be accommodated.

The Basic Program (The Application or User Program)

Besides the basic nervous system that is built into the computer, it is possible to teach it acquired techniques and expertise with respect to specific tasks. These are the computer programs of everyday familiarity. They can be incorporated into the machine's memory simply by writing them in through the keyboard. This means that a programer can develop a program on paper, write it into the computer, and then see if the program does what is wanted. If not, it can be modified right then and tried again. When it is at a working stage in the machine's memory, it is then removed and stored in the subconscious memory (on disc or tape) and only called back into the immediate, conscious memory in the machine when it is to be used to solve a problem. If it is left only in the RAM, it will be lost when the computer is switched off.

An alternative to actually writing the program yourself—and this is a complex task requiring much experience—is to purchase an already prepared program, usually recorded on a floppy disc. The principal problem with these packaged programs is that they may not exactly fit the circumstances in which they are supposed to operate. It can be tempting to purchase a program that is near enough to what is required and to modify it. Again, this is a complicated and expensive business, and only an experienced programmer should contemplate it.

A person using a computer does not need to know anything about the computer program he is using. To use it, you put the appropriate floppy disc into the disc drive and command the computer to transpose the program from the disc into the machine memory. When this has been done, the operator can run the program, type in the data requested, and wait for the program to supply the answers.

To be able to write a program has become synonymous with ability to work with computers. Without doubt, the challenge with these instruments is to master the system that controls them. Anything short of that seems to be, as it were, subservient to their manipulations. This is not so, of course, but one is subservient to the programer who wrote the program, who might not have the same objectives as yours. If that particular constraint of being powerless before a machine can be ignored, there is no reason why one should not have a very profitable collaboration with a computer and yet be quite ignorant of programing and of computer language.

To have had some education in computer programing is an advantage in understanding how any program works, although that is not essential to it. On the other hand, a little education can be a dangerous beginning for writing a program. The technique is complicated, the possibilities for error are infinite, and the damage that a defective program can do is frightening to contemplate. Before anyone engages in writing programs, he should be properly grounded in the science and submit to an assessment of his efficiency.

Computer programs (or more correctly, application programs) are the tools we use to instruct the computer to do certain tasks. They are distinctly different from all other programs because we can write them or modify them. We interact with them. They are the means of communicating with the computer. Programs would be a simple concept and simple items if they were all written in the same language. Life would also be simpler if all operation systems were capable of running all languages. This is not so. Some operating systems can run many languages, others only one.

Computer Languages

A procedure language used in writing programs is a set of MNEMONICS words, or abbreviations of words and signs or collections of words, with strict rules of punctuation and sequence (syntax). There are many of these languages because computer (application) programs are usually written in a language that

the computer can run. For main-frame computers FORTRAN is the most widely used and is very expansive and complicated as befits a language developed for scientific research. For microcomputers, BASIC, FORTRAN, PASCAL, and COBOL are all used, but BASIC is probably the most popular. Typical BASIC commands are:

GOTO   Move computer's point of control to another spot, usually defined by number

IF/THEN   If a particular requirement is carried out, then—usually joined to a GOTO

LOAD   Transfer program or data from a disc to RAM

SAVE   Transfer program or data from RAM to disc, and so on

These languages are referred to as high level because they are far removed from the computer's basic place of operation—the microchip. "Low-level" languages are the ones incorporated in the ROM, and they are therefore close to the lowest point in the computer structure.

These application programs must be compatible with the language of the operating system and the ROM for the system to work. This particular problem is becoming less important because of technical developments that enable incompatible languages to be translated into compatible forms.

Features to Look for in a Computer

THE ONLY SIGNIFICANT GUIDELINE FOR BUYING A COMPUTER IS TO BUY THE SOFTWARE THAT EXACTLY FILLS YOUR NEEDS AND THEN BUY THE COMPUTER THAT WILL RUN IT.

This is the obvious conclusion from all that has been said before. The ultimate extension of the rule is that "If there is no program available to do your task, don't buy a computer."

If there is a program and a choice of computers on which to run it, the final decision can be based on:

1. Capacity of the system to expand to include additional stations comprising keyboards, and one or more peripheral appliances, video terminals or printers, and additional disc drives

2. Capacity to take on additional units of RAM or ROM

3. Compatibility of peripherals with larger computers produced by the same manufacturer. This is more than a secondary consideration, but the chance of buying in the same

manufacturer's range and achieving compatibility is unlikely

4. Price

5. Buy from an established manufacturer with a good reputation; view the package in operation; discuss the degree of satisfaction of the owner. Check that down-time is at a minimum, that backup machine and service facilities are good, and that there is a maintenance program for the machine and the software. Make sure that the supplier will still be in business when things go wrong or when you want to expand or update

6. Availability, price, and effectiveness of peripheral units, especially discs and other bulk storage devices. They are an expensive item and warrant selectivity.

Characteristics of the Software

The standard computer program (application program) is a compilation of commands to the computer (the central processing unit) to carry out a particular task. This might be, for example, to estimate the percentage of the matings by a particular bull that were successful over a particular time period, terminating on a specified date.

A program is written to solve a problem. It may be to arrange the names of a hundred bulls in alphabetical order. In the example cited, the problem is to ascertain the fertility of the bull.

Because of the constraints imposed by the central processing unit, the program must be written as a step-by-step procedure—a sequence of commands—that may turn back on itself and reenter the sequence to form a loop. It may form a whole series of loops and become a very complicated sequence, but it must always begin with a RUN and end with an END.

A program must have material or data on which to work. The data may be in the form of numbers or words. On these data, usually referred to as input, the program carries out the assigned task of storing, searching, sorting, or analyzing, or any combination of these tasks, and produces the results or lists identifiable as the output. Therefore, a discussion of computer programs must be a discussion of input, program, and output.

Input/Data File

How well a program works depends on the proper marshaling and presentation of the data to the program. The important characteristics of the input are as follows.

Individual Animal Versus Herd or Flock Data. For dairy cattle and beef cattle herd health and production programs, there must be a facility to include individual cow data because critical decisions, especially about culling, must be made about individual animals. The same comment really applies to sheep and pigs, but at present sheep programs deal with flocks because of the low individual value of the animals and the high cost of individual animal recording.

Accuracy of Data. The accurate identification of individual animals or groups is an essential prerequisite. This depends largely on the method used to brand or mark the animals and the method of recording events. Structured report forms that set out all the possible responses to questions are most satisfactory. A method that ensures that the recording apparatus is always with the observer is almost essential. A structured pocket diary, a data logger, or a hand-held computer that is programed to receive only certain kinds of data, ensure approximate accuracy.

Limitation of Data—Scope of the Program. This is important from the point of view of economy of computerization, i.e., of computer contact time. Restraint on the part of the programer in not calling for noncritical analyses is vital to having a cost-effective program. On the other hand, the program must cover the full scope of the problem. For example, a report on fertility of a dairy herd will need to contain analyses that indicate the efficiency of estrus detection as well as those that calibrate the success rate of services or breedings. Careful prior mapping of the objectives of the program and the form in which the output is required is the best indicator of the scope required of the input.

The basic subjects included in dairy herd health programs include reproductive efficiency, mastitis, calf survival, and lameness. When production matters are also included, nutrition is much the largest, but cow quality and genetic identity, culling and replacement, financial planning and cash flow are other important subjects.

Fast, Accurate Entry of Data Coding. Almost all data entry for agricultural animals in commercial herds is likely to be by alphanumeric entries via a keyboard for a good long time to come. Accurate, rapid entry therefore depends on the reliability of the keyboard operator. Besides this, there is the matter of coding of the data. For economy's sake, most computers and programs use a code to identify entries. These may be numeric or alphabetical, or alphanumeric—a combination of both. The more friendly a program, the easier to remember are its codes. Thus, a four-letter alphabetical code can bear some similarity to the actual word being encoded. Most veterinary programs these days are leaning toward the user. For example, COSREEL (Russell and Rowlands 1983) has a versatile alphanumeric system claimed to be more easily remembered and recognized than other systems.

Codes are available for diseases identified by the etiological-topographical nomenclature of the standard nomenclature of veterinary diseases and operations put out by the American Veterinary Medical Association. There is also a three-character alphanumeric code for clinical signs (White and Vellake 1980), which is most useful when it is not possible to make a definitive diagnosis. The COSREEL program also encodes clinical signs.

Friendliness of the coding, synonymous with long codes, is contrary to economy, which is synonymous with brevity. Because computer time is not critical with stand-alone computers in rural practices, longer codes are more usual there. This has the added advantage that the operator who is using the same computer for a multiplicity of tasks does not have to remember individual special codes of great complexity for each of these programs.

Fault Correction—Cleaning the Data. As far as possible, the output of the program must be error-free. Failure to ensure this inevitably leads to a failure of farmer confidence, a serious matter at any time, but especially in the early days of a program (Eddy 1982). Much of the problem can be eliminated by putting pressure on the farmer or herdsman to be completely accurate in identifying cows and in recording events. This is much easier if the program itself is error-free; the human is then put on his mettle against the machine.

In the program itself, it is necessary to include input validation subprograms. These check each item of input against what are reasonable values for the parameter, or against previous information about the same cow. Inconsistencies cause an error message to be raised. Some common examples of errors picked up by validation techniques are:

□ return to estrus of a pregnant cow
□ cows that are about to be dried off are not recorded as having been mated or diagnosed pregnant
□ duration of pregnancy as detected by preg-

nancy diagnosis examination is not consistent with the recorded breeding data
□ cows diagnosed as pregnant but not recorded as having been mated

Most of the errors that creep into the data and into the results, if these validation subunits are not instituted, are errors of omission by the herdsman. The fault is in the matter of recording all events, especially estrus observation, breeding dates, drying-off dates, dates and reasons for culling, prices gained at sale, and calving dates. These errors are most likely to occur when the cows are not well branded and their identity is mistaken, when the recording equipment is not carried by the observer, or when notes are transcribed to report sheets or barn sheets. Mistakes can always occur with the machine operator, either by way of misreading or of mis-hitting the keys.

The importance of avoiding errors rather than finding them is the need to have a fast turnaround time. Delaying the program while an error is checked out and corrected is very frustrating, costly, and damaging to credibility.

The Program

A program is a series of commands given to the central processing unit of the computer so that it can satisfactorily solve the problem that you have in mind. In order to create a program it is essential to:

1. Give the commands in the language that the computer (CPU) will understand
2. Use what is called a high-level language, e.g., FORTRAN, PASCAL, or BASIC, devised so that people can understand it and the computer can translate it into the language that the machine understands—the low-level or machine language that may be peculiar to that make of machine only
3. Have a middle-level language in the operating system (e.g., CP/M) that translates most high-level languages into the machine language of any or most computers. Computers that have this capacity to use software written in almost any language have overcome the biggest problem in computerization so far.
4. Write the program as best one can and see if it will run, that is, go through its steps, which have been set out in a logical sequence, and come up with an answer. If it does not work, it is necessary to go back and correct it and run it again. The cycle is repeated until the program works.

5. Validate the program by deriving a credible answer from typical data

6. Convert the answer it produces in machine language back into the high-level language that the operator understands

7. Type in the command "RUN," and the program zips across the video screen like green summer lightning and leaves a pot of gold—the answer to the problem in the bottom right-hand corner

The Steps in the Central Processing Unit at the Run Command

INPUT. Use the data in the data file presented for solving the problem in hand.

Each command in the program is taken in sequence.

The command is translated from its FORTRAN or BASIC or other high-level language form

either

directly into the machine language or machine code in the CPU

or

via an intermediate translator code into the machine code. The translator code makes many high-level languages understandable to the computer.

COMPUTATION. The CPU then directs any search for data that is necessary, moves data about, and carries out mathematical processes like multiplication or measuring time elapsed between two dates.

OUTPUT. The results produced in the CPU are translated back through the high-level language of the input and produce the output—the results in standard English—back into the machine's memory. From here it goes on command to show either on the video screen or the printer.

There are a number of logical stages in creating a program, and they are shown in Figure 13-4 in the form of a flow chart, which is conventional "programese." It helps to do it this way because it is necessary to set the steps out in a logical sequence that can be viewed easily for faults. The step before the actual flow chart is a basic statement of intent in the form of a box and line drawing (Fig. 13-3).

When the flow chart is written and appears logical enough to program, it is then necessary to write the instructions line by line in the program using the appropriate language. It is not proposed to describe how that is done here, and readers are referred to the manuals that accompany their computers if they wish to proceed to that stage.

Desirable Features of Programs. Some of the important characteristics in terms of their desirability have already been dealt with under the heading of input. There is also the inclusion of data cleaning subroutines and programing to limit the scope of data to be recorded. Other important features are listed below. Their relative importance depends to some extent on the kinds of programs that are being used. These are discussed on page 432.

The Transportable Language. Programs written in FORTRAN for main-frame computers are difficult to deal with because they are not really transportable to microcomputers. A program that is written in a transportable language so that it will run on most microcomputers is of enormous value (Esslemont et al. 1982). The inclusion of a translator capability such as a CP/M program has a similar effect but by providing the capacity of the computer to react to commands in many languages.

Backup of Data, Archiving. These are not strictly matters of program. They are points of policy to preserve electronic data against loss by misadventure. At frequent intervals, preferably weekly, all the data stored since the last backup should be copied onto other floppy discs or onto tapes and stored at a separate address. If the computer input has been obtained from written documents, these may be retained as the alternative record.

Each half-year or year, there should be a purging of older files, and only the important raw data and more commonly the analyses and dissections of the data should be extracted and stored as archival material. It is desirable to reduce the bulk of archival storage because it is a much overlooked source of unreliable data.

Rapid Turnaround Time. This is more a factor determined by the efficiency of the data processing bureau. On the other hand, it is possible to bestow a very speedy outcome on it. The inclusion of fault recognition techniques and a rigid exclusion of irrelevant data and analyses are two principal characteristics on which the speed of the program depends.

Acceptability by Farmers. It is logical that better records will provide bigger and better data banks and the information necessary to make the best decisions in farming. It is, however, inescapable that only a small proportion of the veterinary profession is convinced that better decisions make all that much difference to the results of a farming enter-

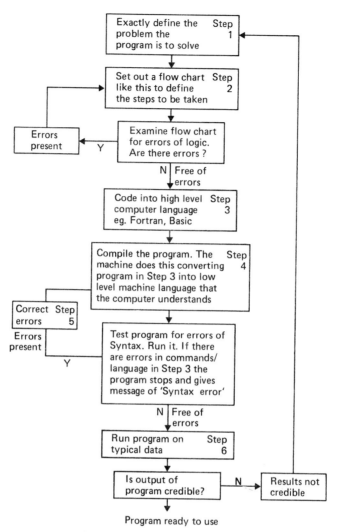

Figure 13-3. Creating a program. (Adapted from Sard, D.M. Computer systems in veterinary medicine. Vet. Rec., *109*:131–133, 1981.)

prise. At least this is what they appear to think, because most farmers do not make decisions; rather, they do what they did before. In a paper entitled "Why Farm Recording Systems are Doomed to Failure" (Hardaker and Anderson 1981), the point is made that only a few perceptive and articulate farmers will embrace and continue to embrace these programs, and that the money currently being expended in promoting them should be invested in simpler, more mundane objectives. The same theme is continued in the promotion of one very popular program, the DAISY (Dairy Information System), but with the practical solution that the enormous workload of a manually operated system can be readily and cheaply absorbed by a microcomputer with a suitable program such as DAISY (Stephens et al. 1982).

If the program is totally accepted by farmers, it might be expected that the future will see the development of programs operated on farms. This does not seem to be happening, and the relative merits of basing these programs on farms or in veterinary practices need to be assessed. The biggest justification for having them in the hands of a practice is that all of the output is passed through the hands of the veterinarian, who can then review and comment on the results. There is also the matter of the cost-effectiveness of the computer. To justify its price, it needs to have maximum usage, and this is more likely to happen in a practice situation than on a single farm.

Adaptation to Various Computer Systems. A really versatile program would be one designed for use on a microcomputer but suitable for use via the microcomputer and for use as a terminal to a main-frame computer, for bigger, more complicated analysis. In this way, the basic data for herds could be maintained on floppy discs at the farm or the veterinarian's office, but the analyses and their results to be used for interfarm comparisons could be passed through the interacting main-frame computer. VIRUS (Veterinary Investigation Recording User System) is a program designed to do this (Martin et al. 1982).

Programs Designed for an Investigative Role. There may be programs designed solely for investigation of disease incidence or the relationship between disease and management. What is more common are programs that are designed to provide farmers with information about disease incidence, feed needs, and comparison of efficiency with other herds, but that are also couched in such terms that the

extraction of other information of a research nature is also possible. The examination of the relationship between genotypic identity and the occurrence of individual diseases is an obvious area where such a program would be useful. Several programs (Blood et al. 1978; Martin et al. 1982) have been designed with this facility in mind.

The Output

The objective of a computer program is to provide a solution to a particular problem, and the output should provide that answer in the most suitable form. It is part of the programing function to design the form of the output. It may be in several forms:

1. Analysis of results, the results of computations

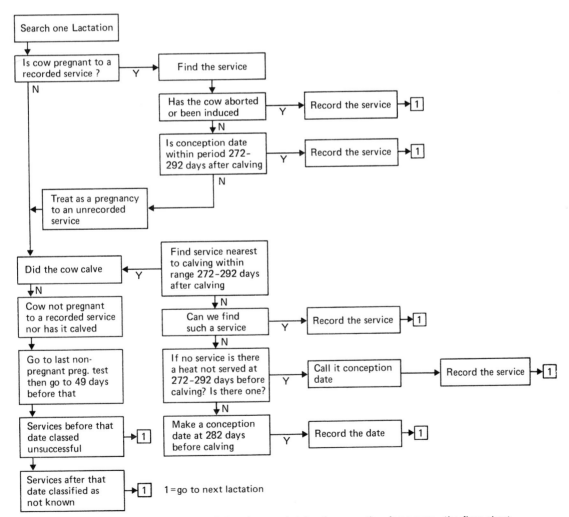

Figure 13-4. Program for defining the exact date of conception for a cow—the flow chart.

2. Arrangement of symbols in a particular order, numerically or alphabetically for example

3. Structured lists of data, e.g., in graphs or histograms

4. Transcription of information. This may be a direct copy of information stored, as in a book

In administrative programs, the output will include:

□ individual itemized accounts for clients

□ monthly and annual analyses of income and expenditure, which may be dissected into categories of kind of service or individual veterinarians

□ lists of staff to be paid, with costs other than salary added to indicate what the total expenditure is

□ annual balance sheets, and so on

These items will probably be in the form of hard copy materials for circulation to clients and staff.

In herd health programs, the principal output will be in the form of periodic reports, i.e., monthly and annual, to provide early warning of impending problems or retrospective analysis of problems that have already occurred. These are the outputs for which the programs were originally planned. In addition, it is customary to use the same data base as was used to generate the reports, to produce lists of animals that will be of value to the farmer, such as lists of cows to calve. It is also common to utilize the data base to generate supernumerary outputs. Thus, the calving roster can be used to predict milk flow, which can be used to predict income, which can be used to predict cash flow.

The output of *computer simulation* models is in the form of results of simulated experiments, which can be used as a basis for advice on management and health.

TYPES OF COMPUTER PROGRAMS ATTRACTIVE TO FOOD ANIMAL VETERINARIANS

Food animal veterinarians are interested in two classes of computer programs—the general administrative programs suited to any professional practice and those programs specifically oriented toward food animal practice.

General Administrative Programs

A standard list includes:

1. *Sundry debtors*. This is a record of fees raised, fees collected, and fees still outstanding, including a dissection into groups depending on the duration of the debt. The credit status of the client is implicit in this record.

2. *Dissection of the fee income*. This is a division of income into categories such as surgery, clinical pathology, referrals, and primary accessions. When matched with accounts payable, which should be similarly categorized, the profitability of each section of the hospital becomes evident. The possible range of categories may tempt the office staff to overdissect; some restraint is needed.

3. *Allocation of income*. The proportion of the total income earned by individual veterinarians, or by sections of the hospital, can be determined.

4. *Diagnostic record*. For epidemiologic purposes, it is desirable to record the prevalence of diseases in the community.

5. *Accounts payable*. This is the purchasing/expenditure side of the practice's financial operations. Each expenditure can be categorized to a section or a function, e.g., equine surgery or anesthesiology, and completes the debit side of the unit's operation.

6. *Drug and materials inventory*. As materials are charged, the amount on hand is adjusted and an alarm raised when a critically low level of the material is reached. Drug sales are adjusted for price by recording the purchase price and adding a proportional handling charge.

7. *Payroll*. The program automatically adjusts expenditure to include payroll charges and costs including workers' compensation and other similar charges.

8. *Vaccination reminders*. Reminders that individual animals are to be revaccinated are automatically produced at the appropriate time.

9. *Appointment scheduling*. Office and on-farm appointment schedules are easily maintained and modified by a computer program.

10. *Annual budgets*.

11. *Cash flow*.

12. *Livestock inventories*.

13. *Agricultural commodity features*.

Food Animal Programs

Below is a summary of the types of program which should be considered as potential investments when approaching the critical moment of buying a computer. Most people find, after buying the machine, that there are many more profitable uses for their new office help. It is important that the following categories be taken into account as well as the previously tested administrative component.

Herd Health Programs

There are now many of these programs available commercially, and care is suggested in assessing them. The criteria are set out in detail in the section on characteristics of the software. They vary largely in their scope and whether they will run on microcomputers. The scope of the programs is included in:

1. *Simple herd or flock health programs* deal strictly with disease matters, e.g., the Melbourne dairy herd health program (Cannon et al. 1978; Williamson et al. 1980).

2. *Special herd or flock health programs* have been devised for special purposes, e.g., the VIRUS program (Martin et al. 1982), which includes the parentage of each cow and is designed to make possible a search for genetic variations in susceptibility to disease, which is linked with capacity to produce milk.

3. *Planned animal health and production programs* link health and production parameters so that they are related to each other in assessments and predictions of performance (Malmo 1982).

4. *Integrated health and production programs.* In most parts of the world at the present time, farmers receive advice from a number of different sources about how they should conduct the management of their farms. Because each adviser looks at the farm from a different point of view, it is common for the advice to overlap, and it is not uncommon for it to conflict and be contradictory. The result is a waste of time and a decline in credibility. What is most required in farmer advice is an integration program that combines all of the streams of advice into a single stream. The existence of such programs has not been established.

5. *Metabolic profile programs* are based on the Compton protocol of periodic examination of blood samples from cows in a herd in an attempt to predict the nutritional and metabolic status of the herd with respect to key metabolites. A computer program to interpret the results of these laboratory examinations is described (Rowlands and Pocock 1971). A more complicated program incorporates health and production parameters with a similar biochemical surveillance (Kelly and Whitaker 1982).

The patterns of most herd health programs are determined by the objectives of:

□ collecting all the critical data about each cow's health and production performance, one lactation at a time

□ updating these data at specific intervals—usually monthly, but in large herds, especially where dairying is seasonal, at weekly intervals

□ then searching through these data and measuring the number of events, the time intervals between the events, and the biological sequence of the events

□ matching the data about each cow with predetermined targets for performance in individual cows and making a decision about each cow that is relevant at that time. It may be decided, for example, to dry off the cow, to cull it, or to examine it for pregnancy

□ collecting all of the individual cow data, summing the data into a herd result, and comparing this result to targets for herd performance

A good herd health program, especially if it includes good protection against errors, is complicated and expensive to produce. There are usually two inputs of data each month, and for these the current lactation record must be brought up into the computer's RAM. The data is added and the time intervals, such as calving to first estrus and calving to conception, are automatically estimated and recorded. If the event is out of sequence, that is recorded also. The output is a monthly or annual report. All of this could be done manually, but the computer is many times faster and much less error-prone.

Animal Production Programs

1. *Nutritional advice.* There are many of these programs, especially in the area of hand-feeding. Estimation of pasture growth and availability as discussed in other sections of this book has now become an important part of pastoral dairy farming and has been incorporated in the grass budgeting/feed planning exercises, which are part of a planned animal health and production program.

2. *Cow quality mating advisory service.* Artificial breeding organizations now run programs that make it possible to match individual cows with bulls who have strengths in characteristics in which the cow is thought to need some boosting.

3. *Breeding advisory service.* The commonest program dealing with reproductive efficiency is the basic program that advises when individual cows should be bred to maintain the calving and subsequent milk supply at the most opportune time—usually the time at which milk production is most profitable (not necessarily the time of highest price).

Herd and Flock Improvement Services. When these are based on computer programs, it is relatively easy to rank animals for productivity within the unit and to conduct interfarm comparisons. In this way, selection for productivity gets a great deal of statistical support. All species organizations appear to have plenty of access to these programs. Beef cattle depend on rate of gain as a measure of productivity; dairy cattle are quantified on their milk production and sheep on their wool or their body weight gain.

Programs to Extract Information from Data Banks. The data collected by herd health and similar disease control programs can be of much more use than the original limited objective intended if it is collected and stored by computer. The computer is capable of economically sorting the information into other categories and analyzing it for other purposes. Some of these "fringe benefits" can be of very great importance and are as follows:

1. *Epidemiologic data.* A large benefit to be derived from a massive data bank accumulated for other purposes is the acquisition of epidemiologic information concerning the occurrence and incidence of individual diseases. This has a great deal of significance in terms of where disease control and research funds should be directed. If it is included in a national study of animal diseases, it can become a continuing exercise of national and international importance (Pilchard 1979). A program to extract epidemiologic information from the data of a series of diagnostic laboratories (Elder 1976) and one for storing and retrieving pathologic diagnoses in a laboratory (Smith et al. 1972) or in a series of laboratories (Hall et al. 1980) have been developed.

2. *Prognosis in the common diseases.* One of the biggest deficiencies in veterinary medicine is that of a store of vital statistics that make it possible to predict the outcome of a particular case with a reasonable degree of accuracy. A large data bank accumulated from herd health programs and other sources of clinical data might then predict that of 100 cases of a particular disease, a specified number would die and another group would make incomplete recoveries. If this were also relatable to the number of cases that were usually encountered per 100 head of cows per year, it would be possible to accurately predict wastage due to the disease. This is also the sort of information on which simulation models are based, and without them, that exciting development cannot begin.

Computer Simulation Models

A simulation model in our context is usually a mathematical model of a system. In veterinary science, a system is usually a collection of components that react with or depend on each other. For example, mastitis—as a system—could be represented as follows:

Streptococcus agalactiae
↓
Teat Skin
↓
Teat Sphincter
↓
Mastitis
↓
Milk Production
↓
Control Program

The model is a simulation model because it attempts to mimic exactly what happens in the real system. The simulation is limited to numerical parameters.

The purpose of models is to permit the conduct of experiments without using the usual experimental tools, especially animals. They are represented in the models, but only as numbers, and they are subjected to the insults and hazards that a cow would be subjected to in a standard commercial herd. The incidents that are inflicted on the cow are arranged to occur randomly but at a level of occurrence that the model predicates for that particular run.

Computer simulation models have gained enormous popularity because of the speed with which they can operate and the great complexity that it is possible to incorporate into them. Computers permit the model to be run on a number of occasions and with great speed. That is how they are used. The model is run with the controlling variables, for example the weather, set at a particular level. The results are noted, the variable that is under consideration is set at another level, the model is run, and the results are again recorded and then compared with the results of the first and other runs. In fact, an experiment is conducted on the herd without actually touching the animals.

In a run of a model of a herd, the computer deals with each cow, each day or week or month, and imprints on her record all of those things that can happen to her in a day—how much food she eats, whether she gets mastitis, comes on heat, has a calf, has milk fever, is treated, culled, or dies. With its enormous speed, a main-frame computer can deal individually with 100 cows daily for four years and include about 350 variables (things that can influence the productivity of the cow) within a few minutes. Such an experiment conducted physically would take at least four years and cost thousands of times as much. The final result of the runs of the model will be the productivity and the profitability of the various management strategies included in the experiment.

Models of Individual Diseases

□ Mastitis (Morris 1976)
□ Reproductive efficiency (Oltenacu et al. 1981)
□ Foot and mouth disease control
□ Trypanosomiasis (Habtemariam et al. 1983)
□ Tuberculosis control
□ Brucellosis control (Beck 1977)

Animal Production Models

□ Dairy herd
□ Beef herd
□ Sheep flock
□ Nutrition of dairy cattle (Brown et al. 1981)
□ Genetics (Freeman 1981)
□ Integrated management systems (Bywater 1981)
□ Pasture growth
□ Heifer replacement

Teaching Models. Many veterinary schools have these to provide practice experience in the use of models and in running simulated control programs. They include mastitis control and vaccination as a disease control tool (Hugh-Jones 1981).

Model Construction. Models are composed of a series of interlocking computer programs, with one main or central program connecting the others. Each of these others, the subroutines, has access to a data file. The latter are composed of data relating to a hypothetical herd, and they set out what happens to each cow each day, week, or month; these figures are based on what does happen, on the average, to cows in real herds. The data files that dictate these occurrences are derived from published papers, from hard data available from government or other research agencies in the area, and from the personal experience of the modeler.

The critical feature of any model is the validity of the data in data files on which the model bases its decisions. Because the data is likely to be generated by observations in a particular geographical area, and often with a particular standard of management, a model is often limited in its range and is likely to be accurate only within that area. This leads to the standard construction procedure of designing and building the model and then validating it against real data in the area in which it is to operate, and with the values and against the actual results in that area.

When the data files are in place, it is possible to run and test the program for its capacity to work through the command and response sequences, which are its continuity. As shown in Figure 13-5, the operator will be asked to define the problem that is to be solved and set the variables that will affect the results. What will happen subsequently is that the model will

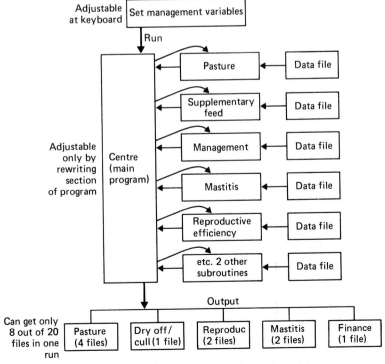

Figure 13-5. Running the S.L. dairy herd model.

be asked what the result will be if the variables are set at a different level. For example, in a model of reproductive efficiency, the model is run once with estrus detection done by casual observation. The results in terms of financial profitability over a five-year period are noted. The model is then run again, but with the variable of estrus detection set at excellent with the use of tail paint. The results for the same time interval as the first run are noted, and a comparison is made between the two.

The beauty of models is that a large number of variables can be available for manipulation. Accordingly, in a reproductive efficiency model, it will be possible to compare the results of casual estrus detection versus tail paint in a circumstance, e.g., nutritional stress, when anestrus is at a high level and at a time when the price of tail paint is escalated by a factor of 10. It is this capacity to include a number of variables into a problem to be solved that is so characteristic of computer simulation models.

The other important characteristic is what is known as its stochastic nature. This is the element of probability that is introduced. A deterministic model does not admit to probability, only to certainty, and therefore does not admit the possibility that all of the bad events may, in fact, occur during the one time period and cause, for example, a complete lack of cash flow.

When the particular run of a model is initialized, that is, its variables have been set, the model is run. Each cow is run through each of the subroutines in turn so that the randomly selected events for that day or month can be imprinted on the cow's record. A sample of the selection of events that can happen to a cow in a model is shown in Figure 13-6. A graphic description of the modular structure of a typical model is shown in Figure 13-7. The record of the cow is passed through a series of loops representing time intervals as shown in Figure 13-8. During each loop in a mastitis

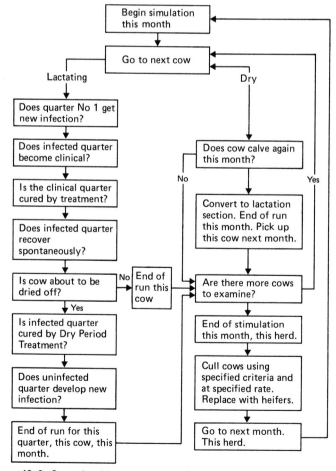

Figure 13-6. Spread-epidemiological segment of RSM bovine mastitis model.

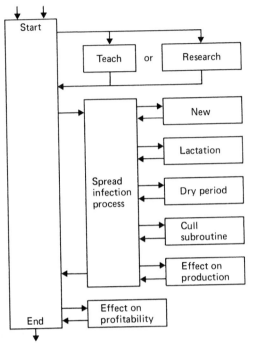

Figure 13-7. Modular structure of computer simulation model of RSM bovine mastitis.

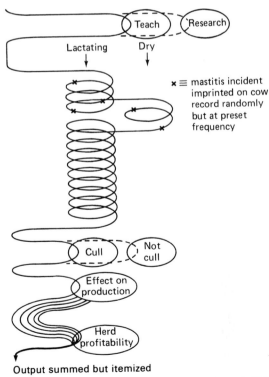

Output summed but itemized

Figure 13-8. Passage of a lactation through RSM mastitis model.

model, the cow may:

- acquire a new in-lactation mammary infection or develop clinical mastitis
- which may, under treatment, be cured or not
- or it may recover spontaneously
- or the cow may be dried off and may acquire a new dry-period infection
- or the infected quarter may be cured by dry-period treatment
- or the cow may be culled
- or calve
- and may exert an effect on average production and profitability.

All of this scanning and imprinting of each cow each month for 100 cows for one year will take 0.5 second of computer connect time and will consist of 1200 loops.

In the much more complex model outlined in Figure 13-9, each cow is run through the entire model every day. For 100 cows, this will mean 36,500 loops per year. In each loop, each cow may be affected by any one of eight incidents in the mastitis subroutine, any of 30 incidents in the reproductive subroutine, and so on through the cull and nutrition subroutines. In this model, there are 20 management variables capable of being initialized at the beginning of the run and 330 other variables capable of manipulation, but only by reprograming that subroutine.

Examples of the initializing variables (variables capable of being set for the beginning of the run) in such a program are:

- starting and finishing dates for this run
- choice of one of four mastitis strategies
- choice of one of five drying-off policies

If the number of culls for mastitis exceeds the replacements available, will the farmer let the herd numbers decline or will he buy in replacements?

- Choice of one of four estrus detection methods
- Is induction of parturition used as a management technique?

The final step in a run is for the model to estimate a finite dollars-and-cents sum to be put on the value of the productivity at the end. When all the cows have been processed, the individual cow's figures are summed and the herd figures printed. The sequence is featured in Figure 13-9.

The output of the model will be a series of figures showing the productivity and/or profitability for that run and the variables used in it. Because the model generates a lot of incidental results on which the productivity figures are based, it is possible to check these

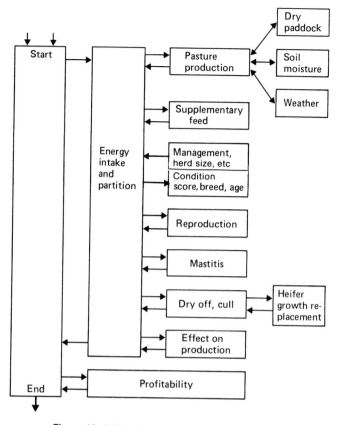

Figure 13-9. S.L. simulation model of a dairy farm.

for possible reasons for the variations in productivity that have already been noticed (see Fig. 13-5).

As described earlier, the method of using the model is to compare the results when the herd is submitted to factors known to affect its performance, with the factors set at different levels for each run. Usually, the frequently used variables—e.g., is irrigation used, is induction of parturition practiced, what proportion of the herd is submitted to artificial insemination—are available for manipulation at the beginning of the model. However, it may be desirable to change the pressure exerted by a parameter for which no provision has been made. For example, if rainfall as a variable factor is capable of being controlled between 500 and 1000 mm. for a year and it is necessary to know what would happen if the rainfall fell to 20 or exceeded 200 mm., it would be necessary to open the file containing weather data and add new material.

At the heart of all models is a series of equations that produce results relating to milk produced, pasture generated, or financial output resulting. These are based on the hard data produced elsewhere by research projects. Because those results might not be quite relevant to the circumstances in which the model herd is operating, it is necessary to run the assembled programs and observe the validity of the results in the light of what might normally be expected in the circumstances. This is one of the most difficult parts of the exercise. It requires a high degree of familiarity of the modeler with the kind of situation he is modeling. This process of validation may take as long as it took to write the original programs from which the model was developed.

No model is ever complete. As new and more accurate information becomes available, it can be added. Sections of it that were weak initially can be bolstered. Sections that persistently produce results that are at variance with those observed in real herds can be modified in the name of validation and, as financial values of costs and income vary with time, these changes can be introduced into the model.

In terms of deciding what to advise farmers to do, models provide the answer to the problem of giving advice that is firmly based on actual results elsewhere and take into account the effects not only of the variable that is under discussion but of all the variables that are exerting their pressure over the same period of time.

Review Literature

Bywater, A.C. and Dent, J.B. Simulation of the intake and partition of nutrients by the dairy cow. Agricultural Systems, 1:246-279, 1976.

Davidson, J. An introduction to the use of computers in bovine practice. Proc. 14th Ann. Conv. Assoc. Bov. Pract., Seattle, 1981, pp. 53-60.

Fick, G.W. A pasture production model for use in a whole farm simulator. Agricultural Systems, 5:137-163, 1980.

France, J., Neal, St.C. and Marsden, S. A dairy herd cash flow. Agricultural Systems, 8:129-142, 1982.

Gartner, J.A. Replacement policy in dairy herds on farms where heifers compete with the cows for grassland. Part 1. Agricultural Systems, 7:289-318, 1981.

Gartner, J.A. Replacement policy in dairy herds on farms where heifers compete with the cows for grassland. Part 2. Agricultural Systems, 8:163-192, 1982.

Morris, R.S. Use of computer modelling techniques in studying epidemiology and control of animal diseases. Proc. Int. Summer School on Computers and Research in Animal Nutrition and Veterinary Medicine at Elsinore, Denmark.

Oltenacu, P.A., Milligan, R.A., Rounsaville, R.T., et al. Modelling reproduction in a herd of dairy cattle. Agricultural Systems, 5:193-205, 1980.

Sard, D.M. Computer systems in veterinary medicine. Parts 1, 2, 3, 4, and 5. Vet. Rec., 108:322-324, 346-348,

References

Beck, H.C. The use of simulation modelling in the management of brucellosis eradication. Aust. Vet. J., 53: 485-489, 1977.

Blood, D.C., Morris, R.S., Williamson, W.B. et al. A health program for commercial dairy herds. Aust. Vet. J., 54:207-230, 1978.

Brodhauf, H., Hoffman, W.D., Klawiter-Pommer, J.H.T. et al. Searching the literature of veterinary science: A comparative study of the use of ten information systems for retrospective searches. Vet. Rec., 101: 461-463, 1977.

Brown, C.A., Stallings, C.C. and Telega, C.W. Nutritional modelling and its impact on managerial goals in dairy production. J. Dairy Sci., 64:2083-2095, 1981.

Bywater, A.C. Development of integrated management information system for dairy producers. J. Dairy Sci., 64:2113-2124, 1981.

Cannon, R.M., Morris, R.S., Williamson, N.B. A health program for commercial dairy herds. Part 2. Data processing. Aust. Vet. J., 54:216-230, 1978.

Eddy, R.G. Dealing with errors in computerized dairy herd recording. 12th World Conf. Dis. of Cattle, Amsterdam, pp. 628-632, 1982.

Elder, J.K. Retrieval of animal disease information from a computer record system. Aust. Vet. J., 52:196-197, 1976.

Esslemont, R.J., Stephens, A.J. and Ellis, P.R. The design of Daisy the Dairy Information System. 12th World Conf. Dis. of Cattle, Amsterdam, pp. 643-646, 1982.

Freeman, A.E. Breeding inputs to managerial goals in dairy production. J. Dairy Sci., 64:2105-2112, 1981.

Gibson, C.D., Kaneene, J.B., Mather, E.C. et al. Computerized herd health records for dairy cattle. 12th World Conf. Dis. of Cattle, Amsterdam, pp.647-653, 1982.

Habtemariam, T., Ruppanner, R., Riemann, H.P. et al. Epidemic and endemic characteristics of Trypanosomiasis in cattle; a simulation model. Prev. Vet. Med., 1:137-145 (see also pp. 125, 147, 157), 1983.

Hall, S.A., Dawson, P.S. and Davis, G. Vida 2. A computerized diagnostic recording system for Veterinary Investigation Centres in Great Britain. Vet. Rec., 106:260-264, 1980.

Hardaker, J.B. and Anderson, J.R. Why farm recording systems are doomed to failure. Rev. Market. and Agric. Econ., 49:199-202, 1981.

Hugh-Jones, M.E. A simple vaccination model. Bull. Off. Int. Epizoot., 93:1-8, 1981.

Kelly, J.M. and Whitaker, D.A. A dairy herd health and productivity service. 12th World Conf. Dis. of Cattle, Amsterdam, pp. 654-664, 1982.

Malmo, J. Planned animal health and production services for seasonally calving dairy herds. 12th World Conf. Dis. of Cattle, Amsterdam, pp. 670-677, 1982.

Martin, B., Mainland, D.D. and Green, M.A. VIRUS: A computer program for herd health and productivity. Vet. Rec., 110:446-448, 1982.

Morris, R.S. The use of computer modelling in epidemiological and economic studies. Ph.D. Thesis, University of Reading, 1976.

Oltenacu, P.A., Rounsaville, T.R., Milligan, R.A. et al. Systems analysis for designing reproductive management programs to increase production and profit in dairy herds. J. Dairy Sci., 64:2096-2104, 1981.

Pilchard, E.I. The world situation for animal health and disease information. J. Am. Vet. Med. Assoc., 175: 1297-1300, 1979.

Robson, J.K.D. and Richmond, G. Viewdata: Its role in veterinary practice. Vet. Rec., 110:263-264, 1982.

Rowlands, G.J. and Pocock, R.M. Use of a computer as an aid in diagnosis of metabolic problems of dairy herds. J. Dairy Res., 38:353-362, 1971.

Russell, A.M. and Rowlands, G.J. Cosreel: Computerized recording system for herd health information management. Vet. Rec., 112:189-193, 1983.

Sard, D.M. Computer systems in veterinary medicine. Vet. Rec., 109:131-133, 1981.

Smith, J.E., McGavin, M.D. and Gronwall, R. English-language computer-based system for storage and retrieval of pathological diagnosis. Vet. Path., 9: 152-158, 1972.

Stephens, A.J., Esslemont, R.J. and Ellis, P.R. DAISY in veterinary practice. Planned animal health and production services and small computers. Vet. Ann., 22: 6-17, 1982.

White, M.E. and Vellake, E. A coding system for veterinary clinical signs. Cornell Vet., 70:160-182, 1980.

Williamson, N.B., Anderson, G.A., Blood, D.C., et al. Extensions to a veterinary health and management program data system for dairy herds. Aust. Vet. J., 56:474-476, 1980.

Wise, J.K. Market report on veterinary practice computers. J. Am. Vet. Med. Assoc., 181:608, 1972.

Index

Note: Numbers in italics refer to illustrations; numbers followed by (t) indicate tables.